MOSBY'S
ESSENTIALS
FOR NURSING
ASSISTANTS

SHEILA A. SORRENTINO, RN, PhD
Curriculum and Health Care Consultant
Normal, Illinois

BERNIE GOREK, RNC, GNP, MA, NHA
Gerontology Consultant
Greeley, Colorado

THIRD EDITION

With **511** Illustrations

MOSBY

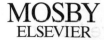

MOSBY
ELSEVIER

11830 Westline Industrial Drive
St. Louis, Missouri 63146
MOSBY'S ESSENTIALS FOR NURSING ASSISTANTS, THIRD EDITION   ISBN-13:978-0-323-03904-8
ISBN-10: 0-323-03904-9

Notice

Nursing is an ever-changing field. Standard safety precautions must be followed, but as new research and clinical experience broaden our knowledge, changes in treatment and drug therapy may become necessary or appropriate. Readers are advised to check the most current product information provided by the manufacturer. It is the responsibility of the licensed health care provider, relying on experience and knowledge of the patient or resident, to determine the best treatment for each individual patient or resident. Neither the publisher nor the author assumes any liability for any injury and/or damage to persons or property arising from this publication.

The Publisher

Previous editions copyrighted 2001, 1997 by Mosby, Inc.

ISBN-13:978-0-323-03904-8
ISBN-10: 0-323-03904-9

Executive Editor: Susan R. Epstein
Senior Developmental Editor: Maria Broeker
Publishing Services Manager: John Rogers
Senior Project Manager: Kathleen L. Teal
Senior Designer: Kathi Gosche

Printed in the United States of America

Last digit is the print number: 9   8   7   6   5   4   3   2   1

To the men and women
who protect our freedoms
Sheila A. Sorrentino

To my sister, Pat
You have much to offer and are loved by many
Bernie Gorek

About the Authors

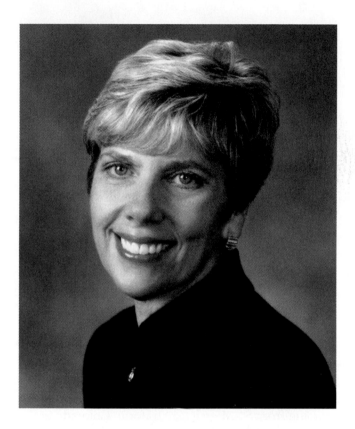

Sheila A. Sorrentino is currently a curriculum and health care consultant focusing on career ladder nursing programs and effective delegation and partnering with assistive personnel in hospitals, long-term care centers, and home care agencies.

Dr. Sorrentino was instrumental in the development and approval of CNA-PN-ADN programs in the Illinois Community College System and has taught in nursing assistant, practical nursing, associate degree, and baccalaureate and higher degree programs. Her career includes experiences as a nursing assistant, staff nurse, charge nurse, head nurse, nursing educator, assistant dean, dean, and consultant.

A Mosby author since 1982, Dr. Sorrentino is the author of *Mosby's Textbook for Nursing Assistants* (sixth edition) and several other textbooks for nursing assistants and other assistive personnel. She was also involved in the development of *Mosby's Nursing Assistant Skills Videos* and *Mosby's Nursing Skills Videos*, winner of the 2003 AJN Book of the Year

Award (electronic media). An earlier version of nursing assistant skills videos won the 1992 International Medical Films Award on caregiving.

Dr. Sorrentino has a bachelor of science degree in nursing, a master of arts in education, a master of science degree in community nursing, and a PhD in higher education administration. She is a member of Sigma Theta Tau and former member and chair of the Central Illinois Higher Education Health Care Task Force. She also served on the Iowa-Illinois Safety Council Board of Directors and the Board of Directors of Our Lady of Victory Nursing Center in Bourbonnais, Illinois. In 1998 she received an alumni achievement award from Lewis University for outstanding leadership and dedication in nursing education. In 2005 she was inducted into the Illinois State University College of Education Hall of Fame. Her presentations at national and state conferences focus on delegation and other issues relating to assistive personnel.

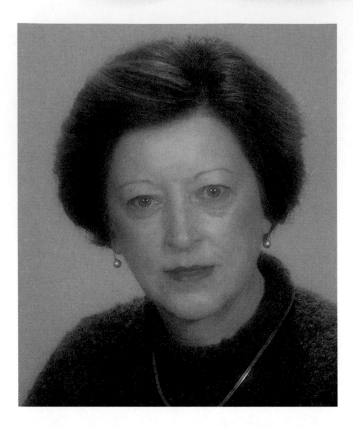

Bernie Gorek is a licensed nursing home administrator in Colorado and a gerontology consultant. She received her RN diploma in nursing from St. Mary's School of Nursing, Rochester, Minnesota, a baccalaureate degree in Health Arts from The College of St Francis, Joliet, Illinois, certification as a gerontological nurse practitioner from The University of Colorado, Denver, Colorado, and a Masters degree in Gerontology from the University of Northern Colorado, Greeley, Colorado, where she received the Dean's Citation for Excellence.

Bernie has had 24 years of experience in gerontological nursing: in a clinical role as a nurse practitioner and in an administrative role as Director of Community Health Services, Director of Nursing Services, and Director of Resident Care and Services at Bonell Good Samaritan Center, Greeley, Colorado. She also has experience as a nursing home administrator in Colorado and Wyoming.

Bernie has been a leader in developing and implementing innovative programs for persons in independent living and long-term health care settings. She was instrumental in the development and implementation of a community nursing assistant training program. She has a Credential for Career and Technical Education from the Colorado State Board of Community Colleges and Occupational Education. She also consults for the School of Nursing at the University of Northern Colorado in various grant writing projects. Bernie served two terms as president of the National Conference of Gerontological Nurse Practitioners.

Reviewers

G. Karla Kirkland, LPN
LPN and Nursing Assistant Instructor
Everett Rehabilitation and Care Center
Sunbridge Healthcare
Everett, Washington

Carolyn M. Ruppel, RN
Nursing Assistant Instructor
MTC/Red Rock Job Corps
Lopez, Pennsylvania

Elaine Townsley, RNC, MSN
Director of Quality Services
ConvaCare Management, Inc.
Searcy, Arkansas

Acknowledgments

As with previous editions of *Mosby's Essentials for Nursing Assistants*, many individuals and agencies have contributed to this new, third edition by providing information, insights, and resources. We are especially grateful and appreciative of the efforts by:

- Jane DeBlois of OSF St. Joseph's Medical Center in Bloomington, Illinois—for being a valuable resource and always responding to information requests in a most timely manner.
- Anne Pauly of Genesis Medical Center in Davenport, Iowa—a colleague of many years who is always ready and willing to answer questions.
- Tammy Taylor of Heartland Community College in Normal, Illinois, and Julie White of Wilbur Wright College in Chicago, Illinois—for providing valuable insights and information and for serving as informal consultants.
- Liz Burns, RN, BSN, Director of Nursing at Bonell Good Samaritan Center in Greeley, Colorado—for her professional expertise and on-going support.
- Zee Zala of Windsor, Colorado—a physical therapist, she shared her professional knowledge and provided practical insights.
- Tess Masters of Aims Community College in Greeley Colorado—for her willingness to provide valuable input based on her classroom experiences with nursing assistant students.
- The artists at Graphic World in St. Louis, Missouri for their talented work.
- G. Karla Kirkland, Carolyn M. Ruppel, and Elaine Townsley for reviewing the manuscript and for their candor and suggestions. They have contributed to the thoroughness and accuracy of this book.
- Tom Wolf, copyeditor, for his insightful queries, efficiency, and appreciation for "language economy."
- Tina Kult, Tyson Sturgeon, Maria Broeker, and Kathy Teal for all their efforts in developing and producing the CD-Companion. It was a challenging but rewarding experience for all.
- And finally, to the talented and dedicated Mosby staff, especially Suzi Epstein, Maria Broeker, Mary Jo Adams, Kathi Gosche, and Kathy Teal. In her role as editor, Suzi once again gave guidance and support and kept the project on track. She also stressed the importance of taking care of self and family. Suzi believes in and supports her authors. Maria Broeker handled numerous details and manuscript needs. Her role in the CD-Companion project was extraordinary and appreciated more than words can say. As always, what would we do without Maria? And Mary Jo provided prompt clerical and secretarial assistance. As project manager, Kathy Teal once again made the production process efficient and produced a user-friendly layout. Along with Maria, Kathy was beyond helpful with the CD-Companion project. And Kathi Gosche created another unique and colorful book and cover design. As always, she made the book distinctive from the rest.
- And to all those who contributed to this effort in any way, we are sincerely grateful.

Sheila A. Sorrentino and Bernie Gorek

Instructor Preface

As with previous editions of *Mosby's Essentials for Nursing Assistants*, this third edition serves to prepare students to function as nursing assistants in hospitals and nursing centers. This textbook serves the needs of students and instructors in community colleges, technical schools, high schools, hospitals, nursing centers, and other agencies. As students complete their education, the book is a valuable resource for competency test review. And as part of one's personal library, the book is a reference for the nursing assistant who seeks to review information for safe care.

Patients and residents are presented as *persons* with dignity and value who have a past, a present, and a future. Caring, understanding the person's rights, and respect for patients and residents as persons with dignity and value are attitudes conveyed throughout the book.

The nursing assistants of today and tomorrow must have a firm understanding of the legal principles affecting their role. Both federal and state laws directly and indirectly define their roles and limitations. Nursing assistant roles and functions also vary among states and agencies. Therefore, emphasis is given to nursing assistant responsibilities and limitations, specifically in Chapter 2, which focuses on the legal and ethical aspects of the role. It includes the reporting of elder abuse.

Nursing assistant functions and role limits also depend on effective delegation. Building on the delegation principles presented in Chapter 2, "Delegation Guidelines" are presented as they relate to procedures. They empower the student to seek information from the nurse and the care plan about critical aspects of the procedure and the observations to report and record. Step 1 of most procedures refers the student to the appropriate *Delegation Guidelines* boxes.

Safety and comfort have been core values of *Mosby's Essentials for Nursing Assistants*. A new feature, "Promoting Safety and Comfort" is integrated throughout the book, but mainly for the procedures. The intent is to focus the student's attention on the need to be safe and cautious and to promote comfort when giving care. Step 1 of most procedures refers the student to the appropriate *Promoting Safety and Comfort* boxes.

Besides legal aspects, delegation, and safety and comfort, work ethics also affect how nursing assistants function. To foster a positive work ethic, Chapter 3 focuses on workplace behaviors and practices.

The goal is for the nursing assistant to be a proud, professional member of the nursing and health teams.

Building on concepts and principles presented in Chapters 1 through 6, *Focus on the Person* is a new feature found at the end of each chapter, beginning in Chapter 7. *PERSON* is spelled out in the first letter of each bullet: **P**roviding comfort, **E**thical behavior, **R**emaining independent, **S**peaking up, **O**BRA and other laws, **N**ursing teamwork. (See Designs and Features section.)

A most exciting new feature is the CD Companion at the back of the book! Using video clips and animations, 26 key procedures are presented, along with interactive exercises. The CD Companion also includes an audio glossary and Body Spectrum program.

ORGANIZATIONAL STRATEGIES

These concepts and principles—the patient or resident as a person, ethical and legal aspects, delegation, safety and comfort, and work ethics—serve as the guiding framework for this book. Other organizational strategies and values include:

- Awareness and understanding of the work setting and the individuals in that setting
- Respect for the patient or resident as a physical, social, psychological, and spiritual being with basic needs and protected rights
- Respect for personal choice and dignity of person
- Appreciating the role of cultural heritage and religion in health and illness practices
- Understanding body structure and function to give safe care and to safely perform psychomotor skills
- That learning proceeds from the simple to the complex
- Certain concepts and functions are foundational—safety, body mechanics, and preventing infection are central to other procedures
- That the nursing process is the basis for planning and delivering nursing care and that nursing assistants must follow the person's care plan

CONTENT ISSUES

With every edition, revision and content decisions are made. When changes are made in laws or in guidelines and standards issued by government or accrediting agencies, the decisions are simple. The content is revised or added as needed. Other content issues are more difficult. The learning needs and abilities of the student, instructor desires, and book length are among the factors considered. With such issues in mind, new and expanded content includes:

Chapter 1 Introduction to Health Care Agencies
- Types of residents in long-term care centers
- Assisted living facilities

Chapter 2 The Nursing Assistant
- Elder abuse

Chapter 3 Work Ethics
- New employee orientation
- Teamwork
- Priority setting—caring for several patients or residents

Chapter 4 Communicating With the Health Team
- Assignment sheets
- Box 4-5 Using Computers
- Problem solving

Chapter 5 Understanding the Person
- The person who is comatose

Chapter 7 Caring For the Older Person
- Growth and development

Chapter 8 Promoting Safety
- Wheelchair and stretcher safety

Chapter 9 Restraint Alternatives and Safe Restraint Use *(new)*

Chapter 10 Preventing Infection
- Hand Hygiene Guideline

Chapter 11 Using Body Mechanics
- Ergonomics
- Chair or wheelchair to bed transfers
  - □ PROCEDURE: TRANSFERRING THE PERSON FROM THE CHAIR OR WHEELCHAIR TO BED
- Transferring the person to and from the toilet
  - □ PROCEDURE: TRANSFERRING THE PERSON TO AND FROM THE TOILET
- Repositioning in a chair or wheelchair

Chapter 12 Assisting With Comfort
- Persons With Dementia: Noise
- Alternative method of putting a pillowcase on the pillow

Chapter 13 Assisting With Hygiene
- Persons With Dementia: Assisting With Hygiene
- Flossing

Chapter 14 Assisting With Grooming
- Caring About Culture: Braiding Hair

Chapter 15 Assisting With Urinary Elimination
- Drainage systems

Chapter 17 Assisting With Nutrition and Fluids
- MyPyramid
- Diabetes meal planning
- Preparing for meals
  - □ PROCEDURE: PREPARING THE PERSON FOR A MEAL
- Box 17-1 The Dysphagia Diet
- Flow rate
- Assisting with IV therapy
- Box 17-4 Signs and Symptoms of IV Therapy Complications

Chapter 18 Assisting With Assessment
- Box 18-1 Temperature Sites
- Pain

Chapter 19 Assisting With Specimens *(new)*

Chapter 21 Assisting With Wound Care
- Box 21-3 Measures to Prevent Circulatory Ulcers

Chapter 22 Assisting With Oxygen Needs
- Box 22-1 Signs and Symptoms of Hypoxia

Chapter 23 Assisting With Rehabilitation and Restorative Care
- Restorative Nursing

Chapter 24 Caring For Persons With Common Health Problems
- Box 24-1 Some Signs and Symptoms of Cancer
- Renal calculi
- Renal failure
- Diverticular disease
- Vomiting
- Box 24-18 Signs and Symptoms of Depression in Older Persons

Chapter 25 Caring For Persons With Confusion and Dementia *(enhanced!)*
- Box 25-1 Changes in the Nervous System From Aging
- Box 25-3 Other Signs and Symptoms of AD
- Validation therapy

Chapter 26 Assisting With Emergency Care
- Chain of Survival
- Automated external defibrillators (AEDs)
- Stroke

FEATURES AND DESIGN

Besides content issues, attention also is given to improving the book's features and designs. To make the book readable and user friendly, new features and design elements are added while others are retained (see Student Preface, p. xv).

- ■ **Illustrations**—the book contains numerous full-color photographs and line art.
- ■ **Objectives**—list the learning objectives for the chapter.
- ■ **Procedures box**—is on the chapter opening page. Procedures found in the chapter are listed. A CD icon precedes those procedures that are also in the CD Companion found at the back of the book.
- ■ **Key Terms with definitions**—are at the beginning of each chapter.
- ■ **Key Terms in bold print**—are throughout the text. The definition is presented in narrative in the text. Unlike other books, students do not have to turn to the margin for the definition, return to the text, and then try to understand the context of the term.
- ■ **Boxes and tables**—list principles, guidelines, signs and symptoms, nursing measures, and other information. They are an efficient way for instructors to highlight content. And they are useful study guides for students.
- ■ **Procedure icons**—in section headings alert the reader to an associated procedure. Procedure boxes contain the same icon
- ■ **Delegation Guidelines**—are associated with procedures. As stated earlier, they focus on the information needed from the nurse and the care plan about critical aspects of the procedure and the observations to report and record. Step 1 of most procedures refers the student to the appropriate *Delegation Guidelines.*
- ■ *Promoting Safety and Comfort*—focus the student's attention on the need to be safe and cautious and promote comfort when giving care. Step 1 of most procedures refers the student to the appropriate Promoting Safety and Comfort boxes. *New!*
- ■ *Procedure boxes divided into Pre-Procedure, Procedure, and Post-Procedure steps*—Labeling and color gradients also differentiate the sections. Including the Pre-Procedure and Post-Procedure steps, rather than referring the student to them as is done in other books, serves to show the procedure as a whole and reinforces learning.
- ■ *Quality of Life*—this section in the procedure boxes reminds the student of six fundamental courtesies:
  - Knock before entering the room.
  - Address the person by name.
  - Introduce oneself by name and title.
  - Explain the procedure to the person before beginning and during the procedure.
  - Protect the person's rights during the procedure.
  - Handle the person gently during the procedure.
- ■ *CD icon*—appears in the procedure box title bar for the skills included in the CD Companion at the back of the book.
- ■ *NNAAP™*—appears in the procedure box title bar for skills included in the National Nurse Aide Assessment Program (NNAAP™).
- ■ *Caring About Culture boxes*—serve to sensitize the student to cultural diversity and how culture influences health and illness practices.
- ■ *Persons With Dementia boxes*—focus on information and insights about caring for persons with dementia.
- ■ *Focus on the Person boxes*—are found at the end of each chapter. Building on concepts and principles presented in Chapters 1 through 6, PERSON is spelled out in the first letter of each bullet beginning in Chapter 7:
  - **P**roviding comfort—suggests ways to meet the person's comfort needs.
  - **E**thical behavior—stresses doing the right thing when dealing with patients, residents, and co-workers.
  - **R**emaining independent—reminds the student to encourage the person to do as much for himself or herself as possible.
  - **S**peaking up—gives the student ideas of what to say and questions to ask when interacting with residents.
  - **O**BRA and other laws—informs the student of OBRA requirements and other laws affecting health care and nursing assistant functions.
  - **N**ursing teamwork—suggests ways to work with and help other nursing team members. The intent is to foster teamwork.
- ■ *Review Questions*—are found at the end of each chapter. A page number is given for where the answers are found.

May this book serve you and your students well. Our intent is to provide you and your students with the information needed to teach and learn safe and effective care during this time of dynamic change in health care.

Sheila A. Sorrentino, RN, BSN, MA, MSN, PhD
Bernie Gorek, RNC, GNP, MA, NHA

Student Preface

This book was designed for you. It was designed to help you learn. The book is a useful resource as you gain experience and expand your knowledge.

This preface gives some study guidelines and helps you use the book. When given a reading assignment do you read from the first page to the last page without stopping? How much do you remember? You will learn more if you use a study system. A useful study system has these steps:

- Survey or preview
- Question
- Read and record
- Recite and review

PREVIEW

Before you start a reading assignment, preview or survey the assignment. This gives you an idea of what the assignment covers. It also helps you recall what you already know about the subject. Carefully look over the assignment. Preview the chapter title, headings, subheadings, and terms or ideas in bold print or italics. Also survey the objectives, key terms, boxes, and review questions at the end of the chapter. Previewing only takes a few minutes. Remember, previewing helps you become familiar with the material.

QUESTION

After previewing, you need to form questions to answer while you read. Questions should relate to what might be asked on a test or how the information applies to giving care. Use the title, headings, and subheadings to form questions. Avoid questions that have one word answers. Questions that begin with what, how, or why are helpful. While reading, you may find that a question does not help you study. If so, just change the question. Remember, questioning sets a purpose for reading. So changing a question only makes this step more useful.

READ AND RECORD

Reading is the next step. Reading is more productive after determining what you already know and what you need to learn. Read to find answers to your questions. The purpose of reading is to:

- Gain new information
- Connect new information to what you know already

Break the assignment into smaller parts. Then answer your questions as you read each part. Also, mark important information—underline, highlight, or make notes. Underlining and highlighting remind you what you need to learn. Go back and review the marked parts later. Making notes results in more immediate learning. To make notes, write down important information in the margins or in a notebook. Use words and statements to jog your memory about the material.

You need to remember what you read. To do so, work with the information. Organize information into a study guide. Study guides have many forms. Diagrams or charts show relationships or steps in a process. Note taking in outline format is also very useful. The following is a sample outline.

1. Main heading
   a. Second level
   b. Second level
      1. Third level
         ii. Third level
2. Main heading

RECITE AND REVIEW

Finally, recite and review. Use your notes and study guides. Answer the questions you formed earlier. Also answer other questions that came up when reading and answering the Review Questions at the end of a chapter. Answer all questions out loud (recite).

Reviewing is more about when to study rather than what to study. You already determined what to study during the preview, question, and reading steps. The best times to review are right after the first study session, 1 week later, and before a quiz or test.

This book was also designed to help you study. Special design features are described on the next pages.

We hope you enjoy learning and your work. You and your work are important. You and the care you give may be bright spots in a person's day!

Sheila A. Sorrentino
Bernie Gorek

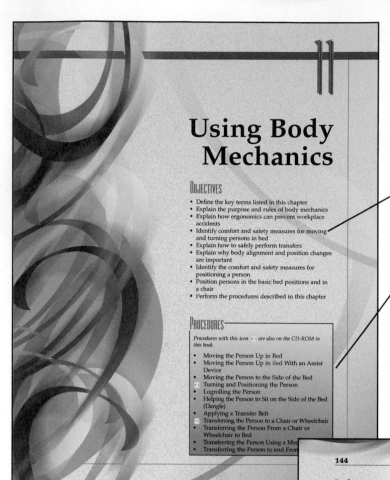

Using Body Mechanics

OBJECTIVES

- Define the key terms listed in this chapter
- Explain the purpose and rules of body mechanics
- Explain how ergonomics can prevent workplace accidents
- Identify comfort and safety measures for moving and turning persons in bed
- Explain how to safely perform transfers
- Explain why body alignment and position changes are important
- Identify the comfort and safety measures for positioning a person
- Position persons in the basic bed positions and in a chair
- Perform the procedures described in this chapter

PROCEDURES

Procedures with this icon are also on the CD-ROM in this book.

- Moving the Person Up in Bed
- Moving the Person Up in Bed With an Assist Device
- Moving the Person to the Side of the Bed
- Turning and Positioning the Person
- Logrolling the Person
- Helping the Person to Sit on the Side of the Bed (Dangle)
- Applying a Transfer Belt
- Transferring the Person to a Chair or Wheelchair
- Transferring the Person From a Chair or Wheelchair to Bed
- Transferring the Person Using a Me...
- Transferring the Person to and Fro...

Objectives tell what is presented in the chapter.

Procedures box lists the procedures presented in the chapter. A CD icon indicates those procedures that are also in the CD Companion found at the back of the book.

---

144 Mosby's Essentials for Nursing Assistants

KEY TERMS

base of support The area on which an object rests
body alignment The way the head, trunk, arms, and legs are aligned with one another; posture
body mechanics Using the body in an efficient and careful way
dorsal recumbent position The back-lying or supine position
Fowler's position A semi-sitting position; the head of the bed is raised between 45 and 60 degrees
friction The rubbing of one surface against another
lateral position The side-lying position
logrolling Turning the person as a unit, in alignment, with one motion
posture Body alignment
prone position Lying on the abdomen with the head turned to one side
semi-prone side position Sims' position
shearing When skin sticks to a surface while muscles slide in the direction the body is moving
side-lying position The lateral position
Sims' position A left side-lying position in which the upper leg is sharply flexed so it is not on the lower leg and the lower arm is behind the person; semi-prone
supine position The back-lying or dorsal recumbent position
transfer belt A belt used to support persons who are unsteady or disabled; a gait belt

You will turn and reposition persons often. You must use your body correctly. This protects you and the person from injury.

BODY MECHANICS

Body mechanics means using the body in an efficient and careful way. Good posture, balance, and the strongest and largest muscles are used. Fatigue, muscle strain, and injury can result from improper use and positioning of the body during activity or rest.

Body alignment (posture) is the way the head, trunk, arms, and legs are aligned with one another. Good alignment lets the body move and function with strength and efficiency. Standing, sitting, and lying down require good alignment.

Base of support is the area on which an object rests. A good base of support is needed for balance (Fig. 11-1). Stand with your feet apart for a wider base of support and more balance.

The strongest and largest muscles are in the shoulders, upper arms, hips, and thighs. Use these muscles to lift and move heavy objects. Otherwise, you place

strain and exertion on smaller and weaker muscles. This causes fatigue and injury. *Back injuries are a major risk.* For good body mechanics:

- Bend your knees and squat to lift a heavy object (Fig. 11-2). Do not bend from your waist. That places strain on small back muscles.
- Hold items close to your body and base of support (see Fig. 11-2). This involves upper arm and shoulder muscles. Holding objects away from your body places strain on small muscles in your lower arms.

All activities require good body mechanics. Follow the rules in Box 11-1.

BOX 11-1 Rules For Body Mechanics
• Keep your body in good alignment with a wide base of support.
• Use the stronger and larger muscles in your shoulders, upper arms, thighs, and hips.
• Keep objects close to your body when you lift, move, or carry them (see Fig. 11-2).
• Avoid unnecessary bending and reaching. Raise the bed so it is close to your waist. Adjust the overbed table so it is at your waist level.
• Face your work area. This prevents unnecessary twisting.
• Push, slide, or pull heavy objects whenever you can rather than lifting them. Pushing is better than pulling.
• Widen your base of support when pushing or pulling. Move your front leg forward when pushing. Move your rear leg back when pulling (Fig. 11-3, p. 146).
• Use both hands and arms to lift, move, or carry heavy objects.
• Turn your whole body when changing the direction of your movement. Move and turn your feet in the direction of the turn, instead of twisting your body.
• Work with smooth and even movements. Avoid sudden or jerky motions.
• Do not lean over the person to give care.
• *Get help from a co-worker if the person cannot assist with turning or moving.* Two or three staff members may be needed to turn or move the person. Assist devices may also be needed. Follow the person's care plan.
• *Get help from a co-worker to move heavy objects or persons.* Do not turn or move them by yourself. Two or three staff members may be needed to turn or move the person. Assist devices also may be needed. Follow the person's care plan.
• Bend your hips and knees to lift heavy objects from the floor (see Fig. 11-2). Straighten your back as the object reaches thigh level. Your leg and thigh muscles work to raise the item off the floor and to waist level.
• Do not lift objects higher than chest level. Do not lift above your shoulders. Use a step stool to reach an object higher than chest level.
• Use assist equipment and devices whenever possible instead of lifting and moving the person manually. Follow the person's care plan.

Key Terms are the important words and phrases in the chapter. Definitions are given for each term. The key terms introduce you to the chapter content. They are also a useful study guide.

Bolded type is used to highlight the key terms in the text. You again see the key term and read its definition. This helps reinforce your learning.

Boxes and tables contain important rules, principles, guidelines, signs and symptoms, nursing measures, and other information in a list format. They identify important information and are useful study guides.

Heading icons alert you to associated procedures. Procedure boxes contain the same icon.

Delegation Guidelines describe what information you need from the nurse and care plan before performing a procedure. They also tell you what information to report and record.

Promoting Safety and Comfort focus your attention on the need to be safe and cautious and promote comfort when giving care.

Color illustrations and photographs visually present key ideas, concepts, or procedure steps. They help you apply and remember the written material.

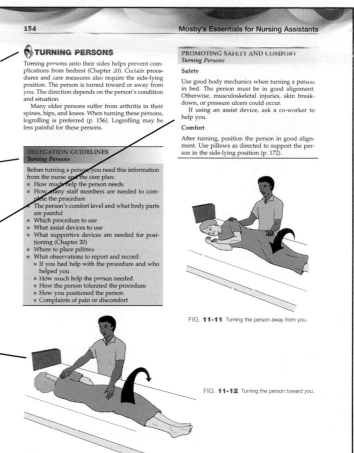

CD icon—appears in the procedure box title bar for the skills included in the CD Companion found at the back of the book.

NNAAP™ in the procedure title bar alerts you to those skills that are part of the National Nurse Aide Assessment Program (NNAAP™). Note: All states do not participate in NNAAP™. Ask your instructor for a list of the skills tested in your state.

Procedures are written in a step-by-step format. They are divided into Pre-Procedure, Procedure, and Post-Procedure sections for easy studying.

Quality of Life in the procedure boxes reminds you of six simple courtesies that show respect for the patient or resident as a person.

Procedure icon in the title bar alerts you to associated content areas. Heading icons and procedure icons are the same.

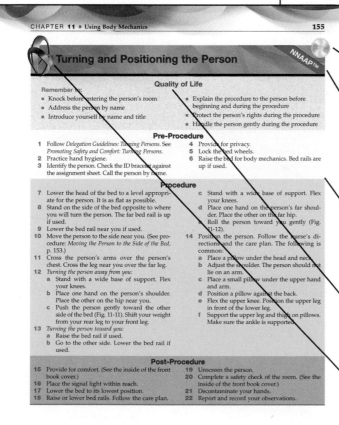

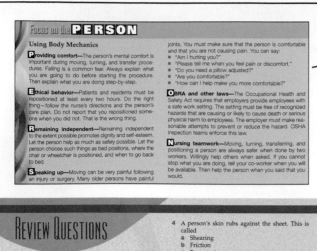

Focus on the Person boxes are found at the end of Chapters 7 through 27. Building on concepts and principles presented in Chapters 1 through 6, PERSON is spelled out in the first letter of each bullet beginning in Chapter 7:

- **P**roviding comfort—suggests ways to meet the person's comfort needs.
- **E**thical behavior—stresses doing the right thing when dealing with patients, residents, and co-workers.
- **R**emaining independent—reminds the student to encourage the person to do as much for himself or herself as possible.
- **S**peaking up—gives the student ideas of what to say and questions to ask when interacting with patients and residents.
- **O**BRA and other laws—informs the student of OBRA requirements and other laws affecting health care and nursing assistant functions.
- **N**ursing teamwork—suggests ways to work with and help other nursing team members. The intent is to foster teamwork.

Review Questions are a useful study guide. They help you to review what you have learned. They can also be used when studying for a test or the competency evaluation. Answers are given at the back of the book beginning on p. 467.

Persons With Dementia boxes focus on information and insights about caring for persons with dementia.

Caring About Culture boxes contain information to help you learn about the various practices of other cultures.

Contents

1 Introduction to Health Care Agencies, 1

Hospitals, 2
Long-Term Care Centers, 2
Hospital and Nursing Center Organization, 4
The Nursing Team, 4
Nursing Care Patterns, 5
Paying For Health Care, 5
The Omnibus Budget Reconciliation Act
  of 1987, 7

2 The Nursing Assistant, 11

OBRA Requirements, 12
Roles and Responsibilities, 13
Job Description, 14
Delegation, 14
Ethical Aspects, 18
Legal Aspects, 18
Reporting Abuse, 19

3 Work Ethics, 22

Health, Hygiene, and Appearance, 23
Getting a Job, 23
Preparing For Work, 27
Teamwork on the Job, 28
Harassment, 30
Resigning From a Job, 30
Losing a Job, 30

4 Communicating With the Health Team, 33

Communication, 34
The Medical Record, 34
The Kardex, 34
The Nursing Process, 39
Resident Care Conferences, 43
Reporting and Recording, 43
Medical Terminology and Abbreviations, 44
Using Computers, 47
Phone Communications, 47
Dealing With Conflict, 48

5 Understanding the Person, 50

Caring For the Person, 51
Needs, 51
Culture and Religion, 52
Behavior Issues, 52
Communicating With the Person, 54
The Family and Visitors, 58

6 Understanding Body Structure and Function, 60

Cells, Tissues, and Organs, 61
The Integumentary System, 62
The Musculoskeletal System, 63
The Nervous System, 66
The Circulatory System, 69
The Respiratory System, 71
The Digestive System, 72
The Urinary System, 74
The Reproductive System, 74
The Endocrine System, 77
The Immune System, 78

7 Caring For the Older Person, 81

Growth and Development, 82
Social Changes, 82
Physical Changes, 84
Needing Nursing Center Care, 85
Sexuality, 86
Ombudsman Program, 87
Focus on the Person, 88

8 Promoting Safety, 90

Accident Risk Factors, 91
Identifying the Person, 91
Preventing Falls, 92
Preventing Burns, 96
Preventing Poisoning, 96
Preventing Suffocation, 96
Preventing Equipment Accidents, 96
Wheelchair and Stretcher Safety, 97
Handling Hazardous Substances, 99
Fire Safety, 100
Using a Fire Extinguisher, 100
PROCEDURE: Using a Fire Extinguisher, 101
Disasters, 102
Workplace Violence, 102
Risk Management, 102
Focus on the Person, 103

9 Restraint Alternatives and Safe Restraint Use, 106

History of Restraint Use, 107
Restraint Alternatives, 107
Safe Restraint Use, 109
Applying Restraints, 115
PROCEDURE: Applying Restraints, 118
Focus on the Person, 120

10 Preventing Infection, 122

Microorganisms, 123
Infection, 123
Medical Asepsis, 124
Hand Hygiene, 125
PROCEDURE: Hand Washing, 127
Isolation Precautions, 128
Gloves, 133
PROCEDURE: Removing Gloves, 134
Gowns and Other Attire, 135
PROCEDURE: Donning and Removing
   a Gown, 135
Masks and Respiratory Protection, 137
PROCEDURE: Donning and Removing
   a Mask, 137
Bloodborne Pathogen Standard, 139
Focus on the Person, 141

11 Using Body Mechanics, 143

Body Mechanics, 144
Ergonomics, 146
Moving Persons in Bed, 146
Moving the Person Up in Bed, 148
PROCEDURE: Moving the Person Up in Bed, 149
Moving the Person Up in Bed With an Assist
   Device, 150
PROCEDURE: Moving the Person Up in Bed
   With an Assist Device, 151
Moving the Person to the Side of the Bed, 152
PROCEDURE: Moving the Person to the Side
   of the Bed, 153
Turning Persons, 154
PROCEDURE: Turning and Positioning
   the Person, 155
Logrolling, 156
PROCEDURE: Logrolling the Person, 157
Sitting on the Side of the Bed (Dangling), 158
PROCEDURE: Helping the Person Sit
   on the Side of the Bed (Dangle), 159
Transferring Persons, 160
Applying Transfer Belts, 160
PROCEDURE: Applying a Transfer Belt, 161
Bed to Chair or Wheelchair Transfers, 162
PROCEDURE: Transferring the Person
   to a Chair or Wheelchair, 163
Chair or Wheelchair to Bed Transfers, 165
PROCEDURE: Transferring the Person From
   a Chair or Wheelchair to Bed, 166
Using Mechanical Lifts, 167
PROCEDURE: Transferring the Person Using
   a Mechanical Lift, 167
Transferring the Person to and From
   the Toilet, 170
PROCEDURE: Transferring the Person
   to and From the Toilet, 171
Positioning, 172
Focus on the Person, 176

12 Assisting With Comfort, 179

The Person's Unit, 180
Bedmaking, 186
The Closed Bed, 189
PROCEDURE: Making a Closed Bed, 189
The Occupied Bed, 195
PROCEDURE: Making an Occupied Bed, 195
The Surgical Bed, 199
PROCEDURE: Making a Surgical Bed, 199
Sleep, 200
Focus on the Person, 201

13 Assisting With Hygiene, 203

Daily Care, 204
Oral Hygiene, 205
Brushing and Flossing Teeth, 205
PROCEDURE: Brushing the Person's Teeth, 206
Mouth Care For the Unconscious Person, 208
PROCEDURE: Providing Mouth Care For
   the Unconscious Person, 209
Denture Care, 210
PROCEDURE: Providing Denture Care, 211
Bathing, 213
The Complete Bed Bath, 214
PROCEDURE: Giving a Complete Bed Bath, 215
The Partial Bath, 220
PROCEDURE: Giving a Partial Bath, 221
Tub Baths and Showers, 222
PROCEDURE: Assisting With a Tub Bath
   or Shower, 224
The Back Massage, 225
PROCEDURE: Giving a Back Massage, 226
Perineal Care, 228
PROCEDURE: Giving Female Perineal Care, 229
PROCEDURE: Giving Male Perineal Care, 231
Focus on the Person, 232

14 Assisting With Grooming, 234

Hair Care, 235
Brushing and Combing Hair, 235
PROCEDURE: Brushing and Combing
   the Person's Hair, 236
Shampooing, 238
PROCEDURE: Shampooing the Person's
   Hair, 239
Shaving, 241
PROCEDURE: Shaving the Person, 242
Nail and Foot Care, 243
PROCEDURE: Giving Nail and Foot Care, 245
Changing Gowns and Clothing, 246
Changing Gowns, 247
PROCEDURE: Changing the Gown of the
   Person With an IV, 247
Dressing and Undressing, 248
PROCEDURE: Undressing the Person, 249
PROCEDURE: Dressing the Person, 253
Focus on the Person, 255

15   Assisting With Urinary Elimination, 256

Normal Urination, 257
Bedpans, 258
PROCEDURE: Giving the Bedpan, 259
Urinals, 261
PROCEDURE: Giving the Urinal, 262
Commodes, 263
PROCEDURE: Helping the Person
  to the Commode, 263
Urinary Incontinence, 264
Catheters, 266
PROCEDURE: Giving Catheter Care, 268
Drainage Systems, 269
PROCEDURE: Emptying a Urinary Drainage
  Bag, 271
The Condom Catheter, 271
PROCEDURE: Applying a Condom
  Catheter, 273
Bladder Training, 274
Focus on the Person, 274

16   Assisting With Bowel Elimination, 276

Normal Bowel Movements, 277
Factors Affecting Bowel Elimination, 277
Common Problems, 278
Bowel Training, 279
Enemas, 280
The Cleansing Enema, 281
PROCEDURE: Giving a Cleansing Enema, 281
The Small-Volume Enema, 284
PROCEDURE: Giving a Small-Volume
  Enema, 285
The Person With an Ostomy, 286
Focus on the Person, 288

17   Assisting With Nutrition and Fluids, 290

Basic Nutrition, 291
Factors Affecting Eating and Nutrition, 295
OBRA Dietary Requirements, 296
Special Diets, 297
Fluid Balance, 299
Meeting Food and Fluid Needs, 300
Preparing for Meals, 300
PROCEDURE: Preparing the Person
  For a Meal, 301
Serving Meal Trays, 302
PROCEDURE: Serving Meal Trays, 303
Feeding the Person, 303
PROCEDURE: Feeding the Person, 305
Meeting Special Needs, 306
Focus on the Person, 309

18   Assisting With Assessment, 311

Vital Signs, 312
Taking Temperatures, 315

PROCEDURE: Taking a Temperature With
  a Glass Thermometer, 315
Electronic Thermometers, 317
PROCEDURE: Taking a Temperature With
  an Electronic Thermometer, 319
Pulse, 320
Taking a Radial Pulse, 321
PROCEDURE: Taking a Radial Pulse, 322
Taking an Apical Pulse, 323
PROCEDURE: Taking an Apical Pulse, 323
Respirations, 324
PROCEDURE: Counting Respirations, 324
Blood Pressure, 325
Measuring Blood Pressure, 326
PROCEDURE: Measuring Blood Pressure, 327
Intake and Output, 329
Measuring Intake and Output, 329
PROCEDURE: Measuring Intake and
  Output, 330
Measuring Weight and Height, 331
PROCEDURE: Measuring Weight and
  Height, 331
Pain, 333
Focus on the Person, 334

19   Assisting With Specimens, 336

Urine Specimens, 337
The Random Urine Specimen, 337
PROCEDURE: Collecting a Random Urine
  Specimen, 338
The Midstream Specimen, 338
PROCEDURE: Collecting a Midstream
  Specimen, 339
The Double-Voided Specimen, 340
PROCEDURE: Collecting a Double-Voided
  Specimen, 340
Testing Urine, 341
PROCEDURE: Testing Urine With Reagent
  Strips, 342
Stool Specimens, 343
PROCEDURE: Collecting a Stool Specimen, 343
Sputum Specimens, 345
PROCEDURE: Collecting a Sputum
  Specimen, 346
Focus on the Person, 347

20   Assisting With Exercise and Activity, 349

Bedrest, 350
Range-of-Motion Exercises, 353
PROCEDURE: Performing Range-of-Motion
  Exercises, 354
Ambulation, 359
PROCEDURE: Helping the Person to Walk, 360
The Falling Person, 361
PROCEDURE: Helping the Falling Person, 361
Focus on the Person, 365

21 Assisting With Wound Care, 367

Skin Tears, 368
Pressure Ulcers, 368
Circulatory Ulcers, 373
Elastic Stockings, 374
PROCEDURE: Applying Elastic Stockings, 375
Elastic Bandages, 376
PROCEDURE: Applying Elastic Bandages, 377
Dressings, 378
Applying Dressings, 378
PROCEDURE: Applying a Dry Non-Sterile Dressing, 379
Binders, 380
Heat and Cold Applications, 381
Focus on the Person, 382
PROCEDURE: Applying Heat and Cold Applications, 385

22 Assisting With Oxygen Needs, 388

Altered Respiratory Function, 389
Promoting Oxygenation, 389
Coughing and Deep Breathing, 390
PROCEDURE: Assisting With Coughing and Deep-Breathing Exercises, 391
Oxygen Therapy, 392
Focus on the Person, 394

23 Assisting With Rehabilitation and Restorative Care, 396

Restorative Nursing, 397
Rehabilitation and the Whole Person, 397
The Rehabilitation Team, 401
Quality of Life, 402
Focus on the Person, 402

24 Caring For Persons With Common Health Problems, 404

Cancer, 405
Musculoskeletal Disorders, 406
Nervous System Disorders, 411
Hearing Loss, 414
Eye Disorders, 417
Respiratory Disorders, 420
Cardiovascular Disorders, 421
Urinary System Disorders, 423
The Endocrine System, 423
Digestive Disorders, 424
Communicable Diseases, 425
Mental Health Disorders, 426
Focus on the Person, 429

25 Caring For Persons With Confusion and Dementia, 432

Confusion, 433
Dementia, 433
Alzheimer's Disease, 434
Care of Persons With AD and Other Dementias, 437
Quality of Life, 441
Focus on the Person, 442

26 Assisting With Emergency Care, 444

Emergency Care, 445
Basic Life Support, 445
Cardiopulmonary Resuscitation for Adults, 446
PROCEDURE: Adult CPR—One rescuer, 449
PROCEDURE: Adult CPR—Two Rescuers, 450
Foreign-Body Airway Obstruction in Adults, 450
PROCEDURE: FBAO—The Responsive Adult, 451
PROCEDURE: FBAO—The Unresponsive Adult, 452
Hemorrhage, 453
Shock, 455
Seizures, 455
Fainting, 455
Stroke, 456
Focus on the Person, 456

27 Caring For the Dying Person, 458

Attitudes About Death, 459
The Stages of Dying, 460
Psychological, Social, and Spiritual Needs, 460
Physical Needs, 460
The Family, 461
Hospice Care, 461
Legal Issues, 461
Signs of Death, 462
Care of the Body After Death, 462
PROCEDURE: Assisting With Postmortem Care, 463
Focus on the Person, 465

Review Question Answers, 467

Appendixes

A National Nurse Aide Assessment Program (NNAAP™) Written Examination Content Outline, 471
National Nurse Aide Assessment Program (NNAAP™) Skills Evaluation, 471

B Minimum Data Set, Version 2.0, 472

C Useful Spanish Vocabulary and Phrases, 483

Glossary, 498

Procedures

Promoting Safety
Using a Fire Extinguisher, 101

Restraint Alternatives and Safe Restraint Use
Applying Restraints, 118

Preventing Infection
Hand Washing, 127
Removing Gloves, 134
Donning and Removing a Gown, 135
Donning and Removing a Mask, 137

Using Body Mechanics
Moving the Person Up in Bed, 149
Moving the Person Up in Bed With an Assist Device, 151
Moving the Person to the Side of the Bed, 153
Turning and Positioning the Person, 155
Logrolling the Person, 157
Helping the Person Sit on the Side of the Bed (Dangle), 159
Applying a Transfer Belt, 161
Transferring the Person to a Chair or Wheelchair, 163
Transferring the Person From a Chair or Wheelchair to Bed, 166
Transferring the Person Using a Mechanical Lift, 167
Transferring the Person to and From the Toilet, 171

Assisting With Comfort
Making a Closed Bed, 189
Making an Occupied Bed, 195
Making a Surgical Bed, 199

Assisting With Hygiene
Brushing the Person's Teeth, 206
Providing Mouth Care for the Unconscious Person, 209
Providing Denture Care, 211
Giving a Complete Bed Bath, 215
Giving a Partial Bath, 221
Assisting With a Tub Bath or Shower, 224
Giving a Back Massage, 226
Giving Female Perineal Care, 229
Giving Male Perineal Care, 231

Assisting With Grooming
Brushing and Combing the Person's Hair, 236
Shampooing the Person's Hair, 239
Shaving the Person, 242
Giving Nail and Foot Care, 245
Changing the Gown of a Person With an IV, 247
Undressing the Person, 249
Dressing the Person, 253

Assisting With Urinary Elimination
Giving the Bedpan, 259
Giving the Urinal, 262

Helping the Person to the Commode, 263
Giving Catheter Care, 268
Emptying a Urinary Drainage Bag, 271
Applying a Condom Catheter, 273

Assisting With Bowel Elimination
Giving a Cleansing Enema, 281
Giving a Small-Volume Enema, 285

Assisting With Nutrition and Fluids
Preparing the Person For a Meal, 301
Serving Meal Trays, 303
Feeding the Person, 305

Assisting With Assessment
Taking a Temperature With a Glass Thermometer, 315
Taking a Temperature With an Electronic Thermometer, 319
Taking a Radial Pulse, 322
Taking an Apical Pulse, 323
Counting Respirations, 324
Measuring Blood Pressure, 327
Measuring Intake and Output, 330
Measuring Weight and Height, 331

Assisting With Specimens
Collecting a Random Urine Specimen, 338
Collecting a Midstream Specimen, 339
Collecting a Double-Voided Specimen, 340
Testing Urine With Reagent Strips, 342
Collecting a Stool Specimen, 343
Collecting a Sputum Specimen, 346

Assisting With Exercise and Activity
Performing Range-of-Motion Exercises, 354
Helping the Person to Walk, 360
Helping the Falling Person, 361

Assisting With Wound Care
Applying Elastic Stockings, 375
Applying Elastic Bandages, 377
Applying a Dry Non-Sterile Dressing, 379
Applying Heat and Cold Applications, 385

Assisting With Oxygen Needs
Assisting With Coughing and Deep Breathing Exercises, 391

Assisting With Emergency Care
Adult CPR—One Rescuer, 449
Adult CPR—Two Rescuers, 450
FBAO—The Responsive Adult, 451
FBAO—The Unresponsive Adult, 452

Caring For the Dying Person
Assisting With Postmortem Care, 463

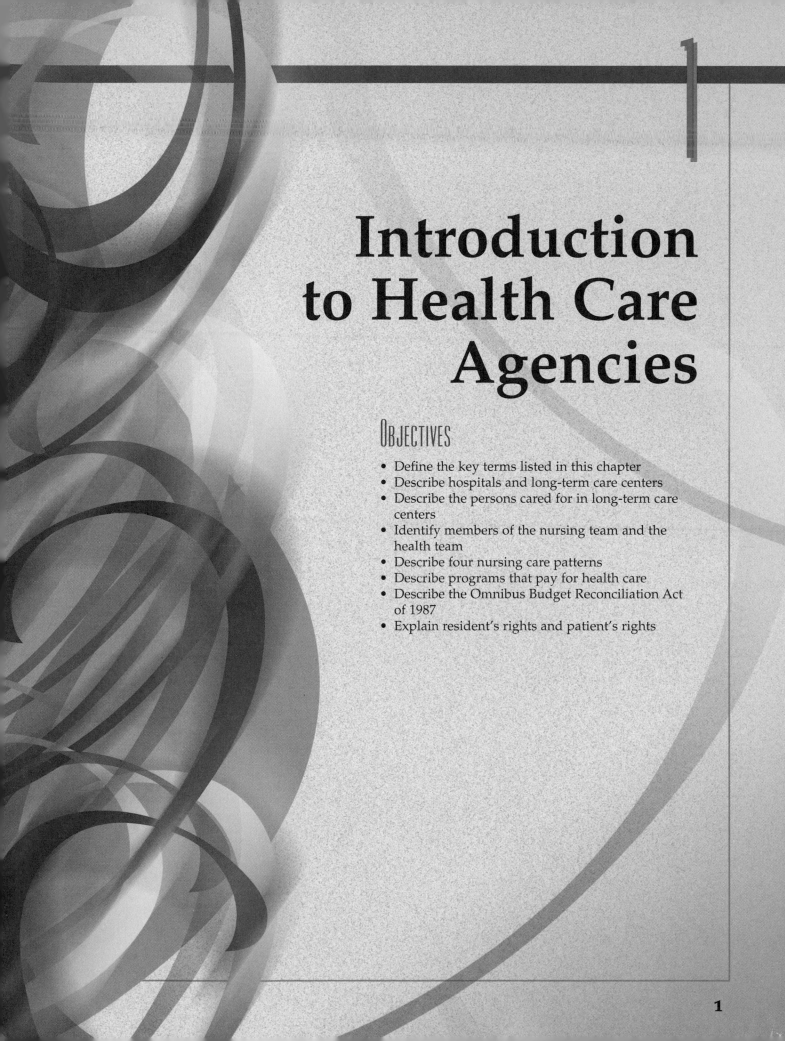

Introduction to Health Care Agencies

OBJECTIVES

- Define the key terms listed in this chapter
- Describe hospitals and long-term care centers
- Describe the persons cared for in long-term care centers
- Identify members of the nursing team and the health team
- Describe four nursing care patterns
- Describe programs that pay for health care
- Describe the Omnibus Budget Reconciliation Act of 1987
- Explain resident's rights and patient's rights

KEY TERMS

assisted living facility Provides housing, support services, and health care to persons needing help with daily activities

board and care home Provides a room, meals, laundry, and supervision; residential care facility

health team Staff members who work together to provide health care; called the interdisciplinary health care team in nursing centers

hospice An agency or program for persons who are dying

licensed practical nurse (LPN) A nurse who has completed a 1-year nursing program and has passed a licensing test; called licensed vocational nurse (LVN) in some states

licensed vocational nurse (LVN) Licensed practical nurse

nursing assistant A person who gives basic nursing care under the supervision of a licensed nurse

nursing center Provides health care services to persons who need regular or continuous care; nursing home or nursing facility

nursing facility (NF) Nursing center or nursing home

nursing home Nursing center or nursing facility

nursing team RNs, LPNs/LVNs, and nursing assistants

Omnibus Budget Reconciliation Act of 1987 (OBRA) A law that requires nursing centers to provide care in a manner and setting that maintains or improves a person's quality of life, health, and safety

registered nurse (RN) A nurse who has completed a 2-, 3-, or 4-year nursing program and has passed a licensing test

residential care facility A board and care home

skilled nursing facility (SNF) A nursing center that provides complex care for persons with severe health problems

subacute care Complex medical care or rehabilitation for persons who no longer need hospital care

Hospitals and long-term care centers provide health care services. Staff members use their talents, knowledge, and skills to meet the person's needs. The *person* is the focus of care.

HOSPITALS

Hospitals provide emergency care, surgery, nursing care, x-ray procedures and treatments, and laboratory testing. They also provide respiratory, physical, occupational, and speech therapies. People of all ages need hospital care. They have babies, surgery, mental health problems, and broken bones. Some people need hospital care to diagnose and treat medical problems or to die.

Persons can have acute, chronic, or terminal illnesses.

- *Acute illness* begins suddenly. The person will likely recover. Heart attack is an example.
- *Chronic illness* is on-going. It often begins slowly and has no cure. The illness can be controlled and complications prevented. Some nervous system disorders result in chronic illness.
- *Terminal illness* ends in death. The person has an illness or injury for which there is no reasonable expectation of recovery. Cancers that do not respond to treatment are examples.

Some hospital stays are less than 24 hours. Some surgeries, diagnostic tests, and therapies do not require 24-hour stays. Other hospital stays can last days, weeks, or months.

Patient's Rights

In April, 2003, The American Hospital Association adopted *The Patient Care Partnership: Understanding Expectations, Rights, and Responsibilities.* The document explains the persons rights and expectations during hospital stays. They include:

- High quality care
- A clean and safe setting
- Being involved in care
- Having privacy protected
- Being prepared to leave the hospital
- Help understanding the hospital bill and filing insurance claims

LONG-TERM CARE CENTERS

Some persons cannot care for themselves. Hospital care is not needed. Long-term care centers are designed to meet their needs. Medical, nursing, dietary, recreational, rehabilitative, and social services are provided.

Persons in long-term care centers are *residents.* They are not patients. The center is their permanent or temporary home.

Most residents are older. They have chronic diseases, poor nutrition, or poor health. Not all residents are old. Some are disabled from birth defects, accidents, or diseases. People are often discharged from hospitals while still recovering from illness or surgery. Some residents return home when well enough. Others need nursing care until death.

Long-term care centers meet the needs of:

- *Alert, oriented residents*—They know who they are, where they are, the year, and the time of day. They have physical problems. Disability level affects the amount of care required. Some require complete care. Others need help with daily activities.

- *Confused and disoriented residents*—They are mildly to severely confused and disoriented. Some simply have trouble remembering where the dining room is or the month and year. Others are more confused and disoriented—they do not know who or where they are. Sometimes the problem is short term. For others, the confusion and disorientation are permanent and become worse.
- *Complete care residents*—Some persons are disabled, confused, and disoriented. They cannot meet their own needs or tell you what they need. They need to be kept clean, safe, and comfortable.
- *Short-term residents*—Some persons need to recover from fractures, illnesses, or surgery. They need to regain strength and mobility to return to their former living situations. Some people cared for at home are admitted to nursing centers for short stays. This is *respite care.* The home caregiver can go on a trip, attend to business matters, or simply rest.
- *Life-long residents*—Birth defects and childhood injuries and diseases can cause disabilities. Mental retardation and Down syndrome are common causes. A disability occurring before 22 years of age is *a developmental disability.* It may be a physical impairment, intellectual impairment, or both. The person has limited function in at least three of these areas: self-care, understanding or expressing language, learning, mobility, self-direction, independent living, and financial support of one's self. The person needs lifelong assistance, support, and special services. Some nursing centers admit developmentally disabled children and adults.
- *Mentally ill residents*—Some people have problems coping or adjusting to stress. Behavior and function are affected. In severe cases, self-care and independent living are impaired. Some residents have physical and mental illnesses.
- *Terminally ill residents*—They may have advanced cancer; liver, kidney, respiratory, or heart disease; or AIDS. Some are alert and oriented; others are comatose. Comatose persons cannot respond to what people say to them. But they may still feel pain. Some have severe pain. Terminally ill persons may need hospice care.

Board and Care Homes

A **board and care home (residential care facility)** provides a room, meals, laundry, and supervision. Each person has a room. They share common areas and eat meals together.

A safe setting is provided but not 24-hour nursing care. Residents usually can dress themselves and meet grooming and elimination needs with little help.

Some homes are for older persons. Others are for people with certain problems. Dementia, mental health problems, and developmental disabilities are examples.

Assisted Living Facilities

An **assisted living facility** provides housing, support services, and health care to persons needing help with daily activities. Most assisted living residents need help taking drugs and with bathing, dressing, elimination, and eating. Many are cognitively impaired. They have problems with thinking, reasoning, and judgment.

Mobility is often required. The person walks or uses a wheelchair or motor scooter. The person must be able to leave the building in an emergency. Stable health also is required. Only limited health care or treatment is needed.

A home-like setting is provided. Residents have a secure setting and 24-hour supervision. They have three meals a day. There are laundry, housekeeping, transportation, social, recreational, and some health services. Services are added or reduced as the person's needs change.

Some assisted living facilities are part of nursing centers or retirement communities. Others are separate facilities. Assisted living facilities must follow state laws and regulations.

Nursing Centers

A **nursing center** provides health care services to residents who need regular or continuous care. **Nursing facility** and **nursing home** are other names. Licensed nurses are required. Medical, nursing, dietary, recreational, rehabilitative, and social services are provided.

Some centers also provide complex care for severe health problems. Such centers are called **skilled nursing facilities (SNFs).** They are part of nursing centers or hospitals (skilled nursing units). Many people are admitted to SNFs from hospitals. They stay for a short time to recover from an illness or surgery or for rehabilitation. Others never return home.

Some nursing centers and hospitals provide subacute care. **Subacute care** is complex medical care or rehabilitation for persons who no longer need hospital care. Such persons may have nervous system injuries, bone or joint injuries or surgeries, or wounds that are not healing. Persons on subacute care units may be called *patients.* Short stays are common.

Hospices
A **hospice** is an agency or program for persons who are dying. The physical, emotional, social, and spiritual needs of the person and family are met. The focus is on comfort, not cure. Hospice care is provided by hospitals, nursing centers, and home care agencies.

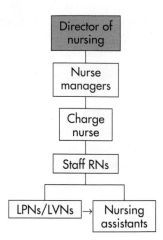

FIG. **1-1** Organization of the nursing department.

Alzheimer's Units (Dementia Care Units)

An Alzheimer's unit is designed for persons with Alzheimer's disease and other dementias (Chapter 25). Such persons suffer increasing memory loss and confusion until they cannot tend to simple personal needs. They often wander about and may become agitated or combative. The unit usually is closed off from the rest of the center. The closed unit provides a safe setting where residents can wander freely.

HOSPITAL AND NURSING CENTER ORGANIZATION

A hospital has a governing body called the *board of trustees*. The board makes policies. It makes sure that good, safe care is given at the lowest possible cost. An administrator manages the hospital. He or she reports to the board. Directors or department heads manage certain areas.

Nursing centers usually are owned by an individual or a corporation. Some are owned by county health departments. Each center has an administrator. Department directors report to the administrator. Nursing centers have nursing, therapy, and food service departments (Fig. 1-1). They also have social service and activity departments.

Hospitals and nursing centers must follow local, state, and federal laws and rules. Safe care must be provided.

Nursing Service

Nursing service is a large department. The director of nursing (DON) is an RN. The DON is responsible for the entire nursing staff and the care given. Nurse managers (usually RNs) assist the DON. They manage and carry out nursing department functions.

Nurse managers oversee a work shift, a nursing area, or a certain function. Functions include staff development, restorative nursing, infection control, or continuous quality improvement. Nurse managers are responsible for all nursing care and the actions of nursing staff in their areas.

Each nursing area has RNs. They provide nursing care and supervise LPNs/LVNs and nursing assistants. Staff RNs report to the nurse manager. LPNs/LVNs report to staff RNs or to the nurse manager. You report to the RN or LPN/LVN supervising your work.

Nursing education is part of nursing service. Nursing education staff:
- Plan and present educational programs
- Provide new and changing information
- Instruct on the use of new equipment
- Teach and train nursing assistants
- Conduct orientation programs for new staff

THE NURSING TEAM

The **nursing team** involves RNs, LPNs/LVNs, and nursing assistants. All focus on the physical, social, emotional, and spiritual needs of the person and family.

Registered Nurses

A **registered nurse (RN)** has completed a 2-, 3-, or 4-year nursing program and has passed a licensing test:
- Community college programs—2 years
- Hospital-based diploma programs—2 or 3 years
- College or university programs—4 years

The graduate nurse takes a licensing test offered by a state board of nursing. The nurse receives a license and becomes *registered* when the test is passed. RNs must have a license recognized by the state in which they work.

RNs assess, make nursing diagnoses, plan, implement, and evaluate nursing care (Chapter 4). They develop care plans, provide care, and delegate nursing care and tasks to the nursing team. They evaluate how care plans and nursing care affect each person. RNs teach persons how to improve or maintain health. They also teach the family.

RNs carry out the doctor's orders. They may delegate them to LPNs/LVNs or nursing assistants. RNs do not diagnose diseases or illnesses. They do not prescribe treatments or drugs. Some RNs study to become clinical nurse specialists or nurse practitioners. These RNs have diagnosing and prescribing functions.

Licensed Practical Nurses and Licensed Vocational Nurses

A **licensed practical nurse (LPN)** has completed a 1-year nursing program and has passed a licensing test. Hospitals, community colleges, vocational schools, and technical schools offer programs. Some programs are 10 to 18 months long. Some high schools offer 2-year programs.

Graduates take a licensing test. When the test is passed, the nurse receives a license and the title of *licensed practical nurse*. Some states use the term **licensed vocational nurse** (**LVN**). Like RNs, practical or vocational nurses must have a license to work.

LPNs/LVNs are supervised by RNs, licensed doctors, and licensed dentists. They have fewer responsibilities than RNs do. LPNs/LVNs have less education than RNs. They need little supervision when the person's condition is stable and care is simple. They assist RNs in caring for acutely ill persons and with complex procedures.

Nursing Assistants

Nursing assistants give basic nursing care under the supervision of a licensed nurse. *Nurse's aide, nursing attendant,* and *health care assistant* are other titles. Nursing assistants give much of the care in nursing centers. To work in nursing centers and skilled nursing units in hospitals, they must have formal training and pass a competency evaluation (Chapter 2).

NURSING CARE PATTERNS

Nursing care is given in many ways. The nursing care pattern depends on how many persons need care, the staff, and the cost.

- *Functional nursing* focuses on tasks and jobs. Each nursing team member has certain tasks and jobs to do. For example, one nurse gives all drugs. One nurse gives all treatments. Nursing assistants give baths, make beds, and serve meals.
- *Team nursing* involves a team of nursing staff led by an RN. The team leader delegates care to other nurses. Some tasks and procedures are delegated to nursing assistants. Delegation is based on the person's needs and team members' abilities. Team members report to the team leader about observations made and the care given.
- *Primary nursing* involves total care. An RN is responsible for the person's total care. The nursing team assists as needed. The RN *(primary nurse)* gives care and plans the person's discharge. The RN teaches and counsels the person and family.
- *Case management* is like primary nursing. A case manager (an RN) coordinates a person's care from admission through discharge and into the home setting. He or she communicates with the doctor and other health team members. There also is communication with the insurance company and community agencies involved in the person's care.

The Health Team

The **health team** involves staff members who work together to provide health care. (Called the *interdisciplinary health care team* in nursing centers.) Their skills and knowledge focus on the person's total care (Box 1-1, p. 6). The goal is to provide quality care.

Many staff members are involved in the care of one person. Coordinated care is needed. An RN usually coordinates the person's care.

PAYING FOR HEALTH CARE

Health care is costly. Most people cannot afford these bills. Some avoid health care because they cannot pay. Others pay doctor bills before buying food or drugs. If the person has insurance, some care costs are covered.

Health care is a major focus of society. The goals are to provide health care to everyone and to reduce care costs. Cost-cutting efforts include managed care and prospective payment systems.

You need to know the following:
- *Private insurance* is bought by individuals and families. It pays for some or all health care costs.
- *Group insurance* is bought by groups for individuals. Many employers and organizations provide health insurance for employees and members under group coverage.
- *Medicare* is a federal health insurance program. It is for persons 65 years of age or older. Some younger people with certain disabilities are covered. Medicare has two parts. Part A pays for some hospital, SNF, hospice, and home care costs. Part B helps pay for doctors' services, outpatient hospital care, physical and occupational therapists, some home care, and many other services. Part B is voluntary. The person pays a monthly premium.
- *Medicaid* is a health care payment program. It is sponsored by federal and state governments. Benefits, rules, and eligibility requirements vary from state to state. Older, blind, and disabled people are usually eligible. So are families with low incomes. There is no insurance premium. The amount paid for each covered service is limited.

Prospective Payment Systems

Prospective payment systems limit the amounts paid by insurers, Medicare, and Medicaid. Prospective means *before* care. The amount paid for services is determined before the person enters a health care agency.
- *Diagnosis-related groups (DRGs)* help reduce Medicare and Medicaid costs.
- *Resource utilization groups (RUGs)* are for SNF payments.
- *Case mix groups (CMGs)* are used to pay rehabilitation centers.

BOX 1-1 **The Health Team**	
Activities director	Assesses, plans, and implements recreational needs
Assistive personnel	Assist nurses in giving nursing care; supervised by a nurse (see nursing assistant)
Audiologist	Tests hearing; prescribes hearing aids; works with hearing-impaired persons
Cleric (clergyman; clergywoman)	Assists with spiritual needs
Dietitian	Assesses and plans for nutritional needs
Licensed practical/vocational nurse (LPN/LVN)	Provides nursing care and gives drugs under the direction of an RN
Medical records and health information technician	Maintains medical records; transcribes medical reports, completes reports
Medical technologist (MT)	Performs laboratory tests
Nurse practitioner	Works with the health team to plan and provide care; does physical exams, health assessments, and health education
Nursing assistant	See assistive personnel
Occupational therapist (OT)	Assists persons to learn or retain skills needed to perform activities of daily living; designs adaptive equipment for activities of daily living
Pharmacist	Fills drug orders written by doctors; monitors and evaluates drug interactions; consults with doctors and nurses about drug actions and interactions
Physical therapist (PT)	Assists persons with musculoskeletal problems; focuses on restoring function and preventing disability
Physician (doctor)	Diagnoses and treats diseases and injuries
Podiatrist	Prevents, diagnoses, and treats foot disorders
Radiographer/radiologic technologist	Takes x-rays and processes film for viewing
Registered nurse (RN)	Assesses, makes nursing diagnoses, plans, implements, and evaluates nursing care; supervises LPNs/LVNs, and nursing assistants
Respiratory therapist	Gives respiratory treatments and therapies
Social worker	Helps persons and families with social, emotional, and environmental issues affecting illness and recovery
Speech-language pathologist	Evaluates speech and language; treats persons with speech, voice, hearing, communication, and swallowing disorders

BOX 1-2   Types of Managed Care

Health Maintenance Organization (HMO)—For a pre paid fee, persons receive needed services offered by the HMO. Some need just an annual physical exam. Others require hospital care. HMOs stress preventing disease and maintaining health. Keeping someone healthy costs far less than treating illness.

Preferred Provider Organization (PPO)—A group of doctors and hospitals that provide health care at reduced rates. Usually the arrangement is between the PPO and an employer or an insurance company. Employees or those insured are given reduced rates for the services used. The person can choose any doctor or hospital in the PPO.

Managed Care

Managed care deals with health care delivery and payment (Box 1-2). Insurers contract with doctors and hospitals for reduced rates or discounts. The insured person uses doctors and agencies providing the lower rates. The person pays for costs not covered by insurance.

Managed care limits the choice of where to go for health care. It also limits the care that doctors provide. Many states require managed care for Medicaid and Medicare coverage.

THE OMNIBUS BUDGET RECONCILIATION ACT OF 1987

In 1987 the U.S. Congress passed the **Omnibus Budget Reconciliation Act (OBRA).** It applies to all 50 states. Nursing centers must provide care in a manner and setting that maintains or improves each person's quality of life, health, and safety. Nursing assistant training and competency evaluation are other requirements (Chapter 2). Resident rights are a major part of OBRA.

Resident Rights

Residents have rights as U.S. citizens. They also have rights relating to their everyday lives and nursing center care. Nursing centers must protect and promote their rights. The center cannot interfere with their rights. Some residents are not competent (not able). They cannot exercise their rights. A spouse, adult child, or legal representative does so for them.

Nursing centers must inform residents of their rights. This is done orally and in writing before or during admission to the center. It is given in the language the person uses and understands. Interpreters are used as needed.

Information

The person has the right to all of his or her records. They include the medical record, contracts, incident reports, and financial records. Record requests can be oral or written.

The person has the right to be fully informed of his or her total health condition. The person must also have information about his or her doctor. This includes the doctor's name, specialty, and how to contact the doctor.

You *do not* give the information described above to the person or family. Report the request to the nurse.

Refusing Treatment

The person can refuse treatment. If a person does not give consent or refuses treatment, it cannot be given. The center must find out what the person is refusing and why. Tell the nurse if a person refuses care measures. Care plan changes may be needed.

Privacy and Confidentiality

The person has the right to personal privacy. This includes using the bathroom in private and all personal care measures. The person's body is exposed only as needed. Only staff involved in the person's care are present. Consent is needed for others to be present.

Residents have the right to visit where others cannot see or hear them. If requested, the center must provide private space. Offices, chapels, dining rooms, and meeting rooms are used as needed.

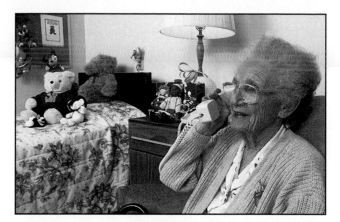

FIG. **1-2** Resident talking privately on the phone.

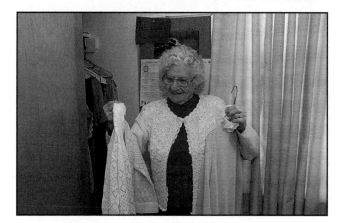

FIG. **1-3** Resident chooses what clothing to wear.

The right to privacy also involves mail and phone calls (Fig. 1-2). No one can interfere with the person sending or getting mail. Consent is needed to open any of the person's mail.

Information about the person's care, treatment, and condition is kept confidential. So are medical and financial records.

Personal Choice

Residents can choose their doctors. They also help plan and decide about their care and treatment. They can choose activities, schedules, and care. They can decide when to get up and go to bed, what to wear, how to spend time, and what to eat (Fig. 1-3). They can choose friends and visitors inside and outside the center. Allow personal choice whenever safely possible.

Disputes and Grievances

The person has the right to voice concerns, questions, and complaints about care. The problem may involve another person. It may be about care that was not given. The center must promptly try to correct the matter. No one can punish the person in any way for voicing the dispute or grievance.

Work

The person does not work for care, care items, or other things or privileges. The person is not required to perform services for the center.

However, the person *can* work or perform services if he or she wants. A person may want to garden, repair things, sew, or cook. Other persons need work for rehabilitation or activity reasons. The desire or need for work is part of the person's care plan.

Taking Part in Resident and Family Groups

The person has the right to form and take part in resident and family groups. Families can meet with other families. These groups can discuss concerns, suggest center improvements, and plan activities. They can support and comfort group members.

Residents have the right to take part in social, cultural, religious, and community events. They have the right to help in getting to and from events of their choice.

Care and Security of Personal Possessions

The person has the right to keep and use personal items. Treat such items with care and respect. The items may not have value to you but are important to the person. They also relate to personal choice, dignity, and quality of life.

The center must protect the person's property. Items are labeled with the person's name. The center must investigate reports of lost, stolen, or damaged items.

Protect yourself and the center from being accused of stealing a person's property. Do not go through a person's closet, drawers, purse, or other space without the person's consent. A nurse may ask you to inspect closets and drawers. If so, have a co-worker with you and the person or legal representative. They are witnesses to your activities.

Freedom From Abuse, Mistreatment, and Neglect

Residents have the right to be free from abuse. This includes verbal, sexual, physical, mental, or financial abuse (Chapter 2). They also have the right to be free from *involuntary seclusion*. This involves:

- Separating a person from others against his or her will
- Keeping the person confined to a certain area
- Keeping the person away from his or her room without consent

No one can abuse, neglect, or mistreat a resident. This includes center staff, volunteers, and staff from other agencies or groups. It also includes other residents, family members, visitors, and legal representatives. Centers must investigate suspected or reported cases of abuse. They cannot employ persons who were convicted of abusing, neglecting, or mistreating others.

Freedom From Restraint

The person has the right not to have body movements restricted. Restraints and certain drugs can restrict body movements (Chapter 9). Some drugs are restraints. They affect mood, behavior, and mental function. Sometimes residents are restrained to protect them from harming themselves or others. A doctor's order is needed for restraint use. Restraints are not used for staff convenience or to discipline a person.

Quality of Life

Residents must be cared for in a manner that promotes dignity and self-esteem. It must also promote physical, psychological, and mental well-being. Protecting the person's rights promotes quality of life. It shows respect for the person.

Speak to the person in a polite and courteous manner (Chapter 3). Give good, honest, and thoughtful care to enhance quality of life. See Box 1-3 for OBRA-required actions that promote dignity and privacy.

Activities. Nursing centers provide activity programs that allow personal choice. They must promote physical, intellectual, social, spiritual, and emotional well-being. Religious services promote spiritual health. Assist residents to and from activity programs. Help them with activities as needed.

Environment. The center's environment must promote quality of life. It must be clean, safe, and as home-like as possible. Personal items enhance quality of life. They allow personal choice and promote a home-like setting.

BOX 1-3	**OBRA-Required Actions to Promote the Resident's Dignity and Privacy**

Courteous and Dignified Interactions

- Use the right tone of voice.
- Use good eye contact.
- Stand or sit close enough as needed.
- Use the person's proper name and title.
- Gain the person's attention before interacting with him or her.
- Use touch if the person approves.
- Respect the person's social status.
- Listen with interest to what the person is saying.
- Do not yell, scold, or embarrass the person.

Courteous and Dignified Care

- Groom hair, beards, and nails as the person wishes.
- Assist with dressing. Clothing is right for time of day and personal choice.
- Promote independence and dignity in dining.
- Respect private space and property.
- Assist with walking and transfers. Do not interfere with independence.
- Assist with bathing and hygiene preferences. Do not interfere with independence.
  - Neat and clean appearance.
  - Clean shaven or groomed beard.
  - Nails trimmed and clean.
  - Dentures, hearing aids, eyeglasses, and other prostheses used correctly.
  - Clothing is clean.
  - Clothing is properly fitted and fastened.
  - Shoes, hose, and socks are properly applied and fastened.
  - Extra clothing for warmth as needed, such as sweater or lap blanket.

Privacy and Self-Determination

- Drape properly during care and procedures. Avoid exposure and embarrassment.
- Drape properly in chair.
- Use curtains or screens during care and procedures.
- Close the door to the room during care and procedures.
- Knock on the door before entering. Wait to be asked in.
- Close the bathroom door when person uses the bathroom.

Maintain Personal Choice and Independence

- Person smokes in allowed areas.
- Person takes part in activities according to interests.
- Person is involved in scheduling activities and care.
- Person gives input into care plan about preferences and independence.
- Person is involved in room or roommate change.

REVIEW QUESTIONS

Circle the **BEST** answer.

1 Persons in nursing centers are called
   a Patients
   b Residents
   c Clients
   d Patrons

2 Which statement is *true*?
   a People in nursing centers are always confused.
   b Most people in nursing centers are older.
   c People in nursing centers always need complete care.
   d People stay in nursing centers until they die.

3 Which agency provides complex care to persons with severe health problems?
   a A board and care home
   b An assisted living facility
   c A skilled nursing facility
   d A hospice

4 Who is responsible for the entire nursing staff?
   a The administrator
   b The director of nursing
   c The team leader
   d The primary nurse

5 You are supervised by
   a Licensed nurses
   b Doctors
   c The health team
   d The nursing team

6 Which is *not* a nursing care pattern?
   a Hospice nursing
   b Team nursing
   c Primary nursing
   d Functional nursing

7 In nursing centers, the health team is called
   a The interdisciplinary health care team
   b The nursing team
   c A diagnosis-related group
   d A resident group

8 Which is a federal health insurance program for persons 65 years of age or older?
   a OBRA
   b Medicaid
   c Medicare
   d Managed care

9 OBRA applies to
   a Hospitals
   b Older people
   c Hospices
   d All 50 states

These statements are about resident rights. Circle **T** if the statement is *true*. Circle **F** if the statement is *false*.

10 T F A person has the right to refuse treatment.
11 T F A person has the right to use the bathroom in private.
12 T F The person's body is exposed for care measures.
13 T F You can open a person's mail.
14 T F You can listen to a person's phone calls.
15 T F A person can decide when he or she will bathe.
16 T F You can punish a person for complaining about a nursing center.
17 T F A person has to work for nursing center meals.
18 T F A person has the right to attend religious services.
19 T F The person's items are treated with care and respect.
20 T F The person's items are labeled with his or her name.
21 T F You can search a person's closet and drawers.
22 T F The person must be free from abuse, mistreatment, and neglect.
23 T F You can decide when to restrain a person.
24 T F The person can take part in activities of his or her choice.
25 T F Nursing centers must be as home-like as possible.

Answers to these questions are on p. 467.

The Nursing Assistant

2

OBJECTIVES

- Define the key terms listed in this chapter
- Describe the educational requirements for nursing assistants
- Explain what nursing assistants can do and their role limits
- Explain why you need a job description
- Describe the delegation process and how to use the "five rights of delegation"
- Give examples of defamation, assault, battery, false imprisonment, invasion of privacy, and fraud
- Describe how to protect the right to privacy
- Explain the purpose of informed consent
- Describe elder abuse

Key Terms

abuse The intentional mistreatment or harm of another person

assault Intentionally attempting or threatening to touch a person's body without the person's consent

battery Touching a person's body without his or her consent

civil law Laws dealing with relationships between people

crime An act that violates a criminal law

criminal law Laws concerned with offenses against the public and against society

defamation Injuring a person's name and reputation by making false statements to a third person

delegate To authorize another person to perform a task

ethics Knowledge of what is right conduct and wrong conduct

false imprisonment Unlawful restraint or restriction of a person's freedom of movement

fraud Saying or doing something to trick, fool, or deceive a person

invasion of privacy When a person's name, picture, or private affairs are exposed or made public without consent

job description A list of responsibilities and functions the agency expects you to perform

law A rule of conduct made by a government body

libel Making false statements in print, writing, or through pictures or drawings

malpractice Negligence by a professional person

neglect Failure to provide the person with goods or services needed to avoid physical harm, mental anguish, or mental illness

negligence An unintentional wrong in which a person did not act in a reasonable and careful manner and caused harm to a person or property

slander Making false statements orally

task A function, procedure, activity, or work that does not require an RN's professional knowledge or judgment

You must protect patients and residents from harm. To do so, you need to know:
- What you can and cannot do
- What is right conduct and wrong conduct
- Your legal limits

Laws, job descriptions, and the person's condition shape your work. So does the amount of supervision you need.

Protecting persons from harm also involves rules and standards of conduct. They form the legal and ethical aspects of care.

OBRA REQUIREMENTS

The Omnibus Budget Reconciliation Act of 1987 (OBRA) applies to every state. Each state must have a nursing assistant training and competency evaluation program (NATCEP). It must be completed by nursing assistants working in nursing centers and hospital long-term care units.

The Training Program

OBRA requires at least 75 hours of instruction. Some states require more hours. The training program includes the knowledge and skills needed to give basic nursing care. Sixteen hours is supervised practical training. It occurs in a laboratory or clinical setting. The student performs nursing care and procedures on another person. A nurse supervises this practical training.

Competency Evaluation

The competency evaluation has a written test and a skills test (Appendix A, p. 471). The written test has multiple-choice questions. For the skills test, you perform certain skills learned in your training program.

You take the competency evaluation after your training program. Your instructor tells you where the tests are given. He or she helps you complete the application. The required fee is sent with your application.

If you listen, study hard, and practice safe care, you should do well on the written and skills tests. If the first attempt was not successful, you can retest. OBRA allows at least three attempts to successfully complete the evaluation.

Nursing Assistant Registry

Each state must have a nursing assistant registry. It is an official record or listing of persons who have successfully completed a NATCEP. The registry has information about each nursing assistant:
- Full name, including maiden name and any married names.
- Last known home address.
- Registration number and its expiration date.
- Date of birth.
- Last known employer, date hired, and date employment ended.
- Date the competency evaluation was passed.
- Information about findings of abuse, neglect, or dishonest use of property. It includes the nature of the offense and supporting evidence. If a hearing was held, the date and its outcome are included. The person has the right to include a statement disputing the finding. All information stays in the registry for at least 5 years.

BOX 2-1	Rules For Nursing Assistants

- You are an assistant to the nurse.
- A nurse assigns and supervises your work.
- You report observations about the person's physical or mental status to the nurse. Report changes at once.
- The nurse decides what should be done for a person. The nurse decides what should not be done for a person. You do not make these decisions.
- Review directions with the nurse before going to the person.
- Perform no function or task that you are not trained to do.
- Perform no function or task that you are not comfortable doing without a nurse's supervision.
- Perform only those functions and tasks that your state and job description allow.

Any agency can access registry information. You also receive a copy of your registry information. The copy is provided when the first entry is made and when information is changed or added. You can correct wrong information.

Other OBRA Requirements

Retraining and a new competency evaluation program are required for nursing assistants who have not worked for 2 consecutive years (24 months). It does not matter how long you worked as a nursing assistant. What matters is how long you did *not* work. States can require:

- A new competency evaluation
- Both retraining and a new competency evaluation

Nursing agencies must provide 12 hours of educational programs to nursing assistants every year. Performance reviews also are required. That is, the nursing assistant's work is evaluated. These requirements help ensure that nursing assistants have current knowledge and skills to give safe, effective care.

ROLES AND RESPONSIBILITIES

OBRA and state laws direct what you can do. To protect persons from harm, you must understand what you can do, what you cannot do, and the legal limits of your role.

Nurses supervise your work. Often you function without a nurse in the room. At other times you help nurses give care. The rules in Box 2-1 will help you understand your role.

Nursing assistant functions and responsibilities

BOX 2-2	Role Limits For Nursing Assistants

- ***Never give medications.*** Licensed nurses give drugs. In some states, nursing assistants can give drugs after completing a state-required medication aide training program.
- ***Never insert tubes or objects into body openings. Do not remove them from the body.*** Exceptions to this rule are the procedures that you will study during your training. Giving enemas is an example.
- ***Never take oral or telephone orders from doctors.*** Politely give your name and title, and ask the doctor to wait. Promptly find a nurse to speak with the doctor.
- ***Never perform procedures that require sterile technique.*** With sterile technique, all objects in contact with the person's body are free of microorganisms. You can assist a nurse with a sterile procedure. However, you will not perform the procedure yourself.
- ***Never tell the person or family the person's diagnosis or medical or surgical treatment plans.*** This is the doctor's responsibility. Nurses may clarify what the doctor has said.
- ***Never diagnose or prescribe treatments or drugs for anyone.*** Only doctors can diagnose and prescribe.
- ***Never supervise other nursing assistants or other staff.*** This is a nurse's responsibility. You will not be trained to supervise others. Supervising others can have serious legal consequences.
- ***Never ignore an order or request to do something that you cannot do or that is beyond your legal limits.*** Promptly explain to the nurse why you cannot carry out the order or request. The nurse assumes you are doing what you were told to do unless you explain otherwise. You cannot neglect the person's care.

---

vary among states and agencies. Before you perform a task or procedure make sure that:

- Your state allows nursing assistants to perform the task or procedure
- The procedure is in your job description
- You have the necessary training and education
- A nurse is available to answer questions and to supervise you

You perform tasks and procedures that meet hygiene, safety, comfort, nutrition, exercise, and elimination needs. You observe the person. This includes measuring temperatures, pulses, respirations, and blood pressures. You assist with admitting and discharging patients and residents. Promoting psychological comfort also is part of your role.

Box 2-2 describes the tasks and procedures that you never perform. State laws differ. You must know what you can do in the state in which you are working. State laws and rules limit nursing assistant functions. Nursing assistant job descriptions reflect those laws and rules.

JOB DESCRIPTION

The **job description** is a list of responsibilities and functions the agency expects you to perform (Fig. 2-1). Always request a written job description when you apply for a job. Ask questions about it during your job interview. Before accepting a job, tell the employer what functions you did not learn. Also advise the employer of functions you cannot do for moral or religious reasons. Clearly understand what is expected before taking a job. Do not take a job that requires you to:

- Act beyond the legal limits of your role
- Function beyond your training limits
- Perform acts that are against your morals or religion

No one can force you to do something beyond the legal limits of your role. Jobs may be threatened for refusing to follow a nurse's orders. Often staff obey out of fear. That is why you must understand your roles and responsibilities. You also need to know the functions you can safely perform, the things you should never do, and your job description.

DELEGATION

In nursing, a **task** is a function, procedure, activity, or work that does not require an RN's professional knowledge or judgment. **Delegate** means to authorize another person to perform a task. The person must be competent to perform the task in a given situation. For example, you know how to give a bed bath. However, Mr. Jones is a new resident. The RN wants to spend time with him and assess his nursing needs. The RN gives the bath.

Who Can Delegate

RNs can delegate tasks to LPNs/LVNs and nursing assistants. In some states, LPNs/LVNs can delegate tasks to nursing assistants. Delegation decisions must protect the person's health and safety.

The delegating nurse must make sure that the task was completed safely and correctly. If the RN delegates, the RN is responsible for the delegated task. If the LPN/LVN delegates, the LPN/LVN is responsible for the delegated task. The RN also supervises LPNs/LVNs. Therefore the RN also is responsible for the tasks that LPNs/LVNs delegate to nursing assistants. The RN is responsible for all nursing care.

Nursing assistants cannot delegate. You cannot delegate any task to other nursing assistants. You can ask someone to help you. But you cannot ask or tell someone to do your work.

Delegation Process

Delegated tasks must be within the legal limits of what you can do. The nurse must know:

- What tasks your state allows nursing assistants to perform
- The tasks in your job description
- What you were taught in your training program
- What skills you learned and how they were evaluated
- About your work experiences

The nurse discusses these areas with you. The nurse needs to learn about you, your abilities, and your concerns. You may be a new employee or new to the nursing unit. Or the nurse may be new. In any case, the nurse needs to know about you. You need to know about the nurse.

Agency policies and your job description state what tasks nurses can delegate to you. The person's needs, the task, and the staff member doing the task must fit. The person's needs and the task may require a nurse's knowledge, judgment, and skill. You may be asked to assist.

Delegation decisions must result in the best care for the person. A person's health and safety are at risk with poor delegation decisions.

The Five Rights of Delegation

The National Council of State Boards of Nursing's "five rights of delegation" sum up the delegation process:

- *The right task.* Can the task be delegated? Is the nurse allowed to delegate the task? Is the task in your job description?
- *The right circumstances.* What are the person's physical, mental, emotional, and spiritual needs at this time?
- *The right person.* Do you have the training and experience to safely perform the task for this person?
- *The right directions and communication.* The nurse must give clear directions. The nurse tells you what to do and when to do it, what observations to make, and when to report back. The nurse allows questions and helps you set priorities.
- *The right supervision.* The nurse guides, directs, and evaluates the care you give. The nurse demonstrates tasks as needed and is available to answer questions. The less experience you have with a task, the more supervision you need. Complex tasks require more supervision than do basic tasks. Also, the person's circumstances affect how much supervision you need. The nurse assesses how the task affected the person and how well you performed the task. The nurse tells you what you did well and what you can do to improve your work.

POSITION DESCRIPTION/PERFORMANCE EVALUATION

Job Title: Certified Nursing Assistant (CNA),   Supervised by: Licensed Nurse
Skilled Nursing Facility

Prepared by: _____   Date: _____   Approved by: _____   Date: _____

Job Summary: Provides direct and indirect resident care activities under the direction of an RN or LPN. Assists residents with activities of daily living, provides for personal care and comfort, and assists in the maintenance of a safe and clean environment for an assigned group of residents.

DUTIES AND RESPONSIBILITIES:

E=Exceeds the Standard   M=Meets the Standard   NI=Needs Improvement

Demonstrates Competency in the Following Areas:	E	M	NI
Assists in the preparation for admission of residents.	2	1	0
Assists in and accompanies residents in the admission, transfer, and discharge procedures.	2	1	0
Provides morning care, which may include bed bath, shower or whirlpool, oral hygiene, combing hair, back massage, dressing resident, changing bed linen, cleaning overbed table and bedside stand, straightening room, and other general care as necessary throughout the day.	2	1	0
Provides evening care, which includes hand/face washing as needed, oral hygiene, back massage, pericare, freshening linen, cleaning overbed table, straightening room, and other general care as needed.	2	1	0
Notifies RN/LPN when resident complains of pain.	2	1	0
Assists with post-mortem care.	2	1	0
Assists nurses in treatment procedures.	2	1	0
Provides general nursing care such as positioning residents, lifting and turning residents, applying/utilizing special equipment, assisting in use of bedpan or commode, and ambulating the residents.	2	1	0
Performs all aspects of resident care in an environment that optimizes resident safety and reduces the likelihood of medical/health care errors.	2	1	0
Takes and records temperature, pulse, respiration, weight, blood pressure, and intake-output.	2	1	0
Makes rounds with outgoing shift. Knows whereabouts of assigned residents.	2	1	0
Makes rounds with oncoming shift to ensure the unit is left in good condition.	2	1	0
Adheres to policies and procedures of the center and the Department of Nursing.	2	1	0
Participates in socialization activities on the unit.	2	1	0
Turns and positions residents as ordered and/or as needed, making sure no rough surfaces are in direct contact with the body. Moves and turns with proper and safe body mechanics and with available resources.	2	1	0
Checks for reddened areas or skin breakdown and reports to RN or LPN.	2	1	0
Ensures residents are dressed properly and assists, as necessary. Ensures that clothing is properly stored in bedside stand or on hangers in closet. Ensures that all residents are clean and dry at all times.	2	1	0
Checks unit for adequate linen. Cleans linen cart. Provides clean linen and clothing. Makes beds.	2	1	0
Treats residents and their families with respect and dignity.	2	1	0
Follows center policies and procedures when caring for persons who are restrained.	2	1	0
Prepares residents for meals. Serves and removes food trays. Assists with meals or feeds residents, if necessary.	2	1	0
Distributes drinking water and other nourishments to residents.	2	1	0

FIG. 2-1 Nursing assistant job description. Note that the job description is also a performance evaluation tool. (Modified from Medical Consultants Network, Inc., Englewood, Colorado.) *Continued*

POSITION DESCRIPTION/PERFORMANCE EVALUATION—cont'd

	E	M	NI
Performs general care activities for residents in isolation.	2	1	0
Answers residents' signal lights promptly. Anticipates residents' needs, and makes rounds to assigned residents.	2	1	0
Assists residents with handling and care of clothing and other personal property (including dentures, eyeglasses, contact lenses, hearing aids, and prosthetic devices).	2	1	0
Transports residents to and from various departments, as requested.	2	1	0
Reports and, when appropriate, records any changes observed in condition or behavior of residents and unusual incidents.	2	1	0
Participates in and contributes to Resident Care Conferences.	2	1	0
Follows directions, both oral and written, and works cooperatively with other staff members.	2	1	0
Establishes and maintains interpersonal relationships with residents, family members, and other center personnel while assuring confidentiality of resident information.	2	1	0
Has the ability to acquire knowledge of and develop skills in basic nursing procedures and simple charting.	2	1	0
Attends in-service education programs, as assigned, to learn new treatments, procedures, skills, etc.	2	1	0
Maintains personal health in order to prevent absence from work due to health problems.	2	1	0

Professional Requirements:

	E	M	NI
Meets dress code standards. Appearance is neat and clean.	2	1	0
Completes annual education requirements.	2	1	0
Maintains regulatory requirements.	2	1	0
Meets center's standards for attendance.	2	1	0
Consistently completes and maintains assigned duties.	2	1	0
Wears identification while on duty.	2	1	0
Practices careful, efficient, and non-wasteful use of supplies and linen. Follows established charge procedure for resident charge items.	2	1	0
Attends annual review and department in-services, as scheduled.	2	1	0
Attends at least 75% of staff meetings. Reads and returns all monthly staff meeting minutes.	2	1	0
Represents the center in a positive and professional manner.	2	1	0
Actively participates in the Continuous Quality Improvement (CQI) activities.	2	1	0
Complies with all center policies regarding ethical business practices.	2	1	0
Communicates the mission, ethics, and goals of the center, as well as the focus statement of the department.	2	1	0
Possesses a genuine interest and concern for older and disabled persons.	2	1	0

TOTAL POINTS _____ _____ _____

Regulatory Requirements:

- High School graduate or equivalent
- Current Certified Nursing Assistant (CNA) certification
- Current Basic Cardiac Life Support for Healthcare Providers certification within three (3) months of hire date

FIG. **2-1, cont'd** Nursing assistant job description. Note that the job description is also a performance evaluation tool. (Modified from Medical Consultants Network, Inc., Englewood, Colorado.)

Language Skills:

• Ability to read and communicate effectively in English

• Additional languages preferred

Skills:

• Basic computer knowledge

Physical Demands:

• See "Physical Demands" policy.

I have received, read, and understand the Position Description/Performance Evaluation above.

Name/Signature	Date Signed

FIG. **2-1, cont'd** Nursing assistant job description.

Your Role in Delegation

You must perform delegated tasks safely. This protects the person from harm. Use the "five rights of delegation" when deciding to accept or refuse a delegated task (Box 2-3).

Accepting a Task

When you agree to perform a task, you are responsible for your own actions. What you do or fail to do can harm the person. *You must complete the task safely.* Ask for help when you are unsure or have questions about a task. Report to the nurse what you did and the observations you made.

Refusing a Task

You have the right to say "no." Sometimes refusing to follow the nurse's directions is your right and duty. You should refuse to perform a task when:

■ The task is beyond the legal limits of your role
■ The task is not in your job description
■ You were not prepared to perform the task
■ The task could harm the person
■ The person's condition has changed
■ You do not know how to use the supplies or equipment
■ Directions are unethical, illegal, or against agency policies
■ Directions are unclear or incomplete
■ A nurse is not available for supervision

Use common sense. This protects you and the person. Ask yourself if what you are doing is safe for the person.

Never ignore an order or a request to do something. Tell the nurse about your concerns. You must not refuse a task because you do not like it or do not want to do it. You must have sound reasons. Otherwise, you risk losing your job.

BOX 2-3 | **The Five Rights of Delegation For Nursing Assistants**

The Right Task

• Does your state allow you to perform the task?
• Were you trained to do the task?
• Do you have experience performing the task?
• Is the task in your job description?

The Right Circumstances

• Do you have experience performing the task given the person's condition and needs?
• Do you understand the purpose of the task for the person?
• Can you perform the task safely under the current circumstances?
• Do you have the equipment and supplies to safely complete the task?
• Do you know how to use the equipment and supplies?

The Right Person

• Are you comfortable performing the task?
• Do you have concerns about performing the task?

The Right Directions and Communication

• Did the nurse give clear directions and instructions?
• Did you review the task with the nurse?
• Do you understand what the nurse expects?

The Right Supervision

• Is a nurse available to answer questions?
• Is a nurse available if the person's condition changes or if problems occur?

Modified from the National Council of State Boards of Nursing, Inc., Chicago.

BOX 2-4	Rules of Conduct For Nursing Assistants

- Respect each person as an individual.
- Perform no act that is not within the legal limits of your role.
- Perform only those acts you have been prepared to do.
- Take no drug without the prescription and supervision of a doctor.
- Carry out the directions and instructions of the nurse to your best possible ability.
- Complete each task safely.
- Be loyal to your employer and co-workers.
- Act as a responsible citizen at all times.
- Know the limits of your role and knowledge.
- Keep the person's information confidential.
- Protect the person's privacy.
- Consider the person's needs to be more important than your own.
- Perform no action that will cause the person harm.
- Do not accept gifts from patients, residents, or families.

ETHICAL ASPECTS

Ethics is knowledge of what is right conduct and wrong conduct. Morals are involved. It also deals with choices or judgments about what should or should not be done. An ethical person behaves and acts in the right way and does not harm anyone.

Ethical behavior also involves not being *prejudiced* or *biased*. To be prejudiced or biased means to make judgments and have views before knowing the facts. Judgments and views usually are based on one's values and standards. They are based in culture, religion, education, and experiences. For example, children want their mother to have nursing home care. In your culture, children care for older parents at home.

Codes of ethics are rules or standards of conduct. Nursing organizations have codes of ethics for RNs and LPNs/LVNs. The rules of conduct in Box 2-4 can guide your thinking and behavior. See Chapter 3 for ethics in the workplace. Also see Ethical Behavior in *Focus on the PERSON* boxes at the end of each chapter beginning in Chapter 7.

LEGAL ASPECTS

A **law** is a rule of conduct made by a government body. The U.S. Congress and state legislatures make laws. Laws protect the public welfare. They are enforced by the government.

Criminal laws are concerned with offenses against the public and against society. An act that violates a criminal law is a **crime** (murder, rape, kidnapping). A person found guilty of a crime is fined or sent to prison.

Civil laws deal with relationships between people. Examples include contracts and nursing practice. A person found guilty of breaking a civil law usually has to pay a sum of money to the injured person.

Tort comes from a French word meaning *wrong*. Torts are part of civil law. A tort is a wrong committed against a person or the person's property. Torts are intentional or unintentional.

Unintentional Torts

Negligence is an unintentional wrong. The negligent person did not act in a reasonable and careful manner. As a result, the person or property was harmed. The person did not do what a reasonable and careful person would have done. Or he or she did what a reasonable and careful person would not have done. Harm was not intended.

Malpractice is negligence by a professional person. A person has professional status because of training, education, and the service provided. Nurses, doctors, dentists, and lawyers are examples.

You are legally responsible *(liable)* for your own actions. What you do or do not do can lead to a lawsuit if a person or property is harmed. A nurse may ask you to do something beyond the legal limits of your role. The nurse is liable as your supervisor. *However, you are responsible for your actions.* Sometimes refusing a task is your right and duty (p. 17).

Intentional Torts

Intentional torts are acts meant to be harmful.

- **Defamation** is injuring a person's name and reputation by making false statements to a third person. **Libel** is making false statements in print, writing, or through pictures or drawings. **Slander** is making false statements orally.
- **Assault** is intentionally attempting or threatening to touch a person's body without the person's consent. The person fears bodily harm.
- **Battery** is touching a person's body without his or her consent. The person must consent to any procedure, treatment, or other act that involves touching the body. The person has the right to withdraw consent at any time.
- **False imprisonment** is the unlawful restraint or restriction of a person's freedom of movement. It involves:
  - Threatening to restrain a person
  - Restraining a person
  - Preventing a person from leaving the agency

BOX 2-5	Protecting the Right to Privacy

- Keep all information about the person confidential.
- Cover the person when he or she is being moved in hallways.
- Screen the person as in Figure 2-2. Close the door when giving care. Also close drapes and window shades.
- Expose only the body part involved in a treatment or procedure.
- Do not discuss the person or the person's treatment with anyone except the nurse supervising your work. "Shop talk" is a common cause of invasion of privacy.
- Ask visitors to leave the room when care is given.
- Do not open the person's mail.
- Allow the person to visit with others in private.
- Allow the person to use the phone in private.

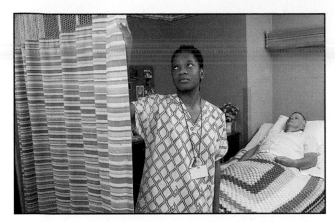

FIG. **2-2** Pulling the curtain around the bed helps protect the person's privacy.

- **Invasion of privacy** is when a person's name, picture, or private affairs are exposed or made public without consent. Only staff involved in the person's care should see, handle, or examine his or her body. See Box 2-5 for measures to protect privacy. The Health Insurance Portability and Accountability Act of 1996 (HIPAA) protects the privacy and security of a person's health information. *Protected health information* refers to identifying information and information about the person's health care. Failure to comply with HIPAA rules can result in fines, penalties, and criminal action including jail time. You must follow agency policies and procedures. Direct any questions about the person or the person's care to the nurse. Also follow the rules for computer use (Chapter 4).
- **Fraud** is saying or doing something to trick, fool, or deceive a person. The act is fraud if it does or could cause harm to a person or the person's property. Telling a person or family that you are a nurse is fraud. So is giving wrong or incomplete information on a job application.

Informed Consent

A person has the right to decide what will be done to his or her body and who can touch his or her body. The doctor is responsible for informing the person about all aspects of treatment. Consent is informed when the person clearly understands all aspects of treatment.

Persons under legal age (usually 18 years of age) cannot give consent. Nor can mentally incompetent persons. Such persons are unconscious, sedated, or confused or have certain mental health problems. Consent is given by a responsible party. A husband, wife, daughter, son, or a legal representative can give consent.

REPORTING ABUSE

Abuse is the intentional mistreatment or harm of another person. Abuse is a crime. It can occur at home or in a health care agency. Abuse has one or more of these elements:

- Willful causing of injury
- Unreasonable confinement
- Intimidation (to make afraid with threats of force or violence)
- Punishment
- Depriving the person of goods or services needed for physical, mental, or psychosocial well-being

Abuse causes physical harm, pain, or mental anguish. Protection against abuse extends to persons in a coma. The abuser is usually a family member or a caregiver. The abuser can be a friend, neighbor, landlord, or other person.

Elder abuse can take these forms:

- *Physical abuse.* Grabbing, hitting, slapping, kicking, pinching, hair-pulling, or beating. It also includes corporal punishment—punishment inflicted directly on the body. Beatings, lashings, or whippings are examples.
- *Neglect.* Failure to provide the person with goods or services needed to avoid physical harm, mental anguish, or mental illness is called **neglect.** This includes failure to provide health care or treatment, food, clothing, hygiene, and other needs. In health care, neglect includes but is not limited to:
  □ Leaving persons lying or sitting in urine or feces
  □ Keeping persons alone in their rooms or other areas
  □ Failing to answer signal lights
- *Verbal abuse.* Using oral or written words or statements that speak badly of, sneer at, criticize, or condemn the person. It also includes unkind gestures.

- *Involuntary seclusion or confinement.* Confining the person to a certain area. People have been locked in closets, basements, attics, and other spaces.
- *Financial exploitation.* To *exploit* means to use unjustly. Financial exploitation means that an older person's resources are misused by another person for that person's profit or benefit. The person's money is stolen or used by another person. It is also misusing a person's property. For example, a daughter sells her father's house without his consent.
- *Emotional abuse.* Humiliation, harassment, ridicule, and threats of punishment are emotional abuse. It includes being deprived of needs such as food, clothing, care, a home, or a place to sleep.
- *Sexual abuse.* The person is harassed about sex or is attacked sexually. The person may be forced to perform sexual acts out of fear of punishment or physical harm.

The abused person may show only some of the signs in Box 2-6. Federal and state laws require the reporting of abuse or suspected abuse. If you suspect abuse, discuss your concerns with the nurse. Give as much information as possible. The nurse contacts health team members as needed. Community agencies that investigate elder abuse also are contacted. Sometimes the help of police or the courts is necessary.

OBRA Requirements

OBRA does not allow nursing centers to employ persons who were convicted of abuse, neglect, or mistreatment of persons in any health care agency. Before hiring a person, the center must thoroughly check the applicant's work history. All references must be checked. Efforts must be made to find out about any criminal prosecutions.

The employer also checks the nursing assistant registry for any findings about abuse, neglect, or mistreatment of residents. It also is checked for misusing or stealing a resident's property. The center must take certain actions if abuse is suspected within the center.

- The incident is reported at once to the administrator and to other officials as required by federal and state laws.
- All claims of abuse are thoroughly investigated.
- The center must prevent further potential for abuse while the investigation is in progress.
- Investigation results are reported to the center administrator and to other officials as required by federal and state laws within 5 days of the incident.
- Corrective actions are taken if the claim is found to be true.

Other Laws

Besides OBRA, other state and federal laws affect what you do as a nursing assistant. See "OBRA and Other Laws" in *Focus on the PERSON* boxes at the end of each chapter beginning in Chapter 7.

BOX 2-6	Signs of Elder Abuse

- Living conditions are unsafe, unclean, or inadequate.
- Personal hygiene is lacking. The person is unclean. Clothes are dirty.
- Weight loss—there are signs of poor nutrition and inadequate fluid intake.
- Assistive devices are missing or broken—eyeglasses, hearing aids, dentures, cane, walker.
- Frequent injuries—conditions behind the injuries are strange or seem impossible.
- Old and new injuries—bruises, welts, scars, and punctures.
- Complaints of pain or itching in the genital area.
- Bleeding and bruising in the genital area.
- Burns on the feet, hands, or buttocks. Cigarettes and cigars cause small circle-like burns.
- Pressure ulcers (Chapter 21) or contractures (Chapter 20).
- The person seems very quiet or withdrawn.
- The person seems fearful, anxious, or agitated.
- The person does not seem to want to talk or answer questions.
- The person is restrained. Or the person is locked in a certain area for long periods of time.
- The person cannot reach toilet facilities, food, water, and other necessary items.
- Private conversations are not allowed. The caregiver is present during all conversations.
- The person seems anxious to please the caregiver.
- Drugs are not taken properly. Drugs are not bought. Or too much or too little of the drug is taken.
- Visits to the emergency room may be frequent.
- The person may change doctors often. Some people do not have a doctor.

REVIEW QUESTIONS

Circle the **BEST** answer.

1. OBRA requires the following for nursing assistants *except*
   a. A license to work
   b. A competency evaluation
   c. Performance reviews
   d. 75 hours of training

2. A task is in your job description. Which is *false?*
   a. Tasks in your job description must always be delegated to you.
   b. Tasks can be delegated to you if the person's circumstances are right.
   c. You must have the necessary education and training to perform delegated tasks.
   d. You must have clear directions before you perform the task.

3. A nurse delegates a task to you. You must
   a. Complete the task
   b. Decide to accept or refuse the task
   c. Delegate the task if you are busy
   d. Ignore the request if you do not know what to do

4. You are responsible for
   a. Completing tasks safely
   b. Delegation
   c. The "five rights of delegation"
   d. Delegating tasks to nursing assistants

5. You can refuse to perform a task for these reasons *except*
   a. The task is beyond the legal limits of your role.
   b. The task is not in your job description.
   c. You do not like the task.
   d. A nurse is not available to supervise you.

6. You decide to refuse a task. What should you do?
   a. Delegate the task to someone else.
   b. Communicate your concerns to the nurse.
   c. Ignore the request.
   d. Talk to the nurse's supervisor.

7. Ethical standards
   a. Are federal laws
   b. Are state laws
   c. Are about right conduct and wrong conduct
   d. Are rules stating what you can and cannot do

8. These statements are about negligence. Which is *false?*
   a. It is an unintentional tort.
   b. The negligent person did not act in a reasonable manner.
   c. Harm was caused to a person or to property.
   d. A prison term is likely.

9. The intentional attempt or threat to touch a person's body without the person's consent is
   a. Assault
   b. Battery
   c. Defamation
   d. False imprisonment

10. Which will *not* protect the person's right to privacy?
    a. Informed consent
    b. Screening the person when giving care
    c. Exposing only the body part involved in the treatment or procedure
    d. Asking visitors to leave the room when care is given

11. A person asks if you are a nurse. You answer "yes." This is
    a. Negligence
    b. Fraud
    c. Libel
    d. Slander

12. Who is responsible for obtaining the person's informed consent?
    a. The doctor
    b. The RN
    c. The LPN/LVN
    d. The nursing assistant

13. Which is *not* a sign of elder abuse?
    a. Stiff joints and joint pain
    b. Old and new bruises
    c. Poor personal hygiene
    d. Frequent injuries

14. You suspect a person was abused. What should you do?
    a. Tell the family.
    b. Call a state agency.
    c. Tell a nurse.
    d. Ask the person if he or she was abused.

Answers to these questions are on p. 467.

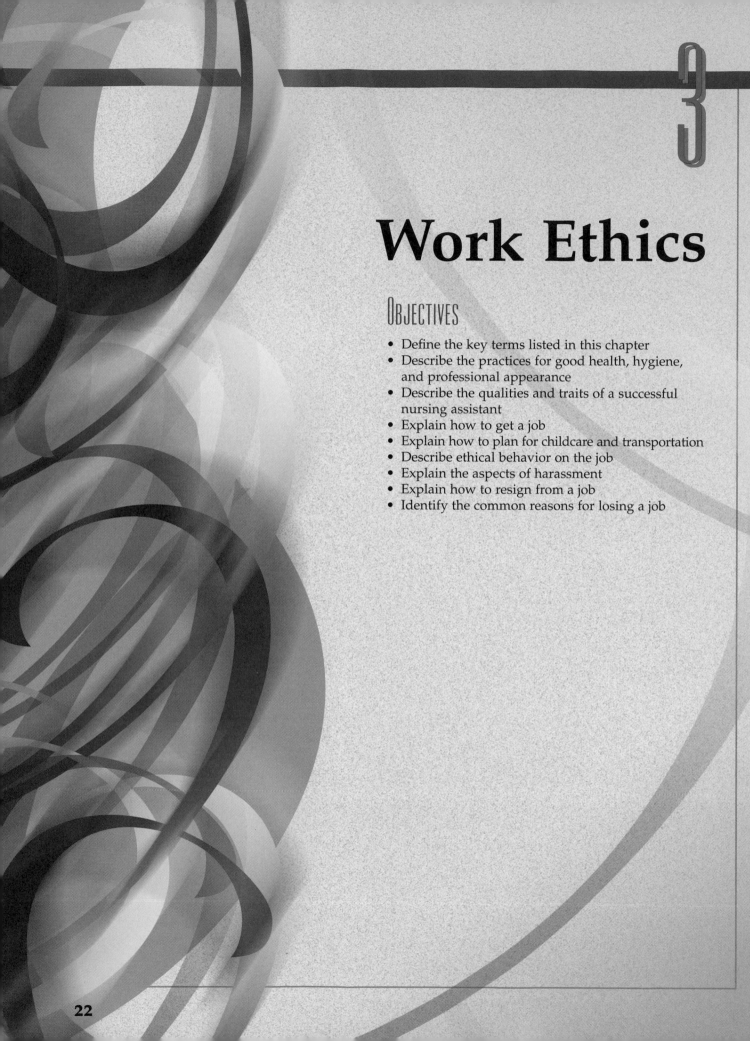

Work Ethics

OBJECTIVES

- Define the key terms listed in this chapter
- Describe the practices for good health, hygiene, and professional appearance
- Describe the qualities and traits of a successful nursing assistant
- Explain how to get a job
- Explain how to plan for childcare and transportation
- Describe ethical behavior on the job
- Explain the aspects of harassment
- Explain how to resign from a job
- Identify the common reasons for losing a job

KEY TERMS

confidentiality Trusting others with personal and private information
gossip To spread rumors or talk about the private matters of others
harassment To trouble, torment, offend, or worry a person by one's behavior or comments
priority The most important thing at the time
teamwork Staff members work together as a group; each person does his or her part to provide safe and effective care; staff members help each other as needed
work ethics Behavior in the workplace

Ethics deals with right conduct and wrong conduct. In the workplace, certain behaviors (conduct), choices, and judgments are expected. **Work ethics** deals with behavior in the workplace. Your conduct reflects your choices and judgments. Work ethics involves:

- How you look
- What you say
- How you behave
- How you treat and work with others

HEALTH, HYGIENE, AND APPEARANCE

Patients, residents, and families expect the health team to look and act healthy. Your health, appearance, and hygiene need careful attention.

Your Health

You must be physically and mentally healthy to function at your best.

- *Diet.* Good nutrition involves eating a balanced diet (Chapter 17).
- *Sleep and rest.* Most adults need about 7 hours of sleep daily.
- *Body mechanics.* You will bend, carry heavy objects, and move and turn persons. You need to use your muscles correctly (Chapter 11).
- *Exercise.* Regular exercise is needed for muscle tone, circulation, and weight control.
- *Your eyes.* You will read instructions and take measurements. Wrong readings can cause the person harm. Have your eyes checked. Wear needed eyeglasses or contact lenses. Provide enough light when reading or doing fine work.
- *Smoking.* Smoking causes lung, heart, and circulatory disorders. Smoke odors stay on your breath, hands, clothing, and hair. Hand washing and good personal hygiene are needed.

- *Drugs.* Some drugs affect thinking, feeling, behavior, and function. Working under the influence of drugs affects the person's safety. Take only those drugs ordered by a doctor. Take them in the prescribed way.
- *Alcohol.* Alcohol is a drug that affects thinking, balance, coordination, and mental alertness. Never report to work under the influence of alcohol. Do not drink alcohol while working.

Hygiene

Your hygiene needs careful attention. Bathe daily and use a deodorant or antiperspirant to prevent body odors. Brush your teeth after meals and use a mouthwash. Shampoo often. Style hair in an attractive and simple way. Keep fingernails clean, short, and neatly shaped.

Menstrual hygiene is important. Change tampons or sanitary napkins often, especially if flow is heavy. Wash your genital area with soap and water at least twice a day. Also practice good hand washing.

Your Appearance

Good health and hygiene practices help you look and feel well. Follow the practices in Box 3-1 on p. 24 to look neat, clean, and professional (Fig. 3-1, p. 24).

GETTING A JOB

There are easy ways to find out about jobs:

- Newspaper classified ads
- Local state employment service
- Agencies you would like to work at
- Phone book yellow pages
- People you know—your instructor, family, and friends
- The Internet
- Your school's or college's job placement counselors
- Your clinical experience site

What Employers Look For

If you owned a business, who would you want to hire? Your answer helps you better understand the employer's point of view. Employers want employees who:

- Are dependable
- Are well-groomed
- Have the needed job skills and training
- Have values and attitudes that fit with the agency
- Have the qualities and traits described in Box 3-2 (p. 25)

BOX 3-1	Practices For a Professional Appearance

- Practice good hygiene.
- Wear uniforms that fit well. They are modest in length and style. Follow the agency's dress code.
- Keep uniforms clean, pressed, and mended. Sew on buttons. Repair zippers, tears, and hems.
- Wear a clean uniform daily.
- Wear your name badge or photo ID at all times when on duty.
- Wear underclothes that are clean and fit properly. Change them daily. Do not wear colored undergarments. They can be seen through white and light-colored uniforms.
- Cover tattoos. They may offend others.
- Do not wear jewelry. Wedding and engagement rings may be allowed. Rings and bracelets can scratch a person. Confused or combative persons can easily pull on jewelry. So can young children.
- Do not wear jewelry in pierced eyebrows, nose, lips, or tongue while on duty.
- Follow the agency's dress code for earrings. Usually small, simple earrings are allowed. For multiple ear piercings, usually only one set of earrings is allowed. The pair is worn in the earlobes, not ear cartilage.

- Wear a wristwatch with a second hand (sweep hand).
- Wear clean stockings and socks that fit well. Change them daily.
- Wear shoes that fit properly, are comfortable, and give needed support. Do not wear sandals or open-toed shoes.
- Clean and polish shoes often. Wash and replace laces as needed.
- Keep fingernails clean, short, and neatly shaped. Long nails can scratch a person.
- Do not wear nail polish or fake nails. Chipped nail polish and fake nails may provide a place for microorganisms to grow.
- Have a simple, attractive hairstyle. Hair is off your collar and away from your face. Use simple pins, combs, barrettes, and bands to keep long hair up and in place.
- Keep beards and mustaches clean and trimmed.
- Use makeup that is modest in amount and moderate in color. Avoid a painted and severe look.
- Do not wear perfume, cologne, or after-shave lotion. They may offend, nauseate, or cause breathing problems in patients and residents.

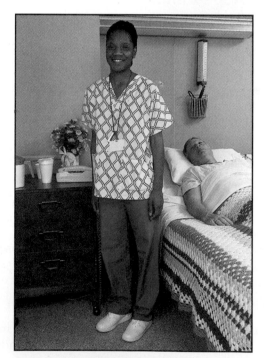

FIG. **3-1** This nursing assistant is well-groomed. Her uniform and shoes are clean. Her hair has a simple style. It is away from her face and off of her collar. She does not wear jewelry.

You must be at work on time and when scheduled. Undependable people cause everyone problems. Other staff take on extra work. Fewer people give care. Quality of care suffers. You want co-workers to work when scheduled. Otherwise, you have extra work and spend less time with patients and residents. Likewise, co-workers also expect you to work when scheduled.

The employer needs proof of required training. Proof of training includes:

- A certificate of course completion
- A high school, college, or technical school transcript
- An official grade report (report card)

Give the employer a *copy* of the document you present. Never give the original to the employer. Keep it for future use. The employer may want a transcript sent directly from the school or college. Your record in the state nursing assistant registry is checked. A criminal background check and drug testing are common requirements.

Job Applications

You get a job application from the *personnel office* or *human resources office*. You can complete the application there. Or you can complete it at home, and return it by mail or in person. You must be well-groomed and behave pleasantly when seeking or returning a job application. It may be your first chance to make a good impression.

To complete a job application, follow the guidelines in Box 3-3. A neat, readable, and complete application gives a good image. A sloppy or incomplete one does not.

Some agencies have job applications on-line. Follow the agency's instructions for completing and sending an on-line application.

BOX 3-2   Qualities and Traits For Good Work Ethics

- **Caring.** Have concern for the person. Help make the person's life happier, easier, or less painful.
- **Dependable.** Report to work on time and when scheduled. Perform delegated tasks. Keep obligations and promises.
- **Considerate.** Respect the person's physical and emotional feelings. Be gentle and kind toward patients, residents, families, and co-workers.
- **Cheerful.** Greet and talk to people in a pleasant manner. Do not be moody, bad-tempered, or unhappy while at work.
- **Empathetic.** Empathy is seeing things from the person's point of view—putting yourself in the person's position. How would you feel if you had the person's problem?
- **Trustworthy.** Patients, residents, and staff members have confidence in you. They believe you will keep information confidential. They trust you not to gossip about patients, residents, or the health team.

- **Respectful.** Patients and residents have rights, values, beliefs, and feelings. They may differ from yours. Do not judge or condemn the person. Treat the person with respect and dignity at all times. Also show respect for the health team.
- **Courteous.** Be polite and courteous to patients, residents, families, visitors, and co-workers. See p. 29 for common courtesies in the workplace.
- **Conscientious.** Be careful, alert, and exact in following instructions. Give thorough care. Do not lose or damage the person's property.
- **Honest.** Accurately report the care given, your observations, and any errors.
- **Cooperative.** Willingly help and work with others. Also take that "extra step" during busy and stressful times.
- **Enthusiastic.** Be eager, interested, and excited about your work. Your work is important.
- **Self-aware.** Know your feelings, strengths, and weaknesses. You need to understand yourself before you can understand patients and residents.

BOX 3-3   Guidelines For Completing a Job Application

- Read and follow the directions. They may ask you to use black ink and to print. Following directions is needed on the job. Employers look at job applications to see if you can follow directions.
- Write neatly. Your writing must be readable. A messy application gives a bad image. Readable writing gives the correct information. The agency cannot contact you if unable to read your phone number. You may miss getting the job.
- Complete the entire form. Something may not apply to you. If so, write "N/A" for non-applicable. Or draw a line through the space. This tells the employer that you read the section. It also shows that you did not skip the item on purpose.
- Report any felony arrests or convictions as directed. Write "no" or "none" as appropriate. Criminal background checks are common requirements.
- Give information about employment gaps. If you did not work for a time, the employer wonders why. Provide this information to give a good impression about your honesty. Some reasons are going to school, raising children, caring for an ill or older family member, or your own illness.
- Tell why you left a job, if asked. Be brief, but honest. People leave jobs for one that pays better. Some leave

for career advancement. Other reasons include those given for employment gaps. If you were fired from a job, give an honest but positive response. Do not talk badly about a former employer.
- Provide references. Be prepared to give the names, titles, addresses, and telephone numbers of at least three references who are not relatives. You should have this information written down before completing an application. (Always ask references if an employer can contact them.) You may get the job faster or over another applicant if the employer can quickly check references. If they are missing or incomplete, the employer waits for all of the information. This wastes your time and the employer's time. Also, the employer wonders if you are hiding something with incomplete reference information.
- Be prepared to provide the following:
  - Social security number
  - Proof of citizenship or legal residence
  - Proof of required training and competency evaluation
  - Identification—driver's license or government-issued ID card
- Give honest responses. Lying on an application is fraud. It is grounds for being fired.

The Job Interview

A job interview is the employer's chance to get to know and evaluate you. You also learn more about the agency. Box 3-4 lists common interview questions. Prepare your answers before the interview. Also prepare a list of your skills for the interviewer.

You must present a good image. You need to be neat, clean, well-groomed, and neatly dressed (Fig. 3-2). Follow the guidelines in Box 3-5.

You must be on time. It shows you are dependable. Go to the agency some day before your interview. Note how long it takes to get there and where to park. Also find the personnel office. A *dry run* (practice run) gives an idea of how long it takes to get from your home to the personnel office.

When you arrive for the interview, tell the receptionist your name and why you are there. Also give the interviewer's name. Then sit quietly in the waiting room. Use the time to review your answers to the common interview questions. Waiting may be part of the interview. The interviewer may ask the receptionist about how you acted. Smile, and be polite and friendly.

Greet the interviewer in a polite manner. A firm handshake is correct for men and women. Address the interviewer as Mr., Mrs., Ms., Miss, or Doctor. Stand until asked to take a seat. When sitting, use good posture. Sit in a professional manner. If offered a beverage, it is correct to accept. Be sure to thank the person.

Look at the interviewer when answering or asking questions. Poor eye contact sends negative information—being shy, insecure, or dishonest or lacking

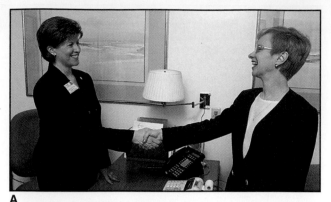

A

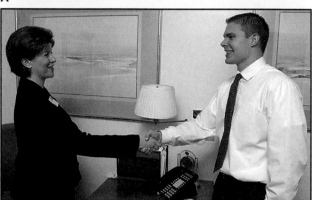

B

FIG. **3-2** **A,** A simple suit is worn for a job interview. **B,** This man wears slacks and a shirt and tie for his interview.

BOX 3-4	**Common Interview Questions**

- Tell me about yourself.
- Tell me about your career goals.
- What are you doing to reach these goals?
- Describe your idea of *professional* behavior.
- Tell me about your last job. Why did you leave?
- What did you like the most about your last job? What did you like the least?
- What would your supervisor and co-workers tell me about you? Your dependability? Your skills? Your flexibility?
- Which functions were the hardest for you? How did you handle this difficulty?
- How do you set priorities?
- How have your past experiences prepared you for this job?
- What would you like to change about your last job?
- How do you handle problems with patients, residents, and co-workers?
- Why do you want to work here?
- Why should this agency hire you?

BOX 3-5	**Grooming and Dressing For an Interview**

- Bathe, brush your teeth, and wash your hair.
- Use a deodorant or antiperspirant.
- Make sure your hands and fingernails are clean.
- Apply makeup in a simple, attractive manner.
- Style your hair so that it is neat and attractive. Wear it as you would for work.
- Do not wear jeans, shorts, tank tops, halter tops, or other casual clothing.
- Iron clothing. Sew on loose buttons and mend garments as needed.
- Wear a simple dress, skirt and blouse, or suit (women). Men should wear a suit or dark slacks and a shirt and tie. A jacket is optional. A long-sleeved white or light blue shirt is best.
- Wear socks (men and women) or hose (women). Hose should be free of runs and snags.
- Make sure shoes are clean and in good repair.
- Avoid heavy perfumes, colognes, and after-shave lotions. A lightly scented fragrance is okay.
- Wear only simple jewelry that complements your clothes. Avoid adornments in body piercings. If you have multiple ear piercings, wear only one set of earrings.
- Stop in the restroom when you arrive for the interview. Check your hair, makeup, and clothes.

interest. Also watch your body language (Chapter 5). What you say is important. However, how you use and move your body also tells a great deal. Avoid distracting habits—biting nails, playing with jewelry or clothing, crossing arms, and swinging legs back and forth.

Give complete and honest answers. Speak clearly and with confidence. Avoid short and long answers. "Yes" and "no" answers give little information. Briefly explain "yes" and "no" responses.

The interviewer will ask about your skills. Share your skills list. He or she may ask about a skill not on your list. Explain that you are willing to learn the skill if your state allows nursing assistants to perform the task.

You can ask questions at the end of the interview (Box 3-6). Review the job description with the interviewer. If you have questions, ask them at this time. Advise him or her of those functions you cannot perform because of training, legal, ethical, or religious reasons.

Ask questions about pay rate, work hours, and uniform requirements. Also ask about the new-employee orientation program. Remember to ask about benefits—health and disability insurance, vacation, and continuing education.

BOX 3-6	Questions to Ask the Interviewer

- Which job functions do you think are the most important?
- What employee qualities and traits are most important to you?
- What nursing care pattern is used here (Chapter 1)?
- Who will I work with?
- When are performance evaluations done? Who does them? How are they done?
- What performance factors are evaluated?
- How does the supervisor handle problems?
- What are the most common reasons that nursing assistants quit their jobs here?
- What are the most common reasons that nursing assistants lose their jobs here?
- How do you see this job in the next year? In the next 5 years?
- What is the greatest reward from this job?
- What is the greatest challenge of this job?
- What do you like the most about nursing assistants who work here?
- What do you like the least about nursing assistants who work here?
- Why should I work here rather than in another agency?
- Why are you interested in hiring me?
- May I have a tour of the agency and the unit I will work on? Will you introduce me to the nurse manager and unit staff?
- Can I have a few minutes to talk to the nurse manager?

You may be offered a job at the end of the interview. Or you are told when to expect a call or letter. Follow-up is acceptable. Ask when you can check on your application. Before leaving, thank the interviewer. Say that you look forward to hearing from him or her. Shake the person's hand before you leave.

A thank-you note or letter is advised. Write it within 24 hours of the interview. Use a computer or typewriter if your writing is hard to read. The thank-you note should include:

- The date
- The interviewer's formal name using Mr., Mrs., Ms., Miss, or Dr.
- A statement thanking the person for the interview
- Comments about the interview, the agency, and your eagerness to hear about the job
- Your signature using your first and last names

Accepting a Job

When you accept a job, agree on a starting date, pay rate, and work hours. Find out where to report on your first day. Ask for such information in writing. You can use the written offer later if questions arise. Also ask for the employee handbook and other agency information. Read everything before you start working.

New Employee Orientation

Agencies have orientation programs for new employees. The policy and procedure manual is reviewed. Your skills are checked to make sure you do them safely and correctly. Also, you are shown how to use the agency's supplies and equipment.

Preceptor programs are common. A *preceptor* is a staff member who guides another staff member. A nurse or nursing assistant will:

- Help you learn the agency's layout
- Introduce you to patients, residents, and staff
- Help you organize your work
- Help you feel part of the nursing team
- Answer questions about the policy and procedure manual

A preceptor program usually lasts 2 to 4 weeks. When the program ends, you should feel comfortable with the setting and your role. If not, ask for more orientation time.

PREPARING FOR WORK

A job is a privilege. You must work when scheduled, be on time, and stay the entire shift. Absences and tardiness (being late) are common reasons for losing a job. Childcare and transportation issues often interfere with getting to work.

Childcare

Someone needs to care for your children when you leave for work, while you are at work, and before you get home. Also plan for emergencies:
- Your childcare provider is ill or cannot care for your children that day.
- A child becomes ill while you are at work.
- You will be late getting home from work.

Transportation

Plan for how to get to and from work. If you drive, keep your car in good working order. Keep plenty of gas in the car. Or leave early enough to get gas.

Carpooling is an option. Carpool members depend on each other. If the driver is late leaving, everyone is late for work. If one person is not ready when the driver arrives, everyone is late for work. Carpool with persons you trust to be ready and on time. When you drive, leave and pick up others on time. As a passenger, be ready to be picked up.

Know your bus or train schedule. Know what other bus or train to take if delays occur. Always carry enough money for fares to and from work.

Always have a back-up plan for getting to work. Your car may not start, the carpool driver may not go to work, or public transportation may not operate.

TEAMWORK ON THE JOB

How you look, how you behave, and what you say affect everyone in the agency. Practice good work ethics—work when scheduled, be cheerful and friendly, perform delegated tasks, help others, and be kind to others.

Remember, you are a member of the nursing team. Teamwork is important for safe and effective care. **Teamwork** means that staff members work together as a group. Each person does his or her part to provide safe and effective care. Also, staff members help each other as needed. (*See* Nursing Teamwork *in Focus on the PERSON boxes at the end of each chapter beginning in Chapter 7*).

Attendance

Report to work when scheduled and on time. The entire unit is affected when just one person is late. Call the agency if you will be late or cannot go to work. Follow the agency's attendance policies.

Be *ready to work* when your shift starts. Store your coat, purse, backpack, and other items. Use the restroom when you arrive at the agency. Arrive on your nursing unit a few minutes early. This gives you time to greet others and settle yourself.

You need to stay the entire shift. You must prepare for childcare emergencies. You may need to work over-time. You need to prepare to stay longer if necessary.

Your Attitude

A good attitude is needed. Show that you enjoy your work. Listen to others. Be willing to learn. Stay busy, and use your time well.

Always think before you speak. These statements signal a bad attitude:
- "That's not my patient (resident)."
- "I can't. I'm too busy."
- "I didn't do it."
- "I don't feel like it."
- "It's not my fault."
- "Don't blame me."
- "It's not my turn. I did it yesterday."
- "Nobody told me."
- "I can't come to work today. I have a headache."
- "That's not my job."
- "You didn't tell me that you needed it right away."
- "I work harder than anyone else."
- "No one appreciates what I do."
- "Is it time to leave yet?"

Gossip

To **gossip** means to spread rumors or talk about the private matters of others. Gossiping is unprofessional and hurtful. To avoid being a part of gossip:
- Remove yourself from a group or situation where gossip is occurring.
- Do not make or repeat any comment that can hurt a person, family member, co-worker, or the agency.
- Do not make or repeat any comment that you do not know to be true.
- Do not talk about patients, residents, visitors, families, co-workers, or the agency at home or in social settings.

Confidentiality

The person's information is private and personal. **Confidentiality** is trusting others with personal and private information. The person's information is shared only among health team members involved in his or her care. The person has the right to privacy and confidentiality. Agency and co-worker information also is confidential.

Avoid talking about patients, residents, the agency, or co-workers when others are present. Share information only with the nurse. Do not talk about patients, residents, the agency, or co-workers in hallways, elevators, dining areas, or outside the agency. Others may overhear you.

Avoid eavesdropping. To eavesdrop means to listen in or overhear what others are saying. It invades a person's privacy.

Many agencies have intercom systems. They allow for communication between the bedside and the nurses' station. Be careful what you say over the intercom. It is like a loud speaker. Others nearby can hear what you are saying.

Hygiene and Appearance

Home and social attire is often improper at work. You cannot wear jeans, halter tops, tank tops, or short skirts. Clothing must not be tight, revealing, or sexual. Females cannot show cleavage, the tops of breasts, or upper thighs. Males must avoid tight pants and exposing their chests. Only the top shirt button is open. Follow the practices in Box 3-1.

Speech and Language

Speech and language used in home and social settings may be improper at work. Words used with family and friends may offend patients, residents, visitors, and co-workers. Remember the following:

- Do not swear or use foul, vulgar, or abusive language.
- Do not use slang.
- Control the volume and tone of your voice. Speak softly and gently.
- Speak clearly. The person may have a hearing problem (Chapter 24).
- Do not shout or yell.
- Do not fight or argue with the person, family, or co-workers.

Courtesies

Courtesies are polite, considerate, or helpful comments or acts. They require little time or energy.

- Address others by Miss, Mrs., Ms., Mr., or Doctor.
- Say "please." Begin or end each request with "please."
- Say "thank you" whenever someone does something for you.
- Apologize when you make a mistake or hurt someone.
- Hold doors open for others. If you are at the door first, open the door and let others pass through. In business, men and women hold doors open for each other.
- Hold elevator doors open for others coming down the hallway.
- Let patients, residents, families, and visitors enter elevators first.

Personal Matters

Personal matters cannot interfere with the job. Otherwise care is neglected. You could lose your job for tending to personal matters at work. To keep personal matters out of the workplace:

- Make personal phone calls only during meals and breaks. Use pay phones or your wireless phone.
- Do not let family and friends visit you on the unit.
- Make appointments (doctor, dentist, lawyer, beauty, and others) for your days off.
- Do not use agency computers, printers, fax machines, copiers, or other equipment for personal use.
- Do not take agency supplies (pens, paper, and others) for your personal use.
- Do not discuss personal problems at work.
- Do not borrow money from or lend it to co-workers.
- Do not sell things or engage in fund-raising at work.
- Do not have personal pagers or wireless phones turned on while at work.

Meals and Breaks

Meal breaks are usually for 30 minutes. Other breaks are usually for 15 minutes. Meals and breaks are scheduled so that some staff are always on the unit.

Staff members depend on each other. Leave for and return from breaks on time. That way other staff can have their turn. Do not take longer than allowed. Tell the nurse when you leave and return to the unit.

Planning Your Work

You assist the nurse with several patients and residents. You perform nursing tasks and routine tasks on the nursing unit. Some tasks need to be done at certain times. Others are done at the start of your shift, during your shift, and at the end of your shift.

The nurse, the Kardex, care plan, and your assignment sheet help you decide what to do and when (Chapter 4). This is called *priority setting*. A **priority** is the most important thing at the time. To set priorities, you need to decide:

- Which person has the greatest or most life-threatening needs
- What tasks the nurse or person needs done first
- What tasks need to be done at a set time
- What tasks need to be done when your shift starts
- What tasks need to be done at the end of your shift
- What tasks can wait until the person goes for a therapy, treatment, test, or meal
- How much time it will take to complete a task
- How much help you will need to complete a task
- Who is available to help you and when

BOX 3-7	Planning Your Work
<ul><li>Discuss priorities with the nurse.</li><li>Know the routine of your shift and nursing unit.</li><li>List care or procedures that are on a schedule. Some persons are turned or offered the bedpan every 2 hours.</li><li>Judge how much time you need for each person, procedure, and task.</li><li>Identify which tasks and procedures can be done while patients or residents are eating, visiting, or involved in activities or therapies.</li><li>Plan care around meal times, visiting hours, and therapies. If working in a nursing center, also consider daily recreation and social activities.</li><li>Identify when you will need help from a co-worker. Ask</li></ul>	<ul><li>a co-worker to help you. Give the time when you will need help.</li><li>Schedule equipment or rooms for the person's use. Some agencies have only one shower or bathtub to a nursing unit.</li><li>Review delegated procedures. Gather needed supplies beforehand.</li><li>Do not waste time. Stay focused on your work.</li><li>Do not leave a messy work area. Make sure rooms are neat and orderly. Also clean utility areas.</li><li>Be a self-starter. Have initiative. Ask others if they need help, follow unit routines, stock supply areas, and clean utility rooms. Stay busy.</li></ul>

Priorities change as the person's needs change. A person's condition can improve or worsen. A new patient or resident may be admitted to your nursing unit. A person may be discharged or transferred to another nursing unit. These and many other factors affect priorities. They can change during your shift. You need to change priorities as needed.

Setting priorities can be hard at first. It will become easier as you gain experience as a nursing assistant. If you have problems setting priorities or getting tasks done, ask the nurse to help you set priorities. Plan your work to give safe, thorough care and to make good use of your time (Box 3-7).

HARASSMENT

Harassment means to trouble, torment, offend, or worry a person by one's behavior or comments. Harassment can be sexual. Or it can involve age, race, ethnic background, religion, or disability. You must respect others. Do not offend others by your gestures, remarks, or use of touch. Do not offend others with jokes or pictures. Harassment is not legal in the workplace.

Sexual Harassment

Sexual harassment involves unwanted sexual behaviors by another. The behavior may be a sexual advance. Or it may be a request for a sexual favor. Some comments or touching are sexual. The behavior affects the person's work and comfort. In extreme cases, the person's job is threatened if sexual favors are not granted.

Victims of sexual harassment may be men or women. Men harass women or men. Women harass men or women. You might feel that you are being harassed. If so, report the matter to the nurse and the human resource officer.

Even innocent remarks and behaviors can be viewed as harassment. Employee orientation programs address harassment. You might not be sure about your own or another person's remarks or behaviors. If so, discuss the matter with the nurse. You cannot be too careful.

RESIGNING FROM A JOB

Whatever the reason for resigning, you need to tell your employer. Do not leave a job without notice. Write a resignation letter or complete a form in the human resource office. Giving 2-weeks notice is a good practice. Include the following in your written notice:

- Reason for leaving
- The last date you will work
- Comments thanking the employer for the opportunity to work in the agency

LOSING A JOB

You must perform your job well and protect patients and residents from harm. Otherwise you could lose your job. Failure to follow an agency policy is often grounds for termination. So is failure to get along with others. Box 3-8 lists the many reasons why you can lose your job.

BOX 3-8 **Common Reasons For Losing a Job**

- Poor attendance—not showing up for work or excessive tardiness (being late)
- Abandonment—leaving the job during your shift
- Falsifying a record—job application or a person's record
- Violent behavior in the workplace
- Having weapons in the work setting—guns, knives, explosives, or other dangerous items
- Having, using, or distributing alcohol in the work setting
- Having, using, or distributing drugs in the work setting (this excludes taking drugs ordered by your doctor)
- Taking a person's drug for your own use or giving it to others
- Harassment
- Using offensive speech and language
- Stealing the agency's or a person's property
- Destroying the agency's or a person's property

- Showing disrespect to patients, residents, visitors, co-workers, or supervisors
- Abusing or neglecting a person
- Invading a person's privacy
- Failing to maintain patient, resident, agency, or co-worker confidentiality (includes access to computer information)
- Using the agency's supplies and equipment for your own use
- Defamation—see Chapter 2 and Gossip, p. 28
- Abusing meal breaks and break periods
- Sleeping on the job
- Violating agency dress code
- Violating any agency policy
- Failing to follow agency procedures for providing care
- Tending to personal matters while on duty

REVIEW QUESTIONS

Circle the **BEST** answer.

1 To perform your job well you need the following *except*
   a Adequate sleep and rest
   b Regular exercise
   c To use drugs and alcohol
   d Good nutrition

2 Good hygiene for work involves the following *except*
   a Bathing daily
   b Using a deodorant or antiperspirant
   c Brushing teeth after meals
   d Keeping fingernails long and polished

3 When should you ask questions about your job description?
   a After completing the application
   b Before completing the application
   c When your interview is scheduled
   d During the interview

4 When completing a job application you should do the following *except*
   a Write neatly and clearly
   b Provide references
   c Give information about employment gaps
   d Leave spaces blank that do not apply to you

5 Which of these qualities and traits do employers look for the *most?*
   a Cooperation
   b Courtesy
   c Dependability
   d Empathy

6 What should you wear to a job interview?
   a A uniform
   b Party clothes
   c A simple dress or suit
   d What is most comfortable

7 Which behavior is poor during a job interview?
   a Good eye contact with the interviewer
   b Shaking hands with the interviewer
   c Asking the interviewer questions
   d Crossing your arms and legs

Review Questions

8 Which response to an interview question is best?
  a "Yes" or "no"
  b Long answers
  c Brief explanations
  d A written response

9 A co-worker tells you that a doctor and nurse are dating. This is
  a Gossip
  b Eavesdropping
  c Confidential information
  d Sexual harassment

10 You are on your meal break. Which is *false?*
  a You can make personal phone calls.
  b Family members can meet you.
  c You can take a few extra minutes if necessary.
  d The nurse needs to know that you are off the unit.

11 You are planning your work. You should do the following *except*
  a Discuss priorities with the nurse
  b Ask others if they need help
  c Stay busy
  d Plan care so that you can watch the person's TV

12 Which is *not* harassment?
  a Using touch to comfort a person
  b Joking about a person's religion
  c Asking for a sexual favor
  d Imitating a person's disability

13 A letter of resignation should include the following *except*
  a Your reason for leaving
  b The last day you will work
  c A thank-you to the employer
  d What problems you had during your work

14 You can lose your job for the following reasons *except*
  a Sharing the person's information with others
  b Arriving at the agency after your shift begins
  c Following the agency's dress code
  d Using the agency's computer for your own use

Answers to these questions are on p. 467.

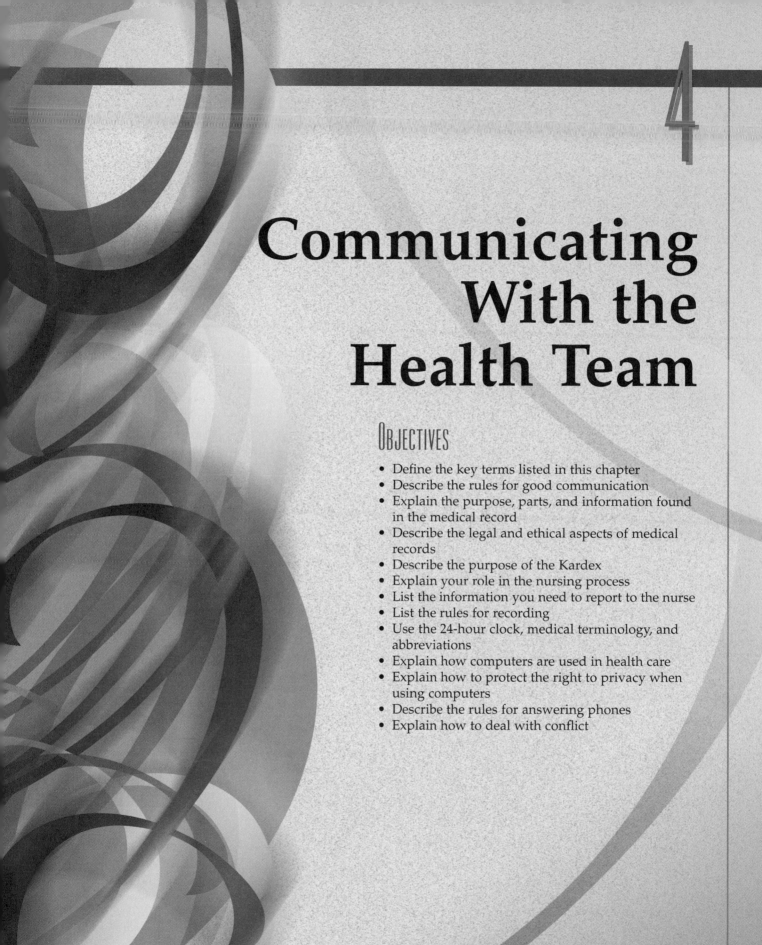

Communicating With the Health Team

OBJECTIVES

- Define the key terms listed in this chapter
- Describe the rules for good communication
- Explain the purpose, parts, and information found in the medical record
- Describe the legal and ethical aspects of medical records
- Describe the purpose of the Kardex
- Explain your role in the nursing process
- List the information you need to report to the nurse
- List the rules for recording
- Use the 24-hour clock, medical terminology, and abbreviations
- Explain how computers are used in health care
- Explain how to protect the right to privacy when using computers
- Describe the rules for answering phones
- Explain how to deal with conflict

KEY TERMS

chart The medical record

communication The exchange of information—a message sent is received and interpreted by the intended person

comprehensive care plan A written guide giving direction for the resident's care (required by OBRA)

medical record A written account of a person's condition and response to treatment and care; chart

nursing care plan A written guide about the person's care

nursing process The method RNs use to plan and deliver nursing care; its five steps are assessment, nursing diagnosis, planning, implementation, and evaluation

objective data Information that is seen, heard, felt, or smelled; signs

observation Using the senses of sight, hearing, touch, and smell to collect information

recording The written account of care and observations; charting

reporting The oral account of care and observations

signs Objective data

subjective data Things a person tells you about that you cannot observe through your senses; symptoms

symptoms Subjective data

 Health team members communicate with each other to give coordinated and effective care. They share information about:

- What was done for the person
- What needs to be done for the person
- The person's response to treatment

COMMUNICATION

Communication is the exchange of information—a message sent is received and interpreted by the intended person. For good communication:

- Use words that mean the same thing to the sender and the receiver. Avoid words with more than one meaning.
- Use familiar words. Do not use terms unfamiliar to the person and family.
- Be brief and concise. Do not add unrelated or unneeded information. Stay on the subject. Avoid wandering in thought. Do not get wordy.
- Give information in a logical and orderly manner. Organize your thoughts. Present them step by step.
- Give facts, and be specific. You report a pulse rate of 110. It is more specific and factual than saying the "pulse is fast."

THE MEDICAL RECORD

The **medical record (chart)** is a written account of a person's condition and response to treatment and care. The record is permanent and a legal document. It can be used in court as evidence of the person's problems, treatment, and care.

Agencies have policies about medical records and who can see them. Policies address who records, when to record, abbreviations, correcting errors, ink color, and signing entries.

Staff involved in a person's care can read and use charts. If you have access, you must keep the information confidential. This is an ethical and legal responsibility. If you are not involved in a person's care, you have no right to see that person's chart. To do so is an invasion of privacy.

The following parts of the medical record relate to your work:

- *Admission sheet*—is completed when the person is admitted to the agency. It has the person's identifying information. Use it to complete forms that require the same information.
- *Nursing history*—is completed by the nurse. The nurse asks about current and past illnesses, signs and symptoms, and drugs.
- *Graphic sheet*—is used to record measurements and observations made daily, every shift, or 3 to 4 times a day (Fig. 4-1). Blood pressure, temperature, pulse, respirations, weight, intake and output, bowel movements, and doctor visits are recorded on the graphic sheet.
- *Progress notes*—describe observations, the care given, and the person's response (Fig. 4-2, p. 36). They are used to record information about special treatments and drugs, teaching and counseling, and procedures performed by the doctor. In long-term care, summaries of care describe the person's progress toward goals and response to care.
- *Flow sheets*—are used to record frequent measurements or observations. The activities of daily living flow sheet is used to record the person's everyday activities (Fig. 4-3, p. 37).

THE KARDEX

The *Kardex* is a type of card file. It summarizes the person's drugs, treatments, diagnosis, routine care measures, equipment, and special needs. The Kardex is a quick, easy source of information about the person (Fig. 4-4, p. 38).

Text continued on p. 39

Med-Forms, Inc.
FORM #MF37079 (Rev 9/95)

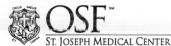

OSF ℠
ST. JOSEPH MEDICAL CENTER
Bloomington, Illinois 61701

DAILY SUMMARY AND GRAPHIC

TEMPERATURE
Write in 105^1 or over

DATE	5 – 7	5 – 8		
HOSPITAL DAY	4	5		
POST OP DAY				

HOUR	2400	0400	0800	1200	1600	2000	2400	0400	0800	1200	1600	2000	2400	0400	0800	1200	1600	2000	2400	0400	0800	1200	1600	2000
B/P			130/80	120/76	130/76	130/80			120/72	120/80	130/80	130/82												

TEMPERATURE scale: 104 / 40, 102.2 / 39, 100.4 / 38, 98.6 / 37, 96.6 / 36

(Temperature graph plotted around 98.6°F / 37°C for both 5-7 and 5-8)

	2400	0400	0800	1200	1600	2000	2400	0400	0800	1200	1600	2000
PULSE			74	80	76	74			74	74	76	72
RESPIRATION			18	18	16	16			18	20	18	16
WEIGHT												
DR. VISIT	@ 0900											

INTAKE	2300-0700	0700-1500	1500-2300	TOTAL	2300-0700	0700-1500	1500-2300	TOTAL	2300-0700	0700-1500	1500-2300	TOTAL	2300-0700	0700-1500	1500-2300	TOTAL
Oral	100	1200	800	2100	100	1050	820	1970								
IV																
Tube Feedings																
PPN/TPN/Lipids																
Blood/Blood Products																
IV Meds																
Chemotherapy																
Unreturned irr. sol.																
TOTAL INTAKE	100	1200	800	2100	100	1050	820	1970								

OUTPUT	2300-0700	0700-1500	1500-2300	TOTAL	2300-0700	0700-1500	1500-2300	TOTAL	2300-0700	0700-1500	1500-2300	TOTAL	2300-0700	0700-1500	1500-2300	TOTAL
Urine	0	1050	800	1850	200	850	750	1800								
GI																
Emesis	100			100												
Drains																
TOTAL OUTPUT	100	1050	800	1950	200	850	750	1800								
Feces		✓				✓										

FIG. **4-1** Graphic sheet. (Courtesy OSF St. Joseph Medical Center, Bloomington, Ill.)

Date	Time	Nursing Margin	Other Depts Margin
3-19	1700	Out with family for dinner. Jane Doe, LPN ————————	
	1930	Returned from outing accompanied by her son. States	
		she had a pleasant time. Mary Smith, CNA ————————	
3-20	0900	IN BED. COMPLAINS OF HEADACHE. T 98.4 ORALLY, RADIAL PULSE	
		72 AND REGULAR, RESPIRATIONS 18 AND UNLABORED. BP 134/84 LEFT	
		ARM LYING DOWN. ALICE JONES, RN NOTIFIED OF RESIDENT COMPLAINT	
		AND VITAL SIGNS. ANN ADAMS, CNA ————————	
	0910	In bed resting. States she has had a headache for about 1/2 hour.	
		Denies nausea and dizziness. No other complaints. PRN	
		Tylenol given. Instructed resident to use signal light if	
		headache worsens or other symptoms occur. Alice Jones, RN ———	
	0945	Resting quietly. Denies headache at this time. T 98.4 orally,	
		radial pulse 70 and regular, respirations 18 and unlabored.	
		BP 132/84 left arm lying down. Alice Jones, RN ————————	

FIG. **4-2** Progress notes. Note that other members of the health team also record on this form.

Activities-of-Daily-Living Flow Sheet

JAN FEB (MAR) APR MAY JUN JUL AUG SEP OCT NOV DEC

ORDER/INSTRUCTION	TIME	1	2	3	4	5	6	7	8	9	10	11	12	13	14	15	16	17	18	19	20	21	22	23	24	25	26	27	28	29	30	31
Bowel Movements L = Large M = Medium S = Small IC = Incontinent	11-7	M																														
	7-3			L																												
	3-11																															
Bladder Elimination I = Independent IC = Incontinent FC = Foley catheter	11-7	I	I	I	I																											
	7-3	I	I	I	I																											
	3-11	I	IC	I	I																											
Weight Bearing Status TT = Toe touch AT = As tol. P = Partial F = Full NWB = No weight bearing	11-7	AT	AT	AT	AT																											
	7-3	AT	AT	AT	AT																											
	3-11	AT	AT	AT	AT																											
Transfer Status ML = Mech lift SBA = Stand by assist; Assist of 1 or 2	11-7	SBA	SBA	SBA	SBA																											
	7-3	SBA	SBA	SBA	SBA																											
	3-11	SBA	SBA	SBA	A-1																											
Activity A = Ambulate GC = Gerichair T = Turn every 2 hrs. W/C = Wheelchair	11-7	T	T	T	T																											
	7-3	A	A	A	A																											
	3-11	A	A	A	A																											
Safety LT = Lap tray BR = Bed rails BA = Bed alarm SB = Seat belt	11-7																															
	7-3																															
	3-11																															
Feeding Status I = Independent S = Set up F = Staff feed SP = Swallow precautions TL = Thickened liquids	Breakfast	S	S	S	S																											
	Lunch	S	S	S	S																											
	Supper	S	S	S	S																											
Amount of food taken in %	Breakfast	75	100	100	75																											
	Lunch	75	75	100	75																											
	Supper	50	50	50	75																											
Bath and Shampoo every *Monday* & *Thursday* on *7-3* shift T = Tub S = Shower B = Bed bath	11-7																															
	7-3		T																													
	3-11																															
Oral Care Own/(Dentures)/No teeth I = Independent S = Set up A = Assist	11-7	S	S	S	S																											
	7-3	S	S	S	S																											
	3-11	S	S	S	S																											
Dressing I = Independent S = Set up A = Assist T = Total care	11-7	A	A	S	S																											
	7-3																															
	3-11	A	A	A	A																											
Grooming: Washing Face and Hands Combing Hair I = Independent S = Set up A = Assist T = Total care	11-7	A	A	A	A																											
	7-3	A	A	A	A																											
	3-11	A	A	A	A																											
Trim Fingernails weekly *Thursday*	11-7																															
	7-3		✓																													
	3-11																															
Lotion Arms and Legs twice daily	11-7																															
	7-3	✓	✓	✓	✓																											
	3-11	✓	✓	✓	✓																											
Shave Men daily Shave (Women) every *Monday* & *Thursday* on *7-3* shift	11-7																															
	7-3		✓																													
	3-11																															
Amount Between-Meal Nourishment taken in %	AM	100	75	100	50																											
	PM	100	100	75	75																											
	HS	50	75	75	75																											
Intake and Output	11-7																															
	7-3																															
	3-11																															
Vital Signs Every *Thursday*	11-7																															
	7-3		✓																													
	3-11																															
Weight Every *Thursday*	11-7		✓																													
	7-3																															
	3-11																															

FIG. **4-3** Some items on an Activities-of-daily-living Flow Sheet.

DIET _Regular_

Hold:

NOURISHMENT/SPECIAL FEEDING
Health shake at Bedtime

INTAKE/OUTPUT
Encourage/Restrict Fluids _2000_ ml/24 Hr.
7-3 _1000_   3-11 _800_   11-7 _200_

FUNCTIONAL STATUS

	SELF	ASSIST	TOTAL	OTHER	SPECIFY
Feeding	☐	☒	☐	☐	
Bathing	☐	☒	☐	☐	
Toileting	☐	☒	☐	☐	
Oral Care	☐	☒	☐	☐	
Positioning	☒	☐	☐	☐	
Transferring	☒	☐	☐	☐	
Wheeling	☐	☐	☐	☐	
Walking	☒	☐	☐	☐	
	☐	☐	☐	☐	

ACTIVITIES
Bedrest & BRP _____
Bedside Commode _____
Up ad Lib _X_
Chair _____
Ambulatory _X_
Ambulate & Assist _____
Turn _____
Dangle _____
Mode of Travel _____

ELIMINATION
Bladder - Cont. (Incont.)
Catheter _____
Date Changed _____
Irrigations _____
Bowel - (Cont.)/ Incont.
Ostomy _____
Irrigations _____

VITALS
Temp. _QID_
Pulse _QID_
Resp. _QID_
BP _QID_
Weight _daily_
Other:
Pulse OX daily

COMMUNICATION DEFICITS   ☐ None
Hearing _Impaired_
Vision _Impaired_
Speech _____
Language _Impaired_

PROSTHESIS   ☐ None
Glasses _X_   Dentures _X_
Contacts _____   Limb _____
Hearing Aid _L ear_

SPECIAL CONDITIONS (Paralysis, Pressure Ulcers, Etc.)

SAFETY/SUPPORTIVE MEASURES
Bed rails: ☐ Nights Only ☐ Constant ☐ No Need
Restraints: ☐ PRN   ☐ Constant

Support Devices: ☐ PRN   ☐ Constant

RESPIRATORY THERAPY
Aerosol
IPPB
Ultrasonic

Rx Med _____

OXYGEN
_2_ Liter/Minute
☒ PRN   ☐ Constant

___ Tent   ___ Catheter
___ Mask   _X_ Cannula

SPECIAL EQUIPMENT/PROCEDURES/ANCILLARY SERVICES/ETC.
Speech therapy 3 times/wk.

DATE	TREATMENTS/MISCELLANEOUS

ORDERED	SCHEDULED	COMPLETED	X-RAY AND SPECIAL DIAGNOSTIC EXAMS
_10-20_	_10-20_	_10-20_	_Chest x-ray_

START DATE	SCHEDULED MEDICATIONS	STOP DATE	RENEW	START DATE	STOP OR RENEW	SITE	IV FLUID & RATE	DATE & TIME CHANGED TUBING	DRESS.	SITE
_10-19_	_Lasix 40 mgm daily_									
_10-19_	_Lanoxin 0.25 mgm daily_									

DATE	ONE TIME ORDERS

DATE	DAILY/REPEATING ORDERS
_10-20_	_Serum potassium daily_

DATE	TIME	PRN MEDICATIONS
_10-19_	_2100_	_Ativan 0.25 mgm_

MISCELLANEOUS

ALLERGIES:
☒ None Known

NURSING ALERTS:

EMERGENCY CONTACT:
Name: _Parker, Marie_   Telephone No. Home: _555-1212_
Relationship: _Wife_   Bus:

ROOM	NAME	PHYSICIAN	ADMITTING DIAGNOSIS/PROBLEM	HOSP. NO.
_310_	_Parker, Edwin_	_Dr. S Epstein_	1. _CHF_ 2. _Dementia_	_1035B_

FIG. **4-4** A sample Kardex. (Modified from Briggs Corp, Des Moines, Iowa.)

THE NURSING PROCESS

The **nursing process** is the method RNs use to plan and deliver nursing care. It has five steps: assessment, nursing diagnosis, planning, implementation, and evaluation. The nursing process deals with the person's nursing needs. All nursing team members do the same things for the person. They have the same goals.

The nursing process is ongoing. It changes as the person's needs change.

Assessment

Assessment involves collecting information about the person. A nursing history is taken. It includes the family's health history. Information from the doctor is reviewed. So are test results and past medical records.

The RN assesses the person's body systems and mental status. You assist the nurse in assessment. You make many observations as you give care and talk to the person.

Observation is using the senses of sight, hearing, touch, and smell to collect information. You *see* how the person lies, sits, or walks. You see flushed or pale skin. You see red and swollen body areas. You *listen* to the person breathe, talk, and cough. Through *touch*, you feel if the skin is hot or cold, or moist or dry. *Smell* is used to detect body, wound, and breath odors. You also smell odors from urine and bowel movements.

Objective data (signs) are seen, heard, felt, or smelled. You can feel a pulse. You can see urine. You cannot feel or see pain, fear, or nausea. **Subjective data (symptoms)** are things a person tells you about that you cannot observe through your senses.

Box 4-1 lists the basic observations you need to make and report to the nurse. Make notes of your observations. Use them to report and record observations. Carry a note pad and pen in your pocket. That way you can note observations as you make them.

OBRA requires the *minimum data set (MDS)* for nursing center residents (Appendix B). The form is completed when the person is admitted to the center. It provides extensive information about the person. Examples are memory, communication, hearing and vision, physical function, and activities. The form is updated before each care conference. A new MDS is completed once a year and whenever the person's condition changes.

BOX 4-1	**Basic Observations**

Ability to Respond

- Is the person easy or hard to arouse?
- Can the person give his or her name, the time, and location when asked?
- Does the person identify others correctly?
- Does the person answer questions correctly?
- Does the person speak clearly?
- Are instructions followed correctly?
- Is the person calm, restless, or excited?
- Is the person conversing, quiet, or talking a lot?

Movement

- Can the person squeeze your fingers with each hand?
- Can the person move arms and legs?
- Are the person's movements shaky or jerky?
- Does the person complain of stiff or painful joints?

Pain or Discomfort

- Where is the pain located? (Ask the person to point to the pain.)
- Does the pain go anywhere else?
- When did the pain begin?
- What was the person doing when the pain began?
- How long does the pain last?

- How does the person describe the pain?
  - Sharp
  - Severe
  - Knife-like
  - Dull
  - Burning
  - Aching
  - Comes and goes
  - Depends on position
- How does the person rate the pain on a scale of 0 to 10? (No pain = 0; worst pain = 10)
- Was a drug given for pain?
- Did the drug help relieve the pain? Is pain still present?
- Can the person sleep and rest?
- What is the position of comfort?

Skin

- Is the skin pale or flushed?
- Is the skin cool, warm, or hot?
- Is the skin moist or dry?
- What color are the lips and nails?
- Is the skin intact? Are there broken areas? If yes, where?
- Are sores or reddened areas present? If yes, where?
- Are bruises present? Where are they located?
- Does the person complain of itching? If yes, where?

Continued

BOX 4-1	Basic Observations — cont'd

Eyes, Ears, Nose, and Mouth

- Is there drainage from the eyes? What color is the drainage?
- Are the eyelids closed?
- Are the eyes reddened?
- Does the person complain of spots, flashes, or blurring?
- Is the person sensitive to bright lights?
- Is there drainage from the ears? What color is the drainage?
- Can the person hear? Is repeating necessary? Are questions answered appropriately?
- Is there drainage from the nose? What color is the drainage?
- Can the person breathe through the nose?
- Is there breath odor?
- Does the person complain of a bad taste in the mouth?
- Does the person complain of painful gums or teeth?

Respirations

- Do both sides of the person's chest rise and fall with respirations?
- Is breathing noisy?
- Does the person complain of difficulty breathing?
- What is the amount and color of sputum?
- What is the frequency of the person's cough? Is it dry or productive?

Bowels and Bladder

- Is the abdomen firm or soft?
- Does the person complain of gas?
- What are the amount, color, and consistency of bowel movements?
- What is the frequency of bowel movements?
- Can the person control bowel movements?

- Does the person have pain or difficulty urinating?
- What is the amount of urine?
- What is the color of urine?
- Is urine clear? Are there particles in the urine?
- Does urine have a foul smell?
- Can the person control the passage of urine?
- What is the frequency of urination?

Appetite

- Does the person like the diet?
- How much of the meal was eaten?
- What food does the person like best?
- Can the person chew food?
- How much liquid was taken?
- What are the person's liquid preferences?
- How often does the person drink liquids?
- Can the person swallow food and fluids?
- Does the person complain of nausea?
- What is the amount and color of material vomited?
- Does the person have hiccups?
- Is the person belching?
- Does the person cough when swallowing?

Activities of Daily Living

- Can the person perform personal care without help?
  - Bathing?
  - Brushing teeth?
  - Combing and brushing hair?
  - Shaving?
- Which does the person use: toilet, commode, bedpan, or urinal?
- Does the person feed himself or herself?
- Can the person walk?
- What amount and kind of help is needed?

Nursing Diagnosis

The RN uses assessment information to make a nursing diagnosis. A *nursing diagnosis* describes a health problem that can be treated by nursing measures. It is different from a medical diagnosis. A *medical diagnosis* is the identification of a disease or condition by a doctor. Cancer, pneumonia, chickenpox, stroke, heart attack, infection, AIDS, and diabetes are examples. Box 4-2 lists some common nursing diagnoses.

Planning

Planning involves setting priorities and goals. Priorities are what is most important for the person. Goals are aimed at the person's highest level of well-being and function: physical, emotional, social, and spiritual.

A *nursing intervention* is an action or measure taken by the nursing team to help the person reach a goal. Nursing intervention, nursing action, and nursing measure mean the same thing. A nursing intervention does not need a doctor's order.

The **nursing care plan** is a written guide about the person's care. It has the person's nursing diagnoses, goals, and measures for each goal. The care plan is a communication tool. Nursing staff use it to see what care to give. The care plan helps ensure that the nursing team gives the same care. It is found in the medical record, on the Kardex, or on computer.

BOX 4-2	**Common Nursing Diagnoses**

- Activity intolerance
- Adjustment, impaired
- Airway clearance, ineffective
- Allergy response, latex
- Anxiety
- Anxiety, death
- Aspiration, risk for
- Body image, disturbed
- Body temperature, imbalanced, risk for
- Bowel incontinence
- Breathing pattern, ineffective
- Communication, verbal, impaired
- Confusion, acute
- Confusion, chronic
- Constipation
- Denial, ineffective
- Dentition, impaired
- Diarrhea
- Disuse syndrome, risk for
- Diversional activity, deficient
- Failure to thrive, adult
- Falls, risk for
- Family processes, interrupted
- Fatigue
- Fear
- Fluid volume, deficient
- Fluid volume, excess
- Grieving, anticipatory
- Health maintenance, ineffective
- Hopelessness
- Identity, personal, disturbed
- Incontinence, urinary, functional
- Incontinence, urinary, reflex
- Incontinence, urinary, stress
- Incontinence, urinary, total
- Incontinence, urinary, urge
- Incontinence, urinary, risk for urge
- Infection, risk for
- Injury, risk for
- Loneliness, risk for
- Memory, impaired

- Mobility, bed, impaired
- Mobility, wheelchair, impaired
- Mobility, physical, impaired
- Nausea
- Nutrition, less than body requirements, imbalanced
- Nutrition, more than body requirements, imbalanced
- Oral mucous membrane, impaired
- Pain, acute
- Pain, chronic
- Powerlessness
- Relocation stress syndrome
- Relocation stress syndrome: risk for
- Self-care deficit, bathing/hygiene
- Self-care deficit, dressing/grooming
- Self-care deficit, feeding
- Self-care deficit, toileting
- Self-esteem, chronic low
- Sensory perception, disturbed (Specify type: visual, auditory, kinesthetic, gustatory, tactile, olfactory)
- Sexuality patterns, ineffective
- Skin integrity, impaired
- Skin integrity, risk for impaired
- Sleep deprivation
- Sleep patterns, disturbed
- Social interaction, impaired
- Sorrow, chronic
- Spiritual distress
- Suffocation, risk for
- Suicide, risk for
- Surgical recovery, delayed
- Swallowing, impaired
- Thought processes, disturbed
- Tissue integrity, impaired
- Transfer ability, impaired
- Trauma, risk for
- Urinary elimination, impaired
- Urinary elimination, readiness for enhanced
- Urinary retention
- Walking, impaired
- Wandering

From *NANDA International: nursing diagnoses: definitions and classification 2005-2006*, Philadelphia, NANDA-I.

The Comprehensive Care Plan

OBRA requires a **comprehensive care plan** for each resident. It is a written guide giving direction for the resident's care. The plan identifies the resident's problems, goals for care, and actions to take.

Problems identified on the MDS give *triggers* (clues) for the resident assessment protocols (RAPs). For example, the MDS shows that Mrs. Reece has problems walking. This triggers the RAPs. They provide guidelines to solve the problem. The goal is for Mrs. Reece to walk without help. Actions to help her reach the goal are:

- Physical therapy to work with Mrs. Reece on exercises daily
- Nursing staff to walk Mrs. Reece 50 feet twice daily

The comprehensive care plan must also identify the resident's strengths. For example, Mrs. Reece can brush and comb her hair. This strength increases her independence. The health team must continue to have Mrs. Reece do her own hair care.

Implementation

Implementation means to perform or carry out. The *implementation* step is providing the nursing measures in the care plan. Care is given in this step. The nurse delegates measures that are within your legal limits and job description.

Assignment Sheets

The nurse uses an assignment sheet to communicate delegated measures and tasks to you (Fig. 4-5). Talk to the nurse about unclear assignments. You can also check the care plan and Kardex if you need more information.

Assignment Sheet

Date: 9–10
Shift: Day
Nursing assistant: John Reed
Supervisor: Mary Adams, RN

Breaks: 1000   1400
Lunch: 1230
Unit Tasks: *Pass ice water @ 0900*
Clean utility room @ 1430

*Check the care plan for other care measures and information

Room # 501A Name: Mrs. Ann Lopez	Functional status/other care measures and procedures
VS: Daily at 0700 T _____ P _____ R _____ BP _____ Wt: Weekly (Monday at 0700) _____ Intake _____ BM _____ Bath: Portable tub Shampoo Bed rails	Total assist with ADL Stand-pivot transfers Uses w/c Incontinent of bowel and bladder – uses briefs Bilateral passive ROM exercises to extremities bid Turn and reposition q2h when in bed Wears eyeglasses and dentures Diet: High fiber (Total Assist)
Room # 510B Name: Mr. Mark Monroe	Functional status/other care measures and procedures
VS: bid at 0700 and 1500 0700: T _____ P _____ R _____ BP _____ 1500: T _____ P _____ R _____ BP _____ Wt: Daily at 0700 _____ Intake _____ Output _____ BM _____ Bath: Shower	Independent with ADL Independent with ambulation Attends exercise group every morning Continent of bowel and bladder – q4h bathroom schedule to maintain continence Wears eyeglasses Coughing and deep breathing exercises q4h Diet: Sodium-controlled (Independent)

FIG. **4-5** Sample Assignment Sheet. Note: This Assignment Sheet is a computer printout.

Evaluation

Evaluation means to measure. The *evaluation* step involves measuring if the goals in the planning step were met. Progress is evaluated. Changes in nursing diagnoses, goals, and the care plan may result.

You have a key role in the nursing process. The RN uses your observations for nursing diagnoses and planning. You may help develop the care plan. In the implementation step, you perform nursing measures in the care plan. Your observations are used for the evaluation step.

RESIDENT CARE CONFERENCES

OBRA requires two types of resident care conferences:
- The *interdisciplinary care planning (IDCP) conference* is held regularly to develop, review, and update care plans. The RN, doctor, and other health team members attend. The person and a family member also attend.
- *Problem-focused conferences* are held when one problem affects a person's care. Only staff directly involved in the problem attend. The person and family may be asked to attend.

Residents have the right to take part in their care planning. They may refuse suggestions made by the health team.

REPORTING AND RECORDING

Reporting and recording are accounts of what was done for and observed about the person. **Reporting** is the oral account of care and observations. **Recording** *(charting)* is the written account of care and observations.

Reporting

You report care and observations to the nurse. Follow these rules:
- Be prompt, thorough, and accurate.
- Give the person's name, room, and bed number.
- Give the time your observations were made or the care was given.
- Report only what you observed or did yourself.
- Give reports as often as the person's condition requires. Or give them as often as the nurse asks you to.
- Report any changes from normal or changes in the person's condition. Report these changes at once.
- Use your notes to give a specific, concise, and clear report.

Recording

When recording on the person's chart, communicate clearly and thoroughly. Follow the rules in Box 4-3. Anyone who reads your charting should know what you observed, what you did, and the person's response.

BOX 4-3	Rules For Recording

- Always use ink. Use the ink color required by the agency.
- Include the date and the time for every recording. Use conventional time (AM or PM) or 24-hour clock time according to agency policy (p. 44).
- Make sure writing is readable and neat.
- Use only agency-approved abbreviations (p. 44).
- Use correct spelling, grammar, and punctuation.
- Never erase errors or use correction fluid. Cross out the incorrect part and write "error" or "mistaken entry" over it. Sign your initials to the error or mistaken entry. Then rewrite the part. Follow agency policy for correcting errors.
- Sign all entries with your name and title as required by agency policy.
- Do not skip lines. Draw a line through the blank space of a partially completed line or to the end of a page. This prevents others from recording in a space with your signature.
- Make sure each form is stamped with the person's name and other identifying information.
- Record only what you observed and did yourself.
- Never chart a procedure or treatment until after it is completed.
- Be accurate, concise, and factual. Do not record judgments or interpretations.
- Record in a logical and sequential manner.
- Be descriptive. Avoid terms with more than one meaning.
- Use the person's exact words whenever possible. Use quotation marks to show that the statement is a direct quote.
- Record any changes from normal or changes in the person's condition. Also record that you informed the nurse (include the nurse's name), what you told the nurse, and the time you made the report.
- Do not omit information.
- Record safety measures, such as placing the signal light within reach or reminding someone not to get out of bed. This helps protect you if the person falls.

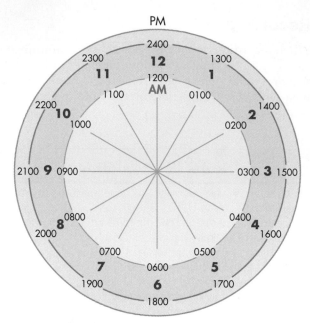

FIG. **4-6** The 24-hour clock.

Recording Time

The 24-hour clock (military time or international time) has four digits (Fig. 4-6). The first two digits are for the hour: 0100 = 1:00 AM; 1300 = 1:00 PM. The last two digits are for minutes: 0110 = 1:10 AM. The AM and PM abbreviations are not used.

As Figure 4-6 shows, the hour is the same for morning times, but AM is not used. For PM times, add 12 to the clock time. If it is 2:00 PM, add 12 and 2 for 1400. For 8:35 PM, add 12 and 835 for 2035.

MEDICAL TERMINOLOGY AND ABBREVIATIONS

Medical terminology and abbreviations are used in health care. Like all words, medical terms are made up of parts or *word elements*. They are combined to form medical terms. A term is translated by separating the word into its elements. Word elements are prefixes, roots, and suffixes (Box 4-4). Most are from Greek or Latin. You may want to buy a medical dictionary so you can learn new words.

BOX 4-4	Medical Terminology		
PREFIX	**MEANING**	**PREFIX**	**MEANING**
a-, an-	without, not, lack of	mono-	one, single
ab-	away from	neo-	new
ad-	to, toward, near	non-	not
ante-	before, forward, in front of	olig-	small, scant
anti-	against	para-	beside, beyond, after
auto-	self	per-	by, through
bi-	double, two, twice	peri-	around
brady-	slow	poly-	many, much
circum-	around	post-	after, behind
contra-	against, opposite	pre-	before, in front of, prior to
de-	down, from	pro-	before, in front of
dia-	across, through, apart	re-	again, backward
dis-	apart, free from	retro-	backward, behind
dys-	bad, difficult, abnormal	semi-	half
ecto-	outer, outside	sub-	under, beneath
en-	in, into, within	super-	above, over, excess
endo-	inner, inside	supra-	above, over
epi-	over, on, upon	tachy-	fast, rapid
eryth-	red	trans-	across
eu-	normal, good, well, healthy	uni-	one
ex-	out, out of, from, away from		
hemi-	half		
hyper-	excessive, too much, high	**ROOT**	
hypo-	under, decreased, less than normal	**(combining**	
in-	in, into, within, not	**vowel)**	**MEANING**
infra-	within	abdomin (o)	abdomen
inter-	between	aden (o)	gland
intro-	into, within	adren (o)	adrenal gland
leuk-	white	angi (o)	vessel
macro-	large	arterio	artery
mal-	bad, illness, disease	arthr (o)	joint
meg-	large	broncho	bronchus, bronchi
micro-	small	card, cardi (o)	heart

BOX 4-4   Medical Terminology—cont'd

ROOT (combining vowel)	MEANING	ROOT (combining vowel)	MEANING
cephal (o)	head	stomat (o)	mouth
chole, chol (o)	bile	therm (o)	heat
chondr (o)	cartilage	thoraco	chest
colo	colon, large intestine	thromb (o)	clot, thrombus
cost (o)	rib	thyr (o)	thyroid
crani (o)	skull	toxic (o)	poison, poisonous
cyan (o)	blue	toxo	poison
cyst (o)	bladder, cyst	trache (o)	trachea
cyt (o)	cell	urethr (o)	urethra
dent (o)	tooth	urin (o)	urine
derma	skin	uro	urine, urinary tract, urination
duoden (o)	duodenum	uter (o)	uterus
encephal (o)	brain	vas (o)	blood vessel, vas deferens
enter (o)	intestines	ven (o)	vein
fibr (o)	fiber, fibrous	vertebr (o)	spine, vertebrae
gastr (o)	stomach		
gloss (o)	tongue	**SUFFIX**	**MEANING**
gluc (o)	sweetness, glucose	-algia	pain
glyc (o)	sugar	-asis	condition, usually abnormal
gyn, gyne, gyneco	woman	-cele	hernia, herniation, pouching
hem, hema, hemo, hemat (o)	blood	-centesis	puncture and aspiration of
hepat (o)	liver	-cyte	cell
hydr (o)	water	-ectasis	dilation, stretching
hyster (o)	uterus	-ectomy	excision, removal of
ile (o), ili (o)	ileum	-emia	blood condition
laparo	abdomen, loin, or flank	-genesis	development, production, creation
laryng (o)	larynx	-genic	producing, causing
lith (o)	stone	-gram	record
mamm (o)	breast, mammary gland	-graph	a diagram, a recording instrument
mast (o)	mammary gland, breast	-graphy	making a recording
meno	menstruation	-iasis	condition of
my (o)	muscle	-ism	a condition
myel (o)	spinal cord, bone marrow	-itis	inflammation
necro	death	-logy	the study of
nephr (o)	kidney	-lysis	destruction of, decomposition
neur (o)	nerve	-megaly	enlargement
ocul (o)	eye	-meter	measuring instrument
oophor (o)	ovary	-metry	measurement
ophthalm (o)	eye	-oma	tumor
orth (o)	straight, normal, correct	-osis	condition
oste (o)	bone	-pathy	disease
ot (o)	ear	-penia	lack, deficiency
ped (o)	child, foot	-phagia	to eat or consume; swallowing
pharyng (o)	pharynx	-phasia	speaking
phleb (o)	vein	-phobia	an exaggerated fear
pnea	breathing, respiration	-plasty	surgical repair or reshaping
pneum (o)	lung, air, gas	-plegia	paralysis
proct (o)	rectum	-ptosis	falling, sagging, dropping, down
psych (o)	mind	-rrhage, -rrhagia	excessive flow
pulmo	lung	-rrhaphy	stitching, suturing
py (o)	pus	-rrhea	profuse flow, discharge
rect (o)	rectum	-scope	examination instrument
rhin (o)	nose	-scopy	examination using a scope
salping (o)	eustachian tube, uterine tube	-stasis	maintenance, maintaining a constant level
splen (o)	spleen	-stomy, -ostomy	creation of an opening
sten (o)	narrow, constriction	-tomy, -otomy	incision, cutting into
stern (o)	sternum	-uria	condition of the urine

Prefixes, Roots, and Suffixes

A *prefix* is a word element placed before a root. It changes the meaning of the word. The prefix *olig* (scant, small amount) is placed before the root *uria* (urine) to make *oliguria.* It means a scant amount of urine. Prefixes are always combined with other word elements. They are never used alone.

The *root* contains the basic meaning of the word. It is combined with another root, with prefixes, and with suffixes. A vowel (an *o* or an *i*) is added between two roots or between a root and a suffix. The vowel makes pronunciation easier.

A *suffix* is placed after a root. It changes the meaning of a word. Suffixes are not used alone. When translating medical terms, begin with the suffix. For example, *nephritis* means inflammation of the kidney. It was formed by combining *nephro* (kidney) and *itis* (inflammation).

Medical terms are formed by combining word elements. Prefixes always come before roots. Suffixes always come after roots. Roots are combined with prefixes, roots, or suffixes. Combining a prefix, root, and suffix is another way to form medical terms.

Endocarditis has the prefix *endo* (inner), the root *card* (heart), and the suffix *itis* (inflammation). *Endocarditis* means inflammation of the inner part of the heart.

Directional Terms

Certain terms describe the position of one body part in relation to another. These terms give the direction of the body part when a person is standing and facing forward (Fig. 4-7):

- *Anterior (ventral)*—at or toward the front of the body or body part
- *Distal*—the part farthest from the center or from the point of attachment
- *Lateral*—away from the midline; at the side of the body or body part
- *Medial*—at or near the middle or midline of the body or body part
- *Posterior (dorsal)*—at or toward the back of the body or body part
- *Proximal*—the part nearest to the center or to the point of origin

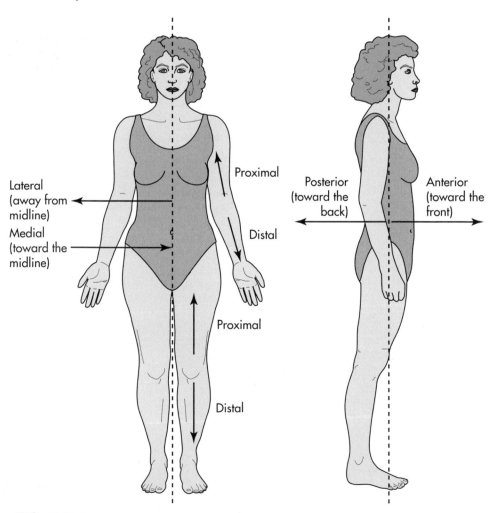

FIG. **4-7** Directional terms describe the position of one body part in relation to another.

Abbreviations

Abbreviations are shortened forms of words or phrases. They save time and space when recording. Each agency has a list of accepted abbreviations. Obtain the list when you are hired. Use only those accepted by the agency. If you are unsure if an abbreviation is acceptable, write the term out in full. This ensures accurate communication.

Common abbreviations are on the inside of this book's back cover for easy use.

USING COMPUTERS

Computer systems collect, send, record, and store information. Many agencies store charts and care plans on computers. Entering information on a computer is easier and faster than charting. Recordings are more accurate, legible, and reliable. Computers save time. Quality care and safety increase. Fewer recording errors are made. Records are more complete. Staff is more efficient.

Computers contain vast amounts of information. Therefore the right to privacy must be protected. Only certain staff members use the computer. If allowed access, you will learn how to use the agency's system. You must follow the agency's policy. Also follow the rules in Box 4-5 and the ethical and legal rules about privacy, confidentiality, and defamation.

BOX 4-5   Using the Agency's Computer

- Follow the rules for recording (see Box 4-3).
- Enter information carefully. Double-check your entries.
- Prevent others from seeing what is on the screen. Do not leave the computer unattended.
- Log off after making an entry.
- Position equipment so the screen cannot be seen in the hallway or by others.
- Do not leave printouts where others can read them or pick them up.
- Destroy or shred computer printouts.
- Do not use e-mail for information or messages that require immediate reporting. Give the report in person. (The person may not read e-mail in a timely manner.)
- Do not use e-mail or messages to report confidential information. This includes addresses, phone numbers, and Social Security numbers. The computer system may not be secure.
- Do not use the agency's computer for your personal use.
- Do not open another person's e-mail or messages.

PHONE COMMUNICATIONS

You may have to answer phones at the nurses' station or in the person's room. Good communication skills are needed. The caller cannot see you. But you give much information by your tone of voice, how clearly you speak, and your attitude. Be professional and courteous. Also practice good work ethics. Follow the agency's policy and the guidelines in Box 4-6.

BOX 4-6   Guidelines For Answering Phones

- Answer the call after the first ring if possible. Be sure to answer by the fourth ring.
- Do not answer the phone in a rushed or hasty manner.
- Give a courteous greeting. Give your name, title, and area. For example: "Good morning. Three center. Jack Parks, nursing assistant."
- Write the following information when taking a message:
  - The caller's name and telephone number (include area code and extension number)
  - The date and time
  - The message
- Repeat the message and phone number back to the caller.
- Ask the caller to "Please hold" if necessary. First find out who is calling. Then ask if the caller can hold. Do not put callers with an emergency on hold.
- Do not lay the phone down or cover the receiver with your hand when not speaking to the caller. The caller may overhear confidential conversations.
- Return to a caller on hold within 30 seconds. Ask if the caller can wait longer or if the call can be returned.
- Do not give confidential information to any caller. Patient, resident, and employee information is confidential. Refer such calls to the nurse.
- Transfer the call if appropriate.
  - Tell the caller that you are going to transfer the call.
  - Give the name of the department if appropriate.
  - Give the caller the phone number in case the call gets disconnected or the line is busy.
- End the conversation politely. Thank the person for calling, and say good-bye.
- Give the message to the appropriate person.

DEALING WITH CONFLICT

People bring their values, attitudes, opinions, experiences, and needs to the work setting. Differences often lead to *conflict*—a clash between opposing interests or ideas. People disagree and argue. There are misunderstandings and unrest.

Conflicts arise over issues or events. Work schedules, absences, and the amount and quality of work performed are examples. The problems must be worked out. Otherwise, unkind words or actions may occur. The work setting becomes unpleasant. Care is affected.

To resolve a conflict, you need to know the real problem. This is part of *problem solving*. The problem solving process involves these steps:

- *Step 1:* Define the problem. *A nurse ignores me.*
- *Step 2:* Collect information. The information must be about the problem. *The nurse does not talk to me. The nurse does not respond when I call her by name. The nurse does not ask me to help her.*
- *Step 3:* Identify possible solutions. *Ignore the nurse. Talk to my supervisor. Talk to co-workers about the problem. Change jobs.*
- *Step 4:* Select the best solution. *Talk to my supervisor.*
- *Step 5:* Carry out the solution. *See next column.*
- *Step 6:* Evaluate the results. *See next column.*

Communication and good work ethics help prevent and resolve conflicts. Identify and solve problems before they become major issues. These guidelines can help you deal with conflict:

- Ask your supervisor for some time to talk privately. Explain the problem. Give facts and specific examples. Ask for advice in solving the problem.
- Approach the person with whom you have a conflict. Ask to talk privately. Be polite and professional.
- Agree on a time and place to talk.
- Talk in a private setting. No one should see or hear you and the other person.
- Explain the problem and what is bothering you. Give facts and specific behaviors. Focus on the problem. Do not focus on the person.
- Listen to the person. Do not interrupt.
- Identify ways to solve the problem. Offer your thoughts. Ask for the co-worker's ideas.
- Set a date and time to review the matter.
- Thank the person for meeting with you.
- Carry out the solutions.
- Review the matter as scheduled.

REVIEW QUESTIONS

Circle the **BEST** answer.

1 To communicate, you should do the following *except*
   a Use terms with many meanings
   b Be brief and concise
   c Present information logically and in sequence
   d Give facts and be specific

2 These statements are about medical records. Which is *false?*
   a The record is used to communicate information about the person.
   b The record is a written account of the person's illness and response to treatment.
   c The record can be used as evidence of the care given.
   d Anyone working in the agency can read the medical record.

3 Where do you describe the care you gave?
   a Admission sheet   c Graphic sheet
   b Nursing history   d Progress notes

4 Which is a sign?
   a Nausea   c Dizziness
   b Headache   d Dry skin

5 Measures in a care plan are carried out. This is
   a A nursing diagnosis   c Implementation
   b Planning   d Evaluation

6 Which statement is *true?*
   a The nursing process is done without the person's input.
   b You are responsible for the nursing process.
   c The nursing process is used to communicate the person's care.
   d Nursing process steps can be done in any order.

7 What is used to communicate the tasks and measures delegated to you?
   a The care plan
   b The Kardex
   c An assignment sheet
   d Care conferences

8 When recording, you do the following *except*
   a Use ink
   b Include the date and time
   c Erase errors
   d Sign all entries with your name and title

9 These statements are about recording. Which action is *false?*
   a Use the person's exact words when possible.
   b Record only what you did and observed.
   c Sign your initials to a mistaken entry.
   d Chart a procedure before completing it.

10 In the evening the clock shows 9:26. In 24-hour clock time, this is
   a 9:26 PM
   b 926
   c 0926
   d 2126

11 A suffix is
   a At the beginning of a word
   b After a root
   c A shortened form of a word or phrase
   d A body position

12 These statements are about using computers. Which is *false?*
   a Computers are used to collect, send, record, and store information.
   b The person's privacy must be protected.
   c You can take computer printouts home.
   d You need to double-check your entries.

13 You answer a person's phone. How should you answer?
   a "Good morning. Mr. Barr's room."
   b "Good morning. Third floor."
   c "Hello."
   d "Good morning. Mr. Barr's room. Joan Bates, nursing assistant, speaking."

14 A co-worker is often late for work. This means extra work for you. To resolve the conflict, you should do the following *except*
   a Explain the problem to your supervisor
   b Discuss the matter with the nursing team
   c Give facts and specific behaviors
   d Suggest ways to solve the problem

Answers to these questions are on p. 467.

Understanding the Person

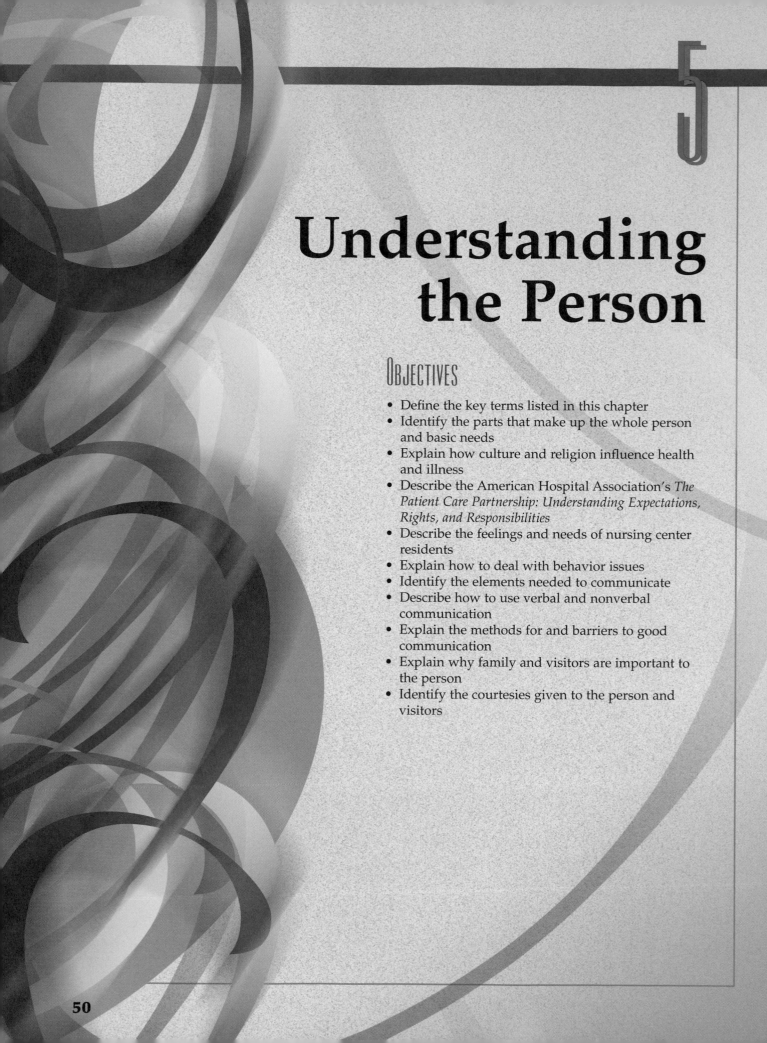

OBJECTIVES

- Define the key terms listed in this chapter
- Identify the parts that make up the whole person and basic needs
- Explain how culture and religion influence health and illness
- Describe the American Hospital Association's *The Patient Care Partnership: Understanding Expectations, Rights, and Responsibilities*
- Describe the feelings and needs of nursing center residents
- Explain how to deal with behavior issues
- Identify the elements needed to communicate
- Describe how to use verbal and nonverbal communication
- Explain the methods for and barriers to good communication
- Explain why family and visitors are important to the person
- Identify the courtesies given to the person and visitors

KEY TERMS

body language Messages sent through facial expressions, gestures, posture, hand and body movements, gait, eye contact, and appearance

culture The characteristics of a group of people—language, values, beliefs, habits, likes, dislikes, customs—passed from one generation to the next

need Something necessary or desired for maintaining life and mental well-being

nonverbal communication Communication that does not use words

optimal level of function A person's highest potential for mental and physical performance

religion Spiritual beliefs, needs, and practices

verbal communication Communication that uses written or spoken words

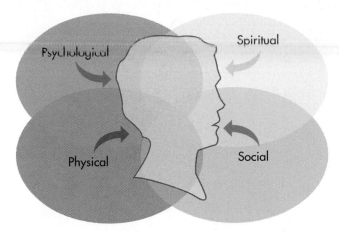

FIG. **5-1** A person is a physical, psychological, social, and spiritual being. The parts overlap and cannot be separated.

The patient or resident is the most important person in the agency. Each person has value. Each has fears, needs, and rights. Each has suffered losses—loss of home, family, friends, and body functions.

CARING FOR THE PERSON

The whole person has physical, social, psychological, and spiritual parts. The parts are woven together and cannot be separated (Fig. 5-1).

Each part relates to and depends on the others. As a social being, a person speaks and communicates with others. Physically, the brain, mouth, tongue, lips, and throat structures must function for speech. Communication is also psychological. It involves thinking and reasoning.

To consider only the physical part is to ignore the person's ability to think, make decisions, and interact with others. It also ignores the person's experiences, life-style, culture, joys, sorrows, and needs.

Hospital Patients

In April 2003, The American Hospital Association (AHA) adopted *The Patient Care Partnership: Understanding Expectations, Rights, and Responsibilities.* The document explains the person's rights and expectations during hospital stays. The relationship between the doctor, the health team, and the patient is stressed.

Nursing Center Residents

Fears and anxieties about living in a nursing center are common. Residents may feel lonely and abandoned by families and friends. Many fear increasing loss of function. Their behavior may reflect fear and other emotions.

You can help residents feel safe, secure, and loved. Protect their rights (Chapter 7). Take an extra minute to visit, to hold a hand, or to give a hug. Treat each person with respect and dignity. Increasing loss of function may be hard to prevent. However, you can help maintain **optimal level of function.** This is the person's highest potential for mental and physical performance. Encourage as much independence as possible. Focus on the person's abilities, not disabilities. Help each person regain or maintain as much physical and mental function as possible. These actions help improve the person's quality of life.

Quality of Life

Patients and residents have the right to quality of life. They must be treated with dignity and respect. Before giving care you must extend the following courtesies:
- Knock before entering the person's room
- Address the person by name
- Introduce yourself by name and title
- Explain the procedure to the person before beginning and during the procedure
- Protect the person's rights during the procedure
- Handle the person gently during the procedure

NEEDS

A **need** is something necessary or desired for maintaining life and mental well-being. According to psychologist Abraham Maslow, basic needs must be met for a person to survive and function. These needs are arranged in order of importance (Fig. 5-2, p. 52).

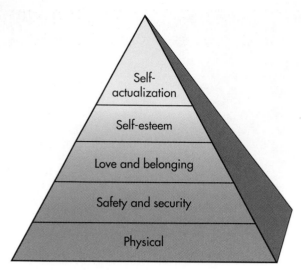

FIG. **5-2** Basic needs for life as described by Maslow. (From Maslow, Abraham H: Frager Robert D (Editor); Fadiman James (Editor) Motivation and personality 3rd edition, 1987. © 1970 by Abraham H. Maslow. Adapted and used by permission of Pearson Education, Inc., Upper Saddle River, NJ.)

Lower-level needs must be met before the higher-level needs. Basic needs, from the lowest level to the highest level, are:

- *Physical needs*—oxygen, food, water, elimination, rest, and shelter are needed for life. They are needed to survive. A person dies within minutes without oxygen. Without food or water, a person feels weak and ill within a few hours. The kidneys and intestines must function. Otherwise toxic wastes build up in the blood. This can cause death. Without enough rest and sleep, a person becomes very tired. Without shelter, the person is exposed to extremes of heat and cold.
- *Safety and security needs*—relate to feeling safe from harm, danger, and fear. Many people are afraid of hospitals and nursing centers. They are in a strange place with strange routines and equipment. Strangers care for them. Some become scared and confused. Fear of pain or discomfort is common. People feel safer and more secure if they know what will happen. For every procedure, they should know:
  - □ Why it is needed
  - □ Who will do it
  - □ How it will be done
  - □ What sensations or feelings to expect
- *Love and belonging needs*—relate to love, closeness, and affection. They also involve meaningful relationships with others. Some people become weaker or die from the lack of love and belonging. This is seen in children and in older persons who have outlived family and friends.

- *Self-esteem needs*—self-esteem means to think well of oneself, and to see oneself as useful and having value. It also relates to being thought well of by others. People often lack self-esteem when ill, injured, older, or disabled.
- *Self-actualization needs*—self-actualization means experiencing one's potential. It involves learning, understanding, and creating to the limit of a person's capacity. This is the highest need. Rarely, if ever, is it totally met. Most people constantly try to learn and understand more. This need can be postponed, and life will continue.

CULTURE AND RELIGION

Culture is the characteristics of a group of people—language, values, beliefs, habits, likes, dislikes, and customs. They are passed from one generation to the next. The person's culture influences health beliefs and practices. Culture also affects behavior during illness.

People come from many cultures, races, and nationalities. Their family practices and food choices may differ from yours. So might their hygiene habits and clothing styles. Some speak a foreign language. Some cultures have beliefs about what causes and cures illness. (*See Caring About Culture: Health Care Beliefs.*) They may perform rituals to rid the body of disease. (*See Caring About Culture: Sick Care Practices.*) Many have beliefs and rituals about dying and death (Chapter 27). Culture also is a factor in communication.

Religion relates to spiritual beliefs, needs, and practices. Religions may have beliefs and practices about diet, healing, days of worship, birth and birth control, and death.

Many people find comfort and strength from religion during illness. They may want to pray and observe religious practices. Assist the person to attend services as needed. Some residents leave the center to attend religious services.

The care plan includes the person's cultural and religious practices. You must respect and accept the person's culture and religion. You will meet people from other cultures and religions. *A person may not follow all beliefs and practices of his or her culture or religion. Some people do not practice a religion. Each person is unique. Do not judge the person by your standards.*

BEHAVIOR ISSUES

People do not choose to be ill, injured, or disabled. Normal, everyday activities may be difficult or impossible. A person may feel angry, frustrated, or useless.

Some patients, residents, and families have the following behaviors. These behaviors are new for some

Caring About Culture

Health Care Beliefs

Some *Mexican-Americans* believe that illness is caused by hot or cold. If hot causes the illness, cold is used for the cure. Likewise, hot is used to cure illnesses caused by cold. Hot and cold are found in body organs, medicines, and food. For example, an earache may occur from cold air entering the body. Hot remedies are used to cure the earache.

The hot-cold balance is also a belief of some *Vietnamese-Americans*. Illnesses, food, drugs, and herbs are either hot or cold. Hot is given to balance cold illnesses. Cold is given for hot illnesses.

From Giger JN, Davidhizar RE: *Transcultural nursing: assessment and intervention*, ed 4, St Louis, 2004, Mosby.

Caring About Culture

Sick Care Practices

Folk practices are common among some *Vietnamese-Americans*. They include *cao gio*—rubbing the skin with a coin to treat the common cold. Skin pinching (*batgio*) is used for headaches and sore throats. Herbs, oils, and soups are used for many signs and symptoms.

Some *Russian-Americans* practice folk medicine. Herbs are taken through drinks or enemas. For headaches, an ointment is placed behind the ears and temples and at the back of the neck. There are treatments for backaches. One involves making a dough of dark rye flour and honey. The dough is placed on the spinal column.

Folk healers are used by some *Mexican-Americans*. Folk healers may be family members skilled in healing practices. Some folk healers are from outside the family. A *yerbero* uses herbs and spices to prevent or cure disease. A *curandero* (*curandera* if female) deals with serious physical and mental illnesses. Witches use magic. A male witch is called a *brujos*. A female witch is called a *brujas*.

From Giger JN, Davidhizar RE: *Transcultural nursing: assessment and intervention*, ed 4, St Louis, 2004, Mosby.

people. For others, they are life-long. They are part of one's personality.

- *Anger*—Anger is a common emotion. Causes include fear, pain, and dying and death. Loss of function and loss of control over health and life are causes. Anger is a symptom of some diseases that affect thinking and behavior. Some people are generally angry. Anger is shown verbally and nonverbally (p. 55). Verbal outbursts, shouting, raised voices, and rapid speech are common. Some people are silent. Others are uncooperative. They may refuse to answer questions. Nonverbal signs include rapid movements, pacing, clenched fists, and a red face. Glaring and getting close to you when speaking are other signs. Violent behaviors can occur.
- *Demanding behavior*—Nothing seems to please the person. The person is critical of others. He or she wants care given at a certain time and in a certain way. Causes include loss of independence, loss of health, loss of control of life, and unmet needs.
- *Self-centered behavior*—The person cares only about his or her own needs. The needs of others are ignored. The person demands the time and attention of others. He or she may become impatient when needs are not met.
- *Aggressive behavior*—The person may swear, bite, hit, pinch, scratch, or kick. Fear, anger, pain, and dementia (Chapter 25) are causes. Protect the person, others, and yourself from harm (Chapter 8).
- *Withdrawal*—The person has little or no contact with others. He or she spends time alone and does not take part in social or group events. This may signal physical illness or depression. Some people are not social and like to be alone.
- *Inappropriate sexual behavior*—Some people make inappropriate sexual remarks. Or they touch others. Some disrobe or masturbate in public. These behaviors may be on purpose. Or they are due to disease, confusion, dementia, or drug side effects.

BOX 5-1	Dealing With Behavior Issues

- Recognize frustrating and frightening situations. Put yourself in the person's situation. How would you feel? How would you want to be treated?
- Treat the person with dignity and respect.
- Answer questions clearly and thoroughly. Ask the nurse to answer questions you cannot answer.
- Keep the person informed. Tell the person what you are going to do and when.
- Do not keep the person waiting. Answer signal lights promptly. If you tell the person that you will do something for him or her, do it promptly.
- Explain the reason for long waits. Ask if you can get or do something to increase the person's comfort.
- Stay calm and professional if the person is angry or hostile. Often the person is not angry at you. He or she is angry at another person or situation.
- Do not argue with the person.
- Listen and use silence. The person may feel better if able to express feelings.
- Report the person's behavior to the nurse. Discuss how you should deal with the person.

A person's behavior may be unpleasant. You cannot avoid the person or lose control. Good communication is needed. If the person's behavior is a problem, it will be part of the care plan. Follow the care plan and the guidelines in Box 5-1.

COMMUNICATING WITH THE PERSON

You communicate with patients and residents all the time. For effective communication between you and the person, you must:

- Follow the rules of communication (Chapter 4).
- Understand and respect the patient or resident as a person.
- View the person as a physical, psychological, social, and spiritual human being.
- Appreciate the person's problems and frustrations.
- Respect the person's rights.
- Respect the person's religion and culture.
- Give the person time to process (understand) information.
- Repeat information as often as needed. Repeat exactly what you said. Do not give the person a new message to process.
- Ask questions to see if the person understood you.
- Be patient. People with memory problems may ask the same question many times. Do not say that you are repeating information.

Verbal Communication

Words are used in **verbal communication.** Words are spoken or written. Most verbal communication involves the spoken word. Follow these rules.

- Face the person.
- Control the loudness and tone of your voice.
- Speak clearly, slowly, and distinctly.
- Do not use slang or vulgar words.
- Repeat information as needed.
- Ask one question at a time. Wait for the answer.
- Do not shout, whisper, or mumble.
- Be kind, courteous, and friendly.

The written word is used if the person cannot speak or hear. The nurse and care plan tell you how to communicate with the person. The devices in Figure 5-3 are often used. The person also may have poor vision. When writing messages, be brief and concise. Use a black felt pen on white paper. Print in large letters. Persons who are deaf may use sign language (Chapter 24).

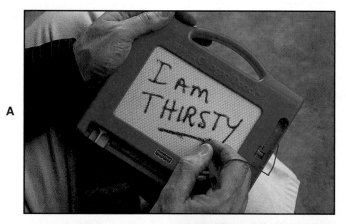

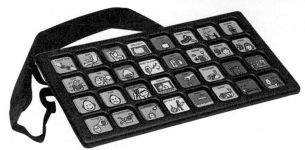

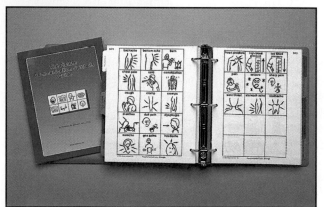

FIG. **5-3** Communication aids. **A,** Magic Slate. **B,** Electronic talking aid. **C,** Communication binder. (**B** Courtesy Mayer-Johnson Co., Solana Beach, Calif.)

Caring About Culture

Touch Practices

Touch practices vary among cultural groups. Touch is used often in *Mexico*. Some people believe that using touch while complimenting a person is important. It is thought to neutralize the power of the evil eye *(mal de ojo)*. Touch also is important in the *Philippine* culture.

Persons from the *United Kingdom* tend not to use touch. Touch is socially acceptable in *Poland*.

In *India*, men shake hands with other men. Men do not shake hands with women. Similar practices occur in *Vietnam*.

People from *China* do not like being touched by strangers. A nod or slight bow is given during introductions.

From D'Avanzo CE, Geissler EM: *Pocket guide to cultural health assessment*, ed 3, St Louis, 2003, Mosby.

Nonverbal Communication

Nonverbal communication does not use words. Gestures, facial expressions, posture, body movements, touch, and smell send messages. Nonverbal messages more accurately reflect a person's feelings than words do. They are usually involuntary and hard to control. A person may say one thing but act another way. Watch the person's eyes, hand movements, gestures, posture, and other actions.

Touch

Touch is a very important form of nonverbal communication. It conveys comfort, caring, love, affection, interest, and reassurance. Touch means different things to different people. The meaning depends on age, gender (male or female), experiences, and culture. *(See Caring About Culture: Touch Practices.)*

Some people do not like to be touched. However, touch can show caring and warmth. Stroking or holding a hand can comfort a person. Touch should be gentle—not hurried, rough, or sexual. To use touch, follow the person's care plan.

Body Language

People send messages through their **body language.**
- Facial expressions *(See Caring About Culture: Facial Expressions.)*
- Gestures
- Posture
- Hand and body movements
- Gait
- Eye contact
- Appearance (dress, hygiene, jewelry, perfume, cosmetics, tattoos, body piercings, and so on)

Caring About Culture

Facial Expressions

Through facial expressions, *Americans* communicate:
- *Coldness*—there is a constant stare. Face muscles do not move.
- *Fear*—eyes are wide open. Eyebrows are raised. The mouth is tense with the lips drawn back.
- *Anger*—eyes are fixed in a hard stare. Upper lids are lowered. Eyebrows are drawn down. Lips are tightly compressed.
- *Tiredness*—eyes are rolled upward.
- *Disapproval*—eyes are rolled upward.
- *Disgust*—narrowed eyes. The upper lip is curled. There are nose movements.
- *Embarrassment*—eyes are turned away or down. The face is flushed. The person pretends to smile. He or she rubs the eyes, nose, or face. He or she twitches hair, beard, or mustache.
- *Surprise*—direct gaze with raised eyebrows.

Italian, Jewish, African-American, and *Hispanic* persons smile readily. They use many facial expressions and gestures for happiness, pain, or displeasure. *Irish, English,* and *Northern European* persons tend to have less facial expression.

In some cultures, facial expressions mean the opposite of what the person is feeling. For example, *Asians* may conceal negative emotions with a smile.

From Giger JN, Davidhizar RE: *Transcultural nursing: assessment and intervention*, ed 4, St Louis, 2004, Mosby.

Slumped posture may mean the person is not happy or feeling well. A person may deny pain. Yet he or she protects a body part by standing, lying, or sitting in a certain way. Many messages are sent through body language.

Your actions, movements, and facial expressions send messages. So does how you stand, sit, walk, and look at a person. Your body language should show interest and enthusiasm. It should show caring and respect for the person. Often you will need to control your body language. Control reactions to odors from fluids, excretions, or the person's body. Many odors are beyond the person's control.

Communication Methods

Certain methods help you communicate with others. They result in better relationships. More information is gained for the nursing process.

Listening

Listening means to focus on verbal and nonverbal communication. You use sight, hearing, touch, and smell. You focus on what the person is saying. You

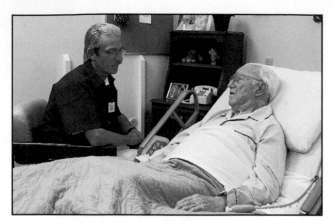

FIG. **5-4** Listen by facing the person. Have good eye contact. Lean toward the person.

observe nonverbal clues. They can support what the person says. Or they can show other feelings. For example, Mr. Kerr says, "I want to go to a nursing home. That way my daughter won't have to care for me." You see tears, and he looks away from you. His verbal says happy. His nonverbal shows sadness.

Listening requires that you care and have interest. Follow these guidelines:

- Face the person.
- Have good eye contact with the person. *(See Caring About Culture: Eye Contact Practices.)*
- Lean toward the person (Fig. 5-4). Do not sit back with your arms crossed.
- Respond to the person. Nod your head. Say "uh huh," "mmm," and "I see." Repeat what the person says. Ask questions.
- Avoid the communication barriers (p. 57).

Direct Questions

Direct questions focus on certain information. You ask the person something you need to know. Some direct questions have "yes" or "no" answers. Others require a brief response. For example:

> *You:* Mr. Kerr, do you want to shave this morning?
> *Mr. Kerr:* Yes.
> *You:* Mr. Kerr, when would you like to do that?
> *Mr. Kerr:* Could we start in 15 minutes? I want to call my son first.
> *You:* Yes, we can start in 15 minutes.

Open-Ended Questions

Open-ended questions lead or invite the person to share thoughts, feelings, or ideas. The person chooses what to talk about. He or she controls the topic and the information given. Answers require a brief response. For example:

- "What do you like about living with your daughter?"
- "Tell me about your grandson."

Caring About Culture

Eye Contact Practices

In the *American* culture, eye contact signals a good self-concept. It also shows openness, interest in others, attention, honesty, and warmth. Lack of eye contact can mean:

- Shyness
- Lack of interest
- Humility
- Guilt
- Embarrassment
- Low self-esteem
- Rudeness
- Dishonesty

For some *Asian* and *American Indian* cultures, eye contact is impolite. It is an invasion of privacy. In certain *Indian* cultures, eye contact is avoided with persons of higher or lower socioeconomic class. It is also given a special sexual meaning.

Direct eye contact is practiced in *Poland* and *Russia*. However, direct eye contact is rude in *Mexican* and *Vietnamese* cultures. In the *United Kingdom*, staring is a part of good listening.

Blinking has meaning. In *Vietnam*, it means that a message is received. It shows understanding in the *United Kingdom*.

From Giger JN, Davidhizar RE: *Transcultural nursing: assessment and intervention*, ed 4, St Louis, 2004, Mosby. From D'Avanzo CE, Geissler EM: *Pocket guide to cultural health assessment*, ed 3, St Louis, 2003, Mosby.

Clarifying

Clarifying lets you make sure that you understand the message. You can ask the person to repeat the message, say you do not understand, or restate the message. For example:

- "Could you say that again?"
- "I'm sorry. I don't understand what you mean."
- "Are you saying that you want to go home?"

Silence

Silence is a powerful way to communicate. Sometimes you do not need to talk or say anything. This is true during sad times. Just being there shows you care. At other times, silence gives time to think, organize thoughts, or choose words. Silence is useful when the person is upset and needs to regain control. Silence on your part shows caring and respect for the person's situation and feelings.

Pauses or long silences can be uncomfortable. You do not need to talk when the person is silent. The person may need silence. *(See Caring About Culture: The Meaning of Silence.)*

Caring About Culture

The Meaning of Silence

In the *English* and *Arabic* cultures, silence is used for privacy. Among *Russian, French, and Spanish* cultures, silence means agreement between parties. In some *Asian* cultures, silence is a sign of respect, particularly to an older person.

From Giger JN, Davidhizar RE: *Transcultural nursing: assessment and intervention,* ed 4, St Louis, 2004, Mosby.

Caring About Culture

Communicating With Persons From Other Cultures

- Ask the nurse about the beliefs and values of the person's culture. Learn as much as you can about the person's culture.
- Do not judge the person by your own attitudes, values, beliefs, and ideas.
- Follow the person's care plan. It includes the person's cultural beliefs and customs.
- Do the following when communicating with foreign speaking persons:
  - Convey comfort by your tone of voice and body language.
  - Do not speak loudly or shout. It will not help the person understand English.
  - Speak slowly and distinctly.
  - Keep messages short and simple.
  - Be alert for words the person seems to understand.
  - Use gestures and pictures.
  - Repeat the message in other ways.
  - Avoid using medical terms and abbreviations.
  - Be alert for signs that the person is pretending to understand. Nodding and answering "yes" to all questions are signs that the person does not understand what you are saying.

Modified from Geissler EM: *Pocket guide to cultural assessment,* ed 3, St Louis, 2003, Mosby.

Communication Barriers

Communication barriers prevent sending and receiving messages:

- *Language.* You and the person must use and understand the same language. If not, messages are not accurately interpreted.
- *Cultural differences.* The person may attach different meanings to verbal and nonverbal communication. *(See Caring About Culture: Communicating With Persons From Other Cultures.)*
- *Changing the subject.* Someone changes the subject when the topic is uncomfortable.
- *Giving opinions.* Opinions involve judging values, behavior, or feelings.
- *Talking a lot when others are silent.* Talking too much is usually due to nervousness and discomfort with silence.
- *Failure to listen.* Do not pretend to listen. It shows lack of interest and caring. You can miss complaints that you must report to the nurse.
- *Pat answers.* "Don't worry. "Everything will be okay." "Your doctor knows best." These make the person feel that you do not care about his or her concerns, feelings, and fears.
- *Illness and disability.* Speech, hearing, vision, cognitive function, and body movements may be affected.

The Person Who Is Comatose

The person who is comatose is unconscious. The person cannot respond to others. Often the person can hear and feel touch and pain. Assume that the person hears and understands you. Use touch and give care gently. Practice these measures:

- Knock before entering the person's room.
- Tell the person your name, the time, and the place every time you enter the room.
- Give care on the same schedule every day.
- Explain what you are going to do. Explain care measures step-by-step as you do them.
- Tell the person when you are finishing care.
- Use touch to communicate care, concern, and comfort.
- Tell the person what time you will be back to check on him or her.
- Tell the person when you are leaving the room.

THE FAMILY AND VISITORS

Family and friends help meet safety and security, love and belonging, and self-esteem needs. They offer support and comfort. They lessen loneliness. Some also help with the person's care. *(See Caring About Culture: Family Roles in Sick Care.)* The presence or absence of family or friends can affect recovery and quality of life.

The person has the right to visit with family and friends in private and without unnecessary interruptions (Fig. 5-5). You may need to give care when visitors are there. Do not expose the person's body in front of them. Politely ask them to leave the room. Show them where to wait. Promptly tell them when they can return.

A partner or other visitor may want to help you with the person's care. If the person gives consent, allow the partner or visitor to stay.

Treat family and visitors with courtesy and respect. They have concerns about the person's condition and care. They need support and understanding. However, do not discuss the person's condition with them. Refer their questions to the nurse.

Visiting rules depend on agency policy and the person's condition. Know your agency's policies and what is allowed for a person.

A visitor may upset or tire a person. Report your observations to the nurse. The nurse will speak with the visitor about the person's needs.

Caring About Culture

Family Roles in Sick Care

In *Vietnam,* all family members are involved in the person's care. A similar practice is common in *China.* Family members bathe, feed, and comfort the person. However, women in *Mexico* cannot give care at home if it involves touching the genitals of adult men.

From D'Avanzo CE, Geissler EM: *Pocket guide to cultural health assessment,* ed 3, St Louis, 2003, Mosby.

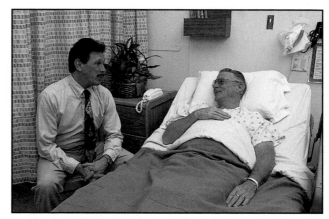

FIG. **5-5** This man has a private visit with his son.

Review Questions

Circle the **BEST** answer.

1 Ms. Jones had surgery. You focus on her
  a Care plan
  b Physical, safety and security, and self-esteem needs
  c As a physical, psychological, social, and spiritual person
  d Cultural and religious practices

2 Which basic need is the *most* essential?
  a Self-actualization
  b Self-esteem
  c Love and belonging
  d Safety and security

3 Ms. Jones says "What are they doing to me?" What basic needs are not being met?
  a Physical needs
  b Safety and security needs
  c Love and belonging needs
  d Self-esteem needs

4 Which is *false?*
  a Culture influences health and illness practices.
  b Culture and religion influence food practices.
  c Religious and cultural practices are allowed in health care agencies.
  d A person must follow all beliefs and practices of his or her religion or culture.

5 A person is angry. You know that
  a The person has a disease that affects thinking and behavior
  b Drug or alcohol abuse is likely
  c The person must calm down
  d Listening and silence are important

6 Which is *false?*
  a Verbal communication uses the written or spoken word.
  b Verbal communication truly reflects a person's feelings.
  c Messages are sent by facial expressions, gestures, posture, and body movements.
  d Touch means different things to different people.

7 To communicate with Mr. Long you should
  a Use medical words and phrases
  b Change the subject often
  c Give your opinions
  d Be quiet when he is silent

8 Which might mean that you are *not* listening?
  a You sit facing the person.
  b You have good eye contact with the person.
  c You sit with your arms crossed.
  d You ask questions.

9 Which is a direct question?
  a "Do you feel better now?"
  b "What are your plans for home?"
  c "What will you do when you get home?"
  d "You said that you can't work."

10 Which promotes communication?
  a "Don't worry."
  b "Everything will be just fine."
  c "This is a good hospital."
  d "Why are you crying?"

11 Ms. Parker is comatose. Which action is *wrong?*
  a Assume that she can hear and feel touch.
  b Explain what you are going to do.
  c Use listening and silence to communicate.
  d Tell her when you are leaving the room.

12 A visitor seems to tire a person. What should you do?
  a Ask the person to leave.
  b Tell the nurse.
  c Stay in the room to observe the person and visitor.
  d Find out the visitor's relationship to the person.

Answers to these questions on are on p. 467.

59

Understanding Body Structure and Function

Objectives

- Define the key terms listed in this chapter
- Identify the basic structures of the cell
- Describe four types of tissue
- Identify the structures of each body system
- Describe the functions of each body system

Key Terms

cell The basic unit of body structure

digestion The process of physically and chemically breaking down food so that it can be absorbed for use by the cells

hormone A chemical substance secreted by the glands into the bloodstream

immunity Protection against a disease or condition; the person will not get or be affected by the disease

metabolism The burning of food for heat and energy by the cells

organ Groups of tissues with the same function

peristalsis Involuntary muscle contractions in the digestive system that move food through the alimentary canal

respiration The process of supplying the cells with oxygen and removing carbon dioxide from them

system Organs that work together to perform special functions

tissue A group of cells with similar functions

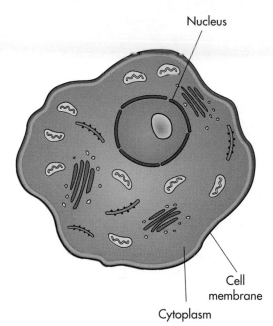

FIG. **6-1** Parts of a cell.

You help patients and residents meet basic needs. Their bodies do not work at peak levels because of illness, disease, injury, or aging. Your care promotes comfort, healing, and recovery. You need to know the body's normal structure and function. It will help you understand signs, symptoms, and the reasons for care and procedures. You will give safer and more efficient care.

CELLS, TISSUES, AND ORGANS

The basic unit of body structure is the **cell**. Cells have the same basic structure. Function, size, and shape may differ. Cells are very small. You need a microscope to see them. Cells need food, water, and oxygen to live and function.

Figure 6-1 shows the cell and its structures. The *cell membrane* is the outer covering. It encloses the cell and helps it hold its shape. The *nucleus* directs the cell activities. It is in the center of the cell. The *cytoplasm* surrounds the nucleus. It contains smaller structures that perform cell functions. *Protoplasm* refers to all structures, substances, and water within the cell. Protoplasm is a semi-liquid substance much like an egg white.

Chromosomes are thread-like structures in the nucleus. Each cell has 46 chromosomes. Chromosomes contain *genes*. Genes control the traits parents give to their children. Height, eye color, and skin color are examples.

The nucleus controls cell reproduction. Cells reproduce by dividing in half. *Mitosis* is the process of cell division. It is needed for tissue growth and repair. During mitosis, the 46 chromosomes arrange themselves in 23 pairs. As the cell divides, the 23 pairs are pulled in half. The two new cells are identical. Each has 46 chromosomes (Fig. 6-2, p. 62).

Groups of cells with similar functions combine to form **tissues:**

■ *Epithelial tissue* covers internal and external body surfaces. Tissue lining the nose, mouth, respiratory tract, stomach, and intestines is epithelial tissue. So are the skin, hair, nails, and glands.

■ *Connective tissue* anchors, connects, and supports other tissues. It is in every part of the body. Bones, tendons, ligaments, and cartilage are connective tissue. Blood is a form of connective tissue.

■ *Muscle tissue* stretches and contracts to let the body move (p. 64).

■ *Nerve tissue* receives and carries impulses to the brain and back to body parts.

Groups of tissues with the same function form **organs.** An organ has one or more functions. Examples of organs are the heart, brain, liver, lungs, and kidneys. **Systems** are formed by organs that work together to perform special functions (Fig. 6-3, p. 62).

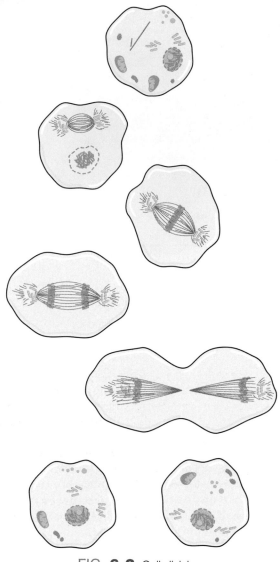

FIG. **6-2** Cell division.

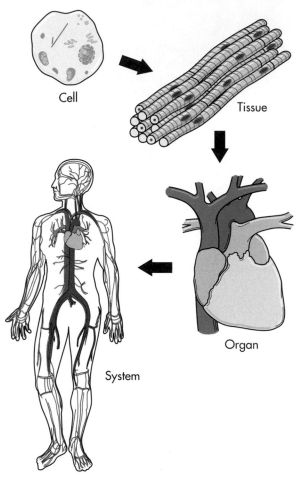

FIG. **6-3** Organization of the body.

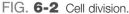

THE INTEGUMENTARY SYSTEM

The *integumentary system,* or skin, is the largest system. *Integument* means covering. The skin covers the body. It has two skin layers (Fig. 6-4):

- The *epidermis* is the outer layer. It has living cells and dead cells. The dead cells were once deeper in the epidermis. They were pushed upward as cells divided. Dead cells constantly flake off. They are replaced by living cells. Living cells also die and flake off. Living cells of the epidermis contain *pigment.* Pigment gives skin its color. The epidermis has no blood vessels and few nerve endings.
- The *dermis* is the inner layer. It has blood vessels, nerves, sweat glands and oil glands, and hair roots.

Oil glands, sweat glands, hair, and *nails* are skin appendages. The entire body, except the palms of the hands and soles of the feet, is covered with hair. Hair in the nose and ears and around the eyes protects these organs from dust, insects, and other objects. Nails protect the tips of fingers and toes. Nails help fingers pick up and handle small objects. Sweat glands help the body regulate temperature. Sweat consists of water, salt, and wastes. Sweat is secreted through pores in the skin. The body is cooled as sweat evaporates. Oil glands secrete an oily substance into the space near the hair shaft. Oil travels to the skin surface. This helps keep the hair and skin soft and shiny.

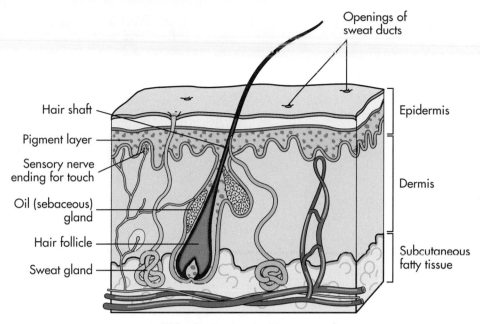

FIG. **6-4** Layers of the skin.

The skin has many functions:
- It is the body's protective covering.
- It prevents bacteria and other substances from entering the body.
- It prevents excess amounts of water from leaving the body.
- It protects organs from injury.
- Nerve endings in the skin sense pleasant and unpleasant stimulation. Nerve endings are over the entire body. They sense cold, pain, touch, and pressure to protect the body from injury.
- It helps regulate body temperature. Blood vessels dilate (widen) when temperature outside the body is high. More blood comes to the body surface for cooling during evaporation. When blood vessels constrict (narrow), the body retains heat. This is because less blood reaches the skin.

THE MUSCULOSKELETAL SYSTEM

The musculoskeletal system provides the framework for the body. It lets the body move. This system also protects and gives the body shape.

Bones

The human body has 206 bones (Fig. 6-5, p. 64). There are four types of bones:
- *Long bones* bear the body's weight. Leg bones are long bones.
- *Short bones* allow skill and ease in movement. Bones in the wrists, fingers, ankles, and toes are short bones.

- *Flat bones* protect the organs. They include the ribs, skull, pelvic bones, and shoulder blades.
- *Irregular bones* are the vertebrae in the spinal column. They allow various degrees of movement and flexibility.

Bones are hard, rigid structures. A membrane called the *periosteum* covers them. Blood vessels in the periosteum supply bone cells with oxygen and food. Inside the hollow centers of the bones is a substance called *bone marrow.* Blood cells are made in the bone marrow.

Joints

A *joint* is the point where two or more bones meet. Joints allow movement. *Cartilage* is the connective tissue at the end of long bones. It cushions the joint so that bone ends do not rub together. The *synovial membrane* lines the joints. It secretes *synovial fluid.* Synovial fluid acts as a lubricant so the joint can move smoothly. Bones are held together at the joint by strong bands of connective tissue called *ligaments.*

There are three types of joints (Fig. 6-6, p. 64):
- *Ball-and-socket joint* allows movement in all directions. The rounded end of one bone fits into the hollow end of the other. Hip and shoulder joints are examples.
- *Hinge joint* allows movement in one direction. The elbow is a hinge joint.
- *Pivot joint* allows turning from side to side. A pivot joint connects the skull to the spine.

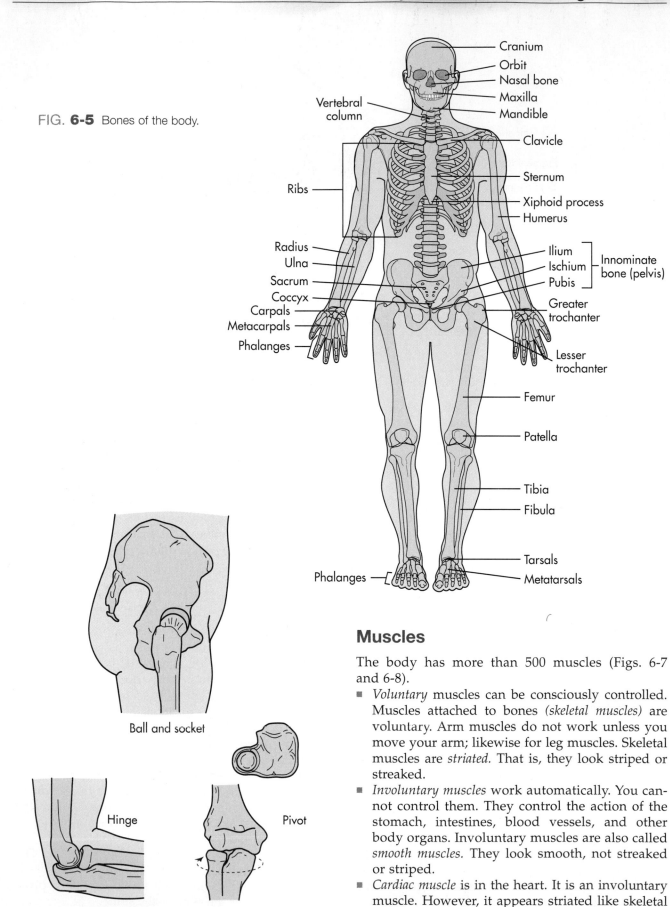

FIG. **6-5** Bones of the body.

FIG. **6-6** Types of joints.

Muscles

The body has more than 500 muscles (Figs. 6-7 and 6-8).

- *Voluntary* muscles can be consciously controlled. Muscles attached to bones *(skeletal muscles)* are voluntary. Arm muscles do not work unless you move your arm; likewise for leg muscles. Skeletal muscles are *striated.* That is, they look striped or streaked.
- *Involuntary muscles* work automatically. You cannot control them. They control the action of the stomach, intestines, blood vessels, and other body organs. Involuntary muscles are also called *smooth muscles.* They look smooth, not streaked or striped.
- *Cardiac muscle* is in the heart. It is an involuntary muscle. However, it appears striated like skeletal muscle.

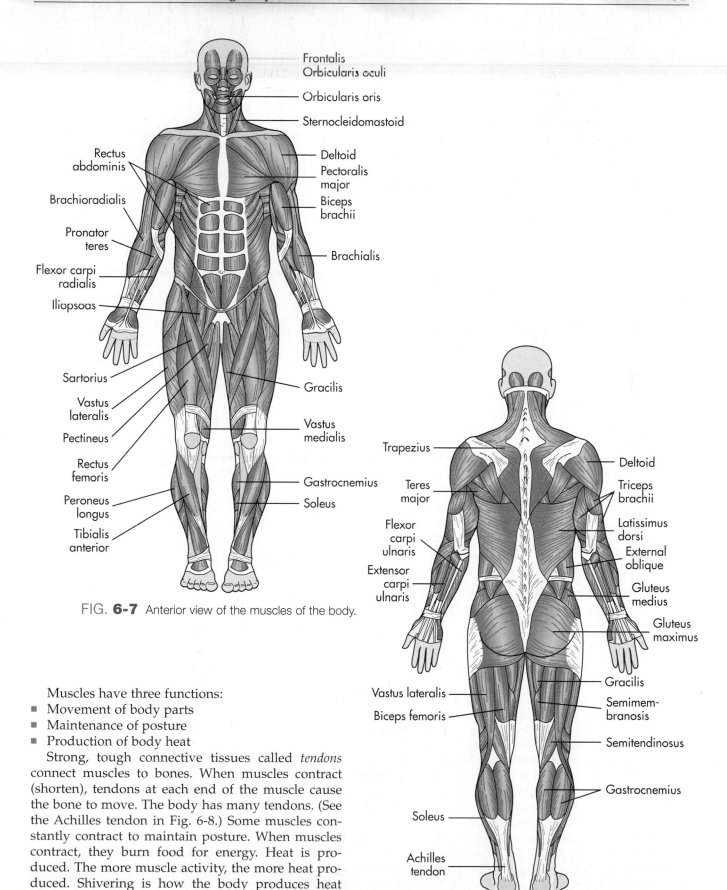

FIG. **6-7** Anterior view of the muscles of the body.

Frontalis
Orbicularis oculi
Orbicularis oris
Sternocleidomastoid
Rectus abdominis
Brachioradialis
Pronator teres
Flexor carpi radialis
Iliopsoas
Sartorius
Vastus lateralis
Pectineus
Rectus femoris
Peroneus longus
Tibialis anterior
Deltoid
Pectoralis major
Biceps brachii
Brachialis
Gracilis
Vastus medialis
Gastrocnemius
Soleus

Trapezius
Teres major
Flexor carpi ulnaris
Extensor carpi ulnaris
Vastus lateralis
Biceps femoris
Soleus
Achilles tendon
Deltoid
Triceps brachii
Latissimus dorsi
External oblique
Gluteus medius
Gluteus maximus
Gracilis
Semimembranosis
Semitendinosus
Gastrocnemius

Muscles have three functions:
- Movement of body parts
- Maintenance of posture
- Production of body heat

Strong, tough connective tissues called *tendons* connect muscles to bones. When muscles contract (shorten), tendons at each end of the muscle cause the bone to move. The body has many tendons. (See the Achilles tendon in Fig. 6-8.) Some muscles constantly contract to maintain posture. When muscles contract, they burn food for energy. Heat is produced. The more muscle activity, the more heat produced. Shivering is how the body produces heat when exposed to cold. Shivering is from rapid, general muscle contractions.

FIG. **6-8** Posterior view of the muscles of the body.

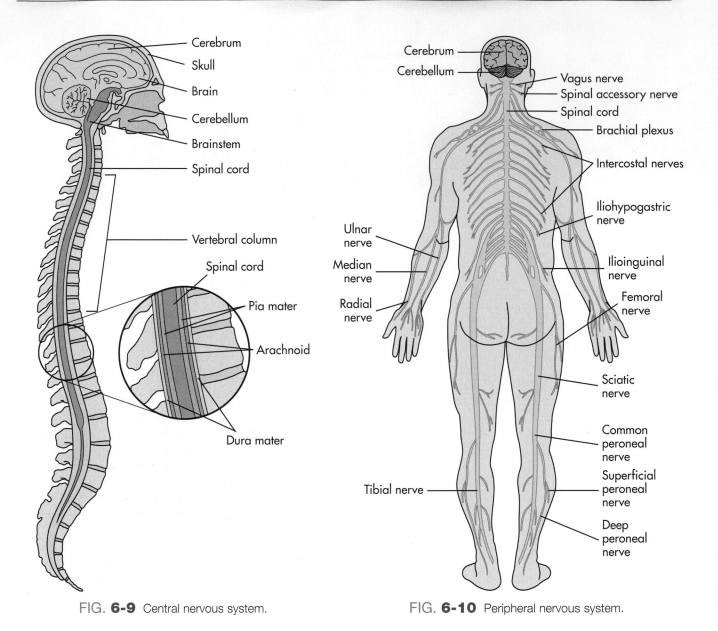

FIG. **6-9** Central nervous system.

FIG. **6-10** Peripheral nervous system.

THE NERVOUS SYSTEM

The nervous system controls, directs, and coordinates body functions. Its two main divisions are:

- The *central nervous system* (CNS). It consists of the *brain* and *spinal cord* (Fig. 6-9).
- The *peripheral nervous system*. It involves the *nerves* throughout the body (Fig. 6-10).

Nerves carry messages or impulses to and from the brain. Nerves connect to the spinal cord. Some nerve fibers have a protective covering called a *myelin sheath.* It insulates the nerve fiber. Nerve fibers covered with myelin conduct impulses faster than those fibers without it.

The Central Nervous System

The brain and spinal cord make up the central nervous system. The skull covers the brain. The main parts of the brain are the *cerebrum,* the *cerebellum,* and the *brainstem* (Fig. 6-11).

The cerebrum is the largest part of the brain. It is the center of thought and intelligence. The cerebrum is divided into two halves—the right and left *hemispheres.* The right hemisphere controls movement and activities on the body's left side. The left hemisphere controls the right side.

The outside of the cerebrum is called the *cerebral cortex.* It controls the highest functions of the brain. These include reasoning, memory, consciousness,

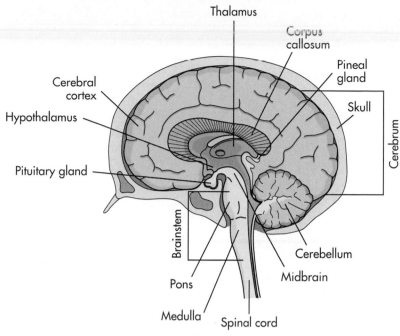

FIG. **6-11** The brain.

speech, voluntary muscle movement, vision, hearing, sensation, and other activities.

The cerebellum regulates and coordinates body movements. It controls balance and the smooth movements of voluntary muscles. Injury to the cerebellum results in jerky movements, loss of coordination, and muscle weakness.

The brainstem connects the cerebrum to the spinal cord. The brainstem contains the *midbrain, pons,* and *medulla.* The midbrain and pons relay messages between the medulla and the cerebrum. The medulla controls heart rate, breathing, blood vessel size, swallowing, coughing, and vomiting. The brain connects to the spinal cord at the lower end of the medulla.

The spinal cord lies within the spinal column. The cord is about 18 inches long. It contains pathways that conduct messages to and from the brain.

The brain and spinal cord are covered by connective tissue called *meninges.* The outer layer lies next to the skull. It is a tough covering called the *dura mater.* The middle layer is the *arachnoid.* The inner layer is the *pia mater.* The space between the middle and inner layers is the *arachnoid space.* The space is filled with *cerebrospinal fluid.* It circulates around the brain and spinal cord. Cerebrospinal fluid protects the central nervous system. It cushions shocks that could easily injure brain and spinal cord structures.

The Peripheral Nervous System

The peripheral nervous system has 12 pairs of *cranial nerves* and 31 pairs of *spinal nerves.* Cranial nerves conduct impulses between the brain and the head, neck, chest, and abdomen. They conduct impulses for smell, vision, hearing, pain, touch, temperature, and pressure. They also conduct impulses for voluntary and involuntary muscles. Spinal nerves carry impulses from the skin, arms and legs, and the internal structures not supplied by cranial nerves.

Some peripheral nerves form the *autonomic nervous system.* This system controls involuntary muscles and certain body functions. The functions include the heartbeat, blood pressure, intestinal contractions, and glandular secretions. These functions are automatic.

The autonomic nervous system is divided into the *sympathetic nervous system* and the *parasympathetic nervous system.* They balance each other. The sympathetic nervous system speeds up functions. The parasympathetic nervous system slows functions. When you are angry, scared, excited, or exercising, the sympathetic nervous system is stimulated. The parasympathetic system is activated when you relax or when the sympathetic system is stimulated for too long.

The Sense Organs

The five senses are sight, hearing, taste, smell, and touch. Receptors for taste are in the tongue. They are called *taste buds.* Receptors for smell are in the nose. Touch receptors are in the dermis of the skin, especially in the toes and fingertips.

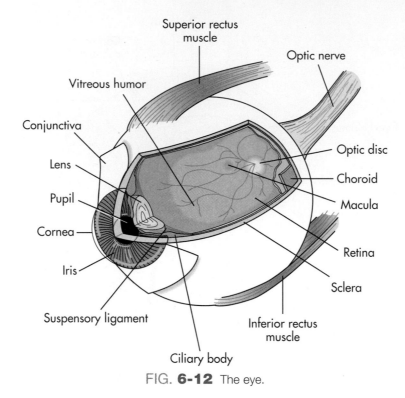

Superior rectus muscle

Optic nerve

Vitreous humor

Conjunctiva

Lens

Pupil

Cornea

Iris

Suspensory ligament

Ciliary body

Optic disc

Choroid

Macula

Retina

Sclera

Inferior rectus muscle

FIG. **6-12** The eye.

The Eye

Receptors for vision are in the eyes (Fig. 6-12). Bones of the skull, eyelids and eyelashes, and tears protect the eyes. The eye has three layers:

- The *sclera,* the white of the eye, is the outer layer. It is made of tough connective tissue.
- The *choroid* is the second layer. Blood vessels, the *ciliary muscle,* and the *iris* make up the choroid. The iris gives the eye its color. The opening in the middle of the iris is the *pupil.* Pupil size varies with the amount of light entering the eye. The pupil constricts (narrows) in bright light. It dilates (widens) in dim or dark places.
- The *retina* is the inner layer. It has receptors for vision and the nerve fibers of the optic nerve.

Light enters the eye through the *cornea.* It is the transparent part of the outer layer that lies over the eye. Light rays pass to the *lens,* which lies behind the pupil. The light is then reflected to the retina. Light is carried to the brain by the optic nerve.

The *aqueous chamber* separates the cornea from the lens. The chamber is filled with a fluid called *aqueous humor.* The fluid helps the cornea keep its shape and position. The *vitreous body* is behind the lens. It is a gelatin-like substance that supports the retina and maintains the eye's shape.

The Ear

The ear functions in hearing and balance (Fig. 6-13). It has three parts: the *external ear, middle ear,* and *inner ear.*

The external ear (outer part) is called the *pinna* or *auricle.* Sound waves are guided through the external ear into the *auditory canal.* Glands in the auditory canal secrete a waxy substance called *cerumen.* The auditory canal extends about 1 inch to the *eardrum.* The eardrum *(tympanic membrane)* separates the external and middle ear.

The middle ear is a small space. It contains the *eustachian tube* and three small bones called *ossicles.* The eustachian tube connects the middle ear and the throat. Air enters the eustachian tube so that there is equal pressure on both sides of the eardrum. The ossicles amplify sound received from the eardrum and transmit the sound to the inner ear.

The inner ear consists of the *semicircular canals* and the *cochlea.* The cochlea contains fluid. The fluid carries sound waves from the middle ear to the *auditory nerve.* The auditory nerve then carries the message to the brain.

The three semicircular canals are involved with balance. They sense the head's position and changes in position. They send messages to the brain.

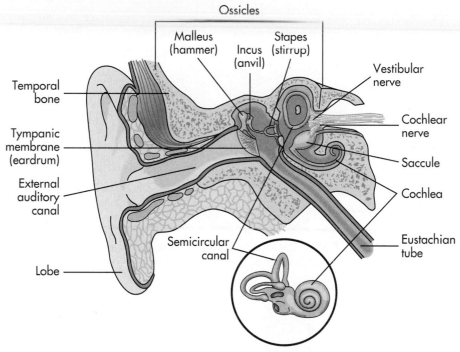

FIG. **6-13** The ear.

THE CIRCULATORY SYSTEM

The circulatory system is made up of the blood, heart, and blood vessels. The heart pumps blood through the blood vessels. The circulatory system functions are:

- Blood carries food, oxygen, and other substances to the cells.
- Blood removes waste products from cells.
- Blood and blood vessels help regulate body temperature. Blood carries heat from muscle activity to other body parts. Blood vessels in the skin dilate to cool the body. They constrict to retain heat.
- The system produces and carries cells that defend the body from microbes that cause disease.

The Blood

The blood consists of blood cells and *plasma.* Plasma is mostly water. It carries blood cells to other body cells. Plasma also carries substances that cells need to function. This includes food (proteins, fats, and carbohydrates), hormones (p. 77), and chemicals.

Red blood cells (RBCs) are called *erythrocytes.* They give the blood its red color because of a substance called *hemoglobin.* As RBCs circulate through the lungs, hemoglobin picks up oxygen. Hemoglobin carries oxygen to the cells. When blood is bright red, hemoglobin in the RBCs is full of oxygen. As blood circulates through the body, oxygen is given to the cells. Cells release carbon dioxide (a waste product). It is picked up by the hemoglobin. RBCs filled with carbon dioxide make the blood look dark red.

The body has about 25 trillion (25,000,000,000,000) RBCs. About 4½ to 5 million cells are in a cubic millimeter of blood (a tiny drop). RBCs live for 3 or 4 months. The liver and spleen destroy them as they wear out. Bone marrow produces about 1 million new RBCs every second.

White blood cells (WBCs) are called *leukocytes.* They have no color. They protect the body against infection. There are 5000 to 10,000 WBCs in a cubic millimeter of blood. At the first sign of infection, WBCs rush to the infection site. There they multiply rapidly. The number of WBCs increases when there is an infection. WBCs are produced by the bone marrow. They live about 9 days.

Platelets (thrombocytes) are needed for blood clotting. They are produced by the bone marrow. There are about 200,000 to 400,000 platelets in a cubic millimeter of blood. A platelet lives about 4 days.

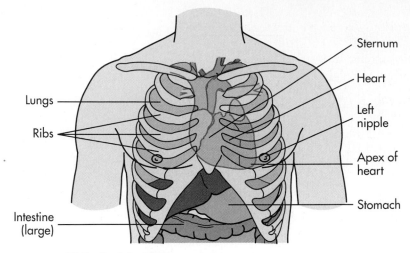

FIG. **6-14** Location of the heart in the chest cavity.

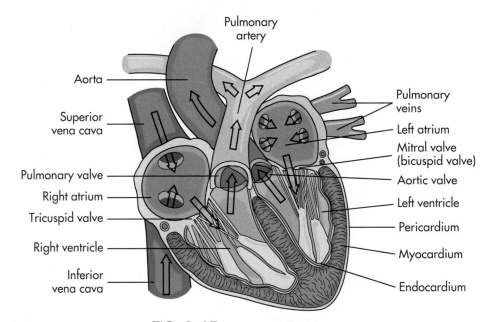

FIG. **6-15** Structures of the heart.

The Heart

The heart is a muscle. It pumps blood through the blood vessels to the tissues and cells. The heart lies in the middle to lower part of the chest cavity toward the left side (Fig. 6-14). The heart is hollow and has three layers (Fig. 6-15):

- The *pericardium* is the outer layer. It is a thin sac covering the heart.
- The *myocardium* is the second layer. It is the thick, muscular part of the heart.
- The *endocardium* is the inner layer. A membrane, it lines the inner surface of the heart.

The heart has four chambers (see Fig. 6-15). Upper chambers receive blood and are called the *atria.* The *right atrium* receives blood from body tissues. The *left atrium* receives blood from the lungs. Lower chambers are called *ventricles.* Ventricles pump blood. The *right ventricle* pumps blood to the lungs for oxygen. The *left ventricle* pumps blood to all parts of the body.

Valves are between the atria and ventricles. The valves allow blood flow in one direction. They prevent blood from flowing back into the atria from the ventricles. The *tricuspid valve* is between the right atrium and right ventricle. The *mitral valve (bicuspid valve)* is between the left atrium and left ventricle.

Heart action has two phases:

- *Diastole.* It is the resting phase. Heart chambers fill with blood.
- *Systole.* It is the working phase. The heart contracts. Blood is pumped through the blood vessels when the heart contracts.

The Blood Vessels

Blood flows to body tissues and cells through the blood vessels. There are three groups of blood vessels: arteries, capillaries, and veins.

Arteries carry blood away from the heart. Arterial blood is rich in oxygen. The *aorta* is the largest artery. It receives blood directly from the left ventricle. The aorta branches into other arteries that carry blood to all parts of the body (Fig. 6-16). These arteries branch into smaller parts within the tissues. The smallest branch of an artery is an *arteriole.*

Arterioles connect to *capillaries.* Capillaries are very tiny vessels. Food, oxygen, and other substances pass from capillaries into the cells. The capillaries pick up waste products from the cells. Veins carry waste products back to the heart.

Veins return blood to the heart. They connect to the capillaries by *venules.* Venules are small veins. Venules branch together to form veins. The many veins also branch together as they near the heart to form two main veins (see Fig. 6-16). The two main veins are the *inferior vena cava* and the *superior vena cava.* Both empty into the right atrium. The inferior vena cava carries blood from the legs and trunk. The superior vena cava carries blood from the head and arms. Venous blood is dark red. It has little oxygen and a lot of carbon dioxide.

Blood flow through the circulatory system is shown in Figure 6-15.

- Venous blood, poor in oxygen, empties into the right atrium.
- Blood flows through the tricuspid valve into the right ventricle.
- The right ventricle pumps blood into the lungs to pick up oxygen.
- Oxygen-rich blood from the lungs enters the left atrium.
- Blood from the left atrium passes through the mitral valve into the left ventricle.
- The left ventricle pumps the blood to the aorta. It branches off to form other arteries.
- The arterial blood is carried to the tissues by arterioles and to the cells by capillaries.
- Cells and capillaries exchange oxygen and nutrients for carbon dioxide and waste products.
- Capillaries connect with venules.
- Venules carry blood that has carbon dioxide and waste products.
- Venules form veins.
- Veins return blood to the heart.

THE RESPIRATORY SYSTEM

Oxygen is needed to live. Air contains oxygen. The respiratory system (Fig. 6-17, p. 72) brings oxygen into the lungs and removes carbon dioxide. **Respiration**

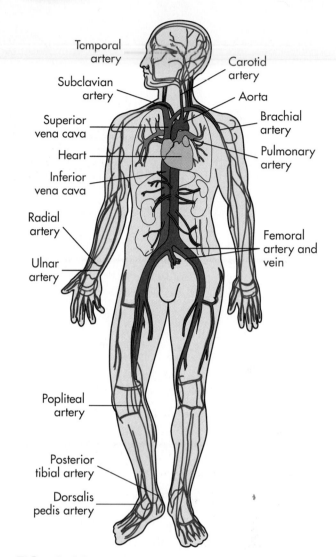

FIG. **6-16** Arterial and venous systems. (Note: The arterial system is in red. The venous system is in blue).

is the process of supplying the cells with oxygen and removing carbon dioxide from them. Respiration involves *inhalation* (breathing in) and *exhalation* (breathing out). The terms *inspiration* (breathing in) and *expiration* (breathing out) are also used.

Air enters the body through the *nose.* The air then passes into the *pharynx* (throat). It is a tube-shaped passageway for air and food. Air passes from the pharynx into the *larynx* (the voice box). A piece of cartilage, the *epiglottis,* acts like a lid over the larynx. The epiglottis prevents food from entering the airway during swallowing. During inhalation, the epiglottis lifts up to let air pass over the larynx. Air passes from the larynx into the *trachea* (the windpipe).

The trachea divides at its lower end into the *right bronchus* and *left bronchus.* Each bronchus enters a lung. Upon entering the lungs, the bronchi divide many times into smaller branches. The smaller branches are called *bronchioles.* Eventually the bronchioles

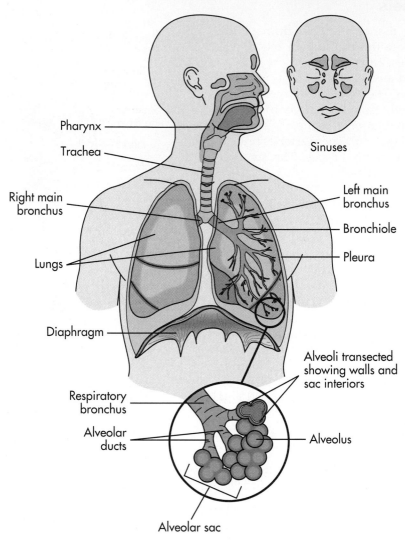

FIG. **6-17** Respiratory system.

subdivide. They end up in tiny one-celled air sacs called *alveoli.*

Alveoli look like small clusters of grapes. Oxygen and carbon dioxide are exchanged between the alveoli and capillaries. Blood in the capillaries picks up oxygen from the alveoli. Then the blood is returned to the left side of the heart and pumped to the rest of the body. Alveoli pick up carbon dioxide from the capillaries for exhalation.

The lungs are separated from the abdominal cavity by a muscle called the *diaphragm.* Each lung is covered by a two-layered sac called the *pleura.* One layer is attached to the lung and the other to the chest wall. The pleura secretes a very thin fluid that fills the space between the layers. The fluid prevents the layers from rubbing together during inhalation and exhalation. A bony framework made up of the ribs, sternum, and vertebrae protects the lungs.

THE DIGESTIVE SYSTEM

The digestive system breaks down food physically and chemically so it can be absorbed for use by the cells. This process is called **digestion.** The digestive system is also called the *gastrointestinal system (GI system).* The system also removes solid wastes from the body.

The digestive system involves the *alimentary canal (GI tract)* and the accessory organs of digestion (Fig. 6-18). The alimentary canal is a long tube. It extends from the mouth to the anus. Its major parts are the mouth, pharynx, esophagus, stomach, small intestine, and large intestine. Accessory organs are the teeth, tongue, salivary glands, liver, gallbladder, and pancreas.

Digestion begins in the *mouth (oral cavity).* It receives food and prepares it for digestion. The *teeth* cut, chop, and grind food into small particles for

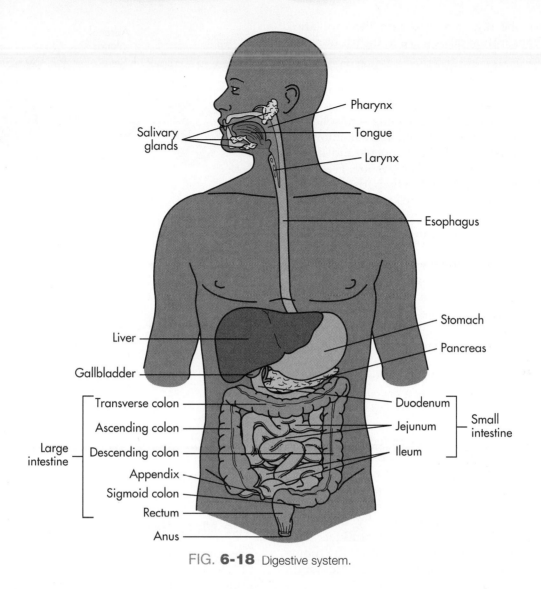

FIG. **6-18** Digestive system.

digestion and swallowing. The *tongue* aids in chewing and swallowing. *Taste buds* on the tongue's surface contain nerve endings. Taste buds allow sweet, sour, bitter, and salty tastes to be sensed. *Salivary glands* in the mouth secrete *saliva*. Saliva moistens food particles to ease swallowing and begins digestion. During swallowing, the tongue pushes food into the pharynx.

The *pharynx* (throat) is a muscular tube. Swallowing continues as the pharynx contracts. Contraction of the pharynx pushes food into the *esophagus.* The esophagus is a muscular tube about 10 inches long. It extends from the pharynx to the stomach. Involuntary muscle contractions called peristalsis move food down the esophagus into the stomach. (**Peristalsis** is the involuntary muscle contractions in the digestive system that move food through the alimentary canal.)

The *stomach* is a muscular sac in the upper left part of the abdominal cavity. Stomach muscles stir and churn food to break it up into even smaller particles. Glands in the stomach's lining secrete *gastric juices.* Food is mixed and churned with the gastric juices to form a semi-liquid substance called *chyme.* Peristalsis pushes chyme into the small intestine.

The *small intestine* is about 20 feet long. It has three parts. The first part is the *duodenum.* There more digestive juices are added to the chyme. One is called *bile.* Bile is a greenish liquid made in the *liver* and stored in the *gallbladder.* Juices from the *pancreas* and small intestine are added to the chyme. Digestive juices chemically break down food so it can be absorbed.

Peristalsis moves the chyme through the two other parts of the small intestine: the *jejunum* and the *ileum.* Tiny projections called *villi* line the small intestine.

Villi absorb the digested food into the capillaries. Most food absorption takes place in the jejunum and ileum.

Some chyme is not digested. Undigested chyme passes from the small intestine into the *large intestine (large bowel* or *colon).* The colon absorbs most of the water from the chyme. The remaining semisolid material is called *feces.* Feces contain a small amount of water, solid wastes, and some mucus and germs. These are the waste products of digestion. Feces pass through the colon into the *rectum* by peristalsis. Feces pass out of the body through the *anus.*

THE URINARY SYSTEM

The urinary system removes waste products from the blood and maintains water balance within the body (Fig. 6-19). The *kidneys* are two bean-shaped organs in the upper abdomen. They lie against the back muscles on each side of the spine. They are protected by the lower edge of the rib cage.

Each kidney has over a million tiny *nephrons* (Fig. 6-20). The nephron is the basic working unit of the kidney. Each nephron has a *convoluted tubule,* a tiny coiled tubule. Each convoluted tubule has a *Bowman's capsule* at one end. The capsule partly surrounds a cluster of capillaries called a *glomerulus.* Blood passes through the glomerulus and is filtered by the capillaries. The fluid part of the blood is squeezed into the Bowman's capsule. The fluid then passes into the tubule. Most water and other needed substances are reabsorbed by the blood. The rest of the fluid and the waste products form *urine* in the tubule. Urine flows through the tubule to a *collecting tubule.* All collecting tubules drain into the kidney's *renal pelvis.*

A tube, the *ureter,* is attached to the renal pelvis. Each ureter is about 10 to 12 inches long. The ureters carry urine from the kidneys to the *bladder.* The bladder is a hollow, muscular sac in the lower part of the abdominal cavity.

Urine is stored in the bladder until the need to urinate is felt. This usually occurs when there is about half a pint (250 ml) of urine in the bladder. Urine passes from the bladder through the *urethra.* The opening at the end of the urethra is the *meatus.* Urine passes from the body through the meatus. Urine is a clear, yellowish fluid.

THE REPRODUCTIVE SYSTEM

Human reproduction results from the union of a female sex cell and a male sex cell. The male and female reproductive systems are different. This allows for the process of reproduction.

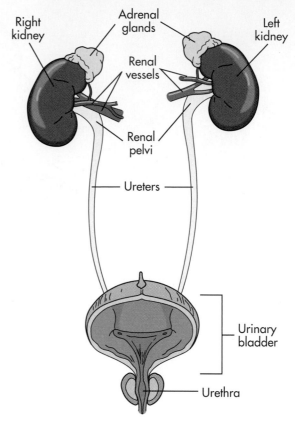

FIG. **6-19** Urinary system.

The Male Reproductive System

The male reproductive system is shown in Figure 6-21. The *testes (testicles)* are the male sex glands. (One testicle is called a *testis).* Sex glands are also called *gonads.* The two testes produce the male sex cells *(sperm cells).*

Testosterone, the male hormone, is produced in the testes. This hormone is needed for reproductive organ function. It also is needed for the development of the male secondary sex characteristics—facial hair; pubic and axillary (underarm) hair; and hair on the arms, chest, and legs. The testes are suspended between the thighs in a sac called the *scrotum.* The scrotum is made of skin and muscle.

Sperm travel from the testis to the *epididymis.* The epididymis is a coiled tube on top and to the side of the testis. From the epididymis, sperm travel through a tube called the *vas deferens.* Each vas deferens joins a *seminal vesicle.* The two seminal vesicles store sperm and produce *semen.* Semen is a fluid that carries sperm. The ducts of the seminal vesicles unite to form the *ejaculatory duct.* It passes through the prostate gland.

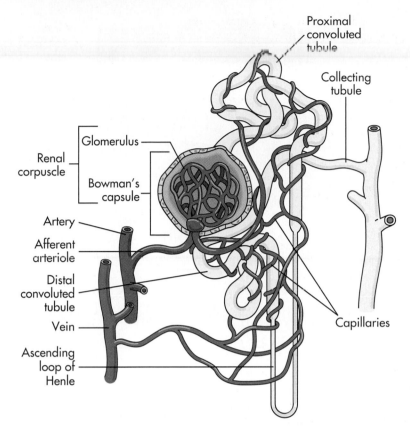

FIG. **6-20** A nephron.

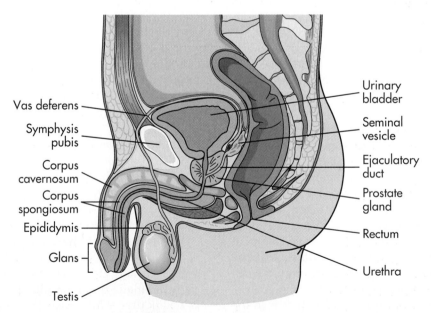

FIG. **6-21** Male reproductive system.

The *prostate gland* lies just below the bladder. It is shaped like a donut. The gland secretes fluid into the semen. As the ejaculatory ducts leave the prostate, they join the *urethra*. The urethra runs through the prostate. The urethra is the outlet for urine and semen. The urethra is contained within the penis.

The *penis* is outside of the body and has *erectile* tissue. When a male is sexually excited, blood fills the erectile tissue. The penis enlarges and becomes hard and erect. The erect penis can enter a female's vagina. The semen, which contains sperm, is released into the vagina.

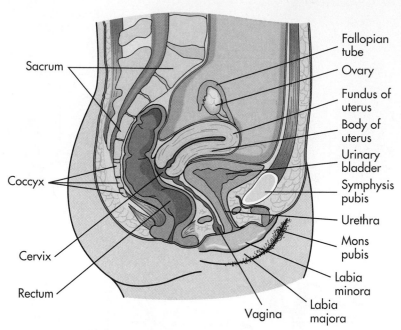

Labels on figure:
Sacrum
Fallopian tube
Ovary
Fundus of uterus
Body of uterus
Urinary bladder
Symphysis pubis
Urethra
Mons pubis
Labia minora
Labia majora
Coccyx
Cervix
Rectum
Vagina

FIG. **6-22** Female reproductive system.

The Female Reproductive System

Figure 6-22 shows the female reproductive system. The female gonads are two almond-shaped glands called *ovaries*. An ovary is on each side of the uterus in the abdominal cavity.

The ovaries contain *ova*, or eggs. Ova are the female sex cells. One ovum (egg) is released monthly during the reproductive years. Release of an ovum is called ovulation.

The ovaries secrete the female hormones *estrogen* and *progesterone*. These hormones are needed for reproductive system function. They also are needed for the development of secondary sex characteristics in the female—increased breast size, pubic and axillary (underarm) hair, and widening and rounding of the hips.

When an ovum is released from an ovary, it travels through a *fallopian tube*. There are two fallopian tubes, one on each side. The tubes are attached at one end to the uterus. The ovum travels through the fallopian tube to the uterus.

The *uterus* is a hollow, muscular organ. It is in the center of the pelvic cavity behind the bladder and in front of the rectum. The main part of the uterus is the *fundus*. The neck or narrow section of the uterus is the *cervix*. Tissue lining the uterus is called the *endometrium*. The endometrium has many blood vessels. If male and female sex cells unite into one cell, that cell implants into the endometrium. There it grows into a baby. The uterus is where the unborn baby *(fetus)* grows and receives nourishment.

The cervix of the uterus projects into a muscular canal called the *vagina*. The vagina opens to the outside of the body. It is just behind the urethra. The vagina receives the penis during intercourse. It also is part of the birth canal. Glands in the vaginal wall keep it moistened with secretions. In young girls, the external vaginal opening is partly closed by a membrane called the *hymen*. The hymen ruptures when the female has intercourse for the first time.

Female external genitalia are called the *vulva* (Fig. 6-23):
- The *mons pubis* is a rounded, fatty pad over a bone called the *symphysis pubis*. The mons pubis is covered with hair in adult females.
- The *labia majora* and *labia minora* are two folds of tissue on each side of the vaginal opening.
- The *clitoris* is a small organ composed of erectile tissue. It becomes hard when sexually stimulated.

The *mammary glands (breasts)* secrete milk after childbirth. The glands are on the outside of the chest. They are made up of glandular tissue and fat (Fig. 6-24). Milk drains into ducts that open onto the nipple.

Menstruation

The endometrium is rich in blood to nourish the cell that grows into an unborn baby *(fetus)*. If pregnancy does not occur, the endometrium breaks up. It is discharged from the body through the vagina. This process is called *menstruation*. Menstruation occurs about every 28 days. Therefore it is also called the *menstrual cycle*.

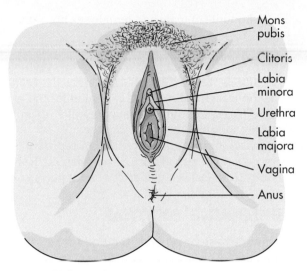

FIG. **6-23** External female genitalia.

Day one of the cycle begins with menstruation. Blood flows from the uterus through the vaginal opening. Menstrual flow usually lasts 3 to 7 days. Ovulation occurs during the next phase. An ovum matures in an ovary and is released. Ovulation usually occurs on or about day 14 of the cycle.

Meanwhile, the ovaries secrete estrogen and progesterone (female hormones). These hormones cause the endometrium to thicken for pregnancy. If pregnancy does not occur, hormones decrease in amount. This causes blood supply to the endometrium to decrease. The endometrium breaks up. It is discharged through the vagina. Another menstrual cycle begins.

Fertilization

To reproduce, a male sex cell (sperm) must unite with a female sex cell (ovum). The uniting of the sperm and ovum into one cell is called *fertilization*. A sperm has 23 chromosomes. An ovum has 23 chromosomes. When the two cells unite, the fertilized cell has 46 chromosomes.

During intercourse, millions of sperm are left in the vagina. Sperm travel up the cervix, through the uterus, and into the fallopian tubes. If a sperm and an ovum unite in a fallopian tube, fertilization results. Pregnancy occurs. The fertilized cell travels down the fallopian tube to the uterus. After a short time, the fertilized cell implants in the thick endometrium and grows during pregnancy.

THE ENDOCRINE SYSTEM

The endocrine system is made up of glands called the *endocrine glands* (Fig. 6-25). They secrete chemical substances called **hormones** into the bloodstream.

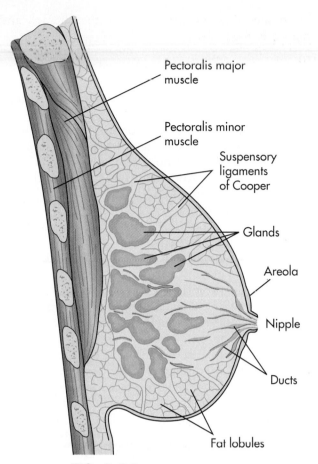

FIG. **6-24** The female breast.

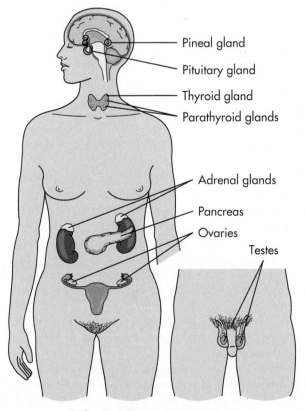

FIG. **6-25** Endocrine system.

Hormones regulate activities of other organs and glands in the body.

The *pituitary gland* is called the *master gland*. About the size of a cherry, it is at the base of the brain behind the eyes. It is divided into the anterior pituitary lobe and the posterior pituitary lobe. The *anterior pituitary lobe* secretes:

- *Growth hormone*—needed for the growth of muscles, bones, and other organs. It is needed throughout life to maintain normal-size bones and muscles. Growth is stunted if a baby does not have enough of the growth hormone. Too much causes excessive growth.
- *Thyroid-stimulating hormone* (TSH)—needed for thyroid gland function.
- *Adrenocorticotropic hormone* (ACTH)—stimulates the adrenal gland.

The anterior lobe also secretes hormones that regulate the growth, development, and function of the male and female reproductive systems.

The *posterior pituitary lobe* secretes *antidiuretic hormone* (ADH) and *oxytocin*. ADH prevents the kidneys from excreting too much water. Oxytocin causes uterine muscles to contract during childbirth.

The *thyroid gland* is in the neck in front of the larynx. The thyroid gland secretes *thyroid hormone* (TH, thyroxine). It regulates metabolism. **Metabolism** is the burning of food for heat and energy by the cells. Too little TH causes slow body processes, slow movements, and weight gain. Too much TH causes increased metabolism, excess energy, and weight loss. Some babies do not have enough TH. Their physical growth and mental growth are stunted.

The four *parathyroid glands* secrete *parathormone*. Two lie on each side of the thyroid gland. Parathormone regulates calcium use. Calcium is needed for nerve and muscle function. Insufficient amounts of calcium cause *tetany*. Tetany is a state of severe muscle contraction and spasm. If untreated, tetany can cause death.

There are two *adrenal glands*. An adrenal gland is on the top of each kidney. The adrenal gland has two parts: *adrenal medulla* and *adrenal cortex*. The adrenal medulla secretes *epinephrine* and *norepinephrine*. These hormones stimulate the body to quickly produce energy during emergencies. Heart rate, blood pressure, muscle power, and energy all increase.

The adrenal cortex secretes three groups of hormones:

- *Glucocorticoids*—regulate carbohydrate metabolism. They also control responses to stress and inflammation.
- *Mineralocorticoids*—regulate the amount of salt and water absorbed and lost by the kidneys.

- Small amounts of male and female sex hormones—see p. 74.

The *pancreas* secretes *insulin*. Insulin regulates the amount of sugar in the blood available for use by the cells. Insulin is needed for sugar to enter the cells. If there is too little insulin, sugar cannot enter the cells. Therefore excess amounts of sugar build up in the blood. This condition is called *diabetes*.

The *gonads* are the glands of human reproduction. Male sex glands (testes) secrete *testosterone*. Female sex glands (ovaries) secrete *estrogen* and *progesterone*.

THE IMMUNE SYSTEM

The immune system protects the body from disease and infection. Abnormal body cells can grow into tumors. Sometimes the body produces substances that cause the body to attack itself. Microorganisms (bacteria, viruses, and other germs) can cause an infection. The immune system defends against threats inside and outside the body.

The immune system gives the body immunity. **Immunity** means that a person has protection against a disease or condition. The person will not get or be affected by the disease:

- *Specific immunity* is the body's reaction to a certain threat.
- *Nonspecific immunity* is the body's reaction to anything that is not a normal body substance.

Special cells and substances function to produce immunity:

- *Antibodies*—normal body substances that recognize abnormal or unwanted substances. They attack and destroy such substances.
- *Antigens*—abnormal or unwanted substances. An antigen causes the body to produce antibodies. The antibodies attack and destroy the antigens.
- *Phagocytes*—white blood cells that digest and destroy microorganisms and other unwanted substances (Fig. 6-26).
- *Lymphocytes*—white blood cells that produce antibodies. Lymphocyte production increases as the body responds to an infection.
- *B lymphocytes (B cells)*—react to specific antigens.
- *T lymphocytes (T cells)*—destroy invading cells. *Killer T cells* produce poisonous substances near the invading cells. Some T cells attract other cells. These other cells destroy the invaders.

When the body senses an antigen (an unwanted substance), the immune system acts. Phagocyte and lymphocyte production increases. Phagocytes destroy the invaders through digestion. Lymphocytes produce antibodies that attack and destroy the unwanted substances.

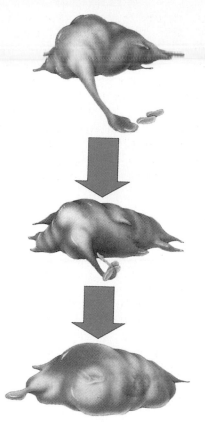

FIG. **6-26** A phagocyte digests and destroys a microorganism. (From Thibodeau GA, Patton KT: *Structure and function of the body,* ed 11, St Louis, 2000, Mosby.)

REVIEW QUESTIONS

Circle the **BEST** answer.

1 The basic unit of body structure is the
 a Cell
 b Neuron
 c Nephron
 d Ovum

2 The outer layer of the skin is called the
 a Dermis
 b Epidermis
 c Integument
 d Myelin

3 Which allows movement?
 a Bone marrow
 b Synovial membrane
 c Joints
 d Ligaments

4 Skeletal muscles
 a Are under involuntary control
 b Appear smooth
 c Are under voluntary control
 d Appear striped and smooth

5 The highest functions of the brain take place in the
 a Cerebral cortex
 b Medulla
 c Brainstem
 d Spinal nerves

6 The ear is involved with
  a Regulating body movements
  b Balance
  c Smoothness of body movements
  d Controlling involuntary muscles

7 The liquid part of the blood is the
  a Hemoglobin
  b Red blood cell
  c Plasma
  d White blood cell

8 Which part of the heart pumps blood to the body?
  a Right atrium
  b Right ventricle
  c Left atrium
  d Left ventricle

9 Which carry blood away from the heart?
  a Capillaries
  b Veins
  c Venules
  d Arteries

10 Oxygen and carbon dioxide are exchanged
  a In the bronchi
  b Between the alveoli and capillaries
  c Between the lungs and the pleura
  d In the trachea

11 Digestion begins in the
  a Mouth
  b Stomach
  c Small intestine
  d Colon

12 Most food absorption takes place in the
  a Stomach
  b Small intestine
  c Colon
  d Large intestine

13 Urine is formed by the
  a Jejunum
  b Kidneys
  c Bladder
  d Liver

14 Urine passes from the body through
  a The ureters
  b The urethra
  c The anus
  d Nephrons

15 The male sex gland is called the
  a Ovary
  b Fallopian tube
  c Testis
  d Scrotum

16 The discharge of the lining of the uterus is called
  a The endometrium
  b Ovulation
  c Fertilization
  d Menstruation

17 The endocrine glands secrete
  a Hormones
  b Mucus
  c Semen
  d Insulin

18 The immune system protects the body from
  a Low blood sugar
  b Disease and infection
  c Falling and loss of balance
  d Stunted growth and loss of fluid

Answers to these questions are on p. 467.

Caring For the Older Person

OBJECTIVES

- Define the key terms listed in this chapter
- Identify the developmental tasks of each age group
- Identify the social changes common in older adulthood
- Describe the physical changes from aging and the care required
- Describe the gains and losses related to long-term care
- Describe the sexual changes and needs of older persons
- Explain how to deal with sexually aggressive persons

KEY TERMS

development Changes in mental, emotional, and social function

developmental task A skill that must be completed during a stage of development

geriatrics The care of aging people

gerontology The study of the aging process

growth The physical changes that are measured and that occur in a steady and orderly manner

menopause The time when menstruation stops and menstrual cycles end

old Between 75 and 84 years of age

old-old 85 years of age and older

ombudsman Someone who supports or promotes the needs and interests of another person

sexuality The physical, psychological, social, cultural, and spiritual factors that affect a person's feelings and attitudes about his or her sex

young-old Between 65 and 74 years of age

People live longer than ever before. They are healthier and more active. Most older people live with a partner, children, or other family. Some live alone or with friends. Others live in nursing centers.

But what does older mean? Late adulthood involves these age ranges:

- **Young-old**—between 65 and 74 years of age
- **Old**—between 75 and 84 years of age
- **Old-old**—85 years of age and older

Gerontology is the study of the aging process. **Geriatrics** is the care of aging people. Aging is normal. It is not a disease. Normal changes occur in body structure and function. They increase the risk for illness, injury, and disability. Psychological and social changes also occur. Most changes are slow. Most people adjust well to these changes. They lead happy, meaningful lives.

GROWTH AND DEVELOPMENT

Throughout life, people grow and develop. **Growth** is the physical changes that are measured and that occur in a steady and orderly manner. Growth is measured in height and weight. Changes in appearance and body functions also measure growth.

Development relates to changes in mental, emotional, and social function. A person behaves and thinks in certain ways in each stage of development. A 2-year-old thinks in simple terms. A 40-year-old thinks in complex ways. The entire person is affected.

Growth and development occur in a sequence, order, and pattern. Certain skills must be completed during each stage. A **developmental task** is a skill that must be completed during a stage of development.

A stage cannot be skipped. Each stage is the basis for the next stage. Each stage has its own characteristics and developmental tasks (Box 7-1).

SOCIAL CHANGES

People cope with aging in their own way. The following social changes occur with aging:

- *Retirement*—Retirement is a reward for a lifetime of work. The person can relax and enjoy life (Fig. 7-1). Some people retire because of poor health or disability. Work helps meet love, belonging, and self-esteem needs. The person feels fulfilled and useful. Friendships and companionship often involve co-workers. Some retired people have part-time jobs or do volunteer work (Fig. 7-2).
- *Reduced income*—Retirement often means reduced income. Social Security may provide the only income. The retired person may still have rent or house payments. Food, clothing, utility bills, and taxes are other expenses. Car expenses, home repairs, drugs, and health care are other costs. Severe money problems can result. Some people have income from savings, investments, retirement plans, and insurance.
- *Social relationships*—Social relationships change throughout life. Children grow up, leave home, and have families. Many live far away. Older family and friends die, move away, or are disabled. Yet most older people have regular contact with family and friends. Others are lonely. Separation from children is a common cause. So is lack of companionship with people their own age. Hobbies, church and community events, and new friends help prevent loneliness. So does taking part in family activities (Fig. 7-3, p. 84).
- *Children as caregivers*—Some children care for older parents. Parents and children change roles. The child cares for the parent. This helps some older persons feel secure. Others feel unwanted, in the way, and useless. Some lose dignity and self-respect. Tensions may occur among the child, parent, and other household members. Lack of privacy is a cause. So are disagreements and criticisms about housekeeping, child rearing, cooking, and friends.
- *Death of a partner*—A person may try to prepare for a partner's death. When death does occur, the loss is crushing. No amount of preparation is ever enough for the emptiness and changes that result. The person loses a friend, lover, companion, and confidant. Grief may be very great. Serious physical and mental problems can result. Some lose the will to live. Some attempt suicide.

BOX 7-1	Stages of Growth and Development

Infancy (Birth to 1 year)

- Learning to walk
- Learning to eat solid foods
- Beginning to talk and communicate with others
- Beginning to have emotional relationships with parents, brothers, and sisters
- Developing stable sleep and feeding patterns

Toddlerhood (1 to 3 years)

- Tolerating separation from parents or primary caregivers
- Gaining control of bowel and bladder function
- Using words to communicate
- Becoming less dependent on parents or primary caregivers

Preschool (3 to 6 years)

- Increasing the ability to communicate and understand others
- Performing self-care
- Learning gender differences and developing sexual modesty
- Learning right from wrong and good from bad
- Learning to play with others
- Developing family relationships

School Age (6 to 9 or 10 years)

- Developing social and physical skills needed for playing games
- Learning to get along with children of the same age and background (peers)
- Learning gender-appropriate behaviors and attitudes
- Learning basic reading, writing, and arithmetic skills
- Developing a conscience and morals
- Developing a good feeling and attitude about oneself

Late Childhood (9 or 10 to 12 years)

- Becoming independent of adults and learning to depend on oneself
- Developing and keeping friendships with peers

- Understanding the physical, psychological, and social roles of one's sex
- Developing moral and ethical behavior
- Developing greater muscular strength, coordination, and balance
- Learning how to study

Adolescence (12 to 18 years)

- Accepting changes in the body and appearance
- Developing appropriate relationships with males and females of the same age
- Accepting the male or female role appropriate for one's age
- Becoming independent from parents and adults
- Developing morals, attitudes, and values needed to function in society

Young Adulthood (18 to 40 years)

- Choosing education and a career
- Selecting a partner
- Learning to live with a partner
- Becoming a parent and raising children
- Developing a satisfactory sex life

Middle Adulthood (40 to 65 years)

- Adjusting to physical changes
- Having grown children
- Developing leisure-time activities
- Adjusting to aging parents

Late Adulthood (65 years and older)

- Adjusting to decreased strength and loss of health
- Adjusting to retirement and reduced income
- Coping with a partner's death
- Developing new friends and relationships
- Preparing for one's own death

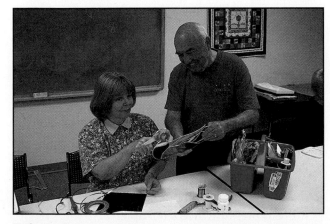

FIG. 7-1 A retired couple enjoying arts and crafts together.

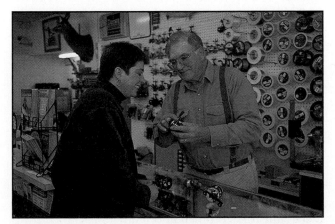

FIG. 7-2 This retired man works at a sports shop.

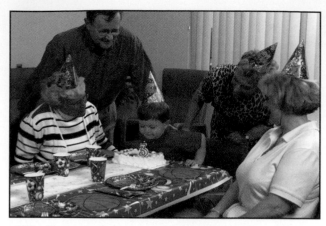

FIG. **7-3** An older woman takes part in family activities.

PHYSICAL CHANGES

Physical changes occur with aging. Body functions slow down. Energy level and body efficiency decline. The changes occur over many years. Often they are not seen for a long time.

The Integumentary System

The skin loses its elasticity and fatty tissue layer. The skin thins and sags. Folds, lines, and wrinkles appear. Oil and sweat secretion decreases. Dry skin occurs. The skin is fragile and easily injured. Skin breakdown and pressure ulcers are risks (Chapter 21).

Brown spots appear on the skin. They are called "age spots" or "liver spots." They are common on the wrists and hands.

The skin has fewer nerve endings. This affects sensing heat, cold, and pain. Loss of the skin's fatty tissue layer also makes the person more sensitive to cold. Protect the person from drafts and cold. Sweaters, lap blankets, socks, and extra blankets are helpful. So are higher thermostat settings.

Dry skin causes itching. It is easily damaged. A shower or bath twice a week is enough for hygiene. Partial baths are taken at other times. Mild soaps or soap substitutes are used to clean the underarms, genitals, and under breasts. Often soap is not used on the arms, legs, back, chest, and abdomen. Lotions, oils, and creams prevent drying and itching. Deodorants usually are not needed. Sweat gland secretion is decreased.

Nails become thick and tough. Feet usually have poor circulation. A nick or cut can lead to a serious infection. Older persons often complain of cold feet. Socks provide warmth. Hot water bottles and heating pads are not used. Burns are great risks.

White or gray hair is common. Hair loss occurs in men. Hair thins on men and women. Facial hair (lip and chin) may occur in women. Hair is drier from decreases in scalp oils. Brushing promotes circulation and oil production. Shampoo frequency depends on personal choice. It is done as needed for hygiene and comfort.

See Chapter 13 for hygiene and Chapter 14 for grooming.

The Musculoskeletal System

Muscles atrophy (shrink). They decrease in strength. Bones lose strength, become brittle, and break easily. Joints become stiff and painful.

Vertebrae shorten. Hip and knee joints flex (bend) slightly. These changes cause gradual loss of height and strength. Mobility also decreases.

Activity, exercise, and diet help prevent bone loss and loss of muscle strength. Walking is good exercise. Exercise groups and range-of-motion exercises are helpful (Chapter 20). A diet high in protein, calcium, and vitamins is needed.

Bones can break easily. Protect the person from injury and prevent falls (Chapter 8). Turn and move the person gently and carefully. Some persons need help and support getting out of bed. Some need help walking.

The Nervous System

Brain cells are lost over time. There is reduced blood flow to the brain. These changes cause dizziness and increase the risk of falls. They also affect personality and mental function. Memory is shorter. Forgetfulness increases. Responses slow. Confusion and fatigue may occur. Recent events are easier to recall than long ago events. Many older people are mentally active and involved in current events. They show fewer personality and mental changes.

Less sleep is needed. Loss of energy and decreased blood flow cause fatigue. Older people may rest or nap during the day. They may go to bed early and get up early. Their sleep periods are shorter.

The Senses

Hearing and vision losses occur (Chapter 24). Taste and smell dull. Touch and sensitivity to pain and pressure are reduced. So is sensing heat and cold. These changes increase the risk for injury. The person may not notice painful injuries or diseases. Or the person feels minor pain. You need to:

- Protect older persons from injury (Chapter 8)
- Follow safety measures for heat and cold (Chapter 21)
- Give good skin care (Chapter 13)
- Prevent pressure ulcers (Chapter 21)

The Circulatory System

The heart muscle weakens. It pumps blood with less force. Activity, exercise, excitement, and illness increase the body's need for oxygen and nutrients. A damaged or weak heart cannot meet the person's needs.

Arteries narrow and are less elastic. Less blood flows through them. Poor circulation occurs in many body parts.

Sometimes circulatory changes are severe. Rest is needed during the day. The person should not walk far, climb many stairs, or carry heavy things. Personal care items, TV, phone, and other needed items are kept nearby. Doctors may order certain exercises and activity limits.

The Respiratory System

Respiratory muscles weaken. Lung tissue becomes less elastic. Difficulty breathing *(dyspnea)* may occur with activity. The person may lack strength to cough and clear the airway of secretions. Respiratory infections and diseases may develop. These can threaten the older person's life.

Normal breathing is promoted. Avoid heavy bed linens over the chest. They prevent normal chest expansion. Turning, repositioning, and deep breathing are important. They help prevent respiratory complications from bedrest. Breathing usually is easier in the semi-Fowler's position (Chapter 12). The person should be as active as possible.

The Digestive System

Salivary glands produce less saliva. This can cause difficulty swallowing *(dysphagia)*. Taste and smell dull. This decreases appetite.

Secretion of digestive juices decreases. As a result, fried and fatty foods are hard to digest. They may cause indigestion.

Loss of teeth and ill-fitting dentures cause chewing problems. Hard to chew foods are avoided. Ground or chopped meat is easier to chew.

Peristalsis decreases. The stomach and colon empty slower. Flatulence and constipation can occur (Chapter 16).

Dry, fried, and fatty foods are avoided. This helps swallowing and digestion problems. Oral hygiene and denture care improve taste.

High-fiber foods are hard to chew and can irritate the intestines. They include apricots, celery, and fruits and vegetables with skins and seeds. Persons with chewing problems or constipation often need foods providing soft bulk. They include whole-grain cereals and cooked fruits and vegetables.

The Urinary System

Kidney function decreases. The kidneys shrink (atrophy) and blood flow to the kidneys is reduced. The removal of waste is less efficient. Urine is more concentrated.

Bladder muscles weaken. Bladder size decreases. The bladder holds less urine. Urinary frequency or urgency may occur. Many older persons have to urinate during the night. Urinary incontinence (inability to control the passage of urine from the bladder) may occur (Chapter 15).

In men, the prostate gland enlarges. This puts pressure on the urethra. Difficulty urinating or frequent urination occurs.

Urinary tract infections are risks. Adequate fluids are needed to help prevent infection. The person needs water, juices, milk, and gelatin. Personal choice in fluids is important. Most fluids should be taken before 1700 (5:00 PM). This reduces the need to urinate during the night.

The Reproductive System

Aging causes changes in the male and female reproductive systems:

- *Female*—The ovaries produce less estrogen and progesterone. Changes in the menstrual cycle and reproduction usually begin around age 40. Most women complete **menopause** (the time when menstruation stops and menstrual cycles end) by their mid-50s. The ovaries and uterus decrease in size. External genitalia shrink and lose elastic tissue. Vaginal walls become thinner, dryer, and lose elastic tissue. This can cause itching and painful intercourse. Breasts are less firm and sag from decreased muscle tone and elasticity.
- *Male*—Fewer healthy sperm are produced. The force of ejaculation is decreased. Testosterone levels decrease. The testes become less firm and smaller. The prostate gland enlarges. In severe cases, it prevents the flow of urine. Surgery is needed. Erections develop more slowly. It takes longer to regain an erection after intercourse.

NEEDING NURSING CENTER CARE

Most older persons are healthy and live in their own homes. Some ill and disabled persons can no longer care for themselves. Nursing centers are designed to meet the needs of older and disabled persons. Health care, nutrition, rehabilitation, psychological, recreation, and social needs are met by nursing center staff. Help is always nearby. A safe, secure, caring setting is provided.

Persons entering nursing centers may experience some or all of these losses:

- Loss of identity as productive members of families and communities
- Loss of possessions (for example: home, household items, car, and so on)
- Loss of independence
- Loss of real-world experiences (for example: shopping, traveling, cooking, driving, hobbies, and so on)
- Loss of health and mobility

These losses may cause a person to feel useless, powerless, and hopeless. The health team helps residents cope with loss and improve their quality of life. You must treat residents with dignity and respect. Also practice good communication skills and follow the person's care plan.

SEXUALITY

Sexuality is the physical, psychological, social, cultural, and spiritual factors that affect a person's feelings and attitudes about his or her sex. It involves the personality and the body. It is part of the whole person. Attitudes and feelings are involved. Sexuality affects how a person behaves, thinks, dresses, and responds to others.

Love, affection, and intimacy are needed throughout life. Attitudes and sex needs change as a person grows older. Things change in life. Divorce, death of a sexual partner, injury, illness, and aging are examples. However, sexual relationships remain important to older persons (Fig. 7-4). They love and fall in love, hold hands, embrace, and have sex.

Frequency of sexual activity often decreases. Weakness, fatigue, pain, and reduced mobility are reasons. One or both partners may be ill or injured.

Some older people do not have sexual intercourse. This does not mean sexual needs or desires are lost.

They can express their needs in other ways. Handholding, touching, caressing, and embracing bring closeness and intimacy.

Sexual partners are lost by death, divorce, and ending a relationship. Or the partner may be in a hospital or nursing center.

Meeting Sexual Needs

The nursing team allows and promotes the meeting of sexual needs. The measures in Box 7-2 may be part of the person's care plan.

Married couples in nursing centers are allowed to share the same room. This is an OBRA requirement. They can share the same bed if their health permits.

The Sexually Aggressive Person

Some patients and residents flirt or make sexual advances or comments. Some expose themselves, masturbate, or touch staff. Often there are reasons for the person's behavior. For men, illness, injury, surgery, or aging often threatens feelings of manhood. The man tries to prove that he is attractive and can perform sexually. Therefore he may behave sexually.

Some sexually aggressive behaviors are from confusion or disorientation. Common causes are nervous system disorders, drugs, fever, dementia, and poor vision. The person may confuse someone with his or her partner. Or the person cannot control behavior. Changes in the brain make control difficult. Sexual behavior in these cases is usually innocent on the person's part.

Sometimes touch serves to gain attention. For example, Mr. Green cannot speak or move his right side. Your buttocks are near him. To get your attention, he touches your buttocks. His behavior is not sexual.

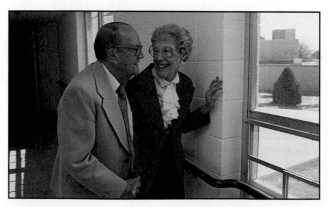

FIG. **7-4** Relationships occur in nursing centers.

BOX 7-2	Promoting Sexuality

- Let the person practice grooming routines. Assist as needed. Women may want to apply makeup, nail polish, lotion, and cologne. Many women shave their legs and underarms and pluck their eyebrows. Men may use after-shave lotion and cologne. Hair care is important to men and women.
- Let the person choose clothing.
- Accept the person's sexual relationships. The person may not share your sexual attitudes, values, practices, or standards. The person may have a homosexual, premarital, or extramarital relationship. Do not judge or gossip about relationships.
- Allow privacy. You can usually tell when people want to be alone. If the person has a private room, close the door for privacy. Some agencies have *Do Not Disturb* signs for doors.

- Let the person and partner know how much time they have alone. For example, remind them about meal times, drugs, or treatments. Tell other staff members that the person wants time alone.
- Knock before you enter any room.
- Consider the person's roommate. Privacy curtains provide little privacy. Arrange for privacy when the roommate is out of the room. Sometimes roommates offer to leave for a while. If the roommate cannot leave, the nurse finds other private areas.
- Allow privacy for masturbation. It is a normal form of sexual expression and release. Close the privacy curtain and the door. Knock before you enter any room. This saves you and the person embarrassment. Sometimes confused persons masturbate in public areas. Lead the person to a private area. Or distract him or her with an activity.

Some persons touch and fondle the genitals for sexual pleasure. This is called *masturbation*. Sometimes masturbation is a sexually aggressive behavior. However, urinary or reproductive system disorders can cause genital soreness or itching. So can poor hygiene or being wet or soiled from urine or feces. Touching the genitals could signal a health problem.

Sexual advances may be intentional. You need to be professional about the matter.

- Ask the person not to touch you. State the places where you were touched.
- Tell the person that you will not do what he or she wants.
- Tell the person what behaviors make you uncomfortable. Politely ask the person not to act that way.
- Allow privacy if the person is becoming aroused. Provide for safety (Chapter 8). Raise bed rails if ordered for the person, place the signal light within reach, and so on. Tell the person when you will return.
- Discuss the matter with the nurse. The nurse can help you understand the behavior.

The care plan has measures to deal with sexually aggressive behaviors. They are based on the cause of the behavior.

OMBUDSMAN PROGRAM

The Older Americans Act is a federal law. It requires a long-term care ombudsman program in every state. An **ombudsman** is someone who supports or

promotes the needs and interests of another person. Long-term care ombudsmen work for a state agency. They do not work for a nursing center. They act on behalf of nursing center and assisted living residents.

Ombudsmen protect the health, safety, welfare, and rights of residents. They:
- Investigate and resolve complaints
- Provide services to assist residents
- Provide information about long-term care services
- Monitor nursing center care and conditions
- Provide support to resident and family groups

Residents have the right to voice grievances and disputes. They also have the right to communicate privately with anyone of their choice. They can share concerns with anyone outside the center. Nursing centers must post the names, addresses, and phone numbers of local and state ombudsmen. This information must be posted where residents can easily see it.

A resident or family member may share a concern with you. You must know state and center policies and procedures for contacting an ombudsman. Ombudsman services are useful when:
- There is concern about a person's care or treatment.
- Someone interferes with a person's rights, health, safety, or welfare.

Focus on the PERSON

Care of the Older Person

Providing comfort—A safe, clean, and comfortable setting is a common standard. To meet this standard, follow the safety measures in Chapter 8. Also make sure each person's room is clean and orderly (Chapter 12). This includes measures to prevent or reduce odors and noise. Also make sure the person, clothes, and linens are clean and dry.

Ethical behavior—The survey team listens to what you say and do. Always practice good work ethics (Chapter 3). Do not use the survey team to share personal complaints. For example, you do not like your work schedule. Or you do not like to do a certain task or procedure. Remember, the focus of the survey is on the standards for quality care. You are not the focus of the survey.

Remaining independent—Most people want to do things for themselves. They do not like to rely on others. During a survey, you might want to do everything possible for the person to prove that you give good care. This is the wrong thing to do. Check the person's care plan for how and when to assist the person. Assist only as needed. Do not do things that the person can do alone.

Speaking up—The survey team may ask you questions about the agency and the care you give. You must answer questions completely and honestly. These questions are examples:
- Do you enjoy working here?
- How many nursing assistants usually work this shift?

- Where are the fire alarms?
- What will you do if there is a fire in a person's room?
- Do you attend resident care conferences?
- Do you share ideas during resident care conferences?

OBRA and other laws—Nursing centers must meet OBRA standards. So must hospitals with long-term care units. A survey team will:
- Review policies, procedures, and medical records
- Interview staff, patients and residents, and families
- Observe how care is given
- Check for cleanliness and safety
- Make sure staff meets state requirements (Are doctors and nurses licensed? Are nursing assistants on the state registry?)

If standards are met, the agency receives a certification. If problems are found, the agency must correct them. The agency can be fined for uncorrected or serious problems. Or it can lose its certification.

Nursing teamwork—Surveyors observe the nursing team. They expect the nursing team to work together to provide quality care. As a nursing team member, you must meet required standards. You also take part in the survey process (see OBRA and other laws). You must:
- Provide quality care
- Protect the person's rights
- Provide for safety
- Help keep the agency clean and safe
- Act in a professional manner
- Have good work ethics
- Follow agency policies and procedures

FOCUS ON THE PERSON

Health care agencies must meet certain standards. Standards are set by federal and state governments. And they are set by accrediting agencies. Standards serve to ensure quality care. Surveys are done to see if the agency meets set standards.

See Focus on the Person: Care of the Older Person.

REVIEW QUESTIONS

Circle the **BEST** answer.

1 Retirement usually means
   a Lowered income
   b Changes from aging
   c Companionship and usefulness
   d Financial security

2 Which prevents loneliness in older persons?
   a Children moving away
   b The death of family and friends
   c Communication problems
   d Contact with other older persons

3 These statements are about a partner's death. Which is *false*?
   a The person loses a lover, friend, companion, and confidant.
   b Preparing for the event lessens grief.
   c The survivor may develop health problems.
   d The survivor's life will likely change.

4 Changes occur in the skin with aging. Care should include the following *except*
   a Providing for warmth
   b Applying lotion
   c Using soap daily
   d Providing good skin care

5 An older person has cold feet. You should
   a Provide socks
   b Apply a hot water bottle
   c Soak the feet in hot water
   d Apply a heating pad

6 Aging causes changes in the musculoskeletal system. Which is *false*?
   a Bones become brittle and can break easily.
   b Bedrest is needed for loss of strength.
   c Joints become stiff and painful.
   d Exercise slows musculoskeletal changes.

7 Reduced blood supply to the brain can result in dizziness. The person is at risk for
   a Confusion
   b Falls
   c Improved memory
   d Fatigue

8 Changes occur in the nervous system. Which is *true*?
   a Less sleep is needed than when younger.
   b The person forgets recent events.
   c Sensitivity to pain increases.
   d Confusion occurs in all older persons.

9 An older person has cardiovascular changes. You should
   a Place needed items nearby
   b Suggest exercises to improve strength
   c Set activity limits for the person
   d Walk long distances with the person

10 Respiratory changes occur with aging. You should
   a Use heavy bed linens
   b Avoid turning the person
   c Position the person for easy breathing
   d Keep the person on bedrest

11 Older persons should avoid dry foods because of
   a Decreases in saliva
   b Loss of teeth or ill-fitting dentures
   c Decreased amounts of digestive juices
   d Decreased peristalsis

12 The doctor ordered increased fluid intake for an older person. You should give most of the fluid before
   a 1700 (5:00 PM)
   b 1900 (7:00 PM)
   c 2100 (9:00 PM)
   d 2300 (11:00 PM)

13 Changes occur in the reproductive system. Which is *false*?
   a Vaginal walls become thinner and dryer.
   b Hormone levels decrease.
   c The testes and ovaries increase in size.
   d The prostate gland increases in size.

14 Mr. Smith is masturbating in the dining room. Which action is *wrong*?
   a Cover him. Take him quietly to his room.
   b Scold him for his behavior.
   c Provide privacy and respect his rights.
   d Report the behavior to the nurse.

15 Residents can do the following *except*
   a Choose their nursing team
   b Contact an ombudsman
   c Voice concerns
   d Make personal choices

Answers to these questions are on p. 467.

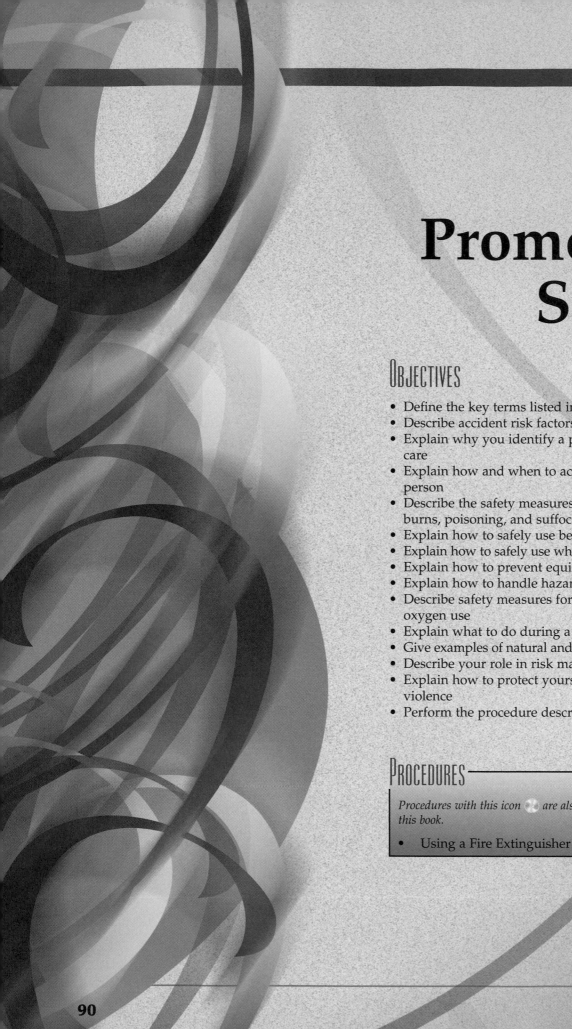

Promoting Safety

OBJECTIVES

- Define the key terms listed in this chapter
- Describe accident risk factors
- Explain why you identify a person before giving care
- Explain how and when to accurately identify a person
- Describe the safety measures to prevent falls, burns, poisoning, and suffocation
- Explain how to safely use bed rails
- Explain how to safely use wheelchairs and stretchers
- Explain how to prevent equipment accidents
- Explain how to handle hazardous substances
- Describe safety measures for fire prevention and oxygen use
- Explain what to do during a fire
- Give examples of natural and human-made disasters
- Describe your role in risk management
- Explain how to protect yourself from workplace violence
- Perform the procedure described in this chapter

PROCEDURES

Procedures with this icon 💿 are also on the CD-ROM in this book.

- Using a Fire Extinguisher

Key Terms

coma A state of being unaware of one's surroundings and being unable to react or respond to people, places, or things

dementia The loss of cognitive and social function caused by changes in the brain

disaster A sudden catastrophic event in which people are injured and killed and property is destroyed

hazardous substance Any chemical in the workplace that can cause harm

suffocation When breathing stops from the lack of oxygen

workplace violence Violent acts directed toward persons at work or while on duty

Persons With Dementia

Accident Risk Factors

Dementia is the loss of cognitive and social function caused by changes in the brain (Chapter 25). *Cognitive* relates to knowledge. Cognitive function involves memory, thinking, reasoning, understanding, judgment, and behavior. Persons with dementia are confused and disoriented. They have a reduced awareness of their surroundings. Judgment is poor. They no longer know what is safe and what are dangers. They may get into closets, cabinets, and other unsafe and unlocked areas. They may eat or drink cleaning supplies, drugs, or other poisons. The health team must meet all their safety needs.

Safety is a basic need. You must protect patients and residents from harm. Common sense and simple safety measures can prevent most accidents. The safety measures in this chapter apply to health care settings. The nursing care plan lists other safety measures needed by the person. The goal is to prevent accidents and injuries without limiting the person's mobility and independence.

ACCIDENT RISK FACTORS

Some people cannot protect themselves. They rely on others for safety. Certain factors increase the risk of falls and injury:

- *Age.* Body changes occur from aging and illness. Older persons have decreased strength, move slowly, and are less steady. Balance may be affected. Older persons are less sensitive to heat and cold. Poor vision, hearing problems, and dulled sense of smell are common.
- *Awareness of surroundings.* **Coma** is a state of being unaware of one's surroundings and being unable to react or respond to people, places, or things. The person relies on others for protection. *See Persons With Dementia: Accident Risk Factors.*
- *Impaired vision.* Persons with poor vision may not see toys, rugs, furniture, or cords. Some have problems reading labels on cleaners, drugs, and other containers. Poisoning can result.
- *Impaired hearing.* Persons with impaired hearing may not hear warning signals or fire alarms. Some cannot hear approaching meal carts, drug carts, stretchers, or people in wheelchairs.
- *Impaired smell and touch.* Illness and aging affect smell and touch. The person may not detect smoke or gas odors. When touch is reduced, burns are a

risk. There are problems sensing heat and cold. Some people have a decreased pain sense. They may be unaware of injury.
- *Impaired mobility.* Some diseases and injuries affect mobility. A person may be aware of danger but cannot move to safety. Some persons cannot walk or propel wheelchairs.
- *Drugs.* Drugs have side effects. They include loss of balance, drowsiness, and lack of coordination. Reduced awareness, confusion, and disorientation also can occur.

IDENTIFYING THE PERSON

Each person has different treatments, therapies, and activity limits. Life and health are threatened if a person is given the wrong care.

The person receives an identification (ID) bracelet when admitted to the agency (Fig. 8-1). The bracelet has the person's name, room and bed number, birth date, age, and other identifying information.

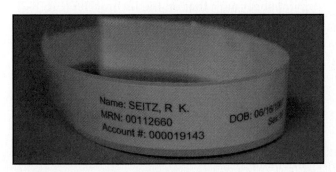

FIG. **8-1** ID bracelet.

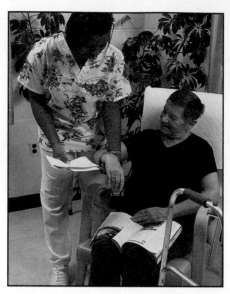

FIG. **8-2** The ID bracelet is checked against the assignment sheet to accurately identify the person.

PROMOTING SAFETY AND COMFORT
Identifying the Person

Safety

Always identify the person right before you begin a task or procedure. Do not identify the person then leave the room to collect equipment and supplies. You could go to the wrong room and give care to the wrong person. And the person for whom the care was intended would not receive it. This too could cause harm.

Comfort

Make sure the person's ID bracelet is not too tight. You should be able to slide 2 fingers under the bracelet. If it is too tight, tell the nurse.

You use the ID bracelet to identify the person before giving care. The assignment sheet states what care to give. To identify the person:
- Compare identifying information on the assignment sheet with that on the ID bracelet (Fig. 8-2). Carefully check the person's full name. Some people have the same first and last names. For example, John Smith is a very common name.
- Call the person by name when checking the ID bracelet. This is a courtesy given as you touch the person and before giving care. Just calling the person by name is not enough to identify him or her. Confused, disoriented, drowsy, hearing-impaired, or distracted persons may answer to any name.

Alert and oriented residents may choose not to wear ID bracelets. This is noted on the person's care plan. Follow the nursing center's policy and the care plan to identify the person.

BOX 8-1	Factors Increasing the Risk of Falls

- A history of falls
- Weakness, being unsteady, balance problems
- Drowsiness and slow reaction time
- Poor vision
- Confusion, disorientation, memory problems, poor judgment
- Decreased mobility
- Foot problems
- Elimination needs (including frequent urination and incontinence—see Chapters 15 and 16)
- Dizziness and lightheadedness
- Joint pain and stiffness
- Low blood pressure
- Fainting
- Depression
- Strange setting
- Care equipment (IV poles, drainage tubes and bags, wheelchairs, walkers, canes, crutches, and so on)

PREVENTING FALLS

The risk of falling increases with age. Persons older than 65 years are at high risk. A history of falls increases the risk of falling again.

Most falls occur in the evening, between 1800 (6:00 PM) and 2100 (9:00 PM). Falls also are more likely during shift changes. During shift changes, staff are busy going off and coming on duty. Confusion can occur about who gives care and answers signal lights. Shift change times vary among agencies.

Agencies have fall prevention programs for persons at risk (Box 8-1). Box 8-2 lists measures that are part of fall prevention programs and care plans. The care plan also lists measures for the person's risk factors.

BOX 8-2	**Safety Measures to Prevent Falls**

Basic Needs

- Fluid needs are met.
- Eyeglasses and hearing aids are worn as needed.
- Tasks and procedures are explained before and while performing them.
- Help is given with elimination needs. It is given at regular times and whenever requested.
- The bedpan, urinal, or commode is kept within easy reach if the person can use the device without help.
- A warm drink, soft lights, or a back massage is used to calm the person who is agitated.
- The person is properly positioned when in bed, a chair, or a wheelchair (Chapter 11).
- Correct procedures and equipment are used for transfers (Chapter 11).
- The person is involved in meaningful activities.

Bathrooms

- Tubs and showers have non-slip surfaces or non-slip bath mats.
- Grab bars are in showers. They also are by tubs.
- Bathrooms have grab bars.
- Safety measures for tub baths and showers are followed (Chapter 13).

Floors

- Scatter, area, and throw rugs are not used.
- Loose floor boards and tiles are reported. So are frayed rugs and carpets.
- Floors and stairs are free of clutter, cords, and other items that can cause tripping.
- Floors are free of spills. Wipe up spills at once.
- Floors are free of excess furniture and equipment.
- Equipment and supplies are kept on one side of the hallway.

Beds, Furniture, and Other Equipment

- The bed is in the lowest horizontal position, except when giving bedside care. The distance from the bed to the floor is reduced if the person falls or gets out of bed.
- A special mattress or mat is on the floor next to the bed if ordered. This reduces the chance of injury if the person falls.
- Bed rails are used according to the care plan (p. 94).
- Furniture is placed for easy movement.
- A telephone and lamp are within the person's reach.
- Crutches, canes, and walkers have non-skid tips.
- Wheel locks on beds, wheelchairs, and stretchers are in working order.

- Bed wheels are locked for transfers.
- Wheelchair and stretcher safety measures are followed (p. 97).
- Cushions are used as ordered to prevent falls (Chapter 11). Follow the care plan.

Lighting

- Rooms, hallways, stairways, and bathrooms have good lighting.
- Night-lights are in bedrooms, hallways, and bathrooms.

Shoes and Clothing

- Non-skid footwear is worn. Socks, bedroom slippers, and long shoelaces are avoided.
- Clothing fits properly. Clothing is not loose. It does not drag on the floor. Belts are tied or secured in place.

Signal Lights and Alarms

- The person is taught how to use the signal light (Chapter 12).
- The signal light is always within the person's reach.
- The person is asked to call for assistance when help is needed getting out of bed or a chair or when walking.
- Signal lights are answered promptly. The person may need help right away. He or she may not wait for help.
- Respond to bed and chair alarms at once. They sense when the person tries to get up (Fig. 8-3, p. 94).

Other

- The person is checked often. Frequent checks are made on persons with poor judgment or memory.
- The person is encouraged to use hand rails and grab bars in bathrooms and shower rooms.
- Non-slip strips are on the floor next to the bed and in the bathroom. They are intact.
- Caution is used when turning corners, entering corridor intersections, and going through doors. You could injure a person coming from the other direction.
- Pull (do not push) wheelchairs, stretchers, carts, and other wheeled equipment through doorways. This allows you to lead the way and to see where you are going.
- A safety check is done before you leave the room and after visitors leave (see the inside of the front book cover). They may have lowered a bed rail, removed the signal light, or moved a walker out of reach. Or they may have brought an item that could harm the person.

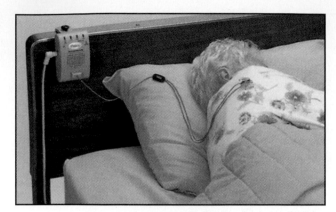

FIG. **8-3** Bed alarm.

Bed Rails

Bed rails (side rails) on hospital beds are raised and lowered. They lock in place with levers, latches, or buttons. Bed rails are half, three quarters, or the full length of the bed. When half-length rails are used, each side may have two rails. One is for the upper part of the bed; the other for the lower part.

The nurse and care plan tell you when to raise bed rails. They are needed by persons who are unconscious or sedated with drugs. Some confused or disoriented people need them. If a person needs bed rails, keep them up at all times except when giving bedside care.

Bed rails present hazards. The person can fall when trying to climb over them. Entrapment is a risk. That is, a person can get caught, trapped, or entangled in bed rail bars or bed rail gaps (Fig. 8-4). Injury or death can occur if the person's head, neck, chest, arm, or leg is trapped. Persons at greatest risk are those who:
- Are older
- Are frail
- Are confused or disoriented
- Are restless
- Have uncontrolled body movements
- Are restrained (Chapter 9)
- Are small in size
- Have poor muscle control

Bed rails prevent the person from getting out of bed. They are considered restraints (Chapter 9) by OBRA and the Centers for Medicare & Medicaid Services (CMS). Bed rails can be used:
- To treat a person's medical symptoms.
- If the person requests them. Some people feel safer with bed rails up. Others use them to change positions in bed.

The person or legal representative must give consent for raised bed rails. The need for bed rails is carefully noted in the person's medical record and care plan.

The procedures in this book include using bed rails. This helps you learn how to use them correctly. The nurse, the care plan, and your assignment sheet tell you which people use bed rails. If a person does

PROMOTING SAFETY AND COMFORT
Bed Rails

Safety

You will raise the bed to give care. Follow these safety measures to prevent the person from falling:
- If the person uses bed rails—always raise the far bed rail if you are working alone. Raise both bed rails if you need to leave the bedside for any reason.
- If the person does not use bed rails—ask a co-worker to help you. The co-worker stands on the far side of the bed. This protects the person from falling off the bed.
- Never leave the person alone when the bed is raised.
- Always lower the bed to its lowest position when you are done giving care.

Comfort

The person has to reach over raised bed rails to access items on the bedside stand and overbed table. Such items include the water pitcher and cup, tissues, and phone. Adjust the overbed table so it is within the person's reach. Ask if the person wants other items nearby. Place them on the overbed table too. Always make sure needed items are within the person's reach.

not use bed rails, omit the "raise bed rails" or "lower bed rails" steps.

If a person uses bed rails, check the person often. Report to the nurse that you checked the person. If you are allowed to chart, record when you checked the person and your observations.

Hand Rails and Grab Bars

Hand rails are in hallways and stairways (Fig. 8-5). They give support to persons who are weak or unsteady when walking.

Grab bars are in bathrooms and in shower and tub rooms. They provide support for sitting down on or getting up from a toilet. They also are used for getting in and out of the shower or tub.

Wheel Locks

Bed legs have wheels. Each wheel has a lock to prevent the bed from moving (Fig. 8-6). Wheels are locked at all times except when moving the bed. Lock bed wheels when:
- Giving bedside care
- You transfer a person to and from the bed

Wheelchair and stretcher wheels also are locked during transfers (p. 97). You or the person can be injured if the bed, wheelchair, or stretcher moves.

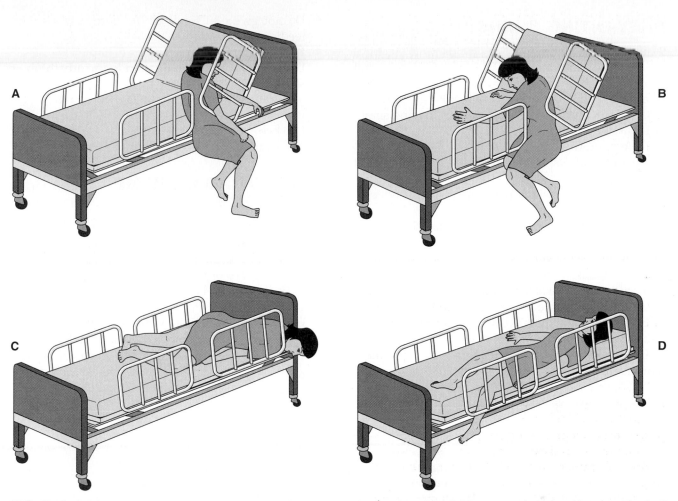

FIG. **8-4** Entrapment is a safety risk with bed rails. Some areas of entrapment are: **A,** The person is trapped between the bed rail bars. **B,** The person is trapped between the bed rail gaps. **C,** The person is trapped between the bed rail and the headboard. **D,** The person is caught between the mattress and the bed rail.

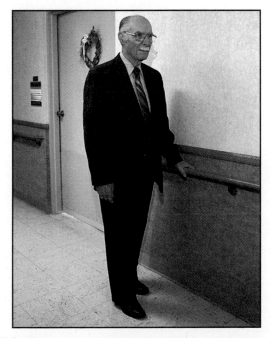

FIG. **8-5** Hand rails provide support when walking.

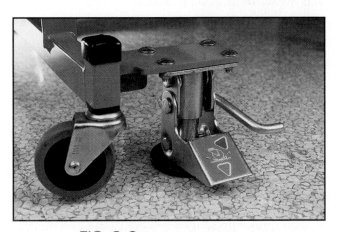

FIG. **8-6** Lock on a bed wheel.

PREVENTING BURNS

Smoking in bed, spilling hot liquids, and electrical devices are common causes of burns. So is very hot bath water. These safety measures can prevent burns:

- Be sure people smoke only in smoking areas.
- Check the person's care plan about leaving smoking materials at the bedside.
- Do not allow smoking in bed.
- Do not allow smoking near oxygen equipment (p. 100).
- Supervise the smoking of persons who cannot protect themselves.
- Do not allow the person to use a heating pad or electric blanket.
- Turn on cold water first, then hot water. Turn off hot water first, then cold water.
- Measure bath water temperature (Chapter 13). Check it before the person gets into the tub.
- Check for "hot spots" in water. Move your hand back and forth.
- Follow the measures to prevent equipment accidents.

PREVENTING POISONING

Drugs and cleaning and personal care products are common poisons. Poisoning in adults may be from confusion or poor vision when reading labels. Make sure patients and residents cannot reach hazardous materials (p. 99). Follow agency policy for storing personal care items. Shampoo, mouthwash, lotion, perfume, and deodorant are examples. These products are harmful when swallowed.

PREVENTING SUFFOCATION

Suffocation is when breathing stops from the lack of oxygen. Death occurs if the person does not start breathing. Common causes include choking, drowning, inhaling gas or smoke, strangulation, and electrical shock. These safety measures help prevent suffocation:

- Follow the measures to prevent equipment accidents.
- Use electrical items correctly.
- Cut food into small, bite-size pieces for persons who cannot do so themselves.
- Make sure dentures are in place.
- Report loose teeth or dentures.
- Make sure the person can chew and swallow the food served.
- Tell the nurse at once if the person has problems swallowing.

- Do not give oral foods or fluids to persons with feeding tubes (Chapter 17).
- Follow aspiration precautions (Chapter 17).
- Do not leave a person unattended in a bathtub or shower.
- Move all persons from the area if you smell smoke.
- Position the person in bed correctly (Chapter 11).
- Use bed rails correctly (p. 94).
- Use restraints correctly (Chapter 9).

PREVENTING EQUIPMENT ACCIDENTS

All equipment is unsafe if broken, not used correctly, or not working properly. Inspect all equipment before use. Check glass and plastic items for cracks, chips, and sharp or rough edges. They can cause cuts, stabs, or scratches. Follow the Bloodborne Pathogen Standard (Chapter 10).

Electrical items must work properly and be in good repair. This includes hospital beds. Frayed cords (Fig. 8-7) and overloaded electrical outlets (Fig. 8-8) can cause fires, electrical shocks, and death.

Warning signs of a faulty electrical item include:

- Shocks
- Loss of power or a power outage
- Dimming or flickering lights
- Sparks
- Sizzling or buzzing sounds
- Burning odor
- Loose plugs

Practice the safety measures in Box 8-3. Complete an incident report (p. 103) if a patient, resident, visitor, or staff member has an equipment-related accident. The Safe Medical Devices Act requires that agencies report equipment-related illnesses, injuries, and deaths.

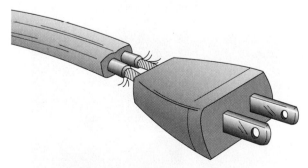

FIG. **8-7** A frayed electrical cord.

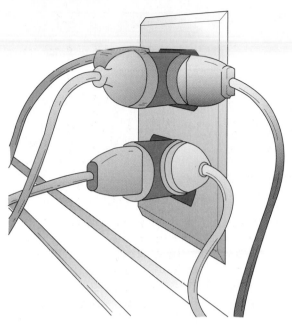

FIG. **8-8** An overloaded electrical outlet.

BOX 8-3	Safety Measures to Prevent Equipment Accidents

- Follow agency policies and procedures.
- Follow the manufacturer's instructions. This includes all caution and warning labels.
- Do not use an unfamiliar item. Ask for needed training. Also ask the nurse to supervise you the first time you use the item.
- Use an item only for its intended purpose.
- Use 3-pronged plugs on all electrical devices (Fig. 8-9).
- Inspect power cords for damage.
- Do not cover power cords with rugs, carpets, linens, or other material.
- Connect a bed power cord directly into a wall outlet. Do not connect a bed power cord to an extension cord or outlet strip.
- Make sure the item works before you begin.
- Show broken or damaged items to the nurse. Follow the nurse's instructions and agency policies for discarding items or sending them for repair.
- Do not try to repair broken items.
- Do not use electrical items owned by the person until they are safety-checked. The maintenance department does this.
- Keep electrical items away from water. Wipe up spills right away.
- Turn off equipment before unplugging it. Sparks occur when electrical items are unplugged while turned on.
- Hold onto the plug (not the cord) when removing it from an outlet.
- Keep cords away from heating vents and other heat sources.
- Turn off equipment when done using the item.
- Unplug all electrical devices when not in use.

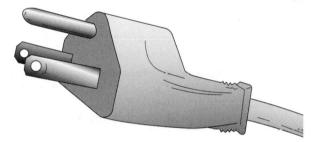

FIG. **8-9** A three-pronged plug.

WHEELCHAIR AND STRETCHER SAFETY

Some people use wheelchairs (Fig. 8-10, p. 98). The handgrips/push handles are used to push wheelchairs. Stretchers are used to transport persons who cannot use wheelchairs.

Follow the safety measures in Box 8-4 on p. 98 when using wheelchairs and stretchers. The person can fall from the wheelchair or stretcher. Or the person can fall during transfers to and from the wheelchair or stretcher.

BOX 8-4	Wheelchair and Stretcher Safety

Wheelchair Safety

- Check the wheel locks. Make sure you can lock and unlock them.
- Check for flat or loose tires. A wheel lock will not work on a flat or loose tire.
- Make sure that wheel spokes are intact. Damaged, broken, or loose spokes can interfere with moving the wheelchair or locking the wheels.
- Make sure casters point forward. This keeps the wheelchair balanced and stable.
- Position the person's feet on the footplates.
- Make sure the person's feet are on the footplates before pushing or repositioning the chair. The person's feet must not touch or drag on the floor when the chair is moving.
- Push the chair forward when transporting the person. Do not pull the chair backward unless going through a doorway (see Box 8-2).
- Lock both wheels before you transfer a person to or from the wheelchair.
- Follow the care plan for keeping the wheels locked when not moving the wheelchair. Locking the wheels prevents the chair from moving if the person wants to move to or from the chair.
- Do not let the person stand on the footplates.
- Do not let the footplates fall back onto the person's legs.

- Make sure the person has needed wheelchair accessories—safety belt, pouch, tray, lapboard, and cushion.
- Remove the armrests (if removable) when the person transfers to the bed, toilet, commode, tub, or car (Chapter 11).
- Swing front rigging out of the way for transfers to and from the wheelchair. Some front riggings detach for transfers.
- Clean the wheelchair according to agency policy.
- Ask a nurse or physical therapist to show you how to propel wheelchairs up steps and ramps and over curbs.
- Follow measures to prevent equipment accidents (p. 96).

Stretcher Safety

- Ask two co-workers to help with the transfer (Chapter 11).
- Lock the stretcher wheels before the transfer.
- Fasten the safety straps when the person is properly positioned on the stretcher.
- Ask a co-worker to help with the transport.
- Raise the side rails. Keep them up during the transport.
- Make sure the person's arms, hands, legs, and feet do not dangle through the side rail bars.
- Stand at the head of the stretcher. Your co-worker stands at the foot of the stretcher.
- Move the stretcher feet first (Fig. 8-11).
- Do not leave the person alone.
- Follow measures to prevent equipment accidents (p. 96).

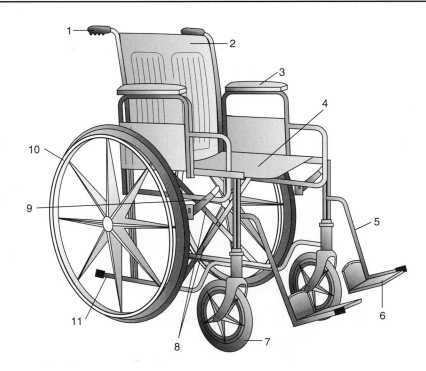

1. Handgrip/push handle
2. Back upholstery
3. Armrest
4. Seat upholstery
5. Front rigging
6. Footplate
7. Caster
8. Crossbrace
9. Wheel lock/brake
10. Wheel and handrim
11. Tipping lever

FIG. **8-10** Parts of a wheelchair.

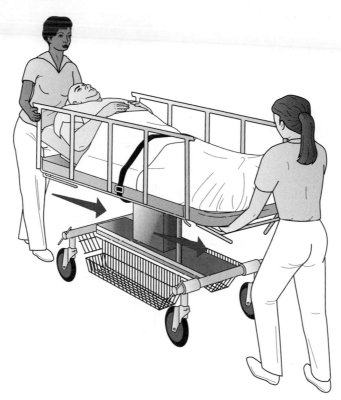

FIG. **8-11** A person is transported by stretcher. The stretcher is moved feet first.

HANDLING HAZARDOUS SUBSTANCES

A **hazardous substance** is any chemical in the workplace that can cause harm. Physical hazards can cause fires or explosions. Health hazards are chemicals that can cause health problems.

The agency provides hazardous substance training for employees. The agency also provides eyewash and total body wash stations in areas where hazardous substances are used. Hazardous substances include:

- Drugs used in cancer therapy (chemotherapy, anticancer drugs)
- Anesthesia gases
- Gases used to sterilize equipment
- Oxygen
- Disinfectants and cleaning solutions
- Radiation used for x-rays and cancer treatments
- Mercury (found in thermometers and blood pressure devices)

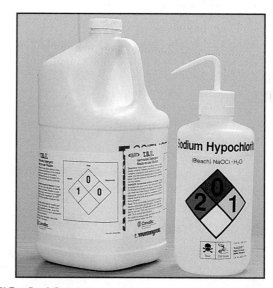

FIG. **8-12** Warning labels on hazardous substances.

Labeling

Hazardous substance containers need warning labels (Fig. 8-12). The manufacturer applies the labels. Warning labels identify:

- The type of hazard
- Safety measures (for example, "Do not use near open flame" or "Avoid skin contact")
- What personal protective equipment to wear (Chapter 10)
- How to use the substance safely
- Storage and disposal information

If a warning label is removed or damaged, do not use the substance. Take the container to the nurse, and explain the problem. Do not leave the container unattended.

Material Safety Data Sheets

Every hazardous substance has a material safety data sheet (MSDS). It gives detailed information about the substance. Check the MSDS before using a hazardous substance, cleaning up a leak or spill, or disposing of the substance. Tell the nurse about a leak or spill right away. Do not leave a leak or spill unattended.

FIRE SAFETY

Faulty electrical equipment and wiring, overloaded circuits, and smoking are major causes of fire. The entire health team must prevent fires. They must act quickly during a fire.

Fire and the Use of Oxygen

Three things are needed for a fire:
- A spark or flame
- A material that will burn
- Oxygen

Air has some oxygen. However, doctors order oxygen therapy for some people (Chapter 22). Safety measures are needed where oxygen is used and stored:
- "No Smoking" signs are placed on the door and near the bed.
- The person and visitors are reminded not to smoke in the room.
- Smoking materials (cigarettes, cigars, and pipes), matches, and lighters are removed from the room.
- Wool blankets and synthetic fabrics that cause static electricity are removed from the person's room. The person wears a cotton gown or pajamas.
- Safety measures to prevent equipment accidents are followed (see Box 8-3).
- Materials that ignite easily are removed from the room. They include oil, grease, alcohol, nail polish remover, and so on.

Preventing Fires

Fire prevention measures were described in relation to burns, equipment-related accidents, and oxygen use. Other measures are listed in Box 8-5.

BOX 8-5	Fire Prevention Measures

- Follow the safety measures for oxygen use.
- Smoke only where allowed.
- Be sure all ashes, cigars, cigarettes, and other smoking materials are out before emptying ashtrays.
- Provide ashtrays to persons who are allowed to smoke.
- Empty ashtrays into a metal container partially filled with sand or water. Do not empty ashtrays into plastic containers or wastebaskets lined with paper or plastic bags.
- Supervise persons who smoke. This is very important for persons who are confused, disoriented, or sedated.
- Follow safety practices when using electrical items.
- Keep matches and lighters out of the reach of persons who are confused or disoriented.
- Do not leave cooking unattended on stoves or in ovens or microwave ovens.
- Store flammable liquids in their original containers. Follow the manufacturer's instructions.
- Do not light matches or lighters or smoke around flammable liquids or materials.

What to Do During a Fire

Know your agency's procedures for fire emergencies. Know where to find fire alarms, fire extinguishers, and emergency exits. Fire drills are held to practice emergency procedures. Remember the word *RACE*:
- *R*—for *rescue*. Rescue persons in immediate danger. Move them to a safe place.
- *A*—for *alarm*. Sound the nearest fire alarm. Notify the switchboard operator.
- *C*—for *confine*. Close doors and windows to confine the fire. Turn off oxygen or electrical items used in the general area of the fire.
- *E*—for *extinguish*. Use a fire extinguisher on a small fire that has not spread to a larger area.

Clear equipment from all normal and emergency exists. *Do not use elevators if there is a fire.*

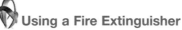 **Using a Fire Extinguisher**

Different extinguishers are used for different kinds of fires: oil and grease fires, electrical fires, and paper and wood fires. A general procedure for using a fire extinguisher follows.

Using a Fire Extinguisher

Procedure

1 Pull the fire alarm.
2 Get the nearest fire extinguisher.
3 Carry it upright.
4 Take it to the fire.
5 Remove the safety pin (Fig. 8-13, *A*).

6 Direct the hose at the base of the fire (Fig. 8-13, *B*).
7 Push the top handle down (Fig. 8-13, *C*).
8 Sweep the hose slowly back and forth at the base of the fire.

A

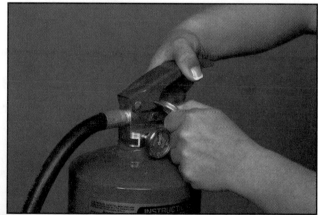

B

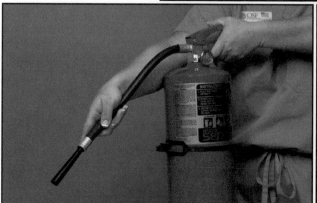

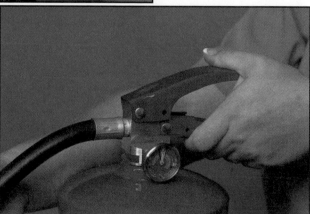

C

FIG. **8-13** Using a fire extinguisher. **A,** Remove the safety pin. **B,** Direct the hose at the base of the fire. **C,** Push the top handle down.

DISASTERS

A **disaster** is a sudden catastrophic event. People are injured and killed. Property is destroyed. Natural disasters include tornadoes, hurricanes, blizzards, earthquakes, volcanic eruptions, floods, and some fires. Human-made disasters include auto, bus, train, and airplane accidents. They also include fires, bombings, nuclear power plant accidents, riots, explosions, gas or chemical leaks, and wars.

Communities, fire and police departments, and agencies have disaster plans. They include procedures to deal with great numbers of people needing treatment. A disaster may damage the agency. The disaster plan includes procedures to evacuate the agency. You should know your agency's disaster plan.

Bomb Threats

Agencies have polices and procedures for bomb threats. You must follow them if a caller makes a bomb threat or if you find an item that looks or sounds strange. Often bomb threats are sent by phone. However, they can be sent by mail, e-mail, messenger, or other means. Or the person can leave a bomb in the agency.

WORKPLACE VIOLENCE

Workplace violence is violent acts directed toward persons at work or while on duty. It includes murders, robbery, beatings, and the use of weapons—firearms, bombs, or knives. It also includes threats—obscene phone calls; threatening oral, written, or body language; and harassment of any nature (being followed, sworn at, or shouted at).

According to OSHA, nurses and nursing assistants are at risk for workplace violence. They have the most contact with patients, residents, and visitors. Risk factors include:
- People with visible or concealed weapons
- Acutely disturbed and violent persons
- Alcohol and drug abuse
- Mentally ill persons who do not follow a treatment program
- Pharmacies have drugs and are a target for robberies
- Gang members and substance abusers are patients, residents, or visitors
- Upset, agitated, and disturbed family and visitors
- Long waits for services
- Being alone with patients and residents during care or transport to other areas
- Low staff levels during meals, emergencies, and at night
- Poor lighting in hallways, rooms, parking lots, and other areas
- Lack of training in recognizing and managing potentially violent situations

OSHA has guidelines for violence prevention programs. Work site hazards are identified. Prevention measures are developed and followed. The staff receives safety and health training.

Practice these measures when dealing with agitated or aggressive persons:
- Stand away from the person. Judge the length of the person's arms and legs. Stand far enough away so the person cannot hit or kick you.
- Stand close to the door. Do not become trapped in the room.
- Know where to find panic buttons, signal lights, alarms, closed-circuit monitors, and other security devices.
- Keep your hands free.
- Stay calm. Talk to the person in a calm manner. Do not raise your voice or argue, scold, or interrupt the person.
- Do not touch the person.
- Tell the person that you will get a nurse to speak to him or her.
- Leave the room as soon as you can. Make sure the person is safe.
- Tell the nurse or security officer about the matter.
- Complete an incident report according to agency policy.

RISK MANAGEMENT

Risk management involves identifying and controlling risks and safety hazards affecting the agency. This includes accident and fire protection, negligence and malpractice, abuse, and federal and state requirements. The intent is to:
- Protect everyone in the agency (patients, residents, visitors, and staff)
- Protect agency property from harm or danger
- Protect the person's valuables
- Prevent accidents and injuries

Personal Belongings

The person's belongings must be kept safe. Often they are sent home with the family. A personal belongings list is completed. Each item is listed and described. The staff member and person sign the completed list.

A valuables envelope is used for money and jewelry. Each jewelry item is listed and described on the envelope. Describe what you see. For example, describe a ring as having a white stone with six prongs in a yellow setting. Do not assume the stone is a diamond in a gold setting. For valuables:

- Count money with the person.
- Put money and each jewelry item in the envelope with the person watching. Sign the envelope just like you do the personal belongings list.
- Give the envelope to the nurse. The nurse puts it in a safe or gives it to the family.

Dentures, eyeglasses, hearing aids, watches, and radios are kept at the bedside. Items kept at the bedside are listed in the person's record. Some people keep money for personal items. The amount kept is noted in the person's record.

In nursing centers, clothing and shoes are labeled with the person's name. So are radios, blankets, and other items brought from home.

Reporting Accidents and Errors

Report accidents and errors at once. This includes:

- Accidents involving patients, residents, visitors, or staff
- Errors in care (includes giving the wrong care, giving care to the wrong person, or not giving care)

- Broken or lost items owned by the person (for example, dentures, hearing aids, eyeglasses, and money)
- Hazardous substance accidents
- Workplace violence incidents

An *incident report* is completed as soon as possible after the incident. Incident reports are reviewed by risk management and a committee of health care workers. They look for patterns and trends of accidents or errors. For example, are falls occurring on the same shift and on the same unit? Are lost or missing items being reported on the same shift or same unit? There may be new policies or procedures to prevent future incidents.

FOCUS ON THE PERSON

Safety is a basic need. You can meet this basic need by doing the right thing (ethics) and following laws that promote safety.

People want to be independent. Let the person do as much for himself or herself as safely possible. Good communication between you, the person, and the nursing team is needed. This will help ensure that the person feels safe and independent.

See Focus on the Person: Safety.

Focus on the PERSON

Safety

Providing comfort—Feeling safe and secure promotes physical and mental comfort. Would you feel comfortable if you were afraid of falling? Would new equipment or a procedure frighten you? Always follow the safety measures in this chapter and the person's care plan. Also, always explain what you are going to do. Do this before starting a task or procedure. When performing a task or procedure, explain what you are doing step-by-step. These measures help meet the person's basic need to feel safe and secure.

Ethical behavior—Negligence occurs when the person or his or her property is harmed (Chapter 2). An error may not cause harm. However, you must still report the error according to agency policy. Reporting the error is the right thing to do. It is wrong not to report the error. Remember, ethics involves right and wrong conduct.

Remaining independent—Most people want to do things for themselves. They do not want to rely on others for simple, everyday things. To help the person remain independent, always keep needed items within the person's reach. Let the person do as much as he or she safely can. For example, some people use the handrims to propel their wheelchairs. Others use their feet to move the chair. Still others used motor-propelled wheelchairs with hand, chin, mouth, or other controls.

Speaking up—Often accidents and injuries occur when the person tries to get needed items. The person has to reach too far and falls out of bed or from a chair. Or the person tries to get up without help. Promote safety by asking the person these questions:

- "What things would you like near you?"
- "Can I move this closer to you?"
- "Can you reach the signal light?"
- "Can you reach your cane?" (Walker and wheelchair are other examples.)
- "Do you need to use the bathroom now?"
- "Is there anything else you need before I leave the room?"

OBRA and other laws—The Occupational Safety and Health Administration (OSHA) is an agency of the federal government. OSHA and other federal and state agencies have the power to issue standards, rules, and regulations. These are called agency-made laws. Employers and employees must comply with them. OSHA conducts inspections to make sure an agency is following OSHA policies. If not following them, OSHA can fine the agency. Fines can be between $5000 and $70,000 for each violation.

Nursing teamwork—The entire staff must protect the person from harm. If you see something unsafe, tell the nurse at once. Do not assume the nurse knows or that the matter is being tended to. Also know your role during shift changes. Nursing staff going off-duty and those of the on-coming shift must work together to meet the needs of patients and residents.

REVIEW QUESTIONS

Circle **T** if the statement is true and **F** if it is false.

1 **T F** Keeping electrical cords and appliances in good repair prevents suffocation.

2 **T F** To correctly identify a person, call him or her by name.

3 **T F** Older persons are at risk for accidents because of changes in the body.

4 **T F** Needing to urinate is a major cause of falls.

5 **T F** Socks and bedroom slippers help prevent falls.

6 **T F** Good lighting helps prevent falls.

7 **T F** Bed rails are always raised when the bed is raised.

8 **T F** The signal light must always be within the person's reach.

9 **T F** Hazardous substances must have warning labels.

10 **T F** In a disaster, people are injured and killed. Property is destroyed.

11 **T F** Smoking is allowed where oxygen is used.

Circle the **BEST** answer.

12 Who has the greatest risk of falling?
 a A person who wears eyeglasses
 b A person who wears a hearing aid
 c A person with memory problems
 d A person who is 59 years old

13 A person in a coma
 a Has suffered an electrical shock
 b Has dementia
 c Is unaware of his or her surroundings
 d Has stopped breathing

14 Which is likely to cause falls?
 a Wiping up spills right away
 b Wearing non-skid shoes
 c Using hand rails and grab bars
 d Keeping bed rails up

15 Which does *not* prevent falls?
 a Meeting elimination needs
 b Answering signal lights promptly
 c Keeping persons at risk for falls in their rooms
 d Using bed rails according to the care plan

16 Burns are caused by the following *except*
 a Smoking
 b Faulty electrical items
 c Very hot bath water
 d Oxygen

17 Mrs. Ford often tries to get up without help. Which action is *unsafe?*
 a Reminding her to use the signal light
 b Checking on her often
 c Helping her to the bathroom at regular intervals
 d Keeping her bed rails up

18 To prevent equipment accidents, you should
 a Fix broken items
 b Use two-pronged plugs
 c Check glass and plastic items for damage
 d Complete an incident report

19 Mr. Wallace is a new resident. Before shaving him with his electric shaver
 a You need to inspect it
 b The maintenance staff needs to do a safety check
 c You need to check for a frayed cord
 d You need an outlet

20 You are using equipment. Which action is *unsafe?*
 a Following the manufacturer's instructions
 b Keeping electrical items away from water and spills
 c Pulling on the cord to remove a plug from an outlet
 d Turning off electrical items after using them

21 Mr. Wallace uses a wheelchair. Which measure is *unsafe?*
 a The wheels are locked for transfers.
 b He can stand on the footplates.
 c You push forward when transporting him.
 d The casters point forward.

22 Stretcher safety involves the following *except*
 a Locking the wheels for transfers
 b Fastening the safety straps
 c Raising the side rails
 d Moving the stretcher head first

23 You spilled a hazardous substance. Which action is *unsafe?*
 a Reading the material safety data sheet
 b Leaving the spill to find a nurse
 c Wearing any needed personal protective equipment to clean up the spill
 d Completing an incident report

REVIEW QUESTIONS

24 Which is *not* needed to start a fire?
a A spark or flame
b A material that will burn
c Oxygen
d Carbon monoxide

25 The fire alarm sounds. Which action is *unsafe*?
a Turning off oxygen
b Using elevators
c Closing doors and windows
d Moving patients and residents to a safe place

26 A person is agitated and aggressive. Which action is *unsafe*?
a Standing away from the person
b Standing close to the door
c Using touch to show you care
d Talking to the person without raising your voice

27 In nursing centers, personal property is
a Labeled with the person's name
b Sent home with the family
c Put in a safe
d Shared with other residents

28 You gave Mrs. Ford the wrong treatment. Which is *true*?
a Report the error at the end of the shift.
b Take action only if Mrs. Ford was injured.
c You are guilty of negligence.
d You must complete an incident report.

Answers to these questions are on p. 468.

9

Restraint Alternatives and Safe Restraint Use

OBJECTIVES

- Define the key terms listed in this chapter
- Describe the purpose and complications of restraints
- Identify restraint alternatives
- Explain how to use restraints safely
- Perform the procedure described in this chapter

PROCEDURES

Procedures with this icon 💿 are also on the CD-ROM in this book.

- Applying Restraints

KEY TERMS

active physical restraint A restraint attached to the person's body and to a fixed (non-movable) object; it restricts movement or body access

passive physical restraint A restraint near but not directly attached to the person's body; it does not totally restrict freedom of movement and allows access to certain body parts

restraint Any item, object, device, garment, material, or drug that limits or restricts a person's freedom of movement or access to one's body

---

BOX 9-1	Risks of Restraint Use

- Agitation
- Anger
- Cuts and bruises
- Constipation
- Dehydration
- Depression
- Embarrassment and humiliation
- Fractures
- Incontinence (Chapters 15 and 16)
- Infections (pneumonia and urinary tract)
- Mistrust
- Nerve injuries
- Pressure ulcers (Chapter 21)
- Strangulation

Many safety measures are presented in Chapter 8. However, some persons need extra protection. They may present dangers to themselves or others. For example:

- Mrs. Perez forgets to call for help when getting up and with walking. Falling is a risk.
- Mrs. Wilson tries to pull out her feeding tube. The tube is part of her treatment.
- Ms. Walsh scratches and picks at a wound. This can damage the skin or the wound.
- Mr. Ross wanders. He may wander into traffic or get lost in neighborhoods, parks, forests, or other areas. Exposure to hot or cold weather presents other dangers.
- Mr. Winters tries to hit, pinch, and bite the staff. They are at risk for harm.

Every attempt is made to protect the person without using restraints. Sometimes they are needed. A **restraint** is any item, object, device, garment, material, or drug that limits or restricts a person's freedom of movement or access to one's body. Restraints are used only as a *last resort* to protect persons from harming themselves or others.

HISTORY OF RESTRAINT USE

Until the late 1980s, restraints were thought to *prevent* falls. Research shows that restraints *cause* falls. Falls occur when persons try to get free of the restraints. Injuries are more serious from falls in restrained persons than in those not restrained.

Restraints also were used to prevent wandering or interfering with treatment. They were often used for persons who showed confusion, poor judgment, or behavior problems. Their purpose was to protect a person. However, they can cause serious harm, even death (Box 9-1).

OBRA, the Centers for Medicare and Medicaid Services (CMS), and the federal Food and Drug Administration (FDA) have guidelines about restraint use. So do states and accrediting agencies. They do not forbid restraint use. *However, all other appropriate alternatives must be tried first.*

RESTRAINT ALTERNATIVES

Often there are causes and reasons for harmful behaviors. Knowing and treating the cause can prevent restraint use. The nurse tries to find out what the behavior means.

- Is the person in pain?
- Is the person ill or injured?
- Is the person short of breath? Are cells getting enough oxygen?
- Is the person afraid in a new setting?
- Does the person need to use the bathroom?
- Is a dressing or bandage tight or causing other discomfort?
- Is clothing tight or causing other discomfort?
- Is the person's position uncomfortable?
- Is the person too hot or too cold?
- Is the person hungry?
- Is the person thirsty?
- Are body fluids, secretions, or excretions causing skin irritation?
- Does the person have problems communicating?
- Is the person seeing, hearing, or feeling things that are not real (Chapter 24)?
- Is the person confused or disoriented (Chapter 25)?
- Are drugs causing the behaviors?

Restraint alternatives for the person are identified (Box 9-2, p. 108). They become part of the care plan. Care plan changes are made as needed. Restraint alternatives may not protect the person. The doctor may need to order restraints.

BOX 9-2 Alternatives to Restraints

- Diversion is provided. This includes TV, videos, music, games, books, relaxation tapes, and so on.
- Lifelong habits and routines are in the care plan. For example: shower before breakfast; read in the bathroom; walk outside before lunch; watch TV after lunch; and so on.
- Family and friends make videos of themselves for the person to watch.
- Videos are made of visits with family and friends for the person to watch.
- Time is spent in supervised areas (dining room, lounge, and near nurses' station).
- Pillows, wedge cushions, and posture and positioning aids are used.
- The signal light is within reach.
- Signal lights are answered promptly.
- Food, fluid, hygiene, and elimination needs are met.
- The bedpan, urinal, or commode is within the person's reach.
- Back massages are given.
- Family, friends, and volunteers visit.
- The person has companions and sitters.
- Time is spent with the person.
- Extra time is spent with a person who is restless.
- Reminiscing is done with the person.
- A calm, quiet setting is provided.
- The person wanders in safe areas.
- The entire staff is aware of persons who tend to wander. This includes those in housekeeping, maintenance, business office, dietary, and so on.
- Exercise programs are provided.
- Outdoor time is planned during nice weather.
- The person does jobs or tasks he or she consents to.
- Warning devices are used on beds, chairs, and doors.
- Knob guards are used on doors.
- Padded hip protectors are worn under clothing (Fig. 9-1).
- Floor cushions are placed next to beds (Fig. 9-2).
- Roll guards are attached to the bed frame (Fig. 9-3).
- Falls are prevented.
- The person's furniture meets his or her needs (lower bed, reclining chair, rocking chair).
- Walls and furniture corners are padded.
- Observations and visits are made at least every 15 minutes.
- The person is moved closer to the nurses' station.
- Procedures and care measures are explained.
- Frequent explanations are given about required equipment or devices.
- Persons who are confused are oriented to person, time, and place. Calendars and clocks are provided.
- Light is adjusted to meet the person's needs and preferences.
- Staff assignments are consistent.
- Uninterrupted sleep is promoted.
- Noise levels are reduced.

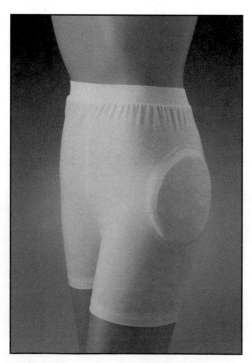

FIG. **9-1** Hip protector. (Courtesy JT Posey Co., Arcadia, Calif.)

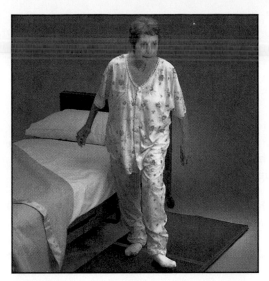

FIG. **9-2** Floor cushion. (Courtesy JT Posey Co., Arcadia, Calif.)

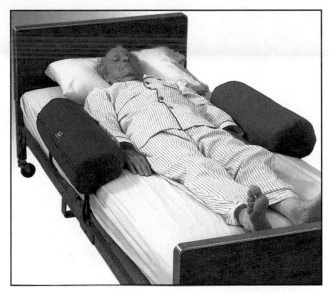

FIG. **9-3** Roll guard. (Courtesy JT Posey Co., Arcadia, Calif.)

SAFE RESTRAINT USE

Restraints can cause serious injury and even death. They are not used to discipline a person or for staff convenience. *Discipline* is any action that punishes or penalizes a person. *Convenience* is any action that:

- Controls the person's behavior
- Requires less effort by the center
- Is not in the person's best interests

Restraints are used only when necessary to treat a person's medical symptoms. Symptoms may be physical, emotional, or behavioral. Sometimes restraints are needed to protect the person or others. That is, a person may behave in ways that are harmful to self or others.

Imagine being restrained:

- Your nose itches. But your hands and arms are restrained. You cannot scratch your nose.
- You need to use the bathroom. Your hands and arms are restrained. You cannot get up. You cannot reach your signal light. You soil yourself with urine or a bowel movement.
- Your phone is ringing. You cannot answer it because your hands and arms are restrained.
- You are thirsty. You cannot reach the water glass because your wrists are restrained.
- You hear the fire alarm. You have on a restraint. You cannot move to a safe place. You must wait until someone rescues you.

What would you try to do? Would you calmly lie or sit there? Would you try to get free from the restraint? Would you cry out for help? What would the nursing staff think? Would they think that you are uncomfortable? Or would they think that you are agitated and uncooperative? Would they think your behavior is improving or getting worse? Would you feel anger, embarrassment, or humiliation?

Put yourself in the person's situation. That will help you understand how the person feels. Treat the person like you would want to be treated—with kindness, caring, respect, and dignity.

Physical and Drug Restraints

According to OBRA and CMS, *physical restraints* include these points:

- May be any manual method, physical or mechanical device, material, or equipment
- Is attached to or next to the person's body
- Cannot be easily removed by the person
- Restricts freedom of movement or access to one's body

Physical restraints are applied to the chest, waist, elbows, wrists, hands, or ankles. They confine the person to a bed or chair. Or they prevent movement of a body part. Some furniture or barriers also prevent free movement.

- Geriatric chairs (Geri-chairs) or chairs with attached trays (Fig. 9-4, p. 110). Such chairs are often used for persons needing support to sit up.
- Placing any chair so close to a wall that the person cannot move.
- Bed rails (Chapter 8).
- Sheets tucked in so tightly that they restrict movement.

Drugs are restraints if they:

- Control behavior or restrict movement
- Are not standard treatment for the person's condition

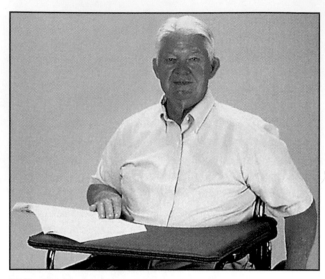

FIG. 9-4 This lap-top tray is a restraint alternative. It is considered a restraint when used to prevent freedom of movement. (Courtesy JT Posey Co., Arcadia, Calif.)

Sometimes drugs can help persons who are confused or disoriented. They may become anxious, agitated, or aggressive. The doctor may order drugs to control these behaviors. The goal is to control the behavior. The drug should not make the person sleepy and unable to function at his or her highest level.

Complications of Restraint Use

Box 9-1 lists complications from restraints. Injuries occur as the person tries to get free of the restraint. Injuries also occur from using the wrong restraint, applying it wrong, or keeping it on too long. Cuts, bruises, and fractures are common. *The most serious risk is death from strangulation.*

There are also mental effects. Restraints affect dignity and self-esteem. Depression, anger, and agitation are common. So are embarrassment, humiliation, and mistrust.

Restraints are medical devices. The Safe Medical Device Act applies if a restraint causes illness, injury, or death. Also, CMS requires the reporting of any death that occurs while a person is in restraints.

Legal Aspects

If a restraint is used, the least restrictive method is used. Used for protection, it allows the greatest amount of movement or body access possible. Remember the following:

- *Restraints must protect the person. They are not used for staff convenience or to discipline a person.* Restraining someone is not easier than properly supervising and observing the person. A restrained person requires more staff time for care, supervision, and observation.
- *A written doctor's order is required.* The doctor gives the reason for the restraint, what body part to restrain, what to use, and how long to use it. This information is on the care plan and your assignment sheet.
- *The least restrictive method is used.* An **active physical restraint** attaches to the person's body and to a fixed (non-movable) object. It restricts movement or body access. Vest, jacket, ankle, wrist, hand, and some belt restraints are active physical restraints. A **passive physical restraint** is near, but not directly attached to, the person's body (bed rails or wedge cushions). It does not totally restrict freedom of movement. It allows access to certain body parts. Passive physical restraints are the least restrictive.
- *Restraints are used only after other measures fail to protect the person* (see Box 9-2). Some people can harm themselves or others. The care plan must include measures to protect the person and prevent harm to others. See fall prevention measures in Chapter 8.
- *Unnecessary restraint is false imprisonment* (Chapter 2). You must clearly understand why a restraint is needed. If not, politely ask about its use. If you apply an unneeded restraint, you could face false imprisonment charges.
- *Informed consent is required.* Restraints cannot be used without consent. The person must understand the reason for the restraint and its risks. If unable to give informed consent, the person's legal representative is given the information. The doctor or nurse provides the necessary information and obtains the consent.

Safety Guidelines

The restrained person must be kept safe. Follow the safety measures in Box 9-3. Also remember these key points:

- *Observe for increased confusion and agitation.* Restraint use can increase confusion and agitation. Whether confused or alert, people are aware of restricted movements. They may try to get out of the restraint or struggle or pull at it. Some restrained persons beg others to free or to help release them. These behaviors often are viewed as signs of confusion. Some people become more confused because they do not understand what is happening to them. Restrained persons need repeated explanations and reassurance. Spending time with them has a calming effect.

■ *Protect the person's quality of life.* Restraints are used for as short a time as possible. The care plan must show how to reduce restraint use. The person's needs are met with as little restraint as possible. You must meet the person's physical and psychosocial needs. Visit with the person and explain the reason for restraints.

■ *Follow the manufacturer's instructions.* They explain how to apply and secure the restraint for the person's safety. The restraint must be snug, but not tight. Tight restraints affect circulation and breathing. The person must be comfortable and able to move the restrained part to a limited and safe extent. You could be negligent for improperly applying or securing a restraint.

■ *Apply restraints with enough help to protect the person and staff from injury.* Combative and agitated people can hurt themselves and the staff when restraints are applied. Enough staff members are needed to complete the task safely and quickly.

■ *Observe the person at least every 15 minutes or more often as required by the care plan.* Restraints are dangerous. Injuries and deaths can result from improper restraint use and poor observation. Prevent complications. Interferences with breathing and circulation are examples.

■ *Remove the restraint, reposition the person, and meet basic needs at least every 2 hours.* This includes food, fluid, comfort, safety, hygiene, and elimination needs and giving skin care. Perform range-of-motion exercises (Chapter 20) or help the person walk. Follow the care plan.

Text continued on p. 115

BOX 9-3   Safety Measures For Using Restraints

- Use the restraint noted in the care plan. Use the correct size.
- Apply a restraint only after being instructed about its proper use.
- Demonstrate proper application of the restraint to the nurse before applying it.
- Use only restraints that have manufacturer instructions and warning labels.
- Read the manufacturer's warning labels. Note the front and back of the restraint.
- Follow the manufacturer's instructions. Some restraints are safe for bed, chair, and wheelchair use. Others are used only with certain equipment.
- Do not use sheets, towels, tape, rope, straps, bandages, or other items to restrain a person.
- Use intact restraints. Look for tears, cuts, or frayed fabric or straps. Look for missing or loose hooks, loops, or straps, or other damage.
- Do not use restraints to position a person on a toilet.
- Do not use restraints to position a person on furniture that does not allow for correct application. Follow the manufacturer's instructions.
- Follow agency policies and procedures.
- Position the person in good alignment before applying the restraint.
- Pad bony areas and skin. This prevents pressure and injury from the restraint.
- Secure the restraint. It should be snug but allow some movement of the restrained part.
- Follow the manufacturer's instructions to check for snugness. For example:
  - If applied to the chest or waist—Make sure that the person can breathe easily. A flat hand should slide between the restraint and the person's body (Fig. 9-5, p. 112).
  - For wrist and mitt restraints—You should be able to slide 1 or 2 fingers under the restraint.

- Criss-cross vest restraints in front (Fig. 9-6, p. 112). Do not criss-cross restraints in the back unless part of the manufacturer's instructions (Fig. 9-7, p. 113). Criss-crossing vests in the back can cause death from strangulation.
- Tie restraints according to agency policy. The policy should follow the manufacturer's instructions. Quick-release buckles or air-line type buckles are used (Fig. 9-8, p. 113). So are quick-release ties (Fig. 9-9, p. 113).
- Secure straps out of the person's reach.
- Leave 1 to 2 inches of slack in the straps. This allows some movement of the part.
- Secure the restraint to the movable part of the bed frame at waist level (see Fig. 9-9). For chairs, secure straps to the wheelchair or the chair frame (Fig. 9-10, p. 113).
- Make sure that straps will not slide in any direction. If straps slide, they change the restraint's position. The person can get suspended off the mattress or chair (Fig. 9-11, p. 113 and Fig. 9-12, p. 114). Strangulation can result.
- Never secure restraints to the bed rails. The person can reach bed rails to release knots or buckles. Also, injury to the person is likely when raising or lowering bed rails.
- Use bed rail covers or gap protectors according to the nurse's instructions (Fig. 9-13, p. 114). They prevent entrapment between the rails or the bed rail bars (see Fig. 9-11). Entrapment can occur between:
  - The bars of a bed rail
  - The space between half-length (split) bed rails
  - The bed rail and mattress
  - The headboard or footboard and mattress

Continued

BOX 9-3	Safety Measures For Using Restraints—cont'd

- Keep full bed rails up when using a vest, jacket, or belt restraint. Also use bed rail covers or gap protectors. Otherwise the person could fall off the bed and strangle on the restraint. If half-length bed rails are used, the person can get caught between them.
- Position the person in semi-Fowler's position when using a vest, jacket, or belt restraint.
- Position the person in a chair so the hips are well to the back of the chair.
- Apply a belt restraint at a 45-degree angle over the hips (Fig. 9-14, p. 115).
- Do not use back cushions when a person is restrained in a chair. If the cushion moves out of place, slack occurs in the straps. Strangulation could result if the person slides forward or down from the extra slack (see Fig. 9-12).
- Do not cover the restraint with a sheet, blanket, bedspread, or other covering. The restraint must be within plain view at all times.
- Check the person's circulation at least every 15 minutes for safety and comfort. You should feel a pulse at a pulse site below the restraint. Fingers or toes should be warm and pink. Tell the nurse at once if:
  - You cannot feel a pulse
  - Fingers or toes are cold, pale, or blue in color
  - The person complains of pain, numbness, or tingling in the restrained part
  - The skin is red or damaged
- Check the person at least every 15 minutes if a belt, jacket, or vest restraint is used. The person should be able to breathe easily. Also check the position of the restraint, especially in the front and back.

- Monitor persons in the supine position constantly. They are at great risk for aspiration if vomiting occurs (Chapter 17). Call for the nurse at once.
- Do not use a restraint near a fire, a flame, or smoking materials. Restraint fabrics may ignite easily.
- Keep scissors in your pocket. In an emergency, cutting the tie may be faster than untying the knot. Never leave scissors at the bedside or where the person can reach them.
- Remove the restraint and reposition the person every 2 hours. Meet the person's basic needs. You need to:
  - Meet elimination needs.
  - Offer food and fluids.
  - Meet hygiene needs.
  - Give skin care.
  - Perform range-of-motion exercises or help the person walk. Follow the care plan.
  - Provide for comfort. (See the inside of the front book cover.)
  - Chart what was done, the care given, your observations, and when and what you reported to the nurse.
- Keep the signal light within the person's reach. (Chart that this was done.)
- Complete a safety check before leaving the room. (See the inside of the front book cover.)
- Report to the nurse every time you checked the person and released the restraint. Report your observations and the care given. Follow agency policy for recording.

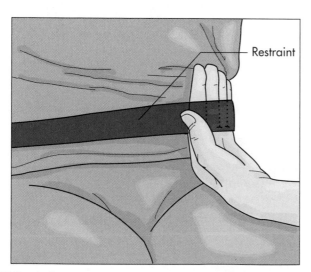

FIG. **9-5** A flat hand slides between the restraint and the person.

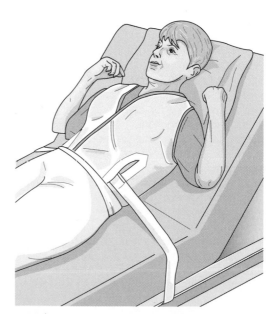

FIG. **9-6** Vest restraint criss-crosses in front. (NOTE: The bed rails are raised after the restraint is applied.)

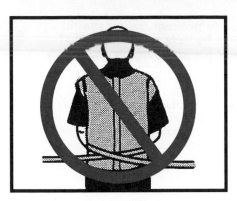

FIG. **9-7** Never criss-cross vest or jacket straps in back. (Courtesy JT Posey Co., Arcadia, Calif.)

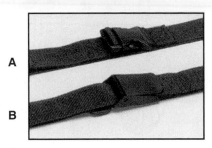

FIG. **9-8** **A,** Quick-release buckle. **B,** Airline-type buckle. (Courtesy JT Posey Co., Arcadia, Calif.)

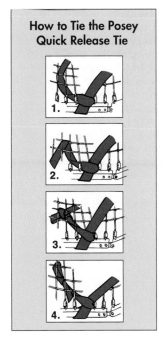

FIG. **9-9** The Posey quick-release tie. (Courtesy JT Posey Co., Arcadia, Calif.)

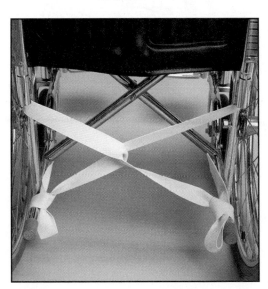

FIG. **9-10** The restraint straps are secured to the wheelchair frame with quick-release ties. (Courtesy JT Posey Co., Arcadia, Calif.)

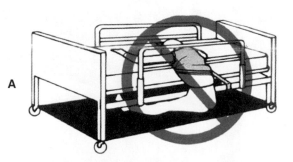

FIG. **9-11** **A,** A person can get suspended and caught between bed rail bars. **B,** The person can get suspended and caught between half-length bed rails. (Courtesy JT Posey Co., Arcadia, Calif.)

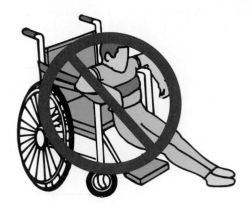

Straps to prevent sliding should always be over the thighs—NOT around the waist or chest. Straps should be at a 45 angle and secured to the chair under the seat, not behind the back. They should be snug but comfortable and not restrict breathing. If a belt or vest is too loose or applied around the waist, the person may slide partially off the seat—resulting in possible suffocation and death.

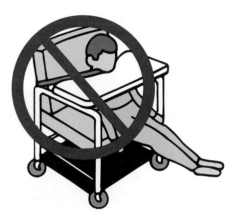

Tray tables (with or without a belt or vest) pose potential danger if the person should slide partly under the table and become caught. This could result in suffocation and death. Make sure the person's hips are positioned at the back of the chair—this may necessitate the use of an anti-slide material (Posey Grip), a pommel cushion, or a restrictive device if the person shows any tendency to slide forward.

FIG. **9-12** Strangulation could result if the person slides forward or down because of extra slack in the restraint. (Courtesy JT Posey Co., Arcadia, Calif.)

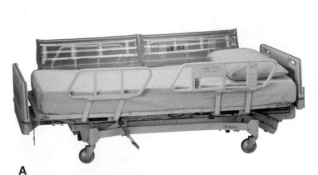

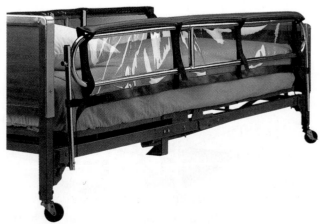

A

B

FIG. **9-13** **A,** Side rail protector. **B,** Guard rail pads. (Courtesy JT Posey Co., Arcadia, Calif.)

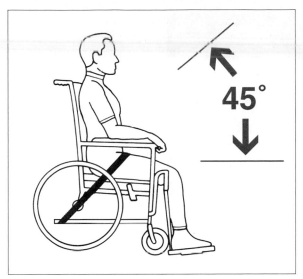

FIG. **9-14** The safety belt is at a 45-degree angle over the hips. (Courtesy JT Posey Co., Arcadia, Calif.)

Reporting and Recording

You might apply restraints or care for a restrained person. Report the following to the nurse. If you are allowed to chart, include this information:

- The type of restraint applied
- The body part or parts restrained
- The reason for the application
- Safety measures taken (for example, bed rails padded and up)
- The time you applied the restraint
- The time you removed the restraint
- The care given when the restraint was removed
- Skin color and condition
- The pulse felt in the restrained part
- Changes in the person's behavior
- Complaints of a tight restraint; difficulty breathing; and pain, numbness, or tingling in the restrained part (Report these complaints to the nurse at once.)

Applying Restraints

Restraints are made of cloth or leather. Cloth restraints are mitts, belts, straps, jackets, and vests. They are applied to the wrists, ankles, hands, waist, and chest. Leather restraints are applied to the wrists and ankles. They are used for extreme agitation and combativeness.

See Persons with Dementia: Applying Restraints.

Persons With Dementia

Applying Restraints

Restraints may increase confusion and agitation in persons with dementia. They do not understand what you are doing. They may resist your efforts to apply a restraint. They may actively try to get free from the restraint. Serious injury and death are risks.

Never use force to apply a restraint. If a person is confused or agitated, ask a co-worker to help apply the restraint. Report problems to the nurse at once.

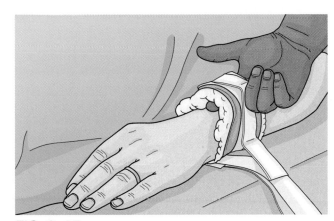

FIG. **9-15** Wrist restraint. The soft part is toward the skin. Note that 1 finger fits between the restraint and the wrist.

Wrist Restraints

Wrist restraints (limb holders) limit arm movement (Fig. 9-15). They may be used when a person continually tries to pull out tubes used for treatment (IV, feeding tube, catheter, or wound drainage tubes). Or the person tries to scratch, pick at, pull at, or peel the skin, a wound, or a dressing. This can damage the skin or the wound.

Mitt Restraints

Hands are placed in mitt restraints. They prevent finger use. They do not prevent hand, wrist, or arm movements. They are used for the same reasons as wrist restraints. Most mitts are padded (Fig. 9-16, p. 116).

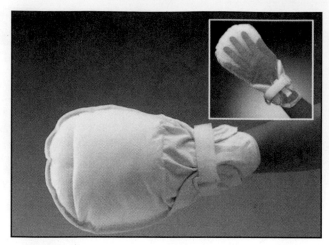

FIG. **9-16** Mitt restraint. (Courtesy JT Posey Co., Arcadia, Calif.)

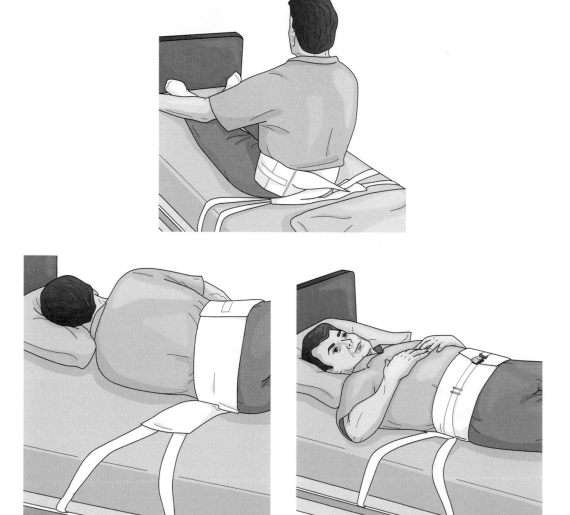

FIG. **9-17** Belt restraint. (NOTE: The bed rails are raised after the restraint is applied.)

Belt Restraints

The belt restraint (Fig. 9-17) is used when injuries from falls are risks. The person cannot get out of bed or out of a chair. However, the person can turn from side to side or sit up in bed.

The belt is applied around the waist and secured to the bed or chair. It is applied over a garment. The person can release the quick-release type. It is less restrictive than those that only staff members can release.

Vest Restraints and Jacket Restraints

Vest and jacket restraints are applied to the chest. They may be used to prevent injuries from falls. And they may be used for persons who need positioning for a medical treatment. The person cannot turn in bed or get out of bed or a chair.

A jacket restraint is applied with the opening in the back. For a vest restraint, the vest crosses in front (see Fig. 9-6). *The straps of vest and jacket restraints always cross in the front.* They must *never* cross in the back. Vest and jacket restraints are never worn backwards. Strangulation or other injury could occur if the person slides down in the bed or chair. The restraint is always applied over a garment. *(NOTE: A vest or jacket restraint may have a positioning slot in the back. Criss-cross the straps according to the manufacturer's instructions.)*

Vest and jacket restraints have life-threatening risks. Death can occur from strangulation. If the person gets caught in the restraint, it can become so tight that the person's chest cannot expand to inhale air. The person quickly suffocates and dies. Restraints must be applied correctly. For vest and jacket restraints, this is critical. You are advised to only assist the nurse in applying them. The nurse should assume full responsibility for applying a vest or jacket restraint.

DELEGATION GUIDELINES
Applying Restraints

Before applying a restraint, you need this information from the nurse and the care plan:
- Why the doctor ordered the restraint
- What type and size to use
- Where to apply the restraint
- How to safely apply the restraint (Have the nurse show you how to apply it. Then demonstrate correct application back to the nurse.)
- How to correctly position the person
- What bony areas to pad and how to pad them
- If bed rail covers or gap protectors are needed
- If bed rails are up or down
- What special equipment is needed
- If the person needs to be checked more often than every 15 minutes
- When to apply and release the restraint
- What observations to report and record, p. 115

PROMOTING SAFETY AND COMFORT
Applying Restraints

Safety

Restraints can cause serious harm, even death. Always follow the manufacturer's instructions. Manufacturers have many types of restraints. The instructions for one type may not apply to another. Also, the manufacturer may have specific instructions when applying restraints to persons who are agitated.

Never use force to apply a restraint. Always ask a co-worker to help apply a restraint to a person who is confused and agitated. Report any problems to the nurse at once.

Check the person at least every 15 minutes or more often as instructed by the nurse and the care plan. Make sure the signal light is within reach. Ask the person to use the signal light at the first sign of problems or discomfort.

Comfort

The person's comfort is always important. It is more so when restraints are used. Remember, restraints limit the person's ability to move. This affects position changes and the ability to reach needed items. Always make sure the person is in good alignment before applying a restraint (Chapter 11). Also make sure the person can reach needed items—water, tissues, phone, bed controls, and so on.

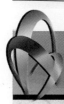

Applying Restraints

Quality of Life

Remember to:

- Knock before entering the person's room
- Address the person by name
- Introduce yourself by name and title
- Explain the procedure to the person before beginning and during the procedure
- Protect the person's rights during the procedure
- Handle the person gently during the procedure

Pre-Procedure

1 Follow *Delegation Guidelines: Applying Restraints*, p. 117. See *Promoting Safety and Comfort: Applying Restraints*, p. 117.
2 Collect the following as instructed by the nurse:
  - Correct type and size of restraints
  - Padding for bony areas
  - Bed rail pads or gap protectors (if needed)

3 Practice hand hygiene.
4 Identify the person. Check the ID bracelet against the assignment sheet. Call the person by name.
5 Provide for privacy.

Procedure

6 Make sure the person is comfortable and in good alignment.
7 Put the bed rail pads or gap protectors on the bed if the person is in bed, if needed. Follow the manufacturer's instructions.
8 Pad bony areas. Follow the nurse's instructions and the care plan.
9 Read the manufacturer's instructions. Note the front and back of the restraint.
10 *For wrist restraints:*
  a Apply the restraint according to the manufacturer's instructions. Place the soft part toward the skin.
  b Secure the restraint so it is snug but not tight. Make sure you can slide 1or 2 fingers under the restraint (see Fig. 9-15). Follow the manufacturer's instructions. Adjust the straps if the restraint is too loose or too tight. Check for snugness again.
  c Tie the straps to the movable part of the bed frame out of the person's reach. Use an agency-approved tie. Leave 1 to 2 inches of slack in the straps.
  d Repeat steps 10 a, b, and c for the other wrist.
11 *For mitt restraints:*
  a Make sure the person's hands are clean and dry.
  b Apply the mitt restraint. Follow the manufacturer's instructions.

  c Tie the straps to the movable part of the bed frame. Use an agency-approved tie. Leave 1 to 2 inches of slack in the straps.
  d Make sure the restraint is snug. Slide 1 or 2 fingers between the restraint and the wrist. Follow the manufacturer's instructions. Adjust the straps if the restraint is too loose or too tight. Check for snugness again.
  e Repeat steps 11 b, c, and d for the other hand.
12 *For a belt restraint:*
  a Assist the person to a sitting position.
  b Apply the restraint with your free hand. Follow the manufacturer's instructions.
  c Remove wrinkles or creases from the front and back of the restraint.
  d Bring the ties through the slots in the belt.
  e Help the person lie down if he or she is in bed.
  f Make sure the person is comfortable and in good alignment.
  g Secure the straps to the movable part of the bed frame out of the person's reach or to the chair or wheelchair. Use an agency-approved tie. Leave 1 to 2 inches of slack in the straps.
  h Make sure the belt is snug. Slide an open hand between the restraint and the person. Adjust the restraint if it is too loose or too tight. Check for snugness again.

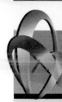

Applying Restraints—cont'd

Procedure—cont'd

13 *For a vest restraint:*
   a Assist the person to a sitting position.
   b Apply the restraint with your free hand. Follow the manufacturer's instructions. The "V" part of the vest crosses in front.
   c Make sure the vest is free of wrinkles in the front and back.
   d Help the person lie down if he or she is in bed.
   e Bring the straps through the slots.
   f Make sure the person is comfortable and in good alignment.
   g Secure the straps to the chair or to the movable part of the bed frame. If secured to the bed frame, the straps are secured at waist level out of the person's reach. Use an agency-approved tie. Leave 1 to 2 inches of slack in the straps.
   h Make sure the vest is snug. Slide an open hand between the restraint and the person. Adjust the restraint if it is too loose or too tight. Check for snugness again.

14 *For a jacket restraint:*
   a Assist the person to a sitting position.
   b Apply the restraint with your free hand. Follow the manufacturer's instructions. Remember, the jacket opening goes in the back.
   c Close the back with the zipper, ties, or hook and loop closures.
   d Make sure the side seams are under the arms. Remove any wrinkles in the front and back.
   e Help the person lie down if he or she is in bed.
   f Make sure the person is comfortable and in good alignment.
   g Secure the straps to the chair or to the movable part of the bed frame. If secured to the bed frame, the straps are secured at waist level out of the person's reach. Use an agency-approved knot. Leave 1 to 2 inches of slack in the straps.
   h Make sure the jacket is snug. Slide an open hand between the restraint and the person. Adjust the restraint if it is too loose or too tight. Check for snugness again.

Post-Procedure

15 Position the person as the nurse directs.
16 Provide for comfort. (See the inside of the front book cover.)
17 Place the signal light within the person's reach.
18 Raise or lower bed rails. Follow the care plan and the manufacturer's instructions for the restraint.
19 Unscreen the person.
20 Complete a safety check of the room. (See the inside of the front book cover.)
21 Decontaminate your hands.
22 Check the person and the restraints at least every 15 minutes. Report and record your observations.
   a For wrist and mitt restraints: check the pulse, color, and temperature of the restrained parts.
   b For vest, jacket, and belt restraints: check the person's breathing. *Call for the nurse at once if the person is not breathing or is having problems breathing.* Make sure the restraint is properly positioned in the front and back.

23 Do the following at least every 2 hours:
   • Remove the restraint.
   • Reposition the person.
   • Meet food, fluid, hygiene, and elimination needs.
   • Give skin care.
   • Perform range-of-motion exercises or help the person walk. Follow the care plan.
   • Provide for comfort. (See the inside of the front book cover.)
   • Reapply the restraints.
24 Complete a safety check of the room. (See the inside of the front book cover.)
25 Report and record your observations and the care given.

FOCUS ON THE PERSON

Patients and residents fear being restrained. They do not want to be "tied down." State and federal laws allow restraints only if medically necessary. When restraints are needed, the entire health team must focus on meeting the person's basic needs.

See Focus on the Person: Restraint Alternatives and Safe Restraint Use.

Focus on the PERSON

Restraint Alternatives and Safe Restraint Use

Providing comfort—The person's comfort is always important. It is especially so when the person is restrained. The person must be in good alignment and in a comfortable position. The restraint must allow for some movement. It must be snug, not tight. If tight, the restraint can interfere with breathing and circulation. Also make sure that any needed items are within the person's reach.

The signal light must also be within the person's reach. This is a safety measure. However, it also promotes physical and mental comfort. It promotes physical comfort because the person knows that he or she can call for help. Being able to call for help promotes mental comfort. The person needs to feel safe and secure.

Safety and security needs also relate to knowing what is happening and why. The nurse explains the reason for the restraint to the person. You need to remind the person why the restraint is needed. When applying restraints, always explain what you are going to do. Tell the person what you are doing step-by-step.

Ethical behavior—You must report exactly what you see, what you do, and what the person says. Do not omit or add wrong information. Doing so could lead the nurse to make wrong judgments. The nurse could ask the doctor to order restraints when they are not needed. Or the reverse could occur—the nurse does not ask for a restraint order when it is needed. Negligence occurs when unethical behavior causes the person harm.

Remaining independent—Mitt and hand restraints limit hand and arm use. Belt, vest, and jacket restraints allow hand and arm use. Make sure needed items are within the person's reach. Water, tissues, and bed and TV controls are examples.

Restraints are removed at least every 2 hours. Food, fluid, hygiene, and elimination needs are met. The person walks or range-of-motion exercises are done. Let the person do as much for himself or herself as safely possible. Also give the person choices. For example, let the person choose if he or she will use the bathroom first or walk first. Let the person choose where to walk and what to eat and drink. Allow choices that are safe for the person. Remember, personal choices promote independence, dignity, and self-esteem.

Speaking up—You may not know the reason for a restraint. If so, politely ask the nurse why it is needed. For example:
- "Why does Mr. Reed need a restraint?"
- "I don't understand. Why did the doctor order the restraint?"

Restraints can increase confusion. Remind the person why the restraint is needed and to call for help when it is needed. Repeat the following as often as needed:
- "Dr. Harris ordered this restraint for you so you don't fall. It will keep you in your wheelchair. If you need to get up, please call for help. I will check on you every 15 minutes. Other staff will check on you too."
- "How does the restraint feel? Is it too tight? Is it too loose?"
- "Please put your signal light on. I want to make sure that you can reach and use it with the restraints on."
- "Please call for help right away if the restraint is tight."
- "Please call for help right away if you feel pain in your fingers or hands. Also call for me if you feel numbness or tingling."
- "Please call for help right away if you are having problems breathing."

OBRA and other laws—Like OSHA, the Centers for Medicare and Medicaid Services (CMS) and the Food and Drug Administration (FDA) have the power to issue rules and regulations. They have rules and regulations for safe restraint use. Agency policies and procedures must include such rules and regulations. The agency can be fined if they are not followed.

Nursing teamwork—You may not be assigned to a restrained person. However, you still must help the nursing team keep the person safe. Make sure you know who is restrained on your unit. Every time you walk past the person or the person's room, check to see if the person is safe and comfortable.

REVIEW QUESTIONS

Circle **T** if the statement is true and **F** if the statement is false.

1 **T F** Restraint alternatives fail to protect a person. The nurse can order a restraint.
2 **T F** Restraints can be used for staff convenience.
3 **T F** A device is a restraint only if it is attached to the person's body.
4 **T F** Bed rails are restraints.
5 **T F** Restraints are used only for specific medical symptoms.
6 **T F** Restraints can be used to protect the person from harming others.
7 **T F** Unnecessary restraint is false imprisonment.
8 **T F** Informed consent is needed for restraint use.
9 **T F** You can apply restraints when you think they are needed.
10 **T F** Restraint straps are secured within the person's reach.
11 **T F** You can use a vest restraint to position a person on the toilet.
12 **T F** Restraints are removed every 2 hours to reposition the person and give skin care.
13 **T F** Restraint straps are tied to bed rails.
14 **T F** A vest restraint crosses in front.
15 **T F** Bed rails are left down when vest restraints are used.

Circle the **BEST** answer.

16 These statements are about restraints. Which is *false*?
   a A restraint can be an object, device, garment, or material.
   b A restraint limits or restricts a person's movement.
   c Some drugs are restraints.
   d A restraint is used when the nurse thinks it is needed.

17 Which is *not* a restraint alternative?
   a Positioning the person's chair close to a wall
   b Answering signal lights promptly
   c Taking the person outside in nice weather
   d Padding walls and corners of furniture

18 Physical restraints
   a Control mental function
   b Control a behavior
   c Confine a person to a bed or chair
   d Decrease care needs

19 The following can occur because of restraints. Which is the *most* serious?
   a Fractures
   b Strangulation
   c Pressure ulcers
   d Urinary tract infection

20 A belt restraint is applied to a person in bed. Where should you tie the straps?
   a To the bed rails
   b To the headboard
   c To the movable part of the bed frame
   d To the footboard

21 Mrs. Hall has a restraint. You should check her and the position of the restraint at least
   a Every 15 minutes
   b Every 30 minutes
   c Every hour
   d Every 2 hours

22 Mrs. Hall has mitt restraints. Which of these is especially important to report to the nurse?
   a Her heart rate
   b Her respiratory rate
   c Why the restraints were applied
   d If you felt a pulse in the restrained extremities

23 Which are *not* used to prevent falls?
   a Wrist restraints
   b Jacket restraints
   c Belt restraints
   d Vest restraints

24 The doctor ordered mitt restraints for Mrs. Hall. You need the following information from the nurse *except*
   a What size to use
   b What other equipment is needed
   c What drugs Mrs. Hall is taking
   d When to apply and release the restraints

25 A person has a vest restraint. It is not too tight or too loose if you can slide
   a A fist between the vest and the person
   b One finger between the vest and the person
   c An open hand between the vest and the person
   d Two fingers between the vest and the person

26 The correct way to apply any restraint is to follow the
   a Nurse's directions
   b Doctor's orders
   c Care plan
   d Manufacturer's instructions

Answers to these questions are on page 468.

10

Preventing Infection

OBJECTIVES

- Define the key terms listed in this chapter
- Identify what microbes need to live and grow
- List the signs and symptoms of infection
- Explain the chain of infection
- Describe the practices of medical asepsis
- Describe disinfection and sterilization methods
- Explain how to care for equipment and supplies
- Explain Isolation Precautions
- Describe Standard Precautions and the Bloodborne Pathogen Standard
- Perform the procedures described in this chapter

PROCEDURES

Procedures with this icon 💿 *are also on the CD-ROM in this book.*

💿 Hand Washing
- Removing Gloves
- Donning and Removing a Gown
- Donning and Removing a Mask

KEY TERMS

asepsis Being free of disease-producing microbes

biohazardous waste Items contaminated with blood, body fluids, secretions, or excretions; *bio* means life, and *hazardous* means dangerous or harmful

carrier A human or animal that is a reservoir for microbes but does not have signs and symptoms of infection

clean technique Medical asepsis

communicable disease A disease caused by pathogens that spread easily; a contagious disease

contagious disease Communicable disease

contamination The process of becoming unclean

disinfection The process of destroying pathogens

infection A disease resulting from the invasion and growth of microbes in the body

medical asepsis Practices used to remove or destroy pathogens and to prevent their spread from one person or place to another person or place; clean technique

microbe A microorganism

microorganism A small (*micro*) living plant or animal (*organism*) seen only with a microscope; a microbe

non-pathogen A microbe that does not usually cause an infection

pathogen A microbe that is harmful and can cause an infection

sterile The absence of *all* microbes

sterilization The process of destroying *all* microbes

Infection is a major safety and health hazard. Minor infections cause short illnesses. Some infections are serious and can cause death. Older and disabled persons are at risk. The health team protects patients, residents, visitors, and themselves from infection.

MICROORGANISMS

A **microorganism (microbe)** is a small (*micro*) living plant or animal (*organism*). It is seen only with a microscope. Microbes are everywhere. They are in the mouth, nose, respiratory tract, stomach, intestines, and on the skin. They are in the air, soil, water, and food. They are on animals, clothing, and furniture.

Some microbes are harmful and can cause infections. They are called **pathogens. Non-pathogens** are microbes that do not usually cause an infection.

Microbes need a *reservoir (host)* to live and grow. The reservoir is where the microbe lives and grows. People, plants, animals, the soil, food, and water are common reservoirs. Microbes need *water* and *nourishment* from the reservoir. Most need *oxygen* to

live. A *warm* and *dark* environment is needed. Most grow best at body temperature. They are destroyed by heat and light.

Multidrug–Resistant Organisms

Multidrug–resistant organisms (MDROs) can resist the effects of antibiotics. Antibiotics are drugs that kill microbes that cause infections. Some microbes can change their structures. This makes them more difficult to kill. They can survive in the presence of antibiotics. Therefore the infections they cause are hard to treat. MDROs are caused by doctors prescribing antibiotics when they are not needed (over-prescribing). Not taking antibiotics for the length of time prescribed also is a cause.

Two common types of MDROs are resistant to many antibiotics:

■ *Methicillin-resistant Staphylococcus aureus (MRSA). Staphylococcus aureus* (commonly called "staph") is normally found in the nose and on the skin. It can cause serious wound infections and pneumonia.

■ *Vancomycin-resistant Enterococcus (VRE). Enterococcus* is normally found in the intestines and in feces. It can be transmitted to others by contaminated hands, toilet seats, care equipment, and other items that the hands touch. When not in its natural site (the intestines), it can cause an infection. It can cause urinary tract, wound, pelvic, and other infections.

INFECTION

An **infection** is a disease resulting from the invasion and growth of microbes in the body. A *local infection* is in a body part. A *systemic infection* involves the whole body. (Systemic means entire.) The person has some or all of the following signs and symptoms:

■ Fever

■ Increased pulse and respiratory rates

■ Pain or tenderness

■ Fatigue

■ Loss of appetite

■ Nausea and vomiting

■ Redness and swelling

■ Discharge or drainage from the infected area

The chain of infection (Fig. 10-1, p. 124) is a process. It begins with a *source*—a pathogen. The pathogen must have a *reservoir* where it can grow and multiply. Humans and animals are common reservoirs. If they do not have signs and symptoms of infection, they are **carriers.** Carriers can pass the pathogen to others. The pathogen must leave the reservoir. That is, it needs a *portal of exit*. Exits are the respiratory, gastrointestinal, urinary, and reproductive tracts, breaks in the skin, and the blood.

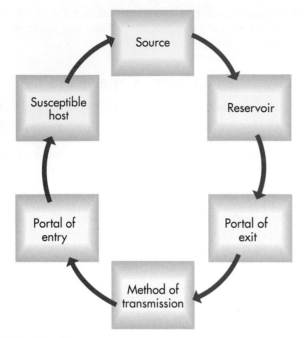

FIG. **10-1** The chain of infection. (Redrawn from Potter PA, Perry AG: *Fundamentals of nursing: concepts, process, and practice*, ed 6, St Louis, 2005, Mosby.)

After leaving the reservoir, the pathogen must be *transmitted* to another host (Fig. 10-2). The pathogen enters the body through a *portal of entry*. Portals of entry and exit are the same. A *susceptible host* (a person at risk for infection) is needed for the microbe to grow and multiply.

The human body can protect itself from infection. The ability to resist infection relates to age, nutrition, stress, fatigue, and health. Drugs, disease, and injury also are factors.

Infection in Older Persons

The immune system protects against disease and infection (Chapter 6). Changes occur in the immune system with aging. Older persons may not show the signs and symptoms of infection (p. 123). They may have only a slight fever or no fever at all. They may not complain of pain. Redness and swelling may be very slight. Confusion and delirium may occur (Chapter 25).

An infection can become life-threatening before the older person has obvious signs and symptoms. Stay alert to the most minor changes in a person's behavior or condition. Report any concerns to the nurse at once.

MEDICAL ASEPSIS

Asepsis is being free of disease-producing microbes. Microbes are everywhere. Measures are needed to achieve asepsis. **Medical asepsis (clean technique)** is the practices used to:

- Remove or destroy pathogens. The number of pathogens is reduced.
- Prevent pathogens from spreading from one person or place to another person or place.

Contamination is the process of becoming unclean. In medical asepsis, an item or area is *clean* when it is free of pathogens. The item or area is contaminated if pathogens are present. A sterile item or area is contaminated when pathogens or non-pathogens are present. **Sterile** means the absence of *all* microbes—pathogens and non-pathogens.

Common Aseptic Practices

Aseptic practices break the chain of infection. To prevent the spread of microbes, wash your hands:

- After urinating or having a bowel movement.
- After changing tampons or sanitary pads.
- After contact with your own or another person's blood, body fluids, secretions, or excretions. This includes saliva, vomitus, urine, feces, vaginal discharge, mucus, semen, wound drainage, pus, and respiratory secretions.
- After coughing, sneezing, or blowing your nose.
- Before and after handling, preparing, or eating food.

Also do the following:

- Provide all persons with their own linens and personal care items.
- Cover your nose and mouth when coughing, sneezing, or blowing your nose.
- Bathe, wash hair, and brush your teeth regularly.
- Wash fruits and raw vegetables before eating or serving them.
- Wash cooking and eating utensils with soap and water after use.

See Persons With Dementia: Common Aseptic Practices.

Persons With Dementia

Common Aseptic Practices

Persons with dementia do not understand aseptic practices. Others must protect them from infection. Assist them with hand washing:

- After elimination
- After coughing, sneezing, or blowing the nose
- Before or after they eat or handle food
- Any time their hands are soiled

Check and clean their hands and fingernails often. They may not or cannot tell you when soiling occurs.

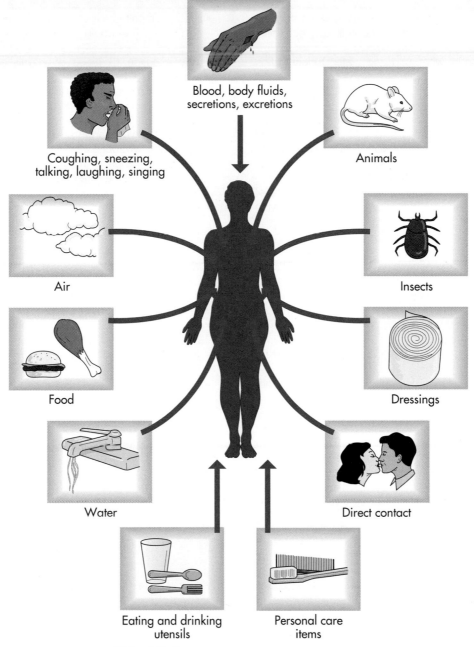

FIG. **10-2** Methods of transmitting microbes.

The labels around the figure are:

Blood, body fluids, secretions, excretions

Coughing, sneezing, talking, laughing, singing

Animals

Air

Insects

Food

Dressings

Water

Direct contact

Eating and drinking utensils

Personal care items

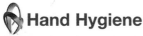 **Hand Hygiene**

Hand hygiene is the easiest and most important way to prevent the spread of infection. You use your hands for almost everything. They are easily contaminated. They can spread microbes to other persons or items. *Practice hand hygiene before and after giving care.* See Box 10-1, p. 126 for the rules of hand hygiene.

Text continued on p. 128

PROMOTING SAFETY AND COMFORT
Hand Hygiene

Safety

You use your hands in almost every task. They can pick up microbes from one person, place, or thing. They transfer them to other people, places, and things. That is why hand hygiene is so very important. You must practice hand hygiene before and after giving care.

Comfort

You will practice hand hygiene very often during your shift. Hand lotions and hand creams help prevent chapping and dry skin. Apply hand lotion or cream as often as needed.

BOX 10-1   **Rules of Hand Hygiene**

- Wash your hands (with soap and water) when they are visibly dirty or soiled with blood, body fluids, secretions, or excretions.
- Wash your hands (with soap and water) before eating and after using a restroom.
- Wash your hands (with soap and water) if exposure to the anthrax spore is suspected or proven.
- Use an alcohol-based hand rub to decontaminate your hands if they are not visibly soiled. (If an alcohol-based hand rub is not available, wash your hands with soap and water.) Follow this rule in the following clinical situations:
  - Before having direct contact with a person.
  - After contact with the person's intact skin (for example, after taking a pulse or blood pressure or after moving a person).
  - After contact with body fluids or excretions, mucous membranes, non-intact skin, and wound dressings if hands are not visibly soiled.
  - When moving from a contaminated body site to a clean body site during care activities.
  - After contact with objects (including equipment) in the person's care setting.
  - After removing gloves.
- Follow these rules for washing your hands with soap and water. See *Hand Washing* procedure.
  - Wash your hands under warm running water. Do not use hot water.
  - Stand away from the sink. Do not let your hands, body, or uniform touch the sink. The sink is contaminated (Fig. 10-3).
  - Keep your hands and forearms lower than your elbows. Your hands are dirtier than your elbows and forearms. If you hold your hands and forearms up, dirty water runs from hands to elbows. Those areas become contaminated.
- Rub your palms together to work up a good lather (Fig. 10-4). The rubbing action helps remove microbes and dirt.
- Pay attention to areas often missed during hand washing—thumbs, knuckles, sides of the hands, little fingers, and under the nails.
- Clean fingernails by rubbing the tips against your palms (Fig. 10-5).
- Use a nail file or orange stick to clean under fingernails (Fig. 10-6). Microbes easily grow under the fingernails.
- Wash your hands for at least 15 seconds. Wash your hands longer if they are dirty or soiled with blood, body fluids, secretions, or excretions. Use your judgment.
- Dry your hands starting at the fingertips. Work up to your forearms. You will dry the cleanest area first.
- Use a clean paper towel for each faucet to turn water off (Fig. 10-7). Faucets are contaminated. The paper towels prevent clean hands from becoming contaminated again.
- Follow these rules when decontaminating your hands with an alcohol-based hand rub:
  - Apply the product to the palm of one hand. Follow the manufacturer's instructions for the amount to use.
  - Rub your hands together.
  - Make sure you cover all surfaces of your hands and fingers.
  - Continue rubbing your hands together until your hands are dry.
- Apply hand lotion or cream after hand hygiene. This prevents skin chapping and drying. Skin breaks can occur in chapped and dry skin. Skin breaks are portals of entry for microbes.

Modified from Centers for Disease Control and Prevention: Guideline for hand hygiene in health-care settings, *Morbidity and Mortality Report,* October 25, 2002, Vol 51, No. RR-16.

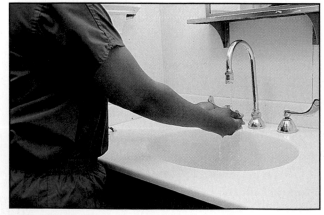

FIG. **10-3** The uniform does not touch the sink. Soap and water are within reach. Hands are lower than the elbows.

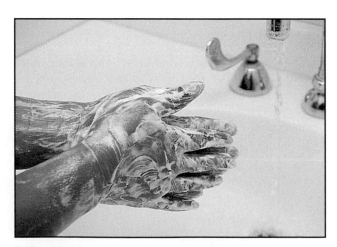

FIG. **10-4** The palms are rubbed together to work up a good lather.

BOX 10-3   Standard Precautions

Hands

- Follow the rules for hand hygiene. See Box 10-1.
- Do not wear fake nails or nail extenders if you will have contact with persons at high risk for infection.

Personal Protective Equipment (PPE)

- Wear PPE when contact with blood or body fluids is likely.
- Do not touch surfaces near the person when giving care.
- Do not contaminate your clothing or skin when removing PPE.
- Remove and discard PPE before leaving the person's room or bed area.

Gloves

- Wear gloves when contact with the following is likely:
  - Blood
  - Potentially infectious materials (body fluids, secretions, and excretions are examples).
  - Mucous membranes
  - Non-intact skin
  - Skin that may be contaminated (for example, when the person has diarrhea)
- Wear gloves that are appropriate for the task:
  - Wear disposable gloves to provide direct care to the person.
  - Wear disposable gloves or utility gloves for cleaning equipment or care settings.
- Remove gloves after contact with the person or the person's care setting.
- Remove gloves after contact with care equipment.
- Do not wear the same pair of gloves to care for more than one person. Remove gloves after contact with a person and before going to another person.
- Do not wash gloves for reuse with different persons.
- Change gloves during care if your hands will move from a contaminated body site to a clean body site.

Gowns and Other PPE Attire

- Wear a gown, apron, or other PPE attire that is appropriate to the task.
- Wear a gown, apron, or other PPE attire to protect your skin and clothing when contact with blood, body fluids, secretions, or excretions is likely.
- Wear a gown for direct contact with a person if he or she has uncontained secretions or excretions.
- Remove the gown, apron, or other PPE attire before leaving the person's room or care setting. Practice hand hygiene before leaving the person's room or care setting.

Mouth, Nose, and Eye Protection

- Wear PPE—masks, goggles, face shields—for procedures and tasks that are likely to cause splashes and sprays of blood, body fluids, secretions, or excretions.

- Wear PPE—mask, goggles, face shield—appropriate for the procedure or task.
- Wear the following for procedures that are likely to cause sprays of respiratory secretions:
  - Gloves
  - Gown
  - Face shield or mask and goggles

Respiratory Hygiene/Cough Etiquette

- Cover the nose and mouth when coughing or sneezing.
- Use tissues to contain respiratory secretions.
- Dispose of tissues in the nearest waste container after use.
- Practice hand hygiene after contact with respiratory secretions.

Care Equipment

- Wear appropriate PPE when handling care equipment that is visibly soiled with blood, body fluids, secretions, or excretions.
- Wear appropriate PPE when handling care equipment that may have been in contact with blood, body fluids, secretions, or excretions.

Care of the Environment

- Follow agency policies and procedures for cleaning and maintaining surfaces. Environmental surfaces and care equipment are examples. Surfaces near the person may need more frequent cleaning and maintenance—door knobs, bed rails, toilet surfaces and areas, and so on.

Textiles and Laundry

- Handle used textiles and fabrics (linens) with minimum agitation. This is done to avoid contamination of the air, surfaces, and other persons.

Worker Safety

- Protect yourself and others from exposure to bloodborne pathogens. Follow federal and state standards and guidelines. See the Bloodborne Pathogen Standard (p. 139).
- Give rescue breathing with a mouthpiece, resuscitation bag, or other ventilation device to prevent contact with the person's mouth and oral secretions. See Chapter 26.

Patient or Resident Placement

- A private room is preferred if the person is at risk for transmitting the infection to others.
- Follow the nurse's instructions if a private room is not available.

Transmission-Based Precautions

Some infections also require Transmission-Based Precautions (Box 10-4). You must understand how certain infections are spread (see Fig. 10-2). This helps you understand the 3 types of Transmission-Based Precautions. The rules in Box 10-5 are a guide for safe care when using isolation precautions.

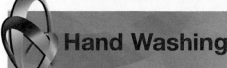

Hand Washing

Procedure

1. See *Promoting Safety and Comfort: Hand Hygiene*, p. 125.
2. Make sure you have soap, paper towels, an orange stick or nail file, and a wastebasket. Collect missing items.
3. Push your watch up your arm 4 to 5 inches. If your uniform sleeves are long push them up too.
4. Stand away from the sink so your clothes do not touch the sink. Stand so the soap and faucet are easy to reach (see Fig. 10-3).
5. Turn on and adjust the water until it feels warm.
6. Wet your wrists and hands. Keep your hands lower than your elbows. Be sure to wet the area 3 to 4 inches above your wrists.
7. Apply about 1 teaspoon of soap to your hands.
8. Rub your palms together and interlace your fingers to work up a good lather (see Fig. 10-4). This step should last at least 15 seconds. (Note: some state competency tests require that you wash your hands for 20 seconds. Others require that you wash your hands for 1 to 2 minutes.)
9. Wash each hand and wrist thoroughly. Clean well between the fingers.
10. Clean under the fingernails. Rub your fingertips against your palms (see Fig. 10-5).
11. Clean under fingernails with a nail file or orange stick (see Fig. 10-6). This step is done for the first hand washing of the day and when your hands are highly soiled.
12. Rinse your wrists and hands well. Water flows from the arms to the hands.
13. Repeat steps 7 through 12, if needed.
14. Dry your wrists and hands with paper towels. Pat dry starting at your fingertips.
15. Discard the paper towels.
16. Turn off faucets with clean paper towels. This prevents you from contaminating your hands (see Fig. 10-7). Use a clean paper towel for each faucet.
17. Discard paper towels into a wastebasket.

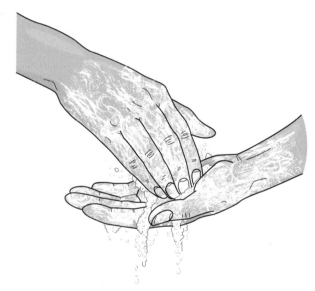

FIG. **10-5** The fingertips are rubbed against the palms to clean under the fingernails.

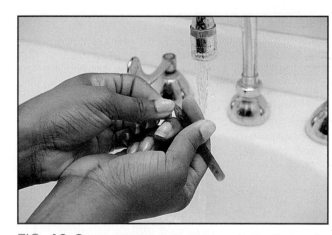

FIG. **10-6** A nail file is used to clean under the fingernails.

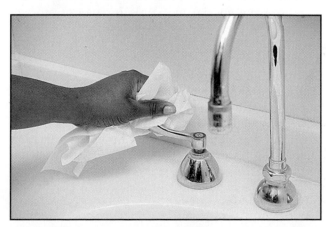

FIG. **10-7** A paper towel is used to turn off the faucet.

Supplies and Equipment

Many single-use and multi-use items are disposable. Single-use items are discarded after use. A person uses multi-use items many times. They include bed-pans, urinals, wash basins, water pitchers, and drinking cups. Label such items with the person's name and room and bed number. Never "borrow" them for another person.

Non-disposable items are cleaned and then disinfected. Then they are sterilized.

Cleaning

Cleaning reduces the number of microbes present. It also removes organic matter such as blood, body fluids, secretions, and excretions. When cleaning equipment:

- Wear personal protective equipment—gloves, mask, gown, and goggles or face shield—when cleaning items contaminated with blood, body fluids, secretions, or excretions.
- Rinse the item in cold water first. Rinsing removes organic matter. Hot water causes organic matter to become thick, sticky, and hard to remove.
- Wash the item with soap and hot water.
- Scrub thoroughly. Use a brush if necessary.
- Rinse the item in warm water. Then dry the item.
- Disinfect or sterilize the item.
- Disinfect equipment and the sink used in the cleaning procedure.
- Discard personal protective equipment.
- Practice hand hygiene.

Disinfection

Disinfection is the process of destroying pathogens. *Germicides* are disinfectants applied to skin, tissues, and non-living objects. Alcohol is a common germicide.

Reusable items are cleaned with *chemical disinfectants*. Such items include blood pressure cuffs, commodes and bedpans, counter tops, wheelchairs and stretchers, and furniture. Wear utility gloves or rubber household gloves to prevent skin irritation. These gloves are *waterproof*. Some disinfectants have special measures for use or storage (Chapter 8).

Sterilization

Sterilization is the process of destroying *all* microbes (pathogens and non-pathogens). Very high temperatures are used. Microbes are destroyed by heat.

Boiling water, radiation, liquid or gas chemicals, dry heat, and *steam under pressure* are sterilization methods. An *autoclave* (Fig. 10-8) is a pressure steam sterilizer. It is used for glass, surgical items, and metal objects. High temperatures destroy plastic and rubber items. They are not autoclaved.

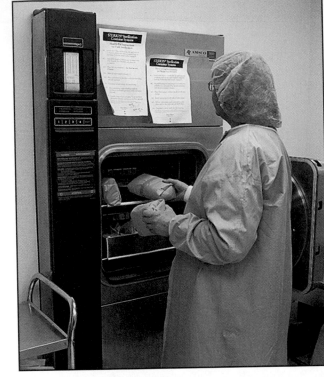

FIG. **10-8** An autoclave.

Other Aseptic Measures

Hand hygiene, cleaning, disinfection, and sterilization are important aseptic measures. So are the measures listed in Box 10-2.

ISOLATION PRECAUTIONS

Blood, body fluids, secretions, and excretions can transmit pathogens. Sometimes barriers are needed to prevent their escape. The pathogens are kept within a certain area, usually the person's room. This requires isolation precautions.

The CDC's Isolation Precautions prevent the spread of **contagious** or **communicable diseases.** They are diseases caused by pathogens that are spread easily.

Isolation Precautions are based on *clean* and *dirty.* *Clean* areas or objects are free of pathogens. They are not contaminated. *Dirty* areas or objects are contaminated with pathogens. If a *clean* area or object has contact with something *dirty,* the clean item is now dirty. *Clean* and *dirty* also depend on how the pathogen is spread.

> **BOX 10-2   Aseptic Measures**
>
> **Controlling Reservoirs (Hosts—You or the Person)**
> - Provide for the person's hygiene needs (Chapter 13).
> - Wash contaminated areas with soap and water. Feces, urine, and blood can contain microbes. So can body fluids, secretions, and excretions.
> - Use leak-proof plastic bags for soiled tissues, linen, and other materials.
> - Keep tables, counters, wheelchair trays, and other surfaces clean and dry.
> - Label bottles with the person's name and the date the bottle was opened.
> - Keep bottles and fluid containers tightly capped or covered.
> - Keep drainage containers below the drainage site.
> - Empty drainage containers and dispose of drainage following the nurse's instructions.
>
> **Controlling Portals of Exit**
> - Provide the person with tissues to use when coughing or sneezing.
> - Wear personal protective equipment as needed (p. 132).
>
> **Controlling Transmission**
> - Do not take equipment (even if unused) from one person's room to use for another person.
> - Hold equipment and linens away from your uniform (Fig. 10-9).
> - Follow the rules for hand hygiene (see Box 10-1).
> - Assist the person with hand washing:
>   - Before and after eating
>   - After elimination
>   - After changing tampons, sanitary napkins, or other personal hygiene products
>   - After contact with blood, body fluids, secretions, or excretions
> - Prevent dust movement. Do not shake linens or equipment.
>
> - Clean from the cleanest area to the dirtiest. This prevents soiling a clean area.
> - Clean away from your body. Do not dust, brush, or wipe toward yourself. Otherwise you transmit microbes to your skin, hair, and clothing.
> - Flush urine and feces down the toilet. Avoid splatters and splashes.
> - Pour contaminated liquids directly into sinks or toilets. Avoid splashing onto other areas.
> - Do not sit on beds. You will pick up microbes. You will transfer them to the next surface that you sit on.
> - Do not use items that are on the floor. The floor is contaminated.
> - Clean and disinfect showers, and shower chairs after each use.
> - Clean and disinfect bedpans, urinals, and commodes after each use.
> - Report pests—ants, spiders, mice, and so on.
>
> **Controlling Portals of Entry**
> - Provide for good skin care and oral hygiene (Chapter 13).
> - Make sure linens are dry and wrinkle-free (Chapter 12).
> - Turn and reposition the person as directed by the nurse and the care plan (Chapter 11).
> - Assist with or clean the genital area after elimination (Chapter 13).
> - Do not let the person lie on tubes or other items.
> - Make sure drainage tubes are properly connected. Otherwise microbes can enter the drainage system.
>
> **Protecting the Susceptible Host**
> - Follow the care plan to meet hygiene needs.
> - Follow the care plan to meet nutrition and fluid needs.
> - Assist with coughing and deep-breathing exercises as directed.

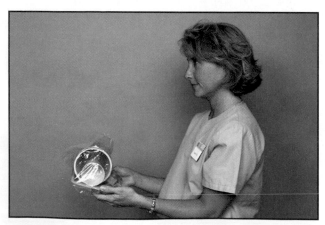

FIG. **10-9** Hold equipment away from your uniform.

Standard Precautions

Standard Precautions are part of the CDC's Isolation Precautions (Box 10-3, p. 130). They reduce the risk of spreading pathogens and known and unknown infections. *Standard Precautions are used for all persons whenever care is given.* They prevent the spread of infection from:
- Blood
- All body fluids, secretions, and excretions (except sweat) even if blood is not visible
- Non-intact skin (skin with open breaks)
- Mucous membranes

BOX 10-4   Transmission-Based Precautions

Airborne Precautions

For known or suspected infections involving microbes transmitted by airborne droplets

Practices

- Standard Precautions are followed.
- A private room is preferred.
- Keep the room door closed and the person in the room.
- Wear respiratory protection (tuberculosis respirator) when entering the room of a person with known or suspected tuberculosis (TB).
- Do not enter the room of a person with known or suspected measles or chickenpox if you are susceptible to these diseases.
- Wear a mask if you must enter the room of a person with known or suspected measles or chickenpox if you are susceptible to these diseases. (A mask is not needed for persons immune to measles or chickenpox.)
- Limit moving and transporting the person from the room. The person wears a mask if moving or transporting from the room is necessary.

Droplet Precautions

- For known or suspected infections involving microbes transmitted by droplets produced by coughing, sneezing, talking, or procedures

Practices

- Standard Precautions are followed.
- A private room is preferred.
- Wear a mask when working within 3 feet of the person. (Wear a mask on entering the room if required by agency policy.)
- Limit moving and transporting the person from the room. The person wears a mask if moving or transporting from the room is necessary.

Contact Precautions

For known or suspected infections involving microbes transmitted by:

- Direct contact with the person (hand or skin-to-skin contact that occurs during care)
- Indirect contact (touching surfaces or care items in the person's room)—gastrointestinal, respiratory, skin, or wound infections

Practices

- Standard Precautions are followed.
- A private room is preferred.
- Wear gloves when entering the room.
- Change gloves after having contact with infective matter that may contain high concentrations of microbes.
- Remove gloves before leaving the person's room.
- Practice hand hygiene immediately after removing gloves. The nurse tells you what agent to use.
- Do not touch potentially contaminated surfaces or items after removing gloves and hand hygiene.
- Wear a gown on entering the room if you will have substantial contact with the person, surfaces, or items in the room.
- Wear a gown on entering the room if the person is incontinent or has diarrhea, an ileostomy, a colostomy, or wound drainage not contained by a dressing.
- Remove the gown before leaving the person's room. Make sure your clothing does not contact potentially contaminated surfaces in the person's room.
- Limit moving or transferring the person from the room. Maintain precautions if the person is moved or transferred from the room.

BOX 10-5   Rules For Isolation Precautions

- Collect all needed items before entering the room.
- Prevent contamination of equipment and supplies. Floors are contaminated. So is any object on the floor or that falls to the floor.
- Use mops wetted with a disinfectant solution to clean floors. Floor dust is contaminated.
- Prevent drafts. Drafts carry pathogens in the air.
- Use paper towels to handle contaminated items.
- Remove items from the room in leak-proof plastic bags.
- Double bag items if the outer part of the bag is or may be contaminated (p. 139).
- Follow agency policy for removing and transporting disposable and reusable items.
- Return reusable dishes, eating utensils, and trays to the food service department. Discard disposable dishes,

eating utensils, and trays in the waste container in the person's room.
- Do not touch your hair, nose, mouth, eyes, or other body parts.
- Do not touch any clean area or object if your hands are contaminated.
- Wash your hands if they are visibly dirty or contaminated with blood, body fluids, secretions, or excretions.
- Place clean items on paper towels.
- Do not shake linen.
- Use paper towels to turn faucets on and off.
- Use a paper towel to open the door to the person's room. Discard it as you leave.
- Tell the nurse if you have any cuts, open skin areas, a sore throat, vomiting, or diarrhea.

You may assist in the care of persons who require Isolation Precautions. If so, review the type used with the nurse. You also need this information from the nurse and the care plan:

- What personal protective equipment to use
- What special safety measures are needed

PROMOTING SAFETY AND COMFORT
Isolation Precautions

Safety

Preventing the spread of infection is important. Isolation Precautions protect everyone—patients, residents, visitors, staff, and you. If you are careless, everyone's safety is at risk.

Comfort

Persons requiring Isolation Precautions usually must stay in their rooms. The person may feel lonely, especially if visitors are few. You can help the person by:

- Treating the person with respect, kindness, and dignity
- Providing newspapers, magazines, books, and other reading matter
- Providing hobby materials if possible
- Urging the person to call family and friends
- Organizing your work so you can stay to visit with the person
- Saying "hello" from the doorway often
  Items brought into the person's room become contaminated. Disinfect or discard items according to agency policy.

Protective Measures

Isolation Precautions involve wearing personal protective equipment (PPE)—gloves, a gown, a mask, and goggles or a face shield (Fig. 10-10). PPE also includes shoes, boots, and leg coverings.

Removing linens, trash, and equipment from the room may require double-bagging. Follow agency procedures when collecting specimens and transporting persons.

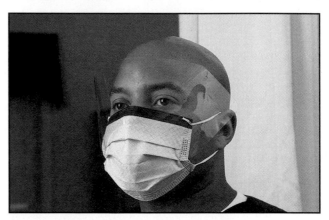

FIG. **10-10** This mask has an eye shield. The eyes and mucous membranes of the mouth and nose are protected.

PROMOTING SAFETY AND COMFORT
Protective Measures

Safety

The PPE needed depends on what tasks, procedures, and care measures you will do while in the room. Sometimes only gloves are needed. The nurse tells you when other PPE are needed.

According to the CDC's isolation guidelines, gloves are always worn when gowns are worn. Sometimes other PPE are needed when gowns are worn. The isolation guidelines shows PPE donned and removed in the following order:

- Donning PPE
  - Gown
  - Mask or respirator
  - Eyewear (goggles or face shield)
  - Gloves
- Removing PPE
  - Gloves (removed at the doorway before leaving the person's room)
  - Goggles or face shield (removed at the doorway before leaving the person's room)
  - Gown (removed at the doorway before leaving the person's room)
  - Mask or respirator (removed outside the room)

Gloves

Small skin breaks on the hands and fingers are common. They are portals of entry for microbes. Disposable gloves act as a barrier. They protect you from pathogens in the person's blood, body fluids, secretions, and excretions. They also protect the person from microbes on your hands.

Wear gloves whenever contact with blood, body fluids, secretions, excretions, mucous membranes, and non-intact skin is likely. Contact may be direct. Or contact may be with items or surfaces contaminated with blood, body fluids, secretions, or excretions.

Wearing gloves is the most common protective measure used with Isolation Precautions. Remember the following when using gloves:

■ The outside of gloves are contaminated.
■ Gloves are easier to put on when your hands are dry.
■ Do not tear gloves when putting them on. Carelessness, long fingernails, and rings can tear gloves.
■ You need a new pair for every person.
■ Remove and discard torn, cut, or punctured gloves at once. Practice hand hygiene. Then put on a new pair.
■ Wear gloves once. Discard them after use.
■ Put on clean gloves just before touching mucous membranes or non-intact skin.
■ Put on new gloves whenever gloves become contaminated with blood, body fluids, secretions, or excretions. A task may require more than 1 pair of gloves.
■ Change gloves when moving from a contaminated body site to a clean body site.
■ Make sure gloves cover your wrists. If you wear a gown, gloves cover the cuffs (Fig. 10-11).
■ Remove gloves so the inside part is on the outside. The inside is *clean.*
■ Decontaminate your hands after removing gloves.

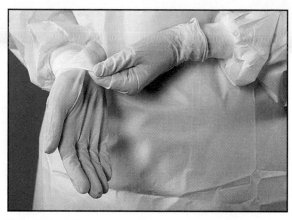

FIG. **10-11** The gloves cover the cuffs of the gown.

PROMOTING SAFETY AND COMFORT
Gloves

Safety

No special method is needed to put on gloves. To remove gloves, see procedure: *Removing Gloves,* p. 134.

Some gloves are made of latex (a rubber product). Latex allergies are common. They can cause skin rashes. Asthma and shock are more serious problems. Report skin rashes and breathing problems to the nurse at once.

If you have a latex allergy, wear latex-free gloves. Some patients and residents are allergic to latex. This information is on the care plan and your assignment sheet.

Comfort

Many nurses and nursing assistants wear gloves for every patient or resident contact. Remember, gloves are needed whenever contact with blood, body fluids, secretions, excretions, mucous membranes, and non-intact skin is likely. You do not need to wear gloves when such contact is unlikely. Back massages and brushing and combing hair are examples. Wearing gloves only when needed helps reduce exposure to latex.

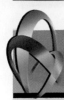

Removing Gloves

Procedure

1 See *Promoting Safety and Comfort: Gloves,* p. 133.
2 Make sure that glove touches only glove.
3 Grasp a glove just below the cuff (Fig. 10-12, *A*). Grasp it on the outside.
4 Pull the glove down over your hand so it is inside out (Fig. 10-12, *B*).
5 Hold the removed glove with your other gloved hand.

6 Reach inside the other glove. Use the first 2 fingers of the ungloved hand (Fig. 10-12, *C*).
7 Pull the glove down (inside out) over your hand and the other glove (Fig. 10-12, *D*).
8 Discard the gloves. Follow agency policy.
9 Decontaminate your hands.

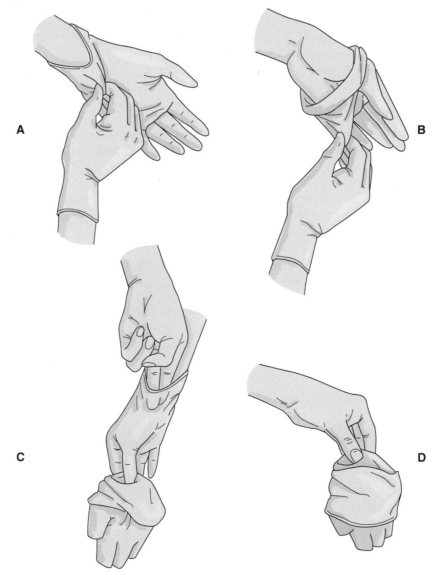

FIG. **10-12** Removing gloves. **A,** Grasp the glove below the cuff. **B,** Pull the glove down over the hand. The glove is inside out. **C,** Insert the fingers of the ungloved hand inside the other glove. **D,** Pull the glove down and over the hand and glove. The glove is inside out.

Gowns and Other Attire

Gowns, aprons, shoe covers, boots, and leg coverings prevent the spread of microbes. They protect your clothes and body from contact with blood, body fluids, secretions, and excretions. They also protect against splashes and sprays.

Gowns must completely cover you from your neck to your knees. The long sleeves have tight cuffs. The gown opens at the back and is tied at the neck and waist. The gown front and sleeves are considered to be *contaminated*.

Gowns are used once. A wet gown is contaminated. It is removed and a dry one put on. Disposable gowns are made of paper. They are discarded after use.

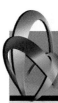

Donning and Removing a Gown

Procedure

1 Remove your watch and all jewelry.
2 Roll up uniform sleeves.
3 Practice hand hygiene.
4 Hold a clean gown out in front of you. Let it unfold. Do not shake the gown.
5 Put your hands and arms through the sleeves (Fig. 10-13, *A*, p. 136).
6 Make sure the gown covers you from your neck to your knees. It must cover your arms to the end of your wrists.
7 Tie the strings at the back of the neck (Fig. 10-13, *B*, p. 136).
8 Overlap the back of the gown. Make sure it covers your uniform. The gown should be snug, not loose (Fig. 10-13, *C*, p. 136).
9 Tie the waist strings. Tie them at the back or the side. Do not tie them in the front.
10 Put on the gloves. Provide care.

11 Remove and discard the gloves. Decontaminate your hands.
12 Remove and discard the goggles or face shield if worn.
13 Remove the gown:
    a Untie the neck and waist strings. Do not touch the front of the gown.
    b Pull the gown down from each shoulder toward the same hand.
    c Turn the gown inside out as it is removed. Hold it at the inside shoulder seams, and bring your hands together (Fig. 10-13, *D*, p. 136).
14 Hold and roll up the gown away from you. Keep it inside out.
15 Discard the gown. Follow agency policy.
16 Remove and discard the mask if worn. (Note: a respirator is removed outside of the room.)
17 Decontaminate your hands.

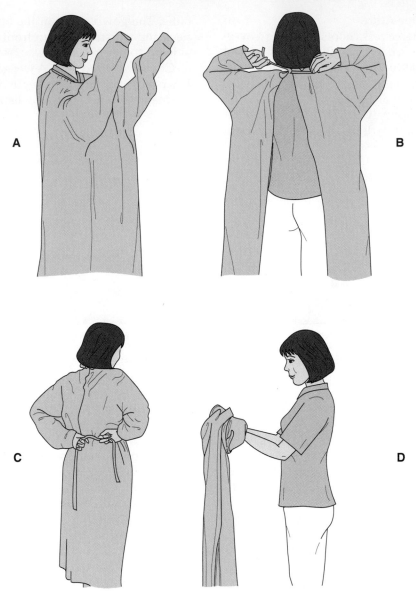

FIG. **10-13** Gowning. **A,** The arms and hands are put through the sleeves. **B,** The strings are tied at the back of the neck. **C,** The gown is overlapped in the back to cover the entire uniform. **D,** The gown is turned inside out as it is removed.

Masks and Respiratory Protection

Masks prevent the spread of microbes from the respiratory tract. Masks are disposable. A wet or moist mask is contaminated. Breathing can cause masks to become wet or moist. Apply a new mask when contamination occurs.

A mask fits snugly over your nose and mouth. Practice hand hygiene before putting on a mask. When removing a mask, touch only the ties or the plastic bands. The front of the mask is contaminated.

Tuberculosis respirators are worn when caring for persons with tuberculosis (TB) (Chapter 24).

Goggles and Face Shields

Goggles and face shields protect your eyes, mouth, and nose from splashing or spraying of blood, body fluids, secretions, and excretions (see Fig. 10-10). Splashes and sprays can occur when giving care, cleaning items, or disposing of fluids.

The outside of goggles or a face shield is contaminated. Use the headband or ear pieces to remove the device.

Discard disposable goggles or face shields after use. Reusable eyewear is cleaned before reuse.

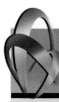

Donning and Removing a Mask

Procedure

1 Practice hand hygiene.
2 Put on a gown if required.
3 Pick up the mask by its upper ties. Do not touch the part that will cover your face.
4 Place the mask over your nose and mouth (Fig. 10-14, *A*, p. 138).
5 Place the upper strings above your ears. Tie them at the back in the middle of your head (Fig. 10-14, *B*, p. 138).
6 Tie the lower strings at the back of your neck (Fig. 10-14, *C*, p. 138). The lower part of the mask is under your chin.
7 Pinch the metal band around your nose. The top of the mask must be snug over your nose. If you wear eyeglasses, the mask must be snug under the bottom of the eyeglasses.
8 Make sure the mask is snug over your face and under your chin.

9 Put on goggles or a face shield if needed and if not part of the mask.
10 Decontaminate your hands. Put on gloves.
11 Provide care. Avoid coughing, sneezing, and unnecessary talking.
12 Change the mask if it becomes moist or contaminated.
13 Remove the mask. (Note: a respirator is removed outside of the room.)
   a Remove the gloves. Also remove the goggles or face shield and gown if worn.
   b Untie the lower strings of the mask.
   c Untie the top strings.
   d Hold the top strings. Remove the mask.
14 Discard the mask. Follow agency policy.
15 Decontaminate your hands.

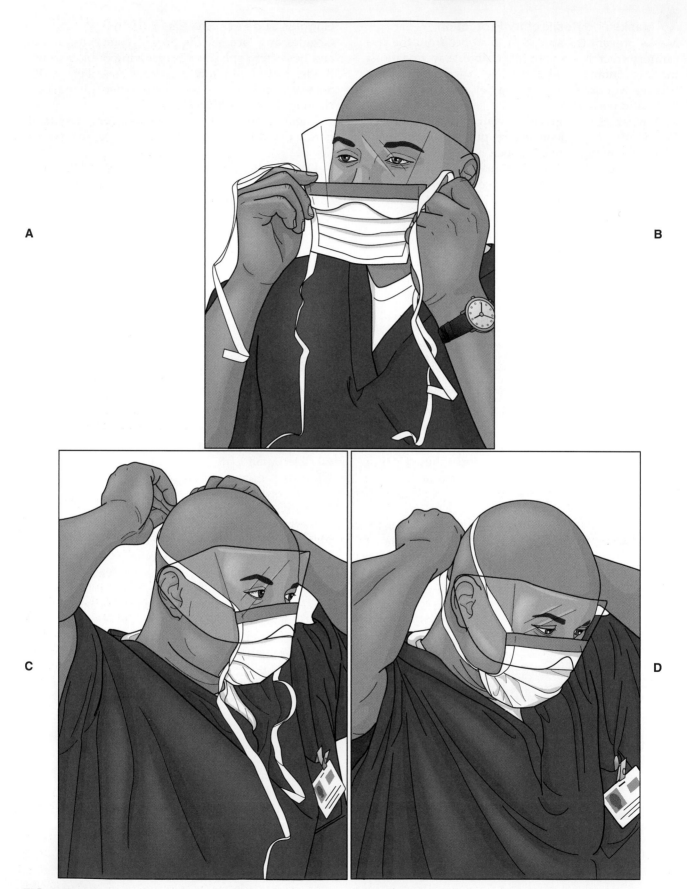

FIG. **10-14** Donning a mask. **A,** The mask covers the nose and mouth. **B,** Upper strings are tied at the back of the head. **C,** Lower strings are tied at the back of the neck.

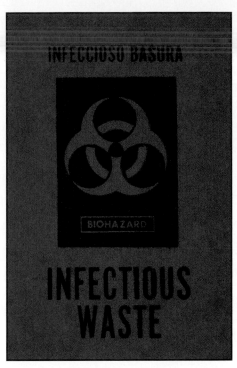

FIG. **10-15** BIOHAZARD symbol.

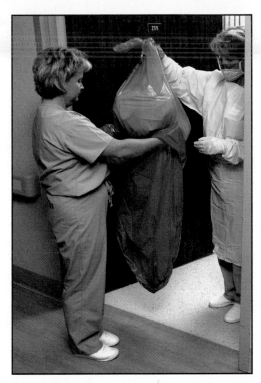

FIG. **10-16** Double bagging. One nursing assistant is in the room by the doorway. The other is outside the doorway. The "dirty" bag is placed inside the "clean" bag.

Bagging Items

Contaminated items are bagged to remove them from the person's room. Leak-proof plastic bags are used. They have the *BIOHAZARD* symbol (Fig. 10-15). **Biohazardous waste** is items contaminated with blood, body fluids, secretions, or excretions. (*Bio* means life. *Hazardous* means dangerous or harmful.)

Bag and transport linens following agency policy. All linen bags need a *BIOHAZARD* symbol. Melt-away bags are common. They dissolve in hot water. Once soiled linen is bagged, no one needs to handle it. Do not overfill the bag. Tie the bag securely. Then place it in a laundry hamper lined with a biohazard plastic bag.

Trash is placed in a container labeled with the *BIOHAZARD* symbol. Follow agency policy for bagging and transporting trash, equipment, and supplies.

Usually one bag is needed. Double bagging involves two bags. Double bagging is not needed unless the outside of the bag is soiled. Two staff members are needed. One is inside the room. The other is at the doorway outside the room. The person in the room places contaminated items into a bag. Then the bag is sealed. The person outside the room holds open another bag. This bag is clean. A wide cuff is made on the clean bag to protect the hands from contamination (Fig. 10-16). The contaminated bag is placed in the clean bag at the doorway.

Meeting Basic Needs

The person has love, belonging, and self-esteem needs. Often they are unmet when Isolation Precautions are used. Visitors and staff often avoid the person. Putting on PPE takes extra effort before entering the room.

The person may feel lonely, unwanted, and rejected. The person knows the disease can be spread to others. He or she may feel dirty and undesirable. Remember, the *pathogen* is undesirable, not the *person*.

Masks, goggles, and face shields can change how you look. Let the person see your face before putting on PPE. Tell the person who you are and what you are going to do.

BLOODBORNE PATHOGEN STANDARD

The Bloodborne Pathogen Standard protects against exposure to the AIDS virus (HIV) and the hepatitis B virus (HBV). It is a regulation of the Occupational Safety and Health Administration (OSHA).

HIV and HBV are found in blood (Chapter 24). They are bloodborne pathogens. They exit the body through blood. They are spread to others by blood and other potentially infectious materials (OPIM). OPIM are contaminated with blood or with a body fluid that may contain blood. This includes semen, vaginal secretions, and saliva. OPIM also includes needles, suction equipment, soiled linens, dressings, and other care items and equipment.

Employee Training

You receive free training upon employment and yearly. Training is also required for new or changed tasks involving exposure to bloodborne pathogens.

Hepatitis B Vaccination

Hepatitis B is a liver disease. It is caused by the hepatitis B virus (HBV). HBV is spread by blood and sexual contact. The hepatitis B vaccine produces immunity against hepatitis B. *Immunity* means that a person has protection against a certain disease. He or she will not get the disease.

You can receive the hepatitis B vaccination within 10 working days of being hired. The agency pays for it. You can refuse the vaccination. If so, you must sign a statement refusing the vaccine. You can have the vaccination at a later time.

Engineering and Work Practice Controls

Engineering controls reduce employee exposure in the workplace. Special containers for contaminated sharps (needles, broken glass) and specimens remove and isolate the hazard from staff. Containers are puncture-resistant, leak-proof, and color-coded in red. They have the *BIOHAZARD* symbol (p. 139).

Work practice controls also reduce exposure risks. All tasks involving blood or OPIM are done in ways to limit splatters, splashes, and sprays. Producing droplets also is avoided. OSHA requires these work practice controls:

- Do not eat, drink, smoke, apply cosmetics or lip balm, or handle contact lenses in areas of occupational exposure.
- Do not store food or drinks where blood or OPIM are kept.
- Practice hand hygiene after removing gloves.
- Wash hands as soon as possible after skin contact with blood or OPIM.
- Never recap, bend, or remove needles by hand. When recapping, bending, or removing contaminated needles is required, use mechanical means (forceps) or a one-handed method.
- Never shear or break contaminated needles.
- Discard contaminated needles and sharp instruments in containers that are closable, puncture-resistant, and leak-proof. Containers are color-

coded red and have the *BIOHAZARD* symbol. Containers must be upright and not allowed to overfill.

Personal Protective Equipment (PPE)

This includes gloves, goggles, face shields, masks, laboratory coats, gowns, shoe covers, and surgical caps. They protect your clothes, undergarments, skin, eyes, mouth, and hair.

PPE is free to employees. Safe handling and use require these measures:
- Remove PPE before leaving the work area.
- Remove PPE when a garment becomes contaminated.
- Place used PPE in marked areas or containers.
- Wear gloves when you expect contact with blood or OPIM.
- Wear gloves when handling or touching contaminated items or surfaces.
- Replace worn, punctured, or contaminated gloves.
- Never wash or decontaminate disposable gloves for reuse.
- Discard utility gloves that show signs of cracking, peeling, tearing, or puncturing.

Equipment

Contaminated equipment is cleaned and decontaminated. Decontaminate work surfaces with a proper disinfectant:
- Upon completing tasks
- At once when there is obvious contamination
- After any spill of blood or OPIM
- At the end of the work shift when surfaces became contaminated since the last cleaning

Use a brush and dustpan or tongs to clean up broken glass. Never pick up broken glass with your hands, not even with gloves. Discard broken glass into a puncture-resistant container.

Laundry

OSHA requires these measures for contaminated laundry:
- Handle it as little as possible.
- Wear gloves or other needed PPE.
- Bag contaminated laundry where it was used.
- Mark laundry bags or containers with the *BIOHAZARD* symbol for laundry sent off-site.
- Place wet, contaminated laundry in leak-proof containers before transport. The containers are color-coded in red or labeled with the *BIOHAZARD* symbol.

Exposure Incidents

An *exposure incident* is any eye, mouth, other mucous membrane, non-intact skin, or parenteral contact with blood or OPIM. *Parenteral* means piercing the mucous membranes or the skin barrier—needle-sticks, human bites, cuts, and abrasions.

Report exposure incidents at once. Medical evaluation and follow-up are free. Your blood is tested for HBV and HIV. If you refuse testing, the blood sample is kept for at least 90 days. Testing is done later if you change your mind.

You are told of any medical conditions that may need treatment. You receive a written opinion of the medical evaluation within 15 days after its completion.

The *source individual* is the person whose blood or body fluids are the source of an exposure incident. His or her blood is tested for HIV and HBV. State laws vary about releasing the results. The agency informs you about laws affecting the source's identity and test results.

FOCUS ON THE PERSON

Microbes are everywhere. Ill, injured, and older persons are at risk for infection. Infection is a risk after surgery. You must do everything you can to help prevent infection.

See Focus on the Person: Preventing Infection.

Focus on the PERSON

Preventing Infection

Providing comfort—Donning and removing PPE take time and effort. Once you don PPE, you must remove it before leaving the room. Therefore you need to organize your time and work so that you do not need to leave the room. Meet the needs of other patients or residents first. Ask a co-worker to answer their signal lights for you. Then gather the care items that you need to bring to the room. Before leaving the room, make sure that the person's needs are met. Also tell the person when you will return to the room.

Ethical behavior—Clean items are easily contaminated. This includes your hands, gloves, and care items. You may be the only one who knows that something is contaminated. You must do the right thing. Always practice Standard Precautions.

Remaining independent—Persons on Isolation Precautions stay in their rooms. They cannot go into the hallway or go to the nurses' station, dining room, or lounge. They must eat in their rooms. These persons depend on the nursing team for needed items. Make sure the person has needed items in the room. They must be within reach for persons who must remain in bed or for those with mobility problems.

Speaking up—Without intending to, people can make the person feel ashamed and guilty for having a contagious disease. Be careful what you say. For example, do not say: "What were you doing?" "How did you get that?" "I'm afraid to touch you." "Don't breathe on me." Always treat the person with respect, kindness, and dignity.

OBRA and other laws—The Centers for Disease Control and Prevention (CDC) is a federal agency. It serves to protect the health and safety of people in the United States. The CDC develops disease prevention and control guidelines and standards to improve health. The CDC's Hand Hygiene Guideline (p. 126) and Isolation Precautions (p. 128) are examples. Survey teams check to make sure that the agency complies with CDC guidelines and standards. They also observe how care is given.

Nursing teamwork—Once in the room, the nursing team member cannot easily leave the room to answer signal lights or obtain needed care items. When a person requires isolation, offer to help your co-worker. Do so willingly and pleasantly. Bring items to the room as needed. Also answer signal lights for your co-worker. Be sure to report to the co-worker what you did for the person and what you observed. Likewise, ask a co-worker to help you if you are going to be with a person needing Isolation Precautions. Ask politely and thank your co-worker for helping you.

REVIEW QUESTIONS

Circle **T** if the statement is true and **F** if it is false.

1 **T F** A pathogen can cause an infection.
2 **T F** An item is sterile if non-pathogens are present.
3 **T F** You hold your hands and forearms up during hand washing.
4 **T F** Unused items in a person's room are used for another person.
5 **T F** A person received the hepatitis B vaccine. The person will develop the disease.

Circle the **BEST** answer.

6 Most pathogens need the following to grow *except*
   a Water
   b Light
   c Oxygen
   d Nourishment

7 Signs and symptoms of infection include the following *except*
   a Fever, nausea, vomiting, rash, and/or sores
   b Pain or tenderness, redness, and/or swelling
   c Fatigue, loss of appetite, and/or a discharge
   d A wound and/or bleeding

8 Which is *not* a portal of exit?
   a Respiratory tract
   b Blood
   c Reproductive system
   d Intact skin

9 When cleaning equipment, do the following *except*
   a Rinse the item in cold water before cleaning
   b Wash the item with soap and hot water
   c Use a brush if necessary
   d Work from dirty to clean areas

10 Isolation Precautions
   a Prevent infection
   b Destroy pathogens
   c Keep pathogens within a certain area
   d Destroy all microbes

11 Standard Precautions
   a Are used for all persons
   b Prevent the spread of pathogens through the air
   c Require gowns, masks, gloves, and goggles
   d Require a doctor's order

12 You wear utility gloves for contact with
   a Blood
   b Body fluids
   c Secretions and excretions
   d Cleaning solutions

13 A mask
   a Can be reused
   b Is clean on the inside
   c Is contaminated when moist
   d Should fit loosely for breathing

14 These statements are about personal protective equipment (PPE). Which is *false*?
   a Wash disposable gloves for reuse.
   b Remove PPE before leaving the work area.
   c Discard cracked or torn utility gloves.
   d Wear gloves when touching contaminated items or surfaces.

15 Contaminated work surfaces are cleaned at the following times *except*
   a After completing a task
   b When there is obvious contamination
   c After blood is spilled
   d After removing gloves

16 The Bloodborne Pathogen Standard involves the following *except*
   a Wearing gloves
   b Discarding sharp items into a biohazard container
   c Storing food and blood in different places
   d Eating and drinking in areas of occupational exposure

Answers to these questions are on p. 468.

Using Body Mechanics

OBJECTIVES

- Define the key terms listed in this chapter
- Explain the purpose and rules of body mechanics
- Explain how ergonomics can prevent workplace accidents
- Identify comfort and safety measures for moving and turning persons in bed
- Explain how to safely perform transfers
- Explain why body alignment and position changes are important
- Identify the comfort and safety measures for positioning a person
- Position persons in the basic bed positions and in a chair
- Perform the procedures described in this chapter

PROCEDURES

Procedures with this icon are also on the CD-ROM in this book.

- Moving the Person Up in Bed
- Moving the Person Up in Bed With an Assist Device
- Moving the Person to the Side of the Bed
- Turning and Positioning the Person
- Logrolling the Person
- Helping the Person to Sit on the Side of the Bed (Dangle)
- Applying a Transfer Belt
- Transferring the Person to a Chair or Wheelchair
- Transferring the Person From a Chair or Wheelchair to Bed
- Transferring the Person Using a Mechanical Lift
- Transferring the Person to and From the Toilet

KEY TERMS

base of support The area on which an object rests

body alignment The way the head, trunk, arms, and legs are aligned with one another; posture

body mechanics Using the body in an efficient and careful way

dorsal recumbent position The back-lying or supine position

Fowler's position A semi-sitting position; the head of the bed is raised between 45 and 60 degrees

friction The rubbing of one surface against another

lateral position The side-lying position

logrolling Turning the person as a unit, in alignment, with one motion

posture Body alignment

prone position Lying on the abdomen with the head turned to one side

semi-prone side position Sims' position

shearing When skin sticks to a surface while muscles slide in the direction the body is moving

side-lying position The lateral position

Sims' position A left side-lying position in which the upper leg is sharply flexed so it is not on the lower leg and the lower arm is behind the person; semi-prone side

supine position The back-lying or dorsal recumbent position

transfer belt A belt used to support persons who are unsteady or disabled; a gait belt

You will turn and reposition persons often. You must use your body correctly. This protects you and the person from injury.

BODY MECHANICS

Body mechanics means using the body in an efficient and careful way. Good posture, balance, and the strongest and largest muscles are used. Fatigue, muscle strain, and injury can result from improper use and positioning of the body during activity or rest.

Body alignment (posture) is the way the head, trunk, arms, and legs are aligned with one another. Good alignment lets the body move and function with strength and efficiency. Standing, sitting, and lying down require good alignment.

Base of support is the area on which an object rests. A good base of support is needed for balance (Fig. 11-1). Stand with your feet apart for a wider base of support and more balance.

The strongest and largest muscles are in the shoulders, upper arms, hips, and thighs. Use these muscles to lift and move heavy objects. Otherwise, you place

strain and exertion on smaller and weaker muscles. This causes fatigue and injury. *Back injuries are a major risk.* For good body mechanics:

- Bend your knees and squat to lift a heavy object (Fig. 11-2). Do not bend from your waist. That places strain on small back muscles.
- Hold items close to your body and base of support (see Fig. 11-2). This involves upper arm and shoulder muscles. Holding objects away from your body places strain on small muscles in your lower arms.

All activities require good body mechanics. Follow the rules in Box 11-1.

BOX 11-1	**Rules For Body Mechanics**

- Keep your body in good alignment with a wide base of support.
- Use the stronger and larger muscles in your shoulders, upper arms, thighs, and hips.
- Keep objects close to your body when you lift, move, or carry them (see Fig. 11-2).
- Avoid unnecessary bending and reaching. Raise the bed so it is close to your waist. Adjust the overbed table so it is at your waist level.
- Face your work area. This prevents unnecessary twisting.
- Push, slide, or pull heavy objects whenever you can rather than lifting them. Pushing is better than pulling.
- Widen your base of support when pushing or pulling. Move your front leg forward when pushing. Move your rear leg back when pulling (Fig. 11-3, p. 146).
- Use both hands and arms to lift, move, or carry heavy objects.
- Turn your whole body when changing the direction of your movement. Move and turn your feet in the direction of the turn, instead of twisting your body.
- Work with smooth and even movements. Avoid sudden or jerky motions.
- Do not lean over the person to give care.
- *Get help from a co-worker if the person cannot assist with turning or moving.* Two or three staff members may be needed to turn or move the person. Assist devices may also be needed. Follow the person's care plan.
- *Get help from a co-worker to move heavy objects or persons. Do not turn or move them by yourself.* Two or three staff members may be needed to turn or move the person. Assist devices also may be needed. Follow the person's care plan.
- Bend your hips and knees to lift heavy objects from the floor (see Fig. 11-2). Straighten your back as the object reaches thigh level. Your leg and thigh muscles work to raise the item off the floor and to waist level.
- Do not lift objects higher than chest level. Do not lift above your shoulders. Use a step stool to reach an object higher than chest level.
- Use assist equipment and devices whenever possible instead of lifting and moving the person manually. Follow the person's care plan.

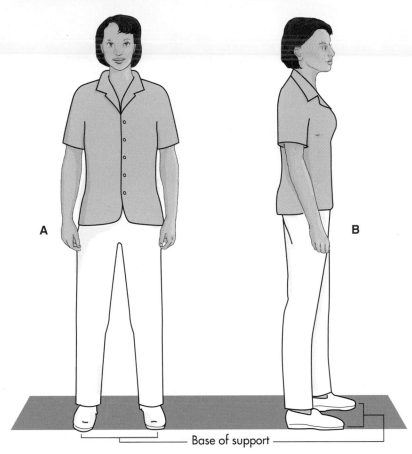

FIG. **11-1 A,** Anterior (front) view of an adult in good body alignment. The feet are apart for a wide base of support. **B,** Lateral (side) view of an adult with good posture and alignment.

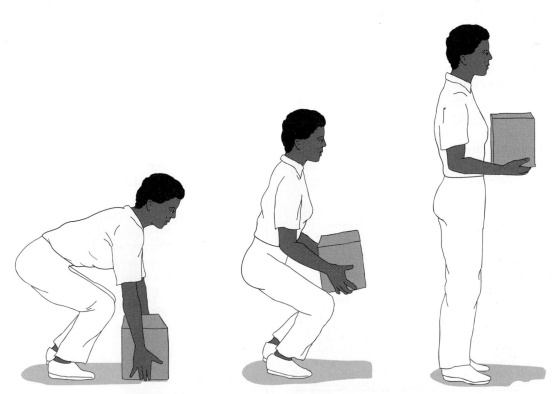

FIG. **11-2** Picking up a box using good body mechanics.

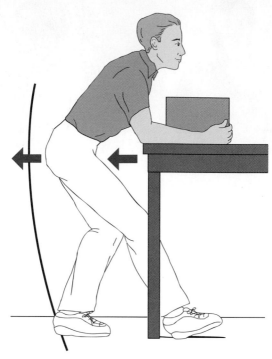

FIG. **11-3** Move your rear leg back when pulling an item.

ERGONOMICS

Ergonomics is the science of designing the job to fit the worker. (*Ergo* means work. *Nomos* means law.) The task, work station, equipment, and tools are changed to reduce stress on the worker's body. The goal is to prevent a serious and disabling work-related musculoskeletal disorder (MSD).

MSDs are injuries and disorders of the muscles, tendons, ligaments, joints, and cartilage. They also involve the nervous system. The arms and back are often affected. MSDs are painful. They can develop slowly over weeks, months, and years. Or they can occur from one event. Pain, numbness, tingling, stiff joints, difficulty moving, and muscle loss can occur.

PROMOTING SAFETY AND COMFORT
Ergonomics

Safety

Back injuries can occur from repeated activities over time or from one event. Use good body mechanics to protect yourself and others from injury. Do not work alone. Have a co-worker help you handle, move, turn, or transfer a person. Follow the rules in Box 11-1.

MOVING PERSONS IN BED

Some persons can move and turn in bed. Others need help from at least one person. Those who are weak, unconscious, paralyzed, on complete bedrest, or in casts need help. Sometimes two or three people or a mechanical lift is needed.

Protect the skin when moving the person. Friction and shearing injure the skin. Both cause infection and pressure ulcers (Chapter 21). Older persons are at risk.

- **Friction** is the rubbing of one surface against another. When moved in bed, the person's skin rubs against the sheet.
- **Shearing** is when the skin sticks to a surface while muscles slide in the direction the body is moving (Fig. 11-4). It occurs when the person slides down in bed or is moved in bed.

Roll or lift the person to reduce friction and shearing. Use assist devices. You can use a *lift sheet (turning sheet)* or a turning pad (p. 150) to move the person in bed and reduce friction. You can also use a large incontinence product, slide board, or slide sheet.

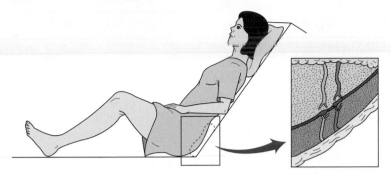

FIG. **11-4** When the head of the bed is raised to a sitting position, skin on the buttocks stays in place. However, internal structures move forward as the person slides down in bed. This causes skin to be pinched between the mattress and the hip bones.

DELEGATION GUIDELINES
Moving Persons in Bed

Before moving a person, you need this information from the nurse and the care plan:
- Position limits and restrictions
- What pillows can be removed
- How far you can lower the head of the bed
- Any limits in the person's ability to move or be repositioned
- What procedure to use:
  - *Moving the Person Up in Bed*
  - *Moving the Person Up in Bed With an Assist Device*
- How many workers are needed to safely move the person
- What equipment is needed—trapeze, lift sheet, mechanical lift
- How to position the person and where to place pillows (p. 172)
- If the person uses bed rails
- What observations to report and record:
  - Who helped you with the procedure
  - How much help the person needed
  - How the person tolerated the procedure
  - How you positioned the person
  - Complaints of pain or discomfort

PROMOTING SAFETY AND COMFORT
Moving Persons in Bed

Safety

Decide how to move the person before starting the procedure. If you need help from co-workers, ask them to help before you begin. Also plan how to protect drainage tubes or containers connected to the person.

Beds are raised horizontally to move persons in bed (Chapter 12). This reduces bending and reaching. You must:
- Use the bed correctly
- Protect the person from falling when the bed is raised
- Follow the rules of body mechanics

Many older persons have osteoporosis or arthritis (Chapter 24). They have fragile bones and joints. Always have help when moving them. Move them carefully to prevent injury or pain.

Comfort

You need to promote the person's comfort during moving procedures. To promote mental comfort, always screen and cover the person to protect the right to privacy. To promote physical comfort:
- Keep the person in good alignment.
- Make sure the person's head does not hit the headboard when he or she is moved up in bed. If the person can be without a pillow, place it upright against the headboard.
- Use pillows to position the person as directed by the nurse and care plan. If a pillow is allowed under the person's head, make sure it is under the head and shoulders.

Moving the Person Up in Bed

When the bed is raised, it is easy to slide down toward the middle and foot of the bed (Fig. 11-5). The person is moved up in bed for good alignment and comfort.

You can sometimes move lightweight adults up in bed alone if they assist or use a trapeze. However, it is best to have help and use an assist device. This protects the person and you from injury.

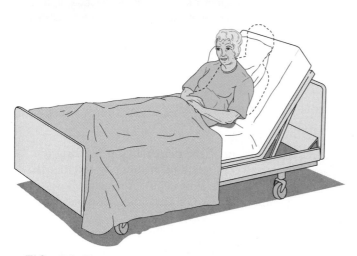

FIG. **11-5** A person in poor alignment after sliding down in bed.

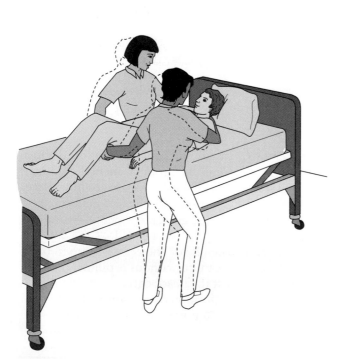

FIG. **11-6** A person is moved up in bed by two nursing assistants. Each has one arm under the person's shoulders and the other under the thighs. They have locked arms under the person. The person's knees are flexed. The nursing assistants shift their weight from the rear leg to the front leg as the person is moved up in bed.

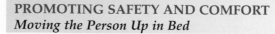

PROMOTING SAFETY AND COMFORT
Moving the Person Up in Bed

Safety

Moving the person up in bed is best done with at least two staff members. Assist devices are used as directed by the nurse and the care plan.

Perform this procedure alone only if:
- The person is small in size
- The person can follow directions
- The person can assist with much of the moving
- The person uses a trapeze
- The person can push against the mattress with his or her feet
- The nurse says it is safe to do so
- You are comfortable doing so

Follow the nurse's directions and the care plan. Ask any questions before you begin the procedure.

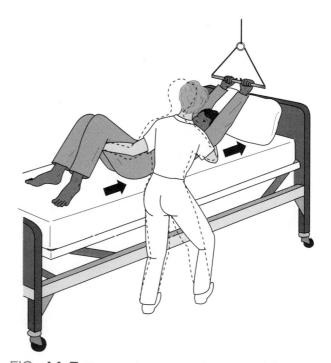

FIG. **11-7** The person grasps a trapeze and flexes the knees. The nursing assistant shifts her body weight from the rear leg to the front leg as she moves the person up in bed. *Note:* Although you can move children and lightweight adults alone with this method, it is best to have help and use an assist device.

Moving the Person Up in Bed

Quality of Life

Remember to:

- Knock before entering the person's room
- Address the person by name
- Introduce yourself by name and title

- Explain the procedure to the person before beginning and during the procedure
- Protect the person's rights during the procedure
- Handle the person gently during the procedure

Pre-Procedure

1 Follow *Delegation Guidelines: Moving Persons in Bed*, p. 147. See *Promoting Safety and Comfort:*
  - *Moving Persons in Bed*
  - *Moving the Person Up in Bed*, p. 148
2 Ask a co-worker to assist you.
3 Practice hand hygiene.

4 Identify the person. Check the ID bracelet against the assignment sheet. Call the person by name.
5 Provide for privacy.
6 Lock the bed wheels.
7 Raise the bed for body mechanics. Bed rails are up if used.

Procedure

8 Lower the head of the bed to a level appropriate for the person. It is as flat as possible.
9 Stand on one side of the bed. Your co-worker stands on the other side.
10 Lower the bed rails if up.
11 Remove pillows as directed by the nurse. Place a pillow upright against the headboard if the person can be without it.
12 Stand with a wide base of support. Point the foot near the head of the bed toward the head of the bed. Face the head of the bed.
13 Bend your hips and knees. Keep your back straight.
14 Place one arm under the person's shoulder and one arm under the thighs. Your co-worker

does the same. Grasp each other's forearms (Fig. 11-6).
15 Ask the person to grasp the trapeze (Fig. 11-7).
16 Have the person flex both knees.
17 Explain the following:
  a You will count "1, 2, 3."
  b The move will be on "3."
  c On "3," the person pushes against the bed with the feet if able. And the person pulls up with the trapeze.
18 Move the person to the head of the bed on the count of "3." Shift your weight from your rear leg to your front leg (see Figs. 11-6 and 11-7). Your co-worker does the same.
19 Repeat steps 12 through 18 if necessary.

Post-Procedure

20 Put the pillow under the person's head and shoulders. Straighten linens.
21 Position the person in good alignment (p. 172).
22 Provide for comfort. (See the inside of the front book cover.)
23 Place the signal light within reach.
24 Raise the head of the bed to a level appropriate for the person.

25 Lower the bed to its lowest position.
26 Raise or lower bed rails. Follow the care plan.
27 Unscreen the person.
28 Complete a safety check of the room. (See the inside of the front book cover.)
29 Decontaminate your hands.
30 Report and record your observations.

MOVING THE PERSON UP IN BED WITH AN ASSIST DEVICE

Assist devices are used to move some persons up in bed. Such assist devices include a drawsheet (lift sheet), flat sheet folded in half, turning pad (Fig. 11-8), slide sheet, and large incontinence product. With these devices, the person is moved more evenly. And the devices reduce shearing and friction. Therefore they are called *friction-reducing devices.*

The device is placed under the person from the head to above the knees or lower. At least two staff members are needed.

Use this procedure for:
- Persons who cannot move up in bed themselves
- Persons who are unconscious or paralyzed
- Persons recovering from spinal cord surgery or spinal cord injuries
- Older persons

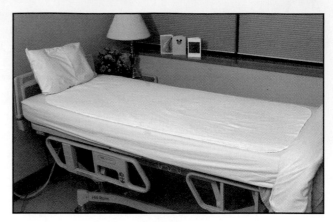

FIG. **11-8** Turning pad.

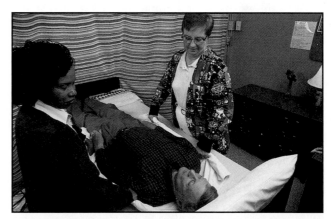

FIG. **11-9** A drawsheet is used to move the person up in bed. The drawsheet extends from the person's head to above the knees. The drawsheet is rolled close to the person and held near the shoulders and hips.

Moving the Person Up in Bed With an Assist Device

Quality of Life

Remember to:

- Knock before entering the person's room
- Address the person by name
- Introduce yourself by name and title

- Explain the procedure to the person before beginning and during the procedure
- Protect the person's rights during the procedure
- Handle the person gently during the procedure

Pre-Procedure

1 Follow *Delegation Guidelines: Moving Persons in Bed*, p. 147. See *Promoting Safety and Comfort: Moving Persons in Bed*, p. 147.

2 Ask a co-worker to help you.

3 Practice hand hygiene.

4 Identify the person. Check the ID bracelet against the assignment sheet. Call the person by name.

5 Provide for privacy.

6 Lock the bed wheels.

7 Raise the bed for body mechanics. Bed rails are up if used.

Procedure

8 Lower the head of the bed to a level appropriate for the person. It is as flat as possible.

9 Stand on one side of the bed. Your co-worker stands on the other side.

10 Lower the bed rails if up.

11 Remove pillows as directed by the nurse. Place a pillow upright against the headboard if the person can be without it.

12 Stand with a broad base of support. Point the foot near the head of the bed toward the head of the bed. Face that direction.

13 Roll the sides of the assist device up close to the person. (Note: Omit this step if the device has handles.)

14 Grasp the rolled-up assist device firmly near the person's shoulders and hips (Fig. 11-9). Or grasp it by the handles. Support the head.

15 Bend your hips and knees.

16 Move the person up in bed on the count of "3." Shift your weight from your rear leg to your front leg.

17 Repeat steps 12 through 16 if necessary.

18 Unroll the lift sheet. (Note: Omit this step if the device has handles.)

Post-Procedure

19 Put the pillow under the person's head and shoulders.

20 Position the person in good alignment (p. 172).

21 Provide for comfort. (See the inside of the front book cover.)

22 Place the signal light within reach.

23 Raise the head of the bed to a level appropriate for the person.

24 Lower the bed to its lowest position.

25 Raise or lower bed rails. Follow the care plan.

26 Unscreen the person.

27 Complete a safety check of the room. (See the inside of the front book cover.)

28 Decontaminate your hands.

29 Report and record your observations.

Moving the Person to the Side of the Bed

Repositioning and care procedures require moving the person to the side of the bed. The person is moved to the side of the bed before turning. Otherwise, after turning, the person lies on the side of the bed—not in the middle.

Sometimes you have to reach over the person. You reach less if the person is close to you.

In one method, the person is moved in segments. Sometimes one person can do this. Use a mechanical lift or the assist device method for older persons and those with arthritis. Also use it for persons recovering from spinal cord injuries or spinal cord surgery. An assist device helps prevent pain, skin damage, and injury to the bones, joints, and spinal cord.

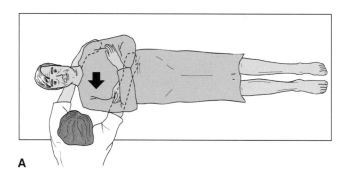

A

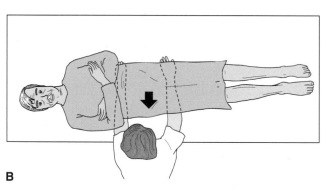

B

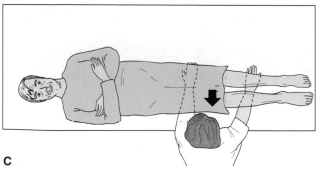

C

FIG. **11-10** The person is moved to the side of the bed in segments. **A,** The upper part of the body is moved. **B,** The lower part of the body is moved. **C,** The legs and feet are moved.

PROMOTING SAFETY AND COMFORT
Moving the Person to the Side of the Bed

Safety

Use the method and equipment best for the person. Get this information from the nurse when delegated tasks involve moving the person to the side of the bed. Such tasks include repositioning, bedmaking, bathing, and range-of-motion exercises.

The wrong method could seriously injure a person. This is very important for persons who are very old, have arthritis, or have spinal cord involvement.

When using an assist device, you need at least 1 co-worker to help you. Depending on the person's size, 3 staff members may be needed. If so, ask 2 co-workers to help you.

If using a slide board or slide sheet, you will need to place it under the person. After moving the person up in bed, remove the device.

To move the person in segments, move the person toward you not away from you. This helps protect you from injury

Comfort

After moving the person to the side of the bed, move the pillow too. Make sure the person's pillow is positioned correctly. It should be under the person's head and shoulders.

Moving the Person to the Side of the Bed

Quality of Life

Remember to:

- Knock before entering the person's room
- Address the person by name
- Introduce yourself by name and title

- Explain the procedure to the person before beginning and during the procedure
- Protect the person's rights during the procedure
- Handle the person gently during the procedure

Pre-Procedure

1 Follow *Delegation Guidelines: Moving Persons in Bed*, p. 147. See *Promoting Safety and Comfort:*
   - *Moving Persons in Bed*, p. 147.
   - *Moving the Person to the Side of the Bed.*
2 Ask a co-worker to help if using an assist device.
3 Practice hand hygiene.

4 Identify the person. Check the ID bracelet against the assignment sheet. Call the person by name.
5 Provide for privacy.
6 Lock the bed wheels.
7 Raise the bed for body mechanics. Bed rails are up if used.

Procedure

8 Lower the head of the bed to a level appropriate for the person. It is as flat as possible.
9 Stand on the side of the bed to which you will move the person.
10 Lower the bed rail near you if bed rails are used. (Both bed rails are lowered for step 15).
11 Remove pillows as directed by the nurse.
12 Stand with your feet about 12 inches apart. One foot is in front of the other. Flex your knees.
13 Cross the person's arms over the person's chest.
14 *Method 1*: Moving the person in segments:
   a Place your arm under the person's neck and shoulders. Grasp the far shoulder.
   b Place your other arm under the mid-back.
   c Move the upper part of the person's body toward you. Rock backward and shift your weight to your rear leg (Fig. 11-10, *A*).

   d Place one arm under the person's waist and one under the thighs.
   e Rock backward to move the lower part of the person toward you (Fig. 11-10, *B*).
   f Repeat the procedure for the legs and feet (Fig. 11-10, *C*). Your arms should be under the person's thighs and calves.
15 *Method 2: Moving the person with a drawsheet:*
   a Roll the drawsheet up close to the person (see Fig. 11-9).
   b Grasp the rolled-up drawsheet near the person's shoulders and hips. Your co-worker does the same. Support the head.
   c Rock backward on the count of "3," moving the person toward you. Your co-worker rocks backward slightly and then forward toward you while keeping the arms straight.
   d Unroll the drawsheet. Remove any wrinkles.

Post-Procedure

16 Position the person in good alignment.
17 Provide for comfort. (See the inside of the front book cover.)
18 Place the signal light within reach.
19 Lower the bed to its lowest position.
20 Raise or lower bed rails. Follow the care plan.

21 Unscreen the person.
22 Complete a safety check of the room. (See the inside of the front book cover.)
23 Decontaminate your hands.
24 Report and record your observations.

TURNING PERSONS

Turning persons onto their sides helps prevent complications from bedrest (Chapter 20). Certain procedures and care measures also require the side-lying position. The person is turned toward or away from you. The direction depends on the person's condition and situation.

Many older persons suffer from arthritis in their spines, hips, and knees. When turning these persons, logrolling is preferred (p. 156). Logrolling may be less painful for these persons.

DELEGATION GUIDELINES
Turning Persons

Before turning a person, you need this information from the nurse and the care plan:
- How much help the person needs
- How many staff members are needed to complete the procedure
- The person's comfort level and what body parts are painful
- Which procedure to use
- What assist devices to use
- What supportive devices are needed for positioning (Chapter 20)
- Where to place pillows
- What observations to report and record:
  - If you had help with the procedure and who helped you
  - How much help the person needed
  - How the person tolerated the procedure
  - How you positioned the person
  - Complaints of pain or discomfort

PROMOTING SAFETY AND COMFORT
Turning Persons

Safety

Use good body mechanics when turning a person in bed. The person must be in good alignment. Otherwise, musculoskeletal injuries, skin breakdown, or pressure ulcers could occur.

If using an assist device, ask a co-worker to help you.

Comfort

After turning, position the person in good alignment. Use pillows as directed to support the person in the side-lying position (p. 172).

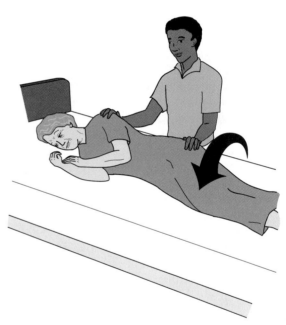

FIG. **11-11** Turning the person away from you.

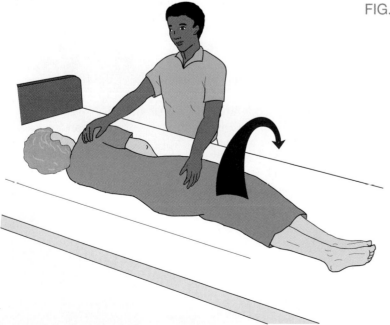

FIG. **11-12** Turning the person toward you.

Turning and Positioning the Person

NNAAP™

Quality of Life

Remember to:

- Knock before entering the person's room
- Address the person by name
- Introduce yourself by name and title

- Explain the procedure to the person before beginning and during the procedure
- Protect the person's rights during the procedure
- Handle the person gently during the procedure

Pre-Procedure

1 Follow *Delegation Guidelines: Turning Persons.* See *Promoting Safety and Comfort: Turning Persons.*
2 Practice hand hygiene.
3 Identify the person. Check the ID bracelet against the assignment sheet. Call the person by name.
4 Provide for privacy.
5 Lock the bed wheels.
6 Raise the bed for body mechanics. Bed rails are up if used.

Procedure

7 Lower the head of the bed to a level appropriate for the person. It is as flat as possible.
8 Stand on the side of the bed opposite to where you will turn the person. The far bed rail is up if used.
9 Lower the bed rail near you if used.
10 Move the person to the side near you. (See procedure: *Moving the Person to the Side of the Bed,* p. 153.)
11 Cross the person's arms over the person's chest. Cross the leg near you over the far leg.
12 *Turning the person away from you:*
  a Stand with a wide base of support. Flex your knees.
  b Place one hand on the person's shoulder. Place the other on the hip near you.
  c Push the person gently toward the other side of the bed (Fig. 11-11). Shift your weight from your rear leg to your front leg.
13 *Turning the person toward you:*
  a Raise the bed rail if used.
  b Go to the other side. Lower the bed rail if used.

  c Stand with a wide base of support. Flex your knees.
  d Place one hand on the person's far shoulder. Place the other on the far hip.
  e Roll the person toward you gently (Fig. 11-12).
14 Position the person. Follow the nurse's directions and the care plan. The following is common:
  a Place a pillow under the head and neck.
  b Adjust the shoulder. The person should not lie on an arm.
  c Place a small pillow under the upper hand and arm.
  d Position a pillow against the back.
  e Flex the upper knee. Position the upper leg in front of the lower leg.
  f Support the upper leg and thigh on pillows. Make sure the ankle is supported.

Post-Procedure

15 Provide for comfort. (See the inside of the front book cover.)
16 Place the signal light within reach.
17 Lower the bed to its lowest position.
18 Raise or lower bed rails. Follow the care plan.
19 Unscreen the person.
20 Complete a safety check of the room. (See the inside of the front book cover.)
21 Decontaminate your hands.
22 Report and record your observations.

LOGROLLING

Logrolling is turning the person as a unit, in alignment, with one motion. The spine is kept straight. The procedure is used to turn:

- Older persons with arthritic spines or knees
- Persons recovering from hip fractures
- Persons recovering from spinal cord injuries or surgery

PROMOTING SAFETY AND COMFORT
Logrolling

Safety

Two or three staff members are needed to logroll a person. Three are needed if the person is tall or heavy. Sometimes an assist device is needed—drawsheets, turning pad, large incontinence product, slide sheet.

Comfort

After spinal cord injury or surgery, the spine must be kept straight. This includes the person's neck. Therefore usually a pillow *is not* allowed under the head and neck. Follow the nurse's directions and the care plan for positioning the person and using pillows.

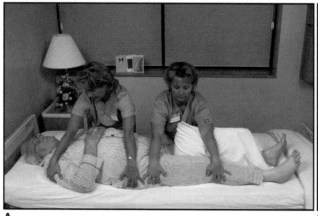
A

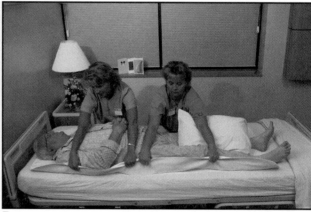
B

FIG. **11-13** Logrolling. **A,** A pillow is between the person's legs. The arms are crossed on the chest. The person is on the far side of the bed. **B,** An assist device is used to logroll a person.

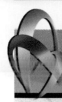

Logrolling the Person

Quality of Life

Remember to:

- Knock before entering the person's room
- Address the person by name
- Introduce yourself by name and title

- Explain the procedure to the person before beginning and during the procedure
- Protect the person's rights during the procedure
- Handle the person gently during the procedure

Pre-Procedure

1 Follow *Delegation Guidelines: Turning Persons,* p. 154. See *Promoting Safety and Comfort:*
- *Turning Persons,* p. 154
- *Logrolling Persons*

2 Ask a co-worker to help you.

3 Practice hand hygiene.

4 Identify the person. Check the ID bracelet against the assignment sheet. Call the person by name.

5 Provide for privacy.

6 Lock the bed wheels.

7 Raise the bed for body mechanics. Bed rails are up if used.

Procedure

8 Make sure the bed is flat.

9 Stand on the side opposite to where you will turn the person. Your co-worker stands on the other side.

10 Lower the bed rails if used.

11 Move the person as a unit to the side of the bed near you. Use the assist device.

12 Place the person's arms across the chest. Place a pillow between the knees.

13 Raise the bed rail if used.

14 Go to the other side.

15 Stand near the shoulders and chest. Your co-worker stands near the hips and thighs.

16 Stand with a broad base of support. One foot is in front of the other.

17 Ask the person to hold his or her body rigid.

18 Roll the person toward you (Fig. 11-13, *A*). Or use the assist device (Fig. 11-13, *B*). Turn the person as a unit.

19 Position the person in good alignment. Use pillows as directed by the nurse and care plan. The following is common (unless the spinal cord is involved):
- a One pillow against the back for support
- b One pillow under the head and neck if allowed
- c One pillow or folded bath blanket between the legs
- d A small pillow under the arm and hand

Post-Procedure

20 Provide for comfort. (See the inside of the front book cover.)

21 Place the signal light within reach.

22 Lower the bed to its lowest position.

23 Raise or lower bed rails. Follow the care plan.

24 Unscreen the person.

25 Complete a safety check of the room. (See the inside of the front book cover.)

26 Decontaminate your hands.

27 Report and record your observations.

DELEGATION GUIDELINES
Dangling

The nurse may ask you to help a person sit on the side of the bed. The procedure is part of other tasks—assisting the person to stand, transferring from bed to chair, partial bed bath, and others. When delegated the dangling procedure or tasks that involve dangling, you need this information from the nurse and the care plan:

- Areas of weakness. For example, if the person's arms are weak, he or she cannot hold onto the side of the mattress for support. If the left side is weak, turn the person onto the stronger right side. The person can use the right arm to help move from the lying to sitting position.
- The amount of help the person needs.
- If you need a co-worker to help you.
- How long the person needs to sit on the side of the bed.
- What exercises the person needs to perform while dangling:
  - Range of motion exercises (Chapter 20)
  - Coughing and deep breathing (Chapter 22)
- If the person will walk or transfer to a chair after dangling.
- What observations to report and record:
  - Pulse and respiratory rates
  - Pale or bluish skin color (cyanosis)
  - Complaints of dizziness, light-headedness, or difficulty breathing
  - How well the activity was tolerated
  - The length of time the person dangled
  - The amount of help needed
  - Other observations and the person's complaints

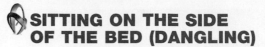

SITTING ON THE SIDE OF THE BED (DANGLING)

Patients and residents may become dizzy or faint when getting up too fast. They may need to sit on the side of the bed for a few minutes before a transfer or walking. Some increase activity in stages—bedrest, to sitting on the side of the bed, and then to sitting in a chair. Walking is the next step. Surgical patients sit on the side of the bed some time after surgery.

While dangling the legs, the person coughs and deep breathes. He or she moves the legs back and forth and in circles. This stimulates circulation.

Two staff members may be needed. Persons with balance and coordination problems need support. If dizziness or fainting occurs, lay the person down.

PROMOTING SAFETY AND COMFORT
Dangling

Safety

Problems with sitting and balance often occur after illness, injury, surgery, and bedrest. Some persons who are disabled also have problems sitting and with balance. Provide support when the person is sitting on the side of the bed. This protects the person from falling and other injuries.

Comfort

Provide for the person's warmth during the dangling procedure. Help the person put on a robe. Or cover the person's shoulders and back with a blanket.

The person may want to perform simple hygiene measures while sitting on the side of the bed. Oral hygiene and washing the face and hands are examples (Chapter 13). These measures refresh the person and stimulate circulation. Follow the nurse's directions and the care plan.

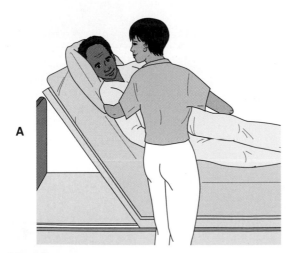
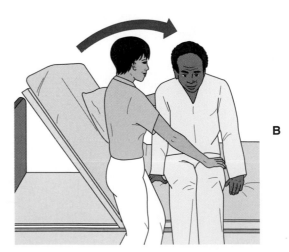

FIG. **11-14** Helping the person sit on the side of the bed. **A,** The person's shoulders and thighs are supported. **B,** The person sits upright as the legs and feet are pulled over the edge of the bed.

Helping the Person Sit on the Side of the Bed (Dangle)

Quality of Life

Remember to:

- Knock before entering the person's room
- Address the person by name
- Introduce yourself by name and title

- Explain the procedure to the person before beginning and during the procedure
- Protect the person's rights during the procedure
- Handle the person gently during the procedure

Pre-Procedure

1 Follow *Delegation Guidelines: Dangling.* See *Promoting Safety and Comfort: Dangling.*
2 Practice hand hygiene.
3 Identify the person. Check the ID bracelet against the assignment sheet. Call the person by name.
4 Provide for privacy.
5 Decide what side of the bed to use.
6 Move furniture to provide moving space.
7 Lock the bed wheels.
8 Raise the bed for body mechanics. Bed rails are up if used.

Procedure

9 Lower the bed rail if up.
10 Position the person in a side-lying position facing you. The person lies on the strong side.
11 Raise the head of the bed to a sitting position.
12 Stand by the person's hips. Face the foot of the bed.
13 Stand with your feet apart. The foot near the head of the bed is in front of the other foot.
14 Slide one arm under the person's neck and shoulders. Grasp the far shoulder. Place your other hand over the thighs near the knees (Fig. 11-14, *A*).
15 Pivot toward the foot of the bed while moving the person's legs and feet over the side of the bed. As the legs go over the edge of the mattress, the trunk is upright (Fig. 11-14, *B*).
16 Ask the person to hold onto the edge of the mattress. This supports the person in the sitting position.
17 Do not leave the person alone. Provide support if necessary.
18 Check the person's condition:
   a Ask how the person feels. Ask if the person feels dizzy or light-headed.
   b Check pulse and respirations.
   c Check for difficulty breathing.
   d Note if the skin is pale or bluish in color (*cyanosis*).
19 Help the person lie down if necessary.
20 Reverse the procedure to return the person to bed.
21 Lower the head of the bed after the person returns to bed. Help him or her move to the center of the bed.
22 Position the person in good alignment.

Post-Procedure

23 Provide for comfort. (See the inside of the front book cover.)
24 Place the signal light within reach.
25 Lower the bed to its lowest position.
26 Raise or lower bed rails. Follow the care plan.
27 Return furniture to its proper places.
28 Unscreen the person.
29 Complete a safety check of the room. (See the inside of the front book cover.)
30 Decontaminate your hands.
31 Report and record your observations.

TRANSFERRING PERSONS

To *transfer* a person means moving the person from one place to another. Persons are often moved from beds to chairs, wheelchairs, and toilets. Some transfers require one, two, or three people.

The rules of body mechanics apply to transfers. Arrange the room so there is enough space for a safe transfer. Correct chair or wheelchair placement is needed for a safe transfer.

DELEGATION GUIDELINES
Transferring Persons

When delegated transferring procedures, you need this information from the nurse and the care plan:

- What procedure to use:
  - *Transferring the Person to a Chair or Wheelchair*
  - *Transferring the Person From a Chair or Wheelchair to Bed*
  - *Transferring the Person Using a Mechanical Lift*
  - *Transferring the Person to and From the Toilet*
- Areas of weakness. For example, if the person's arms are weak, the person cannot hold the side of the mattress for support. If the person has a weak left side, he or she gets out of bed on the stronger right side. The person uses the right arm to help move from the lying to sitting position.
- The equipment needed—transfer belt, wheelchair, mechanical lift, positioning devices, wheelchair cushion, and so on.
- The amount of help the person needs.
- How many co-workers need to help you.
- What observations to report and record:
  - Pulse rate before and after the transfer
  - Complaints of light-headedness, pain, discomfort, difficulty breathing, weakness, or fatigue
  - The amount of help needed to transfer the person
  - How the person helped with the transfer

Applying Transfer Belts

A **transfer belt** is used to support persons who are unsteady or disabled. It helps prevent falls and other injuries. The belt goes around the person's waist. Grasp underneath the belt to support the person during the transfer. The belt is called a *gait belt* when used for walking with a person. Many agencies require staff to use these belts when transferring or walking a person.

PROMOTING SAFETY AND COMFORT
Transferring Persons

Safety

The person wears non-skid footwear for transfers. Such footwear protects the person from falls. Slipping and sliding are prevented. Remember to securely tie shoelaces. Otherwise the person can trip and fall.

Lock bed and wheelchair wheels. This prevents the bed and wheelchair from moving during the transfer. Otherwise, the person can fall. You also are at risk for injury.

Comfort

After the transfer, position the person in good alignment. Make sure the person has needed items within reach.

PROMOTING SAFETY AND COMFORT
Transfer Belts

Safety

Transfer belts are used routinely in nursing centers. If the person needs help, a transfer belt is required. To use one safely, always follow the manufacturer's instructions.

Do not leave excess strap dangling. Tuck the excess strap under the belt.

Comfort

A transfer belt is always applied over clothing. It is never applied over bare skin. Also, it is applied under the breasts. Breasts must not be caught under the belt.

Applying a Transfer Belt

Quality of Life

Remember to:

- Knock before entering the person's room
- Address the person by name
- Introduce yourself by name and title

- Explain the procedure to the person before beginning and during the procedure
- Protect the person's rights during the procedure
- Handle the person gently during the procedure

Procedure

1 See *Promoting Safety and Comfort: Transfer Belts.*
2 Practice hand hygiene.
3 Identify the person. Check the ID bracelet against the assignment sheet. Call the person by name.
4 Provide for privacy.
5 Assist the person to a sitting position.
6 Apply the belt around the person's waist over clothing. Do not apply it over bare skin.

7 Tighten the belt so it is snug. It should not cause discomfort or impair breathing. You should be able to slide 4 fingers (your open, flat hand) under the belt.
8 Make sure that a woman's breasts are not caught under the belt.
9 Place the buckle off center in the front or in the back for the person's comfort (Fig. 11-15). The buckle is not over the spine.

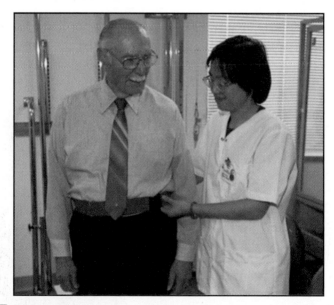

FIG. **11-15** Transfer belt. The belt buckle is positioned off center. The nursing assistant grasps the belt from underneath.

Bed to Chair or Wheelchair Transfers

Safety is important for chair and wheelchair transfers. Help the person out of bed on his or her strong side. If the left side is weak and the right side strong, get the person out of bed on the right side. In transferring, the strong side moves first. It pulls the weaker side along. Transfers from the weak side are awkward and unsafe.

PROMOTING SAFETY AND COMFORT
Chair or Wheelchair Transfers

Safety

The chair or wheelchair must support the person's weight. The number of staff members needed for a transfer depends on the person's abilities, condition, and size. If the person cannot assist, use a mechanical lift (p. 167).

The person must not put his or her arms around your neck. Otherwise the person can pull you forward or cause you to lose your balance. Neck, back, and other injuries from falls are possible.

Using a gait/transfer belt is the *preferred* method for chair or wheelchair transfers. It is safer for the person and you. Putting your arms around the person and grasping the shoulder blades is the other method. It can cause the person discomfort. And it can be stressful for you. Use this method *only* if instructed by the nurse and the care plan.

Wheelchair wheels are locked for a safe transfer. After the transfer, unlock the wheels to position the wheelchair as the person prefers. After positioning the chair, lock the wheels or keep them unlocked according to the care plan. Locked wheels may be considered restraints if the person cannot unlock them to move the wheelchair (Chapter 9). However, falling and other injuries are risks if the person tries to stand when the wheelchair wheels are unlocked.

Comfort

Most wheelchairs and bedside chairs have vinyl seats and backs. Vinyl holds body heat. The person becomes warm and perspires more. You can cover the back and seat with a folded bath blanket. This increases the person's comfort in the chair. Some people have wheelchair cushions or positioning devices. Ask the nurse how to use and place the devices.

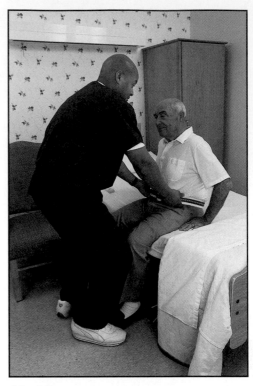

FIG. **11-16** Transferring the person to a chair using a transfer belt. The person's feet and knees are blocked by the nursing assistant's feet and knees. This prevents the person from sliding or falling.

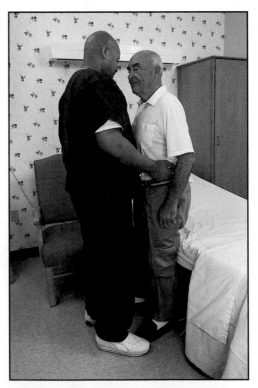

FIG. **11-17** The person is pulled up to a standing position and supported by holding the transfer belt and blocking the person's knees and feet.

Transferring the Person to a Chair or Wheelchair

Quality of Life

Remember to:

- Knock before entering the person's room
- Address the person by name
- Introduce yourself by name and title

- Explain the procedure to the person before beginning and during the procedure
- Protect the person's rights during the procedure
- Handle the person gently during the procedure

Pre-Procedure

1 Follow *Delegation Guidelines: Transferring Persons*, p. 160. See *Promoting Safety and Comfort:*
  - *Transferring Persons*, p. 160
  - *Transfer Belts*, p. 160
  - *Chair or Wheelchair Transfers*
2 Collect:
  - Wheelchair or arm chair
  - Bath blanket
  - Lap blanket
  - Robe and non-skid footwear

  - Paper or sheet
  - Transfer belt (if needed)
  - Seat cushion (if needed)
3 Practice hand hygiene.
4 Identify the person. Check the ID bracelet against the assignment sheet. Call the person by name.
5 Provide for privacy.
6 Decide which side of the bed to use. Move furniture for a safe transfer.

Procedure

7 Place the chair near the bed on the person's strong side. The arm of the chair should almost touch the bed.
8 Place a folded bath blanket or cushion on the seat (if needed).
9 Lock wheelchair wheels. Raise the footplates. Remove or swing the front rigging out of the way.
10 Lower the bed to its lowest position. Lock the bed wheels.
11 Fan-fold top linens to the foot of the bed.
12 Place the paper or sheet under the person's feet. Put footwear on the person.
13 Help the person sit on the side of the bed. His or her feet touch the floor.
14 Help the person put on a robe.
15 Apply the transfer belt (if needed).
16 *Method 1: Using a transfer belt*
  a Stand in front of the person.
  b Have the person hold onto the mattress.
  c Make sure the person's feet are flat on the floor.
  d Have the person lean forward.
  e Grasp the transfer belt at each side. Grasp the belt from underneath.
  f Prevent the person from sliding or falling by doing one of the following:
    1 Brace your knees against the person's knees. Block his or her feet with your feet (Fig. 11-16).

  2 Use the knee and foot of one leg to block the person's weak leg or foot. Place your other foot slightly behind you for balance.
  3 Straddle your legs around the person's weak leg.
  g Explain the following:
    1 You will count "1, 2, 3."
    2 The move will be on "3."
    3 On "3," the person pushes down on the mattress and stands.
  h Ask the person to push down on the mattress and to stand on the count of "3."
  i Pull the person into a standing position as you straighten your knees (Fig. 11-17).
17 *Method 2: No transfer belt* (Note: use this method only if directed by the nurse and the care plan.)
  a Follow step 16, a-c.
  b Place your hands under the person's arms. Your hands are around the person's shoulder blades (Fig. 11-18, p. 164).
  c Have the person lean forward.
  d Prevent the person from sliding or falling by doing one of the following:
    1 Brace your knees against the person's knees. Block his or her feet with your feet.
    2 Use the knee and foot of one leg to block the person's weak leg or foot. Place your other foot slightly behind you for balance.
    3 Straddle your legs around the person's weak leg.

Continued

Transferring the Person to a Chair or Wheelchair—cont'd

NNAAP™

Procedure—cont'd

   e Explain the "count of 3." See step 16, g.

   f Ask the person to push down on the mattress and to stand on the count of "3." Pull the person up into a standing position as you straighten your knees.

18 Support the person in the standing position. Hold the transfer belt, or keep your hands around the person's shoulder blades. Continue to prevent the person from sliding or falling.

19 Turn the person so he or she can grasp the far arm of the chair. The person's legs will touch the edge of the chair (Fig. 11-19).

20 Continue to turn the person until the other armrest is grasped.

21 Lower him or her into the chair as you bend your hips and knees. The person assists by leaning forward and bending the elbows and knees (Fig. 11-20).

22 Make sure the buttocks are to the back of the seat. Position the person in good alignment.

23 Attach the wheelchair front rigging. Position the person's feet on the wheelchair footplates.

24 Cover the person's lap and legs with a lap blanket. Keep the blanket off the floor and the wheels.

25 Remove the transfer belt if used.

26 Position the chair as the person prefers. Lock the wheelchair wheels according to the care plan.

Post-Procedure

27 Provide for comfort. (See the inside of the front book cover.)

28 Place the signal light and other needed items within reach.

29 Unscreen the person.

30 Complete a safety check of the room. (See the inside of the front book cover.)

31 Decontaminate your hands.

32 Report and record your observations.

33 See procedure: *Transferring the Person from the Chair or Wheelchair to Bed*, p. 166, to return the person to bed.

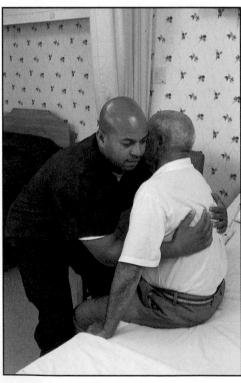

FIG. **11-18** The person is being prepared to stand. The hands are placed under the person's arms and around the shoulder blades.

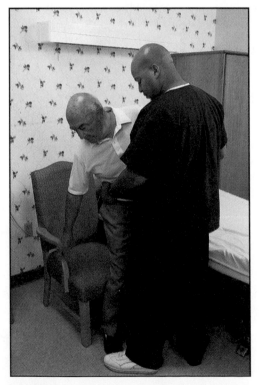

FIG. **11-19** The person is supported as he grasps the far arm of the chair. The legs are against the chair.

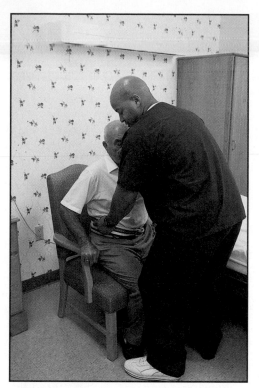

FIG. **11-20** The person holds the armrests, leans forward, and bends the elbows and knees while being lowered into the chair.

Chair or Wheelchair to Bed Transfers

Chair or wheelchair to bed transfers have the same rules as bed to chair transfers. If the person is weak on one side, transfer the person so that the strong side moves first. Therefore the person is transferred to the bed on the opposite side from which the person transferred out of the bed.

For example, Mrs. Lee's right side is weak. Her left side is strong. To transfer her from bed to chair, the chair was positioned on the left side of the bed. This allowed her left side (strong side) to move first. Now you will transfer Mrs. Lee back to bed. If the chair is on the left side of the bed, her right side—the weak side—is near the bed. It is unsafe to move the weak side first. You need to move the chair to the other side of the bed. Mrs. Lee's stronger left side will be near the bed. The stronger left side moves first for a safe transfer.

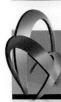

Transferring the Person From a Chair or Wheelchair to Bed

Quality of Life

Remember to:

- Knock before entering the person's room
- Address the person by name
- Introduce yourself by name and title

- Explain the procedure to the person before beginning and during the procedure
- Protect the person's rights during the procedure
- Handle the person gently during the procedure

Pre-Procedure

1 Follow *Delegation Guidelines: Transferring Persons,* p. 160. See *Promoting Safety and Comfort:*
   - *Transferring Persons,* p. 160
   - *Transfer Belts,* p. 160
   - *Chair or Wheelchair Transfers,* p. 162

2 Collect a transfer belt (if needed).
3 Practice hand hygiene.
4 Identify the person. Check the ID bracelet against the assignment sheet. Call the person by name.
5 Provide for privacy.

Procedure

6 Move furniture for moving space.
7 Raise the head of the bed to a sitting position. The bed is in the lowest position.
8 Move the signal light so it is on the strong side when the person is in bed.
9 Position the chair or wheelchair so the person's strong side is next to the bed (Fig. 11-21). Have a co-worker help you if necessary.
10 Lock the wheelchair and bed wheels.
11 Remove and fold the lap blanket.
12 Remove the person's feet from the footplates. Raise the footplates. Remove or swing the front rigging out of the way.
13 Apply the transfer belt (if needed).
14 Make sure the person's feet are flat on the floor.
15 Stand in front of the person.
16 Ask the person to hold onto the armrests. Or place your arms under the person's arms. Your hands are around the shoulder blades.
17 Have the person lean forward.
18 Grasp the transfer belt on each side if using it. Grasp underneath the belt.
19 Prevent the person from sliding or falling by doing one of the following:
   a Brace your knees against the person's knees. Block his or her feet with your feet.

   b Use the knee and foot of one leg to block the person's weak leg or foot. Place your other foot slightly behind you for balance.
   c Straddle your legs around the person's weak leg.
20 Explain the count of "3." (See procedure: *Transferring the Person to a Chair or Wheelchair,* p. 163)
21 Ask the person to push down on the armrests on the count of "3." Pull the person into a standing position as you straighten your knees.
22 Support the person in the standing position. Hold the transfer belt, or keep your hands around the person's shoulder blades. Continue to prevent the person from sliding or falling.
23 Turn the person so he or she can reach the edge of the mattress. The legs will touch the mattress.
24 Continue to turn the person until he or she can reach the mattress with both hands.
25 Lower him or her onto the bed as you bend your hips and knees. The person assists by leaning forward and bending the elbows and knees.
26 Remove the transfer belt.
27 Remove the robe and footwear.
28 Help the person lie down.

Post-Procedure

29 Provide for comfort. (See the inside of the front book cover.)
30 Place the signal light and other needed items within reach.
31 Raise or lower bed rails. Follow the care plan.
32 Arrange furniture to meet the person's needs.

33 Unscreen the person.
34 Complete a safety check of the room. (See the inside of the front book cover.)
35 Decontaminate your hands.
36 Report and record your observations.

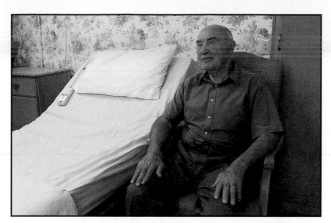

FIG. **11-21** To transfer the person from chair to bed, the chair is positioned so the person's strong side is near the bed.

 Using Mechanical Lifts

Persons who cannot help themselves are transferred with mechanical lifts. So are persons too heavy for the staff to transfer. Lifts are used for transfers to chairs, stretchers, tubs, shower chairs, toilets, commodes, whirlpools, or vehicles.

There are manual and electric lifts. Before using a lift:

■ You must be trained in its use.
■ It must work.

PROMOTING SAFETY AND COMFORT
Mechanical Lifts

Safety

Always follow the manufacturer's instructions. Knowing how to use one lift does not mean that you know how to use others. If you have questions, ask the nurse. If you have not used a certain lift before, ask for needed training. Ask the nurse to help you use it the first time and until you are comfortable using it.

Comfort

The person will be lifted up and off of the bed. Falling from the lift is a common fear. To promote the person's mental comfort, always explain the procedure before you begin. Also show the person how the lift works.

■ The sling, straps, hooks, and chains must be in good repair.
■ The person's weight must not exceed the lift's capacity.

At least two staff members are needed. The following procedure is used as a guide.

 Transferring the Person Using a Mechanical Lift

Quality of Life

Remember to:

■ Knock before entering the person's room
■ Address the person by name
■ Introduce yourself by name and title

■ Explain the procedure to the person before beginning and during the procedure
■ Protect the person's rights during the procedure
■ Handle the person gently during the procedure

Pre-Procedure

1 Follow *Delegation Guidelines: Transferring Persons*, p. 160. See *Promoting Safety and Comfort:*
 • *Transferring Persons*, p. 160
 • *Mechanical Lifts*
2 Ask a co-worker to help you.
3 Collect:
 • Mechanical lift
 • Arm chair or wheelchair

 • Footwear
 • Bath blanket or cushion
 • Lap blanket
4 Practice hand hygiene.
5 Identify the person. Check the ID bracelet against the assignment sheet. Call the person by name.
6 Provide for privacy.

Continued

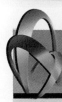

Transferring the Person Using a Mechanical Lift—cont'd

Procedure

7 Raise the bed for body mechanics. Bed rails are used if up.

8 Lower the head of the bed to a level appropriate for the person. It is flat as possible.

9 Stand on one side of the bed. Your co-worker stands on the other side.

10 Lower the bed rails if up.

11 Center the sling under the person (Fig. 11-22, *A*). To position the sling, turn the person from side to side as if making an occupied bed (Chapter 12). Position the sling according to the manufacturer's instructions.

12 Position the person in semi-Fowler's position.

13 Place the chair at the head of the bed. It is even with the headboard and about 1 foot away from the bed. Place a folded bath blanket or cushion in the chair.

14 Lock the bed wheels. Lower the bed to its lowest position.

15 Raise the lift so you can position it over the person.

16 Position the lift over the person (Fig. 11-22, *B*).

17 Lock the lift wheels in position.

18 Attach the sling to the swivel bar (Fig. 11-22, *C*).

19 Raise the head of the bed to a sitting position.

20 Cross the person's arms over the chest. He or she can hold onto the straps or chains but not the swivel bar.

21 Raise the lift high enough until the person and sling are free of the bed (Fig. 11-22, *D*).

22 Have your co-worker support the person's legs as you move the lift and person away from the bed (Fig. 11-22, *E*).

23 Position the lift so that the person's back is toward the chair.

24 Position the chair so you can lower the person into it.

25 Lower the person into the chair. Guide the person into the chair (Fig. 11-22, *F*).

26 Lower the swivel bar to unhook the sling. Remove the sling from under the person unless otherwise indicated.

27 Put footwear on the person. Position the person's feet on wheelchair footplates.

28 Cover the person's lap and legs with a lap blanket. Keep it off the floor and wheels.

29 Position the chair as the person prefers. Lock the wheelchair wheels according to the care plan.

Post-Procedure

30 Provide for comfort. (See the inside of the front book cover.)

31 Place the signal light and other needed items within reach.

32 Unscreen the person.

33 Complete a safety check of the room. (See the inside of the front book cover.)

34 Decontaminate your hands.

35 Report and record your observations.

36 Reverse the procedure to return the person to bed.

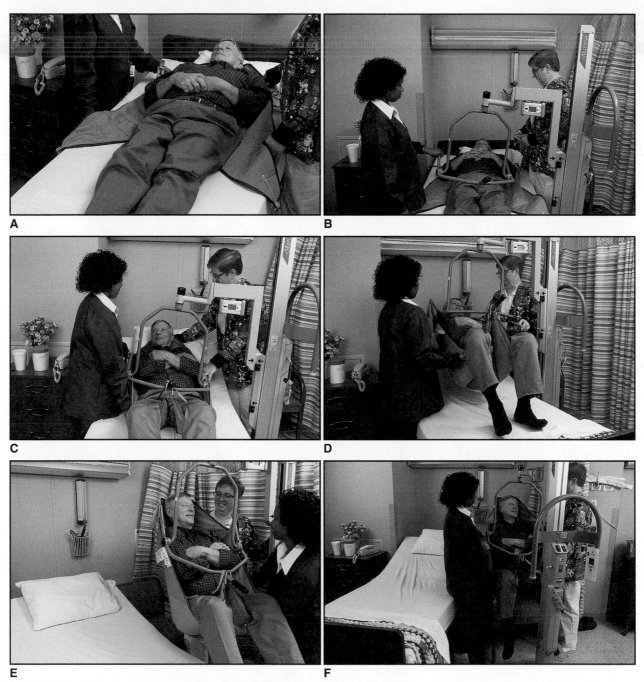

FIG. **11-22** Using a mechanical lift. **A,** The sling is positioned under the person. **B,** The lift is over the person. **C,** The sling is attached to a swivel bar. **D,** The lift is raised until the sling and person are off of the bed. **E,** The person's legs are supported as the person and lift are moved away from the bed. **F,** The person is guided into a chair.

Transferring the Person to and From the Toilet

Using the bathroom promotes dignity, self-esteem, and independence. It is more private than using a bedpan, urinal, or bedside commode. However, getting to the toilet is hard for persons who use wheelchairs. Bathrooms are often small. There is little room for you and a wheelchair. Therefore transfers involving wheelchairs and toilets are often hard. The risk of falls is great.

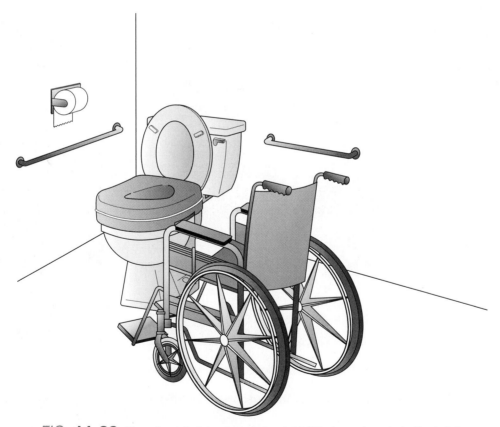

FIG. **11-23** The wheelchair is placed at a right (90-degree) angle to the toilet.

Transferring the Person to and From the Toilet

Quality of Life

Remember to:

- Knock before entering the person's room
- Address the person by name
- Introduce yourself by name and title

- Explain the procedure to the person before beginning and during the procedure
- Protect the person's rights during the procedure
- Handle the person gently during the procedure

Pre-Procedure

1 Follow *Delegation Guidelines: Transferring Persons,* p. 160. See *Promoting Safety and Comfort:*
   - *Transferring Persons,* p. 160
   - *Transfer Belts,* p. 160
   - *Chair or Wheelchair Transfers,* p. 162

2 Practice hand hygiene.

3 Make sure the person has an elevated toilet seat. The toilet seat and wheelchair are at the same level.

4 Check the grab bars by the toilet. If they are loose, tell the nurse. Do not transfer the person to the toilet if the grab bars are not secure.

Procedure

5 Have the person wear non-skid footwear.

6 Position the wheelchair next to the toilet if there is enough room. If not, position the wheelchair at a right (90-degree) angle to the toilet (Fig. 11-23). It is best if the person's strong side is near the toilet.

7 Lock the wheelchair wheels.

8 Raise the footplates. Remove or swing the front rigging out of the way.

9 Apply the transfer belt.

10 Help the person unfasten clothing.

11 Use the transfer belt to help the person stand and to turn to the toilet. (See procedure: *Transferring the Person to a Chair or Wheelchair,* p. 163.) The person uses the grab bars to turn to the toilet.

12 Support the person with the transfer belt while he or she lowers clothing. Or have the person hold onto the grab bars for support. Lower the person's pants and undergarments.

13 Use the transfer belt to lower the person onto the toilet seat.

14 Remove the transfer belt.

15 Tell the person you will stay nearby. Remind the person to use the signal light or call for you when help is needed. Stay with the person if required by the care plan.

16 Close the bathroom door to provide for privacy.

17 Stay near the bathroom. Complete other tasks in the person's room. Check on the person every 5 minutes.

18 Knock on the bathroom door when the person calls for you.

19 Help with wiping, perineal care (Chapter 13), flushing, and hand washing as needed. Wear gloves and practice hand hygiene.

20 Apply the transfer belt.

21 Use the transfer belt to help the person stand.

22 Help the person raise and secure clothing.

23 Use the transfer belt to transfer the person to the wheelchair. (See procedure: *Transferring the Person to a Chair or Wheelchair,* p. 163.)

24 Make sure the person's buttocks are to the back of the seat. Position the person in good alignment.

25 Position the person's feet on the footplates.

26 Cover the person's lap and legs with a lap blanket. Keep the blanket off the floor and wheels.

27 Position the chair as the person prefers. Lock the wheelchair wheels according to the care plan.

Post-Procedure

28 Provide for comfort. (See inside of the front cover.)

29 Place the signal light and other needed items within reach.

30 Unscreen the person.

31 Complete a safety check of the room. (See inside of the front cover.)

32 Practice hand hygiene.

33 Report and record your observations.

POSITIONING

The person must be properly positioned at all times. Regular position changes and good alignment promote comfort and well-being. Breathing is easier. Circulation is promoted. Pressure ulcers (Chapter 21) and contractures (Chapter 20) are prevented.

Whether in bed or chair, the person is repositioned at least every 2 hours. Some people are repositioned more often. You must follow the nurse's instructions and the care plan.

Follow these guidelines to safely position a person:

- Use good body mechanics.
- Ask a co-worker to help you if needed.
- Explain the procedure to the person.
- Be gentle when moving the person.
- Provide for privacy.
- Use pillows as directed for support and alignment.
- Place the signal light within reach after positioning.

DELEGATION GUIDELINES
Positioning

Many delegated tasks involve positioning and repositioning. You need this information from the nurse and the care plan:

- Position or positioning limits ordered by the doctor
- How often to turn and reposition the person
- How many co-workers need to help you
- What skin care measures to perform (Chapter 13)
- What range-of-motion exercises to perform (Chapter 20)
- Where to place pillows
- What positioning devices are needed and how to use them
- What observations to report and record

PROMOTING SAFETY AND COMFORT
Positioning

Safety

Pressure ulcers (Chapter 21) are serious threats from lying or sitting too long in one place. Wet, soiled, and wrinkled linens are other causes. Whenever you reposition a person, make sure linens are clean, dry, and wrinkle-free. Change or straighten linens as needed.

Contractures can develop from staying in one position too long (Chapter 20). A *contracture* is the lack of joint mobility caused by abnormal shortening of a muscle. Repositioning, exercise, and activity help prevent contractures.

Comfort

Pillows and positioning devices are used to position a person. They support body parts and keep the person in good alignment. This promotes comfort. Place pillows and positioning devices as directed by the nurse and the care plan.

Fowler's Position

Fowler's position is a semi-sitting position. The head of the bed is raised between 45 and 60 degrees (Fig. 11-24). For good alignment:

- Keep the spine straight.
- Support the head with a small pillow.
- Support the arms with pillows.

Supine Position

The **supine (dorsal recumbent) position** is the back-lying position (Fig. 11-25). For good alignment:

- The bed is flat.
- The head and shoulders are supported on a pillow.
- Arms and hands are at the sides. You can support the arms with regular pillows. Or you can support the hands on small pillows with the palms down.

The nurse may ask you to place a folded or rolled towel under the lower back and a small pillow under the thighs. A pillow under the lower legs lifts the heels off of the bed. This prevents them from rubbing on the sheets.

Prone Position

A person in the **prone position** lies on the abdomen with the head turned to one side. The bed is flat. Small pillows are placed under the head, abdomen, and lower legs (Fig. 11-26). Arms are flexed at the elbows with the hands near the head.

You also can position a person with the feet hanging over the end of the mattress (Fig. 11-27). A pillow is not needed under the feet.

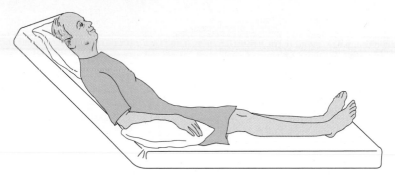

FIG. **11-24** Fowler's position.

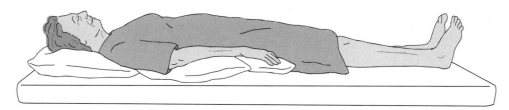

FIG. **11-25** Supine position.

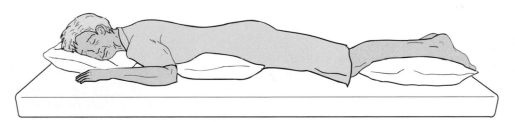

FIG. **11-26** Prone position.

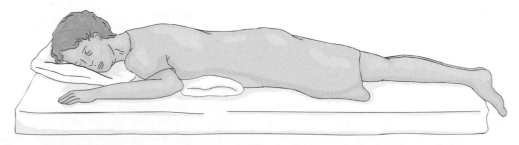

FIG. **11-27** Prone position with the feet hanging over the edge of the mattress.

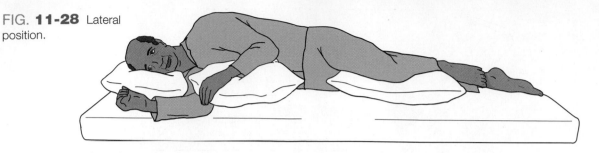

FIG. **11-28** Lateral position.

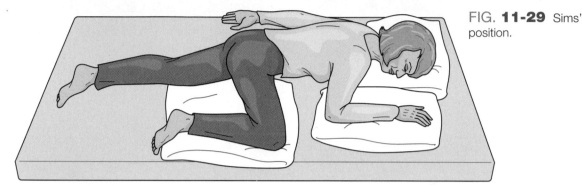

FIG. **11-29** Sims' position.

Lateral Position

A person in the **lateral (side-lying) position** lies on one side or the other (Fig. 11-28):

- The bed is flat
- A pillow is under the head and neck.
- The upper leg is in front of the lower leg. (The nurse may ask you to position the upper leg behind the lower leg, not on top of it.)
- The ankle, upper leg, and thigh are supported with pillows.
- A pillow is positioned against the person's back.
- A small pillow is under the upper hand and arm.

Sims' Position

The **Sims' position** is a left side-lying position. The upper leg is sharply flexed so it is not on the lower leg. The lower arm is behind the person (Fig. 11-29). Sims' position also is called the **semi-prone side position.** For good alignment:

- The bed is flat
- Place a pillow under the person's head and shoulder.
- Support the upper leg with a pillow.
- Place a pillow under the upper arm and hand.

Chair Position

Persons who sit in chairs must hold their upper bodies and heads erect. If not, poor alignment results. For good alignment:

- The person's back and buttocks are against the back of the chair.
- Feet are flat on the floor or wheelchair footplates. Never leave the feet unsupported.

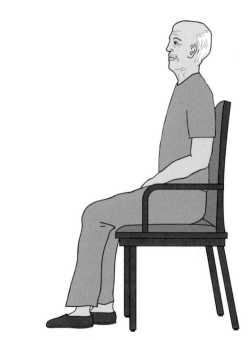

FIG. **11-30** The person is positioned in a chair. The person's feet are flat on the floor, the calves do not touch the chair, and the back is straight and against the back of the chair.

- Backs of the knees and calves are slightly away from the edge of the seat (Fig. 11-30).

The nurse may ask you to put a small pillow between the person's lower back and the chair. Paralyzed arms are supported on pillows. Some residents have positioners (Fig. 11-31). Ask the nurse about their proper use. Wrists are positioned at a slight upward angle.

Some people use postural supports (Fig. 11-32). They help maintain good alignment.

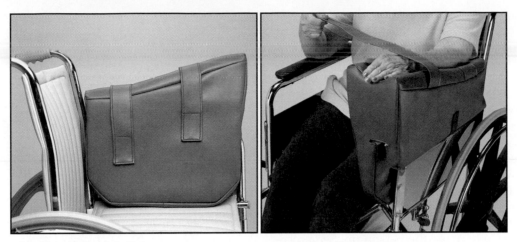

FIG. **11-31** Elevated armrest. (Courtesy JT Posey Co., Arcadia, Calif.)

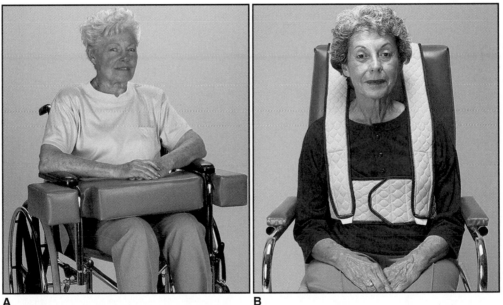

A **B**

FIG. **11-32** Postural supports. **A,** Pelvic holder. **B,** Torso support. (Courtesy JT Posey Co., Arcadia, Calif.)

Repositioning in a Chair or Wheelchair

The person can slide down into the chair. For good alignment and safety, the person's back and buttocks must be against the back of the chair.

Some persons can help with repositioning. Others need help. If the person cannot help, a mechanical lift is needed to reposition the person. Follow the nurse's directions and the care plan for the best way to reposition a person in a chair or wheelchair.

If the person's chair reclines, do the following:

- Ask a co-worker to help you.
- Recline the chair.
- Position a friction-reducing device (drawsheet or slide sheet) under the person.
- Use the device to move the person up. See procedure: *Moving the Person Up in Bed With an Assist Device*, p. 151.

This method can be used if the person is alert and cooperative. The person must be able to follow directions. And the person must have the strength to help.

- Lock the wheelchair wheels.
- Remove or swing the front rigging out of the way.
- Position the person's feet flat on the floor.
- Apply a transfer belt.
- Position the person's arms on the armrests.
- Stand in front of the person. Block his or knees and feet with your knees and feet.
- Grasp the transfer belt on each side while the person leans forward.
- Ask the person to push with his or her feet and arms on the count of "3."
- Move the person back into the chair on the count of "3" as the person pushes with his or her feet and arms (Fig. 11-33).

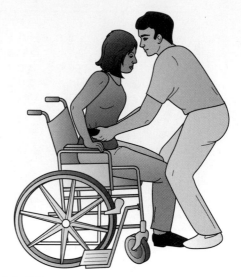

FIG. **11-33** Repositioning the person in a wheelchair. A transfer belt is used to move the person to the back of the chair.

FOCUS ON THE PERSON

Good body mechanics and proper positioning protect the person from injury. So do correct moving, turning, and transferring procedures. You must always protect the person from injury.

See Focus on the Person: Using Body Mechanics.

Focus on the **PERSON**

Using Body Mechanics

Providing comfort—The person's mental comfort is important during moving, turning, and transfer procedures. Falling is a common fear. Always explain what you are going to do before starting the procedure. Then explain what you are doing step-by-step.

Ethical behavior—Patients and residents must be repositioned at least every two hours. Do the right thing—follow the nurse's directions and the person's care plan. Do not report that you repositioned someone when you did not. That is the wrong thing.

Remaining independent—Remaining independent to the extent possible promotes dignity and self-esteem. Let the person help as much as safely possible. Let the person choose such things as bed positions, where the chair or wheelchair is positioned, and when to go back to bed.

Speaking up—Moving can be very painful following an injury or surgery. Many older persons have painful joints. You must make sure that the person is comfortable and that you are not causing pain. You can say:

- "Am I hurting you?"
- "Please tell me when you feel pain or discomfort."
- "Do you need a pillow adjusted?"
- "Are you comfortable?"
- "How can I help make you more comfortable?"

OBRA and other laws—The Occupational Health and Safety Act requires that employers provide employees with a safe work setting. The setting must be free of recognized hazards that are causing or likely to cause death or serious physical harm to employees. The employer must make reasonable attempts to prevent or reduce the hazard. OSHA inspection teams enforce this law.

Nursing teamwork—Moving, turning, transferring, and positioning a person are always safer when done by two workers. Willingly help others when asked. If you cannot stop what you are doing, tell your co-worker when you will be available. Then help the person when you said that you would.

REVIEW QUESTIONS

Circle the **BEST** answer.

1 Good body mechanics involves the following *except*
   a Good posture
   b Balance
   c Using the strongest and largest muscles
   d Having the job fit the worker

2 Good body alignment means
   a The area on which an object rests
   b Having the head, trunk, arms, and legs aligned with one another
   c Using muscles, tendons, ligaments, joints, and cartilage correctly
   d The back-lying or supine position

3 These actions are about body mechanics. Which is *incorrect?*
   a Hold objects away from your body when moving, or carrying them.
   b Face the direction you are working to prevent twisting.
   c Push, pull, or slide heavy objects.
   d Use both hands and arms to lift, move, or carry heavy objects.

4 A person's skin rubs against the sheet. This is called
   a Shearing
   b Friction
   c Ergonomics
   d Posture

5 Which occurs when a person slides down in bed?
   a Shearing
   b Friction
   c Ergonomics
   d Posture

6 Which protects the skin when moving the person in bed?
   a Rolling or lifting the person
   b Sliding the person up in bed
   c Moving the mattress
   d Using ergonomics

7 Whenever you move, turn, transfer, or reposition a person, you must
   a Allow personal choice
   b Protect the person's privacy
   c Use pillows for support
   d Get help from a co-worker

REVIEW QUESTIONS

8 You are delegated tasks that involve moving persons in bed. Which is *true*?
   a The nurse tells you how to position the person.
   b You decide which procedure to use.
   c Bed rails are used at all times.
   d Three workers are needed to complete the task safely.

9 You are using a drawsheet as an assist device. It is placed so that it
   a Covers the person's body
   b Is under the person from the head to above the knees
   c Extends from the mid-back to mid-thigh level
   d Covers the entire mattress

10 Before turning a person onto his or her side, you
   a Move the person to the side of the bed
   b Move the person to the middle of the bed
   c Lock arms with the person
   d Position pillows for comfort

11 The logrolling procedure
   a Is used after spinal cord injuries or surgery
   b Requires a transfer belt
   c Requires a mechanical lift
   d Involves a stretcher and a drawsheet

12 When getting ready to dangle a person, you need to know
   a Which side is stronger
   b If bed rails are used
   c If a mechanical lift is needed
   d If a transfer belt is needed

13 For chair and wheelchair transfers, the person must
   a Wear non-skid footwear
   b Have the bed rails up
   c Use a mechanical lift
   d Have a drawsheet or other assist device

14 Before transferring a person to or from a bed, you must
   a Have the person wear non-skid footwear
   b Lock the bed wheels
   c Apply a transfer belt
   d Position pillows for support

15 A transfer belt is applied
   a To the skin
   b Over clothing
   c Over breasts
   d Under the robe

16 When transferring a person to bed, a chair, or the toilet
   a The person's strong side moves first
   b The weak side moves first
   c Pillows are used for support
   d The transfer belt is removed

17 You are going to use a mechanical lift. You must do the following *except*
   a Follow the manufacturer's instructions
   b Make sure the lift works
   c Compare the person's weight to the lift's weight limit
   d Use a transfer belt

18 To safely transfer a person with a mechanical lift, at least
   a One worker is needed
   b Two workers are needed
   c Three workers are needed
   d Four workers are needed

19 These statements are about transfers to and from a toilet. Which is *false*?
   a The person wears non-skid footwear.
   b Wheelchair wheels must be locked.
   c The person uses the towel bars for support.
   d A transfer belt is used.

20 Patients and residents are repositioned at least every
   a 30 minutes
   b 1 hour
   c 2 hours
   d 3 hours

21 The back-lying position is called
   a Fowler's position
   b The supine position
   c The prone position
   d Sims' position

22 A person is positioned in a chair. The feet
   a Must be flat on the floor
   b Are positioned on footplates
   c Dangle
   d Are positioned on pillows

Answers to these questions are on p. 468.

Assisting
With Comfort

Objectives

- Define the key terms listed in this chapter
- Describe how to control temperature, odors, noise, and lighting for the person's comfort
- Describe the basic bed positions
- Describe how to use furniture and equipment in the person's unit
- Describe four ways to make beds
- Handle linens following the rules of medical asepsis
- Describe the factors that affect sleep and the common sleep disorders
- Identify the nursing measures that promote sleep
- Perform the procedures described in this chapter

Procedures

Procedures with this icon 💿 are also on the CD-ROM in this book.

- Making a Closed Bed
- 💿 Making an Occupied Bed
- Making a Surgical Bed

KEY TERMS

Fowler's position A semi-sitting position; the head of the bed is raised between 45 and 60 degrees

full visual privacy Having the means to be completely free from public view while in bed

insomnia A chronic condition in which the person cannot sleep or stay asleep all night

reverse Trendelenburg's position The head of the bed is raised, and the foot of the bed is lowered

semi-Fowler's position The head of the bed is raised 30 degrees; or the head of the bed is raised 30 degrees and the knee portion is raised 15 degrees

sleep deprivation The amount and quality of sleep are decreased

sleepwalking The sleeping person leaves the bed and walks about

Trendelenburg's position The head of the bed is lowered, and the foot of the bed is raised

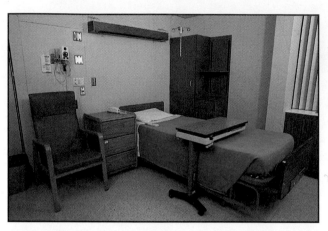

FIG. **12-1** Furniture and equipment in a person's unit.

Comfort is a state of well-being. Age, illness, and activity affect comfort. So do temperature, ventilation, noise, odors, and lighting. A clean, dry, well-made bed promotes comfort. Sleep is promoted when the person is comfortable.

THE PERSON'S UNIT

Patient and resident rooms are designed to provide comfort, safety, and privacy. In nursing centers, resident rooms are as personal and home-like as possible.

The *person's unit* is the space, furniture, and equipment provided for the person by the agency (Fig. 12-1). This area is private. Like a person's home, it is treated with respect.

You need to help keep the person's unit clean, neat, safe, and comfortable. Follow the rules in Box 12-1.

Temperature and Ventilation

Most healthy people are comfortable when the room temperature is 68° F to 74° F. Older and ill persons may need higher room temperatures for comfort. OBRA requires that nursing centers maintain a temperature range of 71° F to 81° F.

Protect older and ill persons from cool areas and drafts.

- Keep room temperatures warm.
- Make sure they wear warm clothing.
- Provide enough blankets for warmth.
- Use bath blankets when giving personal care.
- Offer lap blankets to those in chairs or wheelchairs. Lap blankets cover the legs.
- Move them from drafty areas.

BOX 12-1	Maintaining the Person's Unit

- Place the overbed table and the bedside stand within the person's reach.
- Arrange personal items as the person prefers. Make sure they are easily reached.
- Keep the signal light within reach at all times.
- Make sure the person can reach the phone, TV, and light controls.
- Provide enough tissues and toilet paper.
- Adjust lighting and temperature for the person's comfort.
- Handle equipment carefully to prevent noise.
- Explain the causes of strange noises.
- Use room deodorizers if needed.
- Empty the person's wastebasket at least once a day.
- Respect the person's belongings. An item may not have value to you. Yet it has great meaning for the person. Even a scrap of paper can have great meaning to the person.
- Do not discard items belonging to the person.
- Do not move furniture or the person's belongings. Persons with poor vision rely on memory or feel to find items.
- Straighten bed linens as often as needed.
- Complete a safety check before leaving the room. (See the inside of the front book cover.)

Odors

Bowel movements and urine have embarrassing odors. So do draining wounds and vomitus. Body, breath, and smoking odors may offend others. To reduce odors:

- Empty and clean bedpans, urinals, commodes, and kidney (emesis) basins promptly.
- Change wet or soiled linens and clothing promptly.
- Follow agency policy for wet or soiled linens and clothing.
- Check incontinent persons often (Chapters 15 and 16).
- Clean persons who are wet or soiled from urine, feces, vomitus, wound drainage, or other body fluids.
- Dispose of incontinence and ostomy products promptly (Chapters 15 and 16).
- Keep laundry containers closed.
- Provide good hygiene to prevent body and breath odors (Chapter 13).
- Use room deodorizers as needed. Sometimes odors remain after removing the cause. Do not use sprays around persons with breathing problems. Ask the nurse if you are unsure.

If you smoke, follow the agency's policy. Practice hand washing after handling smoking materials and before giving care. Give careful attention to your uniforms, hair, and breath because of smoke odors.

Noise

Common health care sounds may frighten or irritate patients and residents. The clanging of equipment and the clatter of dishes and trays are examples. So are loud voices, TVs, radios, and music. Phones, signal lights, and intercoms also are annoying. So is noise from equipment needing repair or oil.

To decrease noise:

- Control your voice
- Handle equipment carefully
- Keep equipment working properly
- Answer phones, signal lights, and intercoms promptly

See Persons With Dementia: Noise.

Lighting

Good lighting is needed for safety and comfort. Glares, shadows, and dull lighting can cause falls, headaches, and eyestrain. A bright room is cheerful. Dim light is better for relaxing and rest.

Adjust lighting to meet the person's needs. This includes shades, blinds, and drapes. Adjust the overbed light for soft, medium, or bright lighting. Keep light controls within the person's reach. This protects the right to personal choice.

See Persons With Dementia: Lighting.

Persons With Dementia

Noise

Persons who are confused may react to health care sounds. They may become upset and anxious and show signs of discomfort. Make every effort to provide them with a calm, quiet setting.

Persons With Dementia

Lighting

In dementia care units, lighting is adjusted to help control agitation and aggressive behavior. Soft lights can decrease agitation and help the person relax. Brighter lighting lets the person see surroundings more clearly.

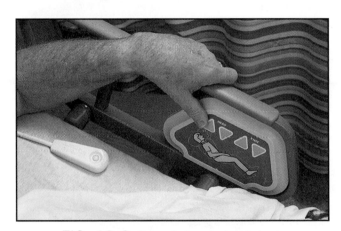

FIG. **12-2** Controls for an electric bed.

Room Furniture and Equipment

Rooms are furnished and equipped to meet basic needs. The right to privacy is also considered.

The Bed

Beds have electrical or manual controls. Beds are raised horizontally to give care. This reduces bending and reaching. The lowest horizontal position lets the person get out of bed with ease. The head of the bed is flat or raised varying degrees.

Electric beds have controls on a side panel, bed rail, or the foot board (Fig. 12-2). Patients and residents are taught how to use the controls. They are warned not to raise the bed to the high position and not to adjust the bed to harmful positions. They are told of any position limits or restrictions.

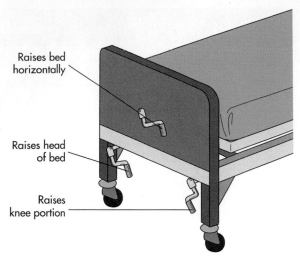

FIG. **12-3** Manually operated hospital bed.

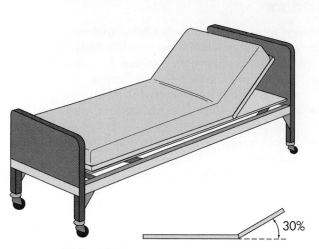

FIG. **12-5** Semi-Fowler's position.

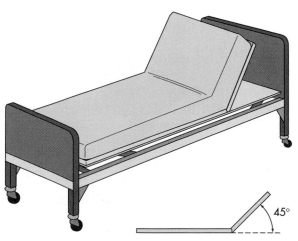

FIG. **12-4** Fowler's position.

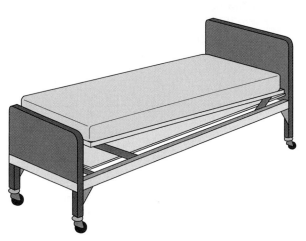

FIG. **12-6** Trendelenburg's position.

Manual beds have cranks at the foot of the bed (Fig. 12-3). The cranks are pulled up for use. They are kept down at all other times. Cranks in the up position are safety hazards. Anyone walking past may bump into them.

There are five basic bed positions.

- *Flat*—This is the usual sleeping position.
- *Fowler's position*—**Fowler's position** is a semi-sitting position. The head of the bed is raised 45 to 60 degrees (Fig. 12-4).
- *Semi-Fowler's position*—In **semi-Fowler's position,** the head of the bed is raised 30 degrees (Fig. 12-5). Some agencies define semi-Fowler's position as when the head of the bed is raised 30 degrees and the knee portion is raised 15 degrees. To give safe care, know the definition used by your agency.

- *Trendelenburg's position*—In **Trendelenburg's position,** the head of the bed is lowered and the foot of the bed is raised (Fig. 12-6). A doctor orders the position. Blocks are placed under the legs at the foot of the bed. Or the bed frame is tilted.
- *Reverse Trendelenburg's position*—In **reverse Trendelenburg's position**, the head of the bed is raised and the foot of the bed is lowered (Fig. 12-7). Blocks are put under the legs at the head of the bed. Or the bed frame is tilted. This position requires a doctor's order.

The Overbed Table

The overbed table (see Fig. 12-1) is placed over the bed by sliding the base under the bed. It is raised or lowered for the person in bed or in a chair. The

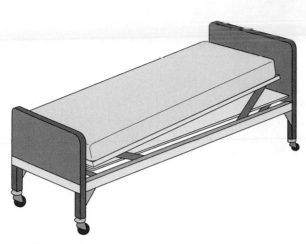

FIG. **12-7** Reverse Trendelenburg's position.

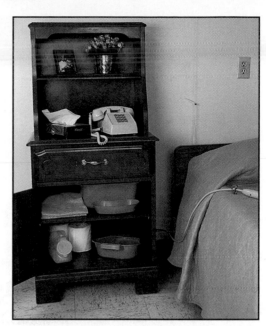

FIG. **12-8** The bedside stand.

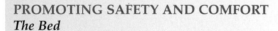

PROMOTING SAFETY AND COMFORT
The Bed

Safety

Beds have bed rails and wheels. See Chapter 8. Bed wheels are locked at all times except when moving the bed. They must be locked when you:

- Give bedside care.
- Transfer a person to and from the bed. The person can be injured if the bed moves.

Use bed rails as the nurse and care plan direct. Otherwise the person could suffer injury or other harm.

Comfort

Some persons spend a lot of time in bed. Make sure the bed is adjusted to meet the person's needs. Tell the nurse if the person complains about the bed or mattress.

overbed table is used for meals, writing, reading, and other activities.

The nursing team uses the overbed table as a work area. Only clean and sterile items are placed on the table. Never place bedpans, urinals, or soiled linen on the overbed table. Clean the table after using it for a work surface.

The Bedside Stand

The bedside stand has a top drawer and a lower cabinet with a shelf (Fig. 12-8). The top drawer is used for money, eyeglasses, books, and other items.

The top shelf is used for the wash basin, which can hold personal care items. These include soap, lotion, towels, washcloth, and a bath blanket. An emesis or kidney basin (shaped like a kidney) can hold oral hygiene items. The kidney basin is stored on the top shelf or in the top drawer. The bedpan and its cover, the urinal, and toilet paper are on the lower shelf.

The top of the stand is often used for tissues and the phone. The person may put a radio, flowers, gifts, cards, and other items there.

Chairs

The person's unit has at least 1 chair. It must be comfortable and sturdy. It must not move or tip during transfers. The person should be able to get in and out of it with ease.

Privacy Curtains

Each person has the right to **full visual privacy**—the means to be completely free from public view while in bed. The privacy curtain is pulled around the bed to provide privacy. *Always* pull it completely around the bed when giving care. Privacy curtains do not block sound or conversations.

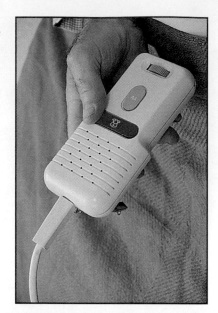

FIG. **12-9** The signal light button is pressed when help is needed.

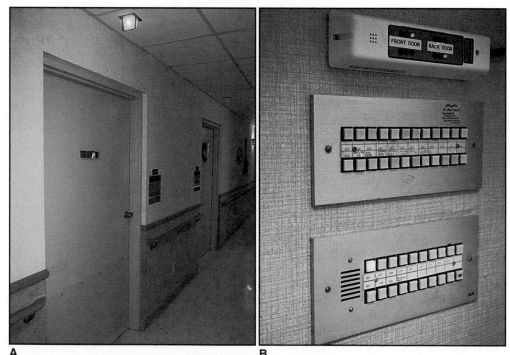

A   **B**

FIG. **12-10** **A,** Light above the room door. **B,** Light panel and intercom at the nurses' station.

The Call System

The call system lets the person signal for help. The signal light is at the end of a long cord (Fig. 12-9). It attaches to the bed or chair. Always keep the signal light within the person's reach—in the room, bathroom, and shower or tub room.

To get help, the person presses a button at the end of the signal light. The signal light connects to a light above the room door. The signal light also connects to a light panel or intercom system at the nurses' station (Fig. 12-10). These tell the nursing team that the person needs help.

An intercom system lets a nursing team member talk with the person from the nurses' station. The person tells what is needed. Hearing-impaired persons may have problems using an intercom. Be

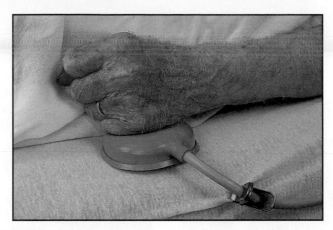

FIG. **12-11** Signal light for a person with limited hand mobility.

careful when using an intercom. Remember confidentiality. Persons nearby can hear what you and the person say.

Some people have limited hand mobility. They may need a special signal light that is turned on by tapping it with a hand or fist (Fig. 12-11).

Some people cannot use signal lights. Examples are persons who are confused or in a coma. Check the care plan for special communication measures. Check these persons often. Make sure their needs are met.

For the person's safety, you must:
- Keep the signal light within the person's reach. Even if the person cannot use the signal light, keep it within reach for use by visitors and staff. They may need to signal for help.
- Place the signal light on the person's strong side.
- Remind the person to signal when help is needed.
- Answer signal lights promptly. Remember, the signal light means that the person needs help.
- Answer bathroom and shower or tub room signal lights at once. These are usually red and have a loud ring.

The Bathroom

A toilet, sink, call system, and mirror are standard equipment. Some bathrooms have showers. For safety, grab bars are by the toilet. The person uses them for support when lowering to or raising from the toilet. Some bathrooms have raised toilet seats. They make wheelchair transfers easier and are helpful for persons with joint problems.

Towel racks, toilet paper, soap, a paper towel dispenser, and wastebasket are in the bathroom. They are placed within easy reach of the person. Usually the signal light is next to the toilet.

Closet and Drawer Space

Closet and drawer space are provided. OBRA requires closet space for each nursing center resident. Such closet space must have shelves and a clothes rack. The person must have free access to the closet and its contents. Items in the closet or drawers are the person's private property.

Other Equipment

Many agencies furnish rooms with other equipment. A TV, radio, and clock provide comfort and relaxation. Many rooms have phones. Residents may bring favorite furniture and items from home.

PROMOTING SAFETY AND COMFORT
Other Equipment

Safety

Nursing center residents are allowed personal choice in arranging items. The choices must be safe and not cause falls or other accidents. You may have to help the person choose the best place for personal items.

Comfort

Nursing center residents have left their homes. Each had furniture, appliances, a private bathroom, and many personal belongings and treasures. Now the person lives in a strange place. It is likely that he or she shares a room with another person. Leaving one's home is a hard part of growing old with poor health. It is important to make the person's unit as home-like as possible.

The person may bring some furniture and personal items. A chair, footstool, lamp, or small table are often allowed. They can bring photos, religious items, and books. Some may have plants to care for.

The center is now the person's home. A home-like setting promotes mental comfort and quality of life.

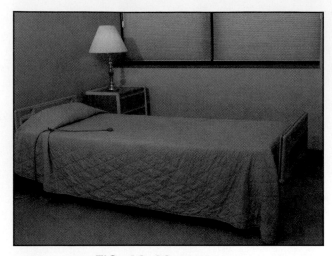

FIG. **12-12** Closed bed.

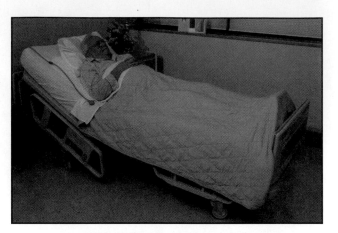

FIG. **12-14** Occupied bed.

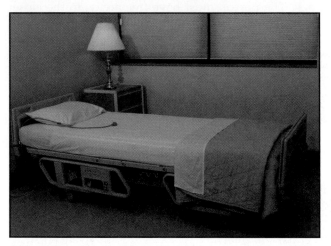

FIG. **12-13** Open bed. Top linens are folded to the foot of the bed.

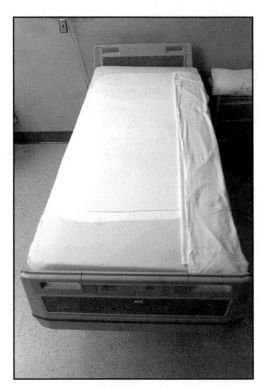

FIG. **12-15** Surgical bed.

BEDMAKING

Beds are made every day. A clean, dry, and wrinkle-free bed increases the person's comfort. It also helps prevent skin breakdown and pressure ulcers (Chapter 21). Beds are made and rooms straightened before visitors arrive.

To keep beds neat and clean:
- Straighten linens whenever loose or wrinkled.
- Straighten loose or wrinkled linens at bedtime.
- Check for and remove food and crumbs after meals.
- Check linens for dentures, eyeglasses, hearing aids, sharp objects, and other items.
- Change linens whenever they become wet, soiled, or damp.
- Follow Standard Precautions and the Bloodborne Pathogen Standard. Contact with blood, body fluids, secretions, or excretions is likely.

Beds are made in these ways:
- A *closed bed* is not in use. Top linens are not folded back. The bed is ready for a new patient or resident (Fig. 12-12). In nursing centers, closed beds are made for residents who are up during the day.
- An *open bed* is in use. Top linens are folded back so the person can get into bed. A closed bed becomes an open bed by folding back the top linens (Fig. 12-13).
- An *occupied bed* is made with the person in it (Fig. 12-14).
- A *surgical bed* is made to transfer a person from a stretcher to the bed. It also is called a *postoperative bed* or *recovery bed* (Fig. 12-15).

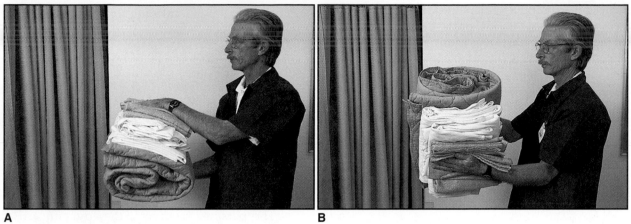

A **B**

FIG. **12-16** Collecting linens. **A,** The arm is placed over the top of the stack of linens. **B,** The stack of linens is turned over onto the arm. Note that linens are held away from the body.

Linens

Collect linens in the order you will use them.
- Mattress pad (if needed)
- Bottom sheet (flat or fitted)
- Plastic drawsheet, (waterproof drawsheet), or waterproof pad (if needed)
- Cotton drawsheet (if needed)
- Top sheet (if needed)
- Blanket
- Bedspread
- Pillowcase(s)
- Bath towel(s)
- Hand towel
- Washcloth
- Gown
- Bath blanket

Use one arm to hold the linens. Use your other hand to pick them up. The item you will use first is at the bottom of your stack. (You picked up the mattress pad first. It is at the bottom. The bath blanket is on top.) You need the mattress pad first. To get it on top, place your arm over the bath blanket. Then turn the stack over onto the arm on the bath blanket (Fig. 12-16). The arm that held the linens is now free. Place the clean linens on a clean surface.

Remove dirty linen one piece at a time. Roll each piece away from you. The side that touched the person is inside the roll and away from you (Fig. 12-17).

In hospitals, beds are usually made in the morning after baths. Top and bottom sheets and pillowcases are changed daily. The mattress pad, drawsheets, blanket, and bedspread are reused for the same person.

In nursing centers, linens are not changed every day. A complete linen change is done on the person's bath day. This is done after the bath or shower when the person is up for the day. Pillowcases, top and

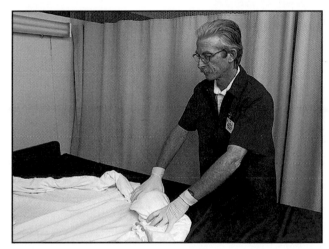

FIG. **12-17** Roll linens away from you when removing them from the bed.

bottom sheets, and drawsheets (if used) may be changed twice a week.

Linens are changed whenever they are soiled, wet, or wrinkled. Wet, damp, or soiled linens are changed right away. Wear gloves and follow Standard Precautions and the Bloodborne Pathogen Standard.

Drawsheets
A *drawsheet* is a small sheet placed over the middle of the bottom sheet.
- A *cotton drawsheet* is made of cotton. It helps keep the mattress and bottom linens clean and dry.
- A *plastic drawsheet (waterproof drawsheet)* is waterproof. It is placed between the bottom sheet and cotton drawsheet. It protects the mattress and bottom linens from dampness and soiling.

The cotton drawsheet protects the person from contact with the plastic and absorbs moisture.

However, discomfort and skin breakdown may occur. Plastic retains heat. Plastic drawsheets are hard to keep tight and wrinkle-free. Many agencies use incontinence products (Chapter 15) to keep the person and linens dry. Others use waterproof pads or disposable bed protectors.

Cotton drawsheets are often used without plastic drawsheets. Plastic-covered mattresses cause some persons to perspire heavily. This increases discomfort. A cotton drawsheet reduces heat retention and absorbs moisture. Cotton drawsheets are often used as assist devices to move persons in bed (Chapter 11). When used for this purpose, do not tuck them in at the sides.

The bedmaking procedures that follow include plastic and cotton drawsheets. This is so you learn how to use them. Ask the nurse about their use in your agency.

Making Beds

When making beds, follow the rules in Box 12-2.

BOX 12-2	**Rules For Bedmaking**

- Use good body mechanics at all times.
- Follow the rules of medical asepsis.
- Follow Standard Precautions and the Bloodborne Pathogen Standard.
- Practice hand hygiene before handling clean linen.
- Practice hand hygiene after handling dirty linen.
- Bring enough linen to the person's room. Do not bring extra linen.
- Extra linen in a person's room is considered contaminated. Do not use it for other people. Put it with the dirty laundry.
- Do not use torn linen.
- Hold linens away from your uniform. Dirty and clean linen must not touch your uniform.
- Never shake linens. Shaking linens spreads microbes.
- Never put dirty linens on the floor or on clean linens. Follow agency policy for dirty linen.
- Keep bottom linens tucked in and wrinkle-free.
- Cover a plastic drawsheet with a cotton drawsheet. A plastic drawsheet must not touch the person's body.
- Straighten and tighten loose sheets, blankets, and bedspreads as needed.
- Make as much of one side of the bed as possible before going to the other side. This saves time and energy.
- Change wet, damp, and soiled linens right away.

DELEGATION GUIDELINES
Making Beds

Before making a bed, you need this information from the nurse and the care plan:

- What type of bed to make—closed, open, occupied, or surgical.
- If you need to use a cotton drawsheet.
- If you need to use a plastic drawsheet, waterproof pad, or incontinence product.
- Position restrictions or limits in the person's movement.
- If the person uses bed rails.
- The person's treatment, therapy, and activity schedule. For example, Mr. Smith needs a treatment in bed. Change linens after the treatment. Mrs. Jones goes to physical therapy. Make the bed while she is out of the room.
- How to position the person and the positioning devices needed.
- If the bed needs to be locked into a certain position.

PROMOTING SAFETY AND COMFORT
Making Beds

Safety

You need to raise the bed for body mechanics. The bed also must be flat.

Wear gloves when removing linen from the person's bed. Also follow the other aspects of Standard Precautions and the Bloodborne Pathogen Standard. Linens may contain blood, body fluids, secretions, or excretions.

After making a bed, lower the bed to its lowest position. Lock the bed wheels. For an occupied bed, raise or lower bed rails according to the care plan.

Comfort

For an occupied bed, cover the person with a bath blanket before removing the top sheet. Do not leave the person uncovered when making the bed. The bath blanket provides for warmth and privacy.

If the person uses a pillow, adjust it as needed during the procedure. After the procedure, position the person as directed by the nurse and the care plan. Always make sure linens are straight and wrinkle-free.

The Closed Bed

A closed bed is made after a person is discharged. It is made for a new patient or resident. The bed is made after the bed frame and mattress are cleaned and disinfected.

In nursing centers, closed beds are made for residents who are up for most or all of the day. Top linens are folded back at bedtime. Clean linens are used as needed.

The Open Bed

A closed bed becomes an open bed by folding the top linens back. The open bed lets the person get into bed with ease. Make this bed for:

- Newly admitted persons arriving by wheelchair
- Patients who are out of bed
- Residents who are out of bed for a short time

Text continued on p. 195

Making a Closed Bed

Quality of Life

Remember to:

- Knock before entering the person's room
- Address the person by name
- Introduce yourself by name and title

- Explain the procedure to the person before beginning and during the procedure
- Protect the person's rights during the procedure
- Handle the person gently during the procedure

Pre-Procedure

1 Follow *Delegation Guidelines: Making Beds.* See *Promoting Comfort and Safety: Making Beds.*
2 Practice hand hygiene.
3 Collect clean linen:
   - Mattress pad (if needed)
   - Bottom sheet (flat sheet or fitted sheet)
   - Plastic drawsheet or waterproof pad (if needed)
   - Cotton drawsheet (if needed)
   - Top sheet
   - Blanket
   - Bedspread
   - Two pillowcases
   - Bath towel(s)
   - Hand towel
   - Washcloth
   - Gown
   - Bath blanket
   - Gloves
   - Laundry bag
4 Place linen on a clean surface.
5 Raise the bed for body mechanics.

Procedure

6 Put on the gloves.
7 Remove linen. Roll each piece away from you. Place each piece in a laundry bag. (Note: Discard incontinence products or disposable bed protectors in the trash. Do not put them in the laundry bag.)
8 Clean the bed frame and mattress if this is part of your job.
9 Remove and discard the gloves. Decontaminate your hands.
10 Move the mattress to the head of the bed.
11 Put the mattress pad on the mattress. It is even with the top of the mattress.

12 Place the bottom sheet on the mattress pad (Fig. 12-18, p. 191).
   a Unfold it lengthwise.
   b Place the center crease in the middle of the bed.
   c Position the lower edge even with the bottom of the mattress.
   d Place the large hem at the top and the small hem at the bottom.
   e Face hem-stitching downward, away from the person.
13 Open the sheet. Fan-fold it to the other side of the bed (Fig. 12-19, p. 191).

Continued

Making a Closed Bed—cont'd

Procedure—cont'd

14　Tuck the top of the sheet under the mattress. The sheet is tight and smooth.

15　Make a mitered corner if using a flat sheet (Fig. 12-20).

16　Place the plastic drawsheet on the bed. It is in the middle of the mattress. Or put the waterproof pad on the bed.

17　Open the plastic drawsheet. Fan-fold it to the other side of the bed.

18　Place a cotton drawsheet over the plastic drawsheet. It covers the entire plastic drawsheet (Fig. 12-21, p. 192).

19　Open the cotton drawsheet. Fan-fold it to the other side of the bed.

20　Tuck both drawsheets under the mattress. Or tuck each in separately.

21　Go to the other side of the bed.

22　Miter the top corner of the flat bottom sheet.

23　Pull the bottom sheet tight so there are no wrinkles. Tuck in the sheet.

24　Pull the drawsheets tight so there are no wrinkles. Tuck both in together or separately (Fig. 12-22, p. 192).

25　Go to the other side of the bed.

26　Put the top sheet on the bed.
　　a　Unfold it lengthwise.
　　b　Place the center crease in the middle.
　　c　Place the large hem even with the top of the mattress.
　　d　Open the sheet. Fan-fold it to the other side.
　　e　Face hem-stitching outward, away from the person.
　　f　Do not tuck the bottom in yet.
　　g　Never tuck top linens in on the sides.

27　Place the blanket on the bed.
　　a　Unfold it so the center crease is in the middle.
　　b　Put the upper hem about 6 to 8 inches from the top of the mattress.
　　c　Open the blanket. Fan-fold it to the other side.
　　d　If steps 33 and 34 are not done, turn the top sheet down over the blanket. Hem-stitching is down, away from the person.

28　Place the bedspread on the bed.
　　a　Unfold it so the center crease is in the middle.
　　b　Place the upper hem even with the top of the mattress.
　　c　Open and fan-fold the spread to the other side.
　　d　Make sure the spread facing the door is even. It covers all top linens.

29　Tuck in top linens together at the foot of the bed. They should be smooth and tight. Make a mitered corner.

30　Go to the other side.

31　Straighten all top linen. Work from the head of the bed to the foot.

32　Tuck in the top linens together at the foot of the bed. Make a mitered corner.

33　Turn the top hem of the spread under the blanket to make a cuff (Fig. 12-23, p. 192).

34　Turn the top sheet down over the spread. Hem-stitching is down. (Steps 33 and 34 are not done in some agencies. The spread covers the pillow. If so, tuck the spread under the pillow.)

35　Put the pillowcase on the pillow as in Figure 12-24 (p. 193) or Figure 12-25 (p. 194). Fold extra material under the pillow at the seam end of the pillowcase.

36　Place the pillow on the bed. The open end of the pillowcase is away from the door. The seam is toward the head of the bed.

Post-Procedure

37　Provide for comfort. (See the inside of the front book cover.) Note: Omit this step if the bed is prepared for a new patient or resident.

38　Attach the signal light to the bed or place the signal light within the person's reach.

39　Lower the bed to its lowest position. Lock the bed wheels.

40　Put the towels, washcloth, gown, and bath blanket in the bedside stand.

41　Complete a safety check of the room. (See the inside of the front book cover.)

42　Follow agency policy for dirty linen.

43　Decontaminate your hands.

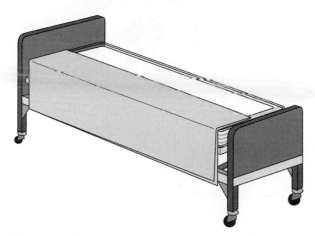

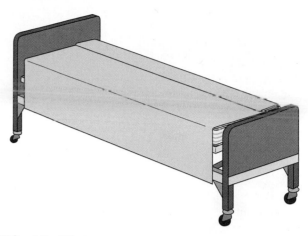

FIG. **12-18** The bottom sheet is on the bed with the center crease in the middle. The lower edge of the sheet is even with the bottom of the mattress.

FIG. **12-19** The bottom sheet is fan-folded to the other side of the bed.

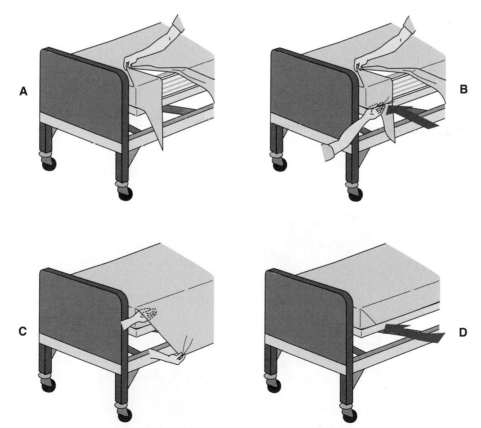

FIG. **12-20** Making a mitered corner. **A,** Bottom sheet is tucked under the mattress at the head of the bed. The side of the sheet is raised onto the mattress. **B,** The remaining portion of the sheet is tucked under the mattress. **C,** The raised portion of the sheet is brought off the mattress. **D,** The entire side of the sheet is tucked under the mattress.

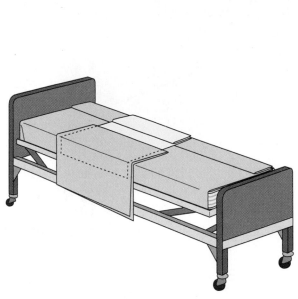

FIG. **12-21** A cotton drawsheet is over the plastic drawsheet. The cotton drawsheet completely covers the plastic drawsheet.

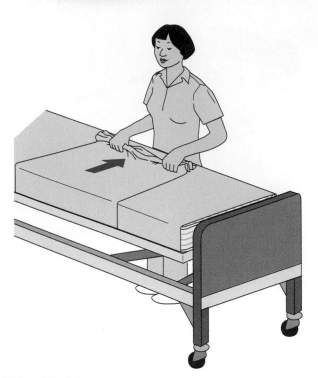

FIG. **12-22** The drawsheet is pulled tight to remove wrinkles.

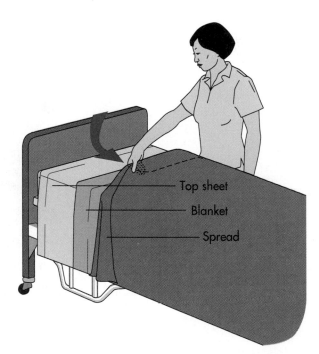

FIG. **12-23** The top hem of the bedspread is turned under the top hem of the blanket to make a cuff.

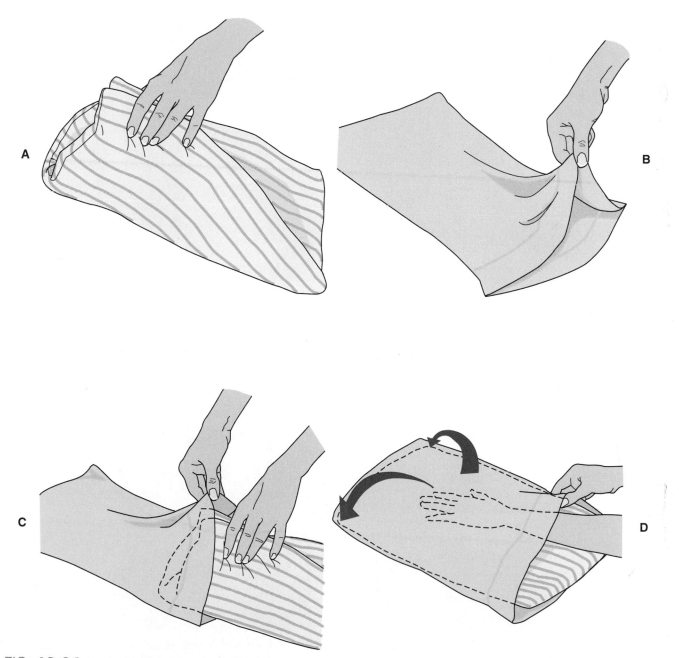

FIG. **12-24** Putting a pillowcase on a pillow. **A,** Open the pillowcase so it is flat on the bed. Grasp the corners of the pillow at the seam end and form a "V" with the pillow. **B,** Open the pillowcase with your free hand. **C,** Guide the "V" end of the pillow into the pillowcase. **D,** Let the "V" end of the pillow fall into the corners of the pillowcase.

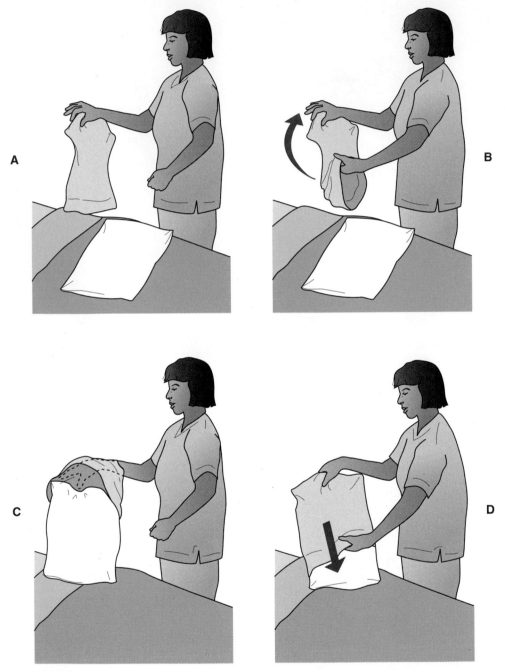

FIG. **12-25** Putting a pillowcase on the pillow. **A,** Grasp the closed end of the pillowcase. **B,** Using your other hand, gather up the pillowcase. The pillowcase should cover your hand holding the closed end. **C,** Grasp the pillow with the hand covered by the pillowcase. **D,** Pull the pillowcase down over the pillow with your other hand.

The Occupied Bed

You make an occupied bed when a person stays in bed. Keep the person in good alignment. Follow restrictions or limits in the person's movement or position.

Explain each procedure step to the person before it is done. This is important even if the person cannot respond to you or is in a coma.

Text continued on p. 199

PROMOTING SAFETY AND COMFORT
The Occupied Bed

Safety

The person lies on one side of the bed and then the other. Protect the person from falling out of bed. If the person uses bed rails, the far bed rail is up. If the person does not use bed rails, have another person help you. You work on one side of the bed. Your co-worker works on the other.

Comfort

To make an occupied bed, the person lays on his or her side. You tuck dirty bottom linens under the person. Then you put clean linens on the bed. These, too, are tucked under the person. The tucked linens create a "bump" in the middle of the bed. To make the other side, the person rolls over the "bump" to the other side of the bed. For the person's, comfort try to make the "bump" as low as possible. Do this by fan-folding dirty and clean bottom linens neatly and flat.

Making an Occupied Bed

NNAAP™

Quality of Life

Remember to:

- Knock before entering the person's room
- Address the person by name
- Introduce yourself by name and title

- Explain the procedure to the person before beginning and during the procedure
- Protect the person's rights during the procedure
- Handle the person gently during the procedure

Pre-Procedure

1. Follow *Delegation Guidelines: Making Beds*, p. 188. See *Promoting Safety and Comfort:*
   - *Making Beds*, p. 188
   - *The Occupied Bed*
2. Practice hand hygiene.
3. Collect the following:
   - Gloves
   - Laundry bag
   - Clean linen (see procedure: *Making a Closed Bed*, p. 189).

4. Place linen on a clean surface.
5. Identify the person. Check the ID bracelet against the assignment sheet. Call the person by name.
6. Provide for privacy.
7. Remove the signal light.
8. Raise the bed for body mechanics. Bed rails are up if used.
9. Lower the head of the bed. It is as flat as possible.

Continued

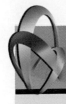

Procedure

10 Decontaminate your hands. Put on gloves.

11 Loosen top linens at the foot of the bed.

12 Remove the bedspread. Then remove the blanket (Fig. 12-26). Place each over the chair.

13 Cover the person with a bath blanket. Use the bath blanket in the bedside stand.
  a Unfold a bath blanket over the top sheet.
  b Ask the person to hold onto the bath blanket. If he or she cannot, tuck the top part under the person's shoulders.
  c Grasp the top sheet under the bath blanket at the shoulders. Bring the sheet down to the foot of the bed. Remove the sheet from under the blanket (Fig. 12-27, p. 198).

14 Lower the bed rail near you if up.

15 Position the person on the side of the bed away from you. Adjust the pillow for comfort.

16 Loosen bottom linens from the head to the foot of the bed.

17 Fan-fold bottom linens one at a time toward the person. Start with the cotton drawsheet (Fig. 12-28, p. 198). If reusing the mattress pad, do not fan-fold it.

18 Place a clean mattress pad on the bed. Unfold it lengthwise. The center crease is in the middle. Fan-fold the top part toward the person. If reusing the mattress pad, straighten and smooth any wrinkles.

19 Place the bottom sheet on the mattress pad. Hem-stitching is away from the person. Unfold the sheet so the crease is in the middle. The small hem is even with the bottom of the mattress. Fan-fold the top part toward the person.

20 Make a mitered corner at the head of the bed. Tuck the sheet under the mattress from the head to the foot.

21 Pull the plastic drawsheet toward you over the bottom sheet. Tuck excess material under the mattress. Do the following for a clean plastic drawsheet (Fig. 12-29, p. 198).
  a Place the plastic drawsheet on the bed. It is in the middle of the mattress top.
  b Fan-fold the top part toward the person.
  c Tuck in the excess fabric.

22 Place the cotton drawsheet over the plastic drawsheet. It covers the entire plastic drawsheet. Fan-fold the top part toward the person. Tuck in excess fabric.

23 Raise the bed rail if used. Go to the other side, and lower the bed rail.

24 Explain to the person that he or she will roll over a "bump". Assure the person that he or she will not fall.

25 Help the person turn to the other side. Adjust the pillow for comfort.

26 Loosen bottom linens. Remove one piece at a time. Place each piece in the laundry bag. (Note: Discard disposable bed protectors and incontinence products in the trash. Do not put them in the laundry bag.)

27 Remove and discard the gloves. Decontaminate your hands.

28 Straighten and smooth the mattress pad.

29 Pull the clean bottom sheet toward you. Make a mitered corner at the top. Tuck the sheet under the mattress from the head to the foot of the bed.

30 Pull the drawsheets tightly toward you. Tuck both under together or separately.

31 Position the person supine in the center of the bed. Adjust the pillow for comfort.

32 Put the top sheet on the bed. Unfold it lengthwise. The crease is in the middle. The large hem is even with the top of the mattress. Hem-stitching is on the outside.

33 Ask the person to hold onto the top sheet so you can remove the bath blanket. Or tuck the top sheet under the person's shoulders. Remove the bath blanket.

34 Place the blanket on the bed. Unfold it so the crease is in the middle and it covers the person. The upper hem is 6 to 8 inches from the top of the mattress.

35 Place the bedspread on the bed. Unfold it so the center crease is in the middle and it covers the person. The top hem is even with the mattress top.

36 Turn the top hem of the spread under the blanket to make a cuff.

37 Bring the top sheet down over the spread to form a cuff.

38 Go to the foot of the bed.

39 Make a toe pleat. Make a 2-inch pleat across the foot of the bed. The pleat is about 6 to 8 inches from the foot of the bed.

40 Lift the mattress corner with one arm. Tuck all top linens under the mattress together. Make a mitered corner.

41 Raise the bed rail if used. Go to the other side, and lower the bed rail if used.

42 Straighten and smooth top linens.

43 Tuck the top linens under bottom of the mattress. Make a mitered corner.

44 Change the pillowcase(s).

Post-Procedure

45 Provide for comfort. (See the inside of the front book cover.)

46 Place the signal light within reach.

47 Lower the bed to its lowest position. Lock the bed wheels.

48 Raise or lower bed rails. Follow the care plan.

49 Put the towels, washcloth, gown, and bath blanket in the bedside stand.

50 Unscreen the person.

51 Complete a safety check of the room. (See the inside of the front book cover.)

52 Follow agency policy for dirty linen.

53 Decontaminate your hands.

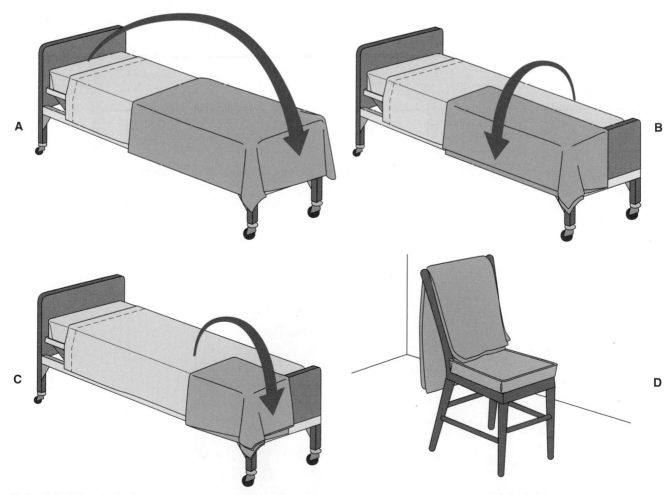

FIG. **12-26** Folding linen for reuse. **A,** Fold the top edge of the blanket down to the bottom edge. **B,** Fold the blanket from far side of the bed to the near side. **C,** Fold the top edge of the blanket down to the bottom edge again. **D,** Place the folded blanket over the back of a chair.

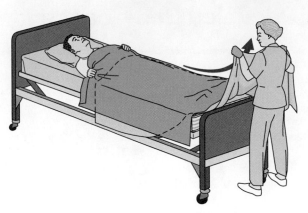

FIG. **12-27** The person holds onto the bath blanket. The top sheet is removed from under the bath blanket.

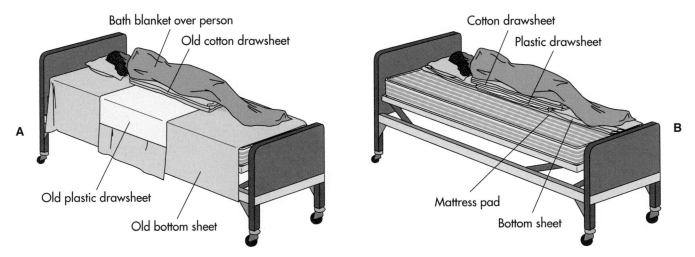

Bath blanket over person
Old cotton drawsheet
Cotton drawsheet
Plastic drawsheet

A

B

Old plastic drawsheet
Old bottom sheet
Mattress pad
Bottom sheet

FIG. **12-28** Occupied bed. **A,** The cotton drawsheet is fan-folded and tucked under the person. **B,** All bottom linens are tucked under the person.

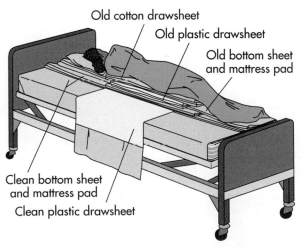

Old cotton drawsheet
Old plastic drawsheet
Old bottom sheet and mattress pad

Clean bottom sheet and mattress pad
Clean plastic drawsheet

FIG. **12-29** A clean bottom sheet and plastic drawsheet are on the bed with both fan-folded and tucked under the person.

The Surgical Bed

Top linens are folded to transfer the person from a stretcher to the bed. Surgical beds are made for persons:

- Who arrive at the agency by ambulance
- Who are taken by stretcher to treatment or therapy areas
- Using portable tubs
- Having surgery (A complete linen change is done.)

PROMOTING SAFETY AND COMFORT
Surgical Beds

Safety

Follow the rules for stretcher use (Chapter 8). After the transfer, lower the bed to its lowest position, and lock the bed wheels. Raise or lower bed rails according to the care plan.

Making a Surgical Bed

Procedure

1 Follow *Delegation Guidelines: Making Beds*, p. 188. See *Promoting Safety and Comfort:*
- *Making Beds*, p. 188
- *Surgical Beds*
2 Practice hand hygiene.
3 Collect the following:
- Clean linen (see procedure: *Making a Closed Bed*, p. 189)
- Gloves
- Laundry bag
- Equipment requested by the nurse
4 Place linen on a clean surface.
5 Remove the signal light.
6 Raise the bed for body mechanics.
7 Remove all linen from the bed. Wear gloves.
8 Make a closed bed (See procedure: *Making a Closed Bed*, p. 189). Do not tuck the top linens under the mattress.

9 Fold all top linens at the foot of the bed back onto the bed. The fold is even with the edge of the mattress (Fig. 12-30).
10 Fan-fold linen lengthwise to the side of the bed farthest from the door (Fig. 12-31).
11 Put the pillowcase(s) on the pillow(s).
12 Place the pillow(s) on a clean surface.
13 Leave the bed in its highest position.
14 Leave both bed rails down.
15 Put the towels, washcloth, gown, and bath blanket in the bedside stand.
16 Move furniture away from the bed. Allow room for the stretcher and for the staff.
17 Do not attach the signal light to the bed.
18 Complete a safety check of the room. (See the inside of the front cover.)
19 Follow agency policy for soiled linen.
20 Decontaminate your hands.

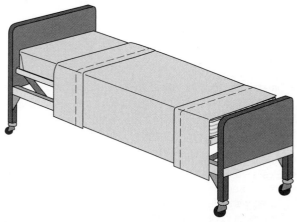

FIG. **12-30** Surgical bed. The bottom of the top linens is folded back onto the bed. The fold is even with the edge of the mattress.

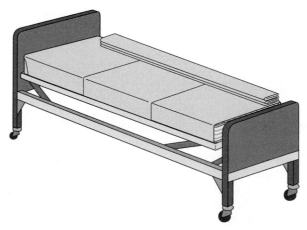

FIG. **12-31** A surgical bed with the top linens fan-folded lengthwise to the opposite side of the bed.

SLEEP

Sleep is a basic need. The mind and body rest. The body saves energy. Body functions slow. Blood pressure, temperature, pulse, and respirations are lower than when awake. Tissue healing and repair occur. Sleep lowers stress, tension, and anxiety. It refreshes and renews the person. The person regains energy and mental alertness. The person thinks and functions better after sleep.

Factors Affecting Sleep

Many factors affect the amount and quality of sleep.
- *Illness.* Illness increases the need for sleep. However, pain, nausea, vomiting, coughing, difficulty breathing, diarrhea, frequent voiding, and itching can interfere with sleep. So can treatments and therapies. Often the person is awakened for treatments or drugs. Fear, anxiety, and worry also affect sleep.
- *Nutrition.* Foods with caffeine (chocolate, coffee, tea, and colas) prevent sleep. Caffeine is a stimulant that prevents sleep. The protein L-tryptophan tends to help sleep. It is found in milk, cheese, and beef.
- *Exercise.* Exercise causes the release of substances into the bloodstream that stimulate the body. Exercise is avoided 2 hours before bedtime.
- *Environment.* People adjust to their usual sleep settings. They get used to the bed, pillows, noises, lighting, and a sleeping partner. Any change in the usual setting can affect sleep.
- *Drugs and other substances.* Sleeping pills promote sleep. Drugs for anxiety, depression, and pain may cause the person to sleep. Alcohol interferes with sleep. Some drugs contain caffeine. The side effects of some drugs cause frequent voiding and nightmares.
- *Emotional problems.* Fear, worry, depression, and anxiety affect sleep. People may have problems falling asleep or they awaken often. Some have problems getting back to sleep.

Sleep Disorders

Sleep disorders involve repeated sleep problems. The amount and quality of sleep are affected. Physical and behavioral problems may result.
- **Insomnia** is a chronic condition in which the person cannot sleep or stay asleep all night. The person:
  - Cannot fall asleep
  - Cannot stay asleep
  - Awakens early and cannot fall back asleep

- **Sleep deprivation** means that the amount and quality of sleep are decreased. Sleep is interrupted.
- **Sleepwalking** is when the sleeping person leaves the bed and walks about. The person is not aware of sleepwalking. He or she has no memory of the event on awakening. The event may last 3 to 4 minutes or longer. Protect the person from injury. Falling is a risk. Guide the person back to bed. Because the person startles easily, awaken him or her gently.

Promoting Sleep

The nurse assesses the person's sleep patterns. Measures are planned to promote sleep (Box 12-3). Follow the care plan. Also report your observations about how the person slept. This helps the nurse evaluate if the person develops a regular sleep pattern.

The person is involved in planning care. The person chooses when to nap or go to bed. The person chooses the measures that promote comfort, rest, and sleep. Follow the care plan and the person's wishes.
See Persons With Dementia: Promoting Sleep.

BOX 12-3   Nursing Measures to Promote Sleep

- Organize care for uninterrupted rest.
- Avoid physical activity before bedtime.
- Allow a flexible bedtime. Bedtime is when the person is tired, not a certain time.
- Provide a comfortable room temperature.
- Let the person take a warm bath or shower.
- Provide a bedtime snack.
- Avoid caffeine (coffee, tea, colas, chocolate) and alcoholic beverages.
- Have the person void before going to bed.
- Make sure incontinent persons are clean and dry.
- Follow bedtime routines. Hygiene, elimination, and prayer are examples.
- Have the person wear loose-fitting nightwear.
- Provide for warmth (blankets, socks) for those who tend to be cold.
- Reduce noise.
- Darken the room—close shades, blinds, and the privacy curtain. Shut off or dim lights.
- Make sure linens are clean, dry, and wrinkle-free.
- Position the person in good alignment and in a comfortable position.
- Support body parts as ordered.
- Give a back massage.
- Let the person read, listen to music, or watch TV.
- Assist with relaxation exercises as ordered.
- Dim lights in hallways and the nursing unit.

Persons With Dementia

Promoting Sleep

Some older persons have dementia. Sleep problems are common in some types of dementia. Night wandering is common. Restlessness and confusion increase at night. This increases the risk of falls. It often helps to quietly and calmly direct the person to his or her room. Night-time wandering in a safe and supervised setting is helpful for some people. The measures listed in Box 12-3 also are tried. Follow the care plan.

FOCUS ON THE PERSON

By assisting with comfort, you promote the person's well-being. Comfort affects the total person—the physical, emotional, social, and spiritual. *See Focus on the Person: Assisting With Comfort.*

Focus on the PERSON

Assisting With Comfort

Providing comfort—Some patients bring their own pillow to the hospital. Some residents bring bedspreads, pillows, blankets, quilts, or afghans from home. Use them to make the bed. These items are the person's property. Handle them with care and respect. Make sure the items are labeled with the person's name. This prevents loss or confusion with another person's property.

Ethical behavior—Some nursing team members just cover the person with the top sheet when making beds or giving personal care. This takes less time than using a bath blanket. However, the top sheet does not provide warmth and privacy like a bath blanket does. Using a bath blanket is the *right* thing. Using the top sheet is the *wrong* thing.

Remaining independent—Personal choice promotes independence. Some agencies have colored or printed linens. If so, let the person choose what color to use. Also let him or her decide how many pillows or blankets to use. If possible, the person chooses the time when you make the bed.

Speaking up—Do not assume that a person is comfortable. You can ask the following:
■ "Are you comfortable?"
■ "What can I do to help you be more comfortable?"
■ "Are you warm enough?"
■ "Do you need another blanket?"
■ "Do you need another pillow?"
■ "Do you want me to adjust your pillow?"

OBRA and other laws—OBRA has requirements for resident rooms. They include a clean, neat, and odor-free room. The noise level must be acceptable to the person. Areas where residents walk or use wheelchairs must be free of clutter and furniture.

Nursing teamwork—Patients and residents use their signal lights when they need help. A person may put on a signal light when you are with another person. The same may happen to another nursing team member. If nursing team members answer signal lights for each other, lights are answered promptly. Patients and residents receive quality care. Everyone is responsible for answering signal lights even if not assigned to the person.

REVIEW QUESTIONS

Circle the **BEST** answer.

1 Which does *not* protect a person from drafts?
   a Wearing enough clothing
   b Being covered with enough blankets
   c Being moved out of a drafty area
   d Warm room temperature

2 Which does *not* prevent or reduce odors?
   a Placing fresh flowers in the room
   b Emptying bedpans promptly
   c Using room deodorizers
   d Cleaning persons who are wet or soiled

3 Which does *not* control noise?
   a Answering signal lights promptly
   b Handling dishes with care
   c Speaking softly
   d Keeping the TV off

4 The head of the bed is raised 30 degrees. This is called
   a Fowler's position
   b Semi-Fowler's position
   c Trendelenburg's position
   d Reverse Trendelenburg's position

5 The overbed table is *not* used
   a For eating   c For the urinal
   b As a working   d To store shaving
     surface   items

6 The bedpan is stored in the
   a Closet   c Overbed table
   b Bedside stand   d Bathroom

7 Signal lights are answered
   a When you have time   c Promptly
   b At the end of your   d When you are by
     shift   the person's room

8 Which requires a linen change?
   a The person will have visitors
   b Wet linen
   c Wrinkled linen
   d Crumbs in the bed

9 When handling linens,
   a Put dirty linens on the floor
   b Hold linens away from your body and uniform
   c Shake linens to remove crumbs
   d Take extra linen to another person's room

10 A resident is out of the room most of the day. What type of bed should you make?
   a A closed bed   c An occupied bed
   b An open bed   d A surgical bed

11 You are using a plastic drawsheet. Which is *true*?
   a A cotton drawsheet must completely cover the plastic drawsheet.
   b Disposable bed protectors are needed.
   c The person's consent is needed.
   d The plastic is in contact with the person's skin.

12 When making an occupied bed you do the following *except*
   a Cover the person with a bath blanket
   b Screen the person
   c Raise the far bed rail if bed rails are used
   d Fan-fold top linens to the foot of the bed

13 A surgical bed is kept
   a In Fowler's position
   b In the lowest position
   c In the highest position
   d In the supine position

14 Which will prevent sleep?
   a Chocolate   c Milk
   b Cheese   d Beef

15 These measures are part of Mr. Smith's care plan. Which should you question?
   a Let Mr. Smith choose his bedtime.
   b Provide hot tea and a cheese sandwich at bedtime.
   c Position him in good alignment.
   d Follow his bedtime rituals.

Circle **T** if the statement is true and **F** if it is false.

16 **T F** Soft, dim lighting is relaxing.
17 **T F** The privacy curtain prevents others from hearing conversations.
18 **T F** The signal light must always be within the person's reach except in the bathroom.
19 **T F** The overbed table and bedside stand should be within the person's reach.
20 **T F** You can adjust the person's room temperature for your comfort.

Answers to these questions are on p. 468.

Assisting With Hygiene

OBJECTIVES

- Define the key terms listed in this chapter
- Describe the care given before and after breakfast, after lunch, and in the evening
- Describe the rules for bathing
- Identify safety measures for tub baths and showers
- Explain the purposes of a back massage
- Explain the purposes of perineal care
- Identify the observations to make while assisting with hygiene
- Perform the procedures described in this chapter

PROCEDURES

Procedures with this icon are also on the CD-ROM in this book.

- Brushing the Person's Teeth
- Providing Mouth Care for the Unconscious Person
- Providing Denture Care
- Giving a Complete Bed Bath
- Giving a Partial Bath
- Assisting With a Tub Bath or Shower
- Giving a Back Massage
- Giving Female Perineal Care
- Giving Male Perineal Care

KEY TERMS

aspiration Breathing fluid or an object into the lungs
oral hygiene Mouth care
perineal care Cleaning the genital and anal areas; pericare

The skin is the body's first line of defense against disease. Intact skin prevents microbes from entering the body and causing an infection. Likewise, mucous membranes of the mouth, genital area, and anus must be clean and intact. Besides cleansing, good hygiene prevents body and breath odors. It is relaxing and increases circulation.

Culture and personal choice affect hygiene. *(See Caring About Culture: Assisting With Hygiene).* The person's preferences are part of the care plan. *See Persons With Dementia: Assisting With Hygiene.*

DAILY CARE

Most people have hygiene routines and habits. For example, teeth are brushed and face and hands washed on awakening. These and other hygiene measures are often done before and after meals and at bedtime.

In hospitals and nursing centers, routine care is given at certain times. You assist with routine hygiene and whenever it is needed. Always protect the right to privacy and personal choice.

Caring About Culture

Assisting With Hygiene

Personal hygiene is very important to *East Indian Hindus.* Their religion requires at least one bath a day. Some believe it is harmful to bathe after a meal. Another belief is that a cold bath prevents blood disease. Some believe that eye injuries can occur if a bath is too hot. Hot water can be added to cold water. However, cold water is not added to hot water when preparing the bath. After bathing, the body is carefully dried with a towel.

(From Giger JN, Davidhizar, RE: Transcultural nursing: assessment and intervention, ed 4, St Louis, 2004, Mosby.)

Persons With Dementia

Assisting With Hygiene

Persons with dementia may resist your efforts to assist with hygiene. Follow the care plan to meet the person's needs.

Before Breakfast

Routine care before breakfast is *early morning care* or *AM care.* The person gets ready for breakfast or morning tests. AM care includes:

- Assisting with elimination
- Cleaning incontinent persons
- Changing wet or soiled linens
- Assisting with hygiene—face and hand washing and oral hygiene
- Assisting with dressing and hair care
- Positioning persons for breakfast—dining room, bedside chair, or in bed
- Making beds and straightening units

After Breakfast

Morning care is given after breakfast. Hygiene measures are thorough. They include:

- Assisting with elimination
- Cleaning incontinent persons
- Changing wet or soiled linens and garments
- Assisting with hygiene—face and hand washing, oral hygiene, bathing, back massage, and perineal care
- Assisting with grooming—hair care, shaving, dressing, or changing gowns or pajamas
- Assisting with activity—range-of-motion exercises and ambulation
- Making beds and straightening units

Afternoon Care

Routine hygiene is done after lunch and the evening meal. If done before visitors arrive, the person is refreshed and can visit without interruption. Afternoon care involves:

- Assisting with elimination
- Cleaning incontinent persons
- Changing wet or soiled linens and garments
- Assisting with hygiene and grooming—face and hand washing, oral hygiene, hair care, changing garments
- Assisting with activity—range-of-motion exercises and ambulation
- Brushing or combing hair if needed
- Straightening beds and units

Evening Care

Care given at bedtime is *evening care* or *PM care*. Evening care is relaxing and promotes comfort. Measures performed before sleep include:

- Assisting with elimination
- Cleaning incontinent persons
- Changing wet or soiled linens and garments
- Assisting with hygiene—face and hand washing, oral hygiene, and back massages
- Helping persons change into sleepwear
- Straightening beds and units

ORAL HYGIENE

Oral hygiene (mouth care) does the following:

- Keeps the mouth and teeth clean
- Prevents mouth odors and infections
- Increases comfort
- Makes food taste better
- Reduces the risk for *cavities (dental caries)* and *periodontal disease (gum disease, pyorrhea)*

Illness, disease, and some drugs often cause a bad taste in the mouth. They may cause a whitish coating in the mouth and on the tongue. Others cause redness and swelling in the mouth and on the tongue. Dry mouth is common from oxygen, smoking, decreased fluid intake, and anxiety. Some drugs cause dry mouth.

Brushing and Flossing Teeth

Many people perform oral hygiene themselves. Others need help gathering and setting up equipment. You may have to brush the teeth of persons who:

- Are very weak
- Cannot use or move their arms
- Are too confused to brush their teeth

Many people floss their teeth. Flossing removes food from between the teeth. It also prevents periodontal disease. Usually done after brushing, it can be done at other times. Some people floss after meals. If done once a day, bedtime is the best time to floss. You need to floss for persons who cannot do so.

DELEGATION GUIDELINES
Oral Hygiene

To assist with oral hygiene, you need this information from the nurse and the care plan:

- The type of oral hygiene to give:
  - *Brushing the Person's Teeth*, p. 206
  - *Providing Mouth Care for an Unconscious Person*, p. 209
  - *Providing Denture Care*, p. 211
- If flossing is needed
- What cleaning agent and equipment to use.
- If lubricant is applied to the lips. If so, what lubricant to use.
- How often to give oral hygiene.
- How much help the person needs.
- What observations to report and record:
  - Dry, cracked, swollen, or blistered lips
  - Mouth or breath odor
  - Redness, swelling, irritation, sores, or white patches in the mouth or on the tongue
  - Bleeding, swelling, or redness of the gums
  - Loose teeth
  - Rough, sharp, or chipped areas on dentures

PROMOTING SAFETY AND COMFORT
Oral Hygiene

Safety

Use a toothbrush with soft bristles. Hard bristles can injure the gums and tongue.

Use sponge swabs for persons who are unconscious and for those with sore mouths. Check the foam pad to make sure it is tight on the stick. The person could choke on the foam pad if it comes off the stick.

Follow Standard Precautions and the Bloodborne Pathogen Standard when giving oral hygiene. You have contact with the person's mucous membranes. Gums may bleed during mouth care. Also the mouth has many microbes. Pathogens spread through sexual contact may be in the mouths of some persons.

Comfort

Assist with oral hygiene on awakening, after meals, and at bedtime. Many people practice oral hygiene before meals. Some persons need mouth care every 2 hours or more often. Always follow the care plan.

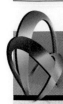

Brushing the Person's Teeth

NNAAP™

Quality of Life

Remember to:

- Knock before entering the person's room
- Address the person by name
- Introduce yourself by name and title

- Explain the procedure to the person before beginning and during the procedure
- Protect the person's rights during the procedure
- Handle the person gently during the procedure

Pre-Procedure

1 Follow *Delegation Guidelines: Oral Hygiene*, p. 205. See *Promoting Safety and Comfort: Oral Hygiene*, p. 205.
2 Practice hand hygiene.
3 Collect the following:
   - Toothbrush
   - Toothpaste
   - Mouthwash (or solution noted on the care plan)
   - Dental floss (if used)
   - Water glass with cool water
   - Straw
   - Kidney basin
   - Hand towel
   - Paper towels
   - Gloves
4 Place the paper towels on the overbed table. Arrange items on top of them.
5 Identify the person. Check the ID bracelet against the assignment sheet. Call the person by name.
6 Provide for privacy.
7 Raise the bed for body mechanics. Bed rails are up if used.

Procedure

8 Lower the bed rail near you if up.
9 Assist the person to a sitting position or to a side-lying position near you.
10 Place the towel over the person's chest.
11 Adjust the overbed table so you can reach it with ease.
12 Decontaminate your hands. Put on the gloves.
13 Hold the toothbrush over the kidney basin. Pour some water over the brush.
14 Apply toothpaste to the toothbrush.
15 Brush the teeth gently (Fig. 13-1).
16 Brush the tongue gently.
17 Let the person rinse the mouth with water. Hold the kidney basin under the person's chin (Fig. 13-2). Repeat this step as needed.
18 Floss the person's teeth (optional):
   a Break off an 18-inch piece of floss from the dispenser.

   b Hold the floss between the middle fingers of each hand (Fig. 13-3, *A*).
   c Stretch the floss with your thumbs.
   d Start at the upper back tooth on the right side. Work around to the left side.
   e Move the floss gently up and down between the teeth (Fig. 13-3, *B*). Move floss up and down against the side of the tooth. Work from the top of the crown to the gum line.
   f Move to a new section of floss after every second tooth.
   g Floss the lower teeth. Use up and down motions as for the upper teeth. Start on the right side. Work around to the left side.
19 Let the person use mouthwash or other solution. Hold the kidney basin under the chin.
20 Wipe the person's mouth. Remove the towel.
21 Remove and discard the gloves. Decontaminate your hands.

Post-Procedure

22 Provide for comfort. (See the inside of the front book cover.)
23 Place the signal light within reach.
24 Lower the bed to its lowest position.
25 Raise or lower bed rails. Follow the care plan.
26 Clean and return equipment to its proper place. Wear gloves.
27 Wipe off the overbed table with the paper towels. Discard the paper towels.

28 Remove the gloves. Decontaminate your hands.
29 Unscreen the person.
30 Complete a safety check of the room. (See the inside of the front book cover.)
31 Follow agency policy for dirty linen.
32 Decontaminate your hands.
33 Report and record your observations.

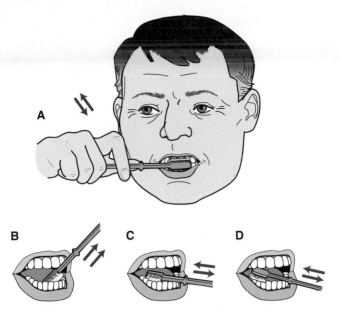

FIG. **13-1** Brushing teeth. **A,** Place the brush at a 45-degree angle to the gums. Brush teeth with short strokes. **B,** Place the brush at a 45-degree angle against the inside of the front teeth. Brush teeth from the gum to the crown of the tooth with short strokes. **C,** Hold the brush horizontally against the inner surfaces of the teeth. Brush back and forth. **D,** Position the brush on the biting surfaces of the teeth. Brush back and forth.

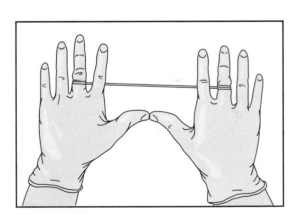

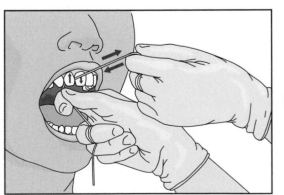

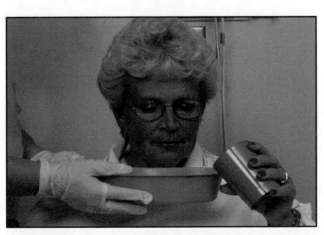

FIG. **13-2** The kidney basin is held under the person's chin.

FIG. **13-3** Flossing. **A,** Floss is held between the middle fingers to floss the upper teeth. **B,** Floss is moved in up and down motions between the teeth. Floss is moved up and down from the crown to the gum line.

Mouth Care For the Unconscious Person

Unconscious persons cannot eat or drink. They may breathe with their mouths open. Many receive oxygen. These factors cause mouth dryness. They also cause crusting on the tongue and mucous membranes. Oral hygiene keeps the mouth clean and moist. It also helps prevents infection.

The care plan tells you what cleaning agent to use. Use sponge swabs to apply the cleaning agent. Apply a lubricant (check the care plan) to the lips after cleaning. It prevents cracking of the lips.

Unconscious persons usually cannot swallow. Protect them from choking and aspiration. **Aspiration** is breathing fluid or an object into the lungs. It can cause pneumonia and death. To prevent aspiration:

- Position the person on one side with the head turned well to the side (Fig. 13-4). In this position, excess fluid runs out of the mouth.
- Use only a small amount of fluid to clean the mouth.
- Do not insert dentures. Dentures are not worn when the person is unconscious.

Keep the person's mouth open with a padded tongue blade. Do not use your fingers. The person can bite down on them. The bite breaks the skin and creates a portal of entry for microbes. Infection is a risk. Many agencies buy padded tongue blades. If not, make one as shown in Figure 13-5.

Unconscious persons cannot speak or respond to you. However, some can hear. Always assume that unconscious persons can hear. Explain what you are doing step by step. Also tell the person when you are done, when you are leaving the room, and when you will return.

Mouth care is given at least every 2 hours. Follow the nurse's directions and the care plan.

PROMOTING SAFETY AND COMFORT
Mouth Care for the Unconscious Person

Safety

Use sponge swabs with care. Make sure the sponge pad is tight on the stick. The person could choke or aspirate on the sponge if it comes off the stick.

Comfort

Unconscious persons are repositioned at least every 2 hours. To promote comfort, combine mouth care with skin care, repositioning, and other comfort measures.

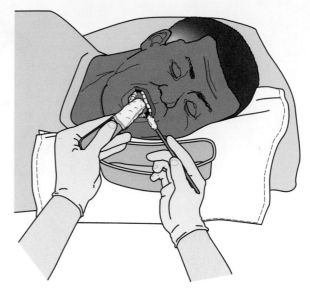

FIG. **13-4** The head of the unconscious person is turned well to the side to prevent aspiration. A padded tongue blade is used to keep the mouth open while cleaning the mouth with swabs.

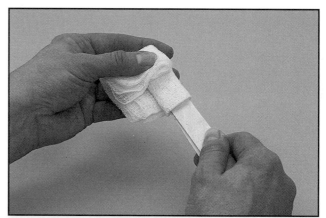

A

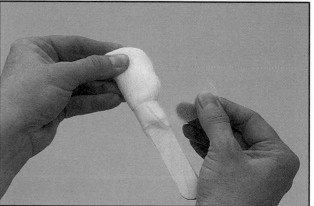

B

FIG. **13-5** Making a padded tongue blade. **A,** Place two wooden tongue blades together. Wrap gauze around the top half. **B,** Tape the gauze in place.

Providing Mouth Care For the Unconscious Person

Quality of Life

Remember to:

■ Knock before entering the person's room

■ Address the person by name

■ Introduce yourself by name and title

■ Explain the procedure to the person before beginning and during the procedure

■ Protect the person's rights during the procedure

■ Handle the person gently during the procedure

Pre-Procedure

1 Follow *Delegation Guidelines: Oral Hygiene,* p. 205. See *Promoting Safety and Comfort:*
   • *Oral Hygiene,* p. 205
   • *Mouth Care for the Unconscious Person*
2 Practice hand hygiene.
3 Collect the following:
   • Cleaning agent (check the care plan)
   • Sponge swabs
   • Padded tongue blade
   • Water glass with cool water
   • Hand towel
   • Kidney basin

   • Lip lubricant
   • Paper towels
   • Gloves
4 Place the paper towels on the overbed table. Arrange items on top of them.
5 Identify the person. Check the ID bracelet against the assignment sheet. Call the person by name.
6 Provide for privacy.
7 Raise the bed for body mechanics. Bed rails are up if used.

Procedure

8 Lower the bed rail near you if up.
9 Decontaminate your hands. Put on the gloves.
10 Position the person in a side-lying position near you. Turn his or her head well to the side.
11 Place the towel under the person's face.
12 Place the kidney basin under the chin.
13 Separate the upper and lower teeth. Use the padded tongue blade. Be gentle. Never use force. If you have problems, ask the nurse for help.
14 Clean the mouth using sponge swabs moistened with the cleaning agent (see Fig. 13-4).
   a Clean the chewing and inner surfaces of the teeth.

   b Clean the gums and outer surfaces of the teeth.
   c Swab the roof of the mouth, inside of the cheeks, and the lips.
   d Swab the tongue.
   e Moisten a clean swab with water. Swab the mouth to rinse.
   f Place used swabs in the kidney basin.
15 Apply lubricant to the lips.
16 Remove the kidney basin and supplies.
17 Wipe the person's mouth. Remove the towel.
18 Remove and discard the gloves. Decontaminate your hands.

Post-Procedure

19 Provide for comfort. (See the inside of the front book cover.)
20 Place the signal light within reach.
21 Lower the bed to its lowest position.
22 Raise or lower bed rails. Follow the care plan.
23 Clean and return equipment to its proper place. Discard disposable items. (Wear gloves.)
24 Wipe off the overbed table with paper towels. Discard the paper towels.

25 Remove the gloves. Decontaminate your hands.
26 Unscreen the person.
27 Complete a safety check of the room. (See inside front cover.)
28 Tell the person that you are leaving the room. Tell him or her when you will return.
29 Follow agency policy for dirty linen.
30 Decontaminate your hands.
31 Report and record observations.

Denture Care

Mouth care is given and dentures cleaned as often as natural teeth. Dentures are slippery when wet. They easily break or chip if dropped onto a hard surface (floors, sinks). Hold them firmly. During cleaning, firmly hold them over a basin of water lined with a towel. This prevents them from falling onto a hard surface.

To use a cleaning agent, follow the manufacturer's instructions. They tell what water temperature to use. Hot water causes dentures to lose their shape (warp). If not worn after cleaning, store dentures in a container with cool water or a denture soaking solution. Otherwise they can dry out and warp.

Dentures are usually removed at bedtime. Some people do not wear their dentures. Others wear dentures for eating and remove them after meals. Remind them not to wrap dentures in tissues or napkins. Otherwise, they are easily discarded.

PROMOTING SAFETY AND COMFORT
Denture Care

Safety

Dentures are the person's property. They are costly. Handle them very carefully. Label the denture cup with the person's name and room and bed number. Report lost or damaged dentures to the nurse at once. Losing or damaging dentures is negligent conduct.

Comfort

Many people do not like being seen without their dentures. Privacy is important. Allow privacy when the person cleans dentures. If you clean dentures, return them to the person as quickly as possible.

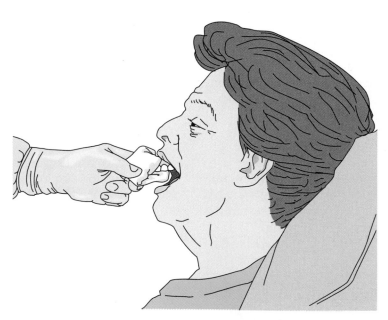

FIG. **13-6** Remove the upper denture by grasping it with the thumb and index finger of one hand. Use a piece of gauze to grasp the slippery denture.

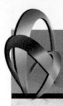

Providing Denture Care

Quality of Life

Remember to:

- Knock before entering the person's room
- Address the person by name
- Introduce yourself by name and title

- Explain the procedure to the person before beginning and during the procedure
- Protect the person's rights during the procedure
- Handle the person gently during the procedure

Pre-Procedure

1 Follow *Delegation Guidelines: Oral Hygiene*, p. 205. See *Promoting Safety and Comfort:*
   - *Oral Hygiene*, p. 205
   - *Denture Care*
2 Practice hand hygiene.
3 Collect the following:
   - Denture brush or toothbrush (for cleaning dentures)
   - Denture cup labeled with the person's name and room and bed number
   - Denture cleaning agent
   - Soft-bristled toothbrush or sponge swabs (for oral hygiene)
   - Toothpaste
   - Water glass with cool water
   - Straw
   - Mouthwash (or other noted solution)
   - Kidney basin
   - Two hand towels
   - Gauze squares
   - Paper towels
   - Gloves
4 Place the paper towels on the overbed table. Arrange items on top of them.
5 Identify the person. Check the ID bracelet against the assignment sheet. Call the person by name.
6 Provide for privacy.
7 Raise the bed for body mechanics.

Procedure

8 Lower the bed rail near you if used.
9 Decontaminate your hands. Put on the gloves.
10 Place a towel over the person's chest.
11 Ask the person to remove the dentures. Carefully place them in the kidney basin.
12 Remove the dentures if the person cannot do so. Use gauze squares to get a good grip on the slippery dentures.
   a Grasp the upper denture with your thumb and index finger (Fig. 13-6). Move it up and down slightly to break the seal. Gently remove the denture. Place it in the kidney basin.
   b Grasp and remove the lower denture with your thumb and index finger. Turn it slightly, and lift it out of the mouth. Place it in the kidney basin.
13 Follow the care plan for raising bed rails.
14 Take the kidney basin, denture cup, denture brush, and denture cleaning agent to the sink.
15 Line the sink with a towel. Fill the sink halfway with water.
16 Rinse each denture under warm running water. (Some state competency tests require cool water.)
17 Return dentures to the kidney basin or denture cup.
18 Apply the denture cleaning agent to the brush.
19 Brush the dentures as in Figure 13-7, p. 212.
20 Rinse dentures under running water. Use warm or cool water as directed by the cleaning agent manufacturer. (Some state competency tests require cool water.)
21 Rinse the denture cup. Place dentures in the denture cup. Cover the dentures with cool water.
22 Clean the kidney basin.
23 Take the denture cup and kidney basin to the overbed table.
24 Lower the bed rail if up.
25 Position the person for oral hygiene.
26 Clean the person's gums and tongue, using toothpaste and the toothbrush (or sponge swab).
27 Have the person use mouthwash (or noted solution). Hold the kidney basin under the chin.
28 Ask the person to insert the dentures. Insert them if the person cannot.
   a Hold the upper denture firmly with your thumb and index finger. Raise the upper lip with the other hand. Insert the denture. Gently press on the denture with your index fingers to make sure it is in place.
   b Hold the lower denture with your thumb and index finger. Pull the lower lip down slightly. Insert the denture. Gently press down on it to make sure it is in place.

Continued

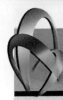

Providing Denture Care—cont'd

NNAAP™

Procedure—cont'd

29 Place the denture cup in the top drawer of the bedside stand if the dentures are not worn. The dentures must be in water or in a denture soaking solution.

30 Wipe the person's mouth. Remove the towel.
31 Remove the gloves. Decontaminate your hands.

Post-Procedure

32 Assist with hand washing.
33 Provide for comfort. (See the inside of the front book cover.)
34 Place the signal light within reach.
35 Lower the bed to its lowest position.
36 Raise or lower bed rails. Follow the care plan.
37 Clean and return equipment to its proper place. Discard disposable items. Wear gloves for this step.

38 Wipe off the overbed table with the paper towels. Discard the paper towels.
39 Remove the gloves. Decontaminate your hands.
40 Unscreen the person.
41 Complete a safety check of the room. (See the inside of the front book cover.)
42 Follow agency policy for dirty linen.
43 Decontaminate your hands.
44 Report and record your observations.

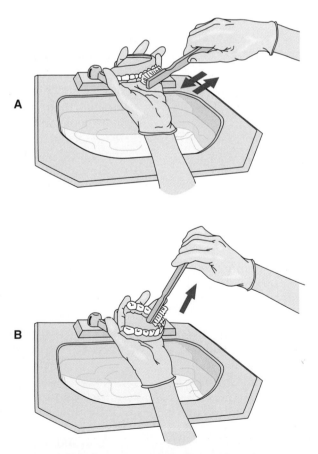

FIG. **13-7** Cleaning dentures. **A,** Brush the outer surfaces of the upper denture with back-and-forth motions. Note that the denture is held over the sink. The sink is filled halfway with water and is lined with a towel. **B,** Position the brush vertically to clean the inner surfaces of the denture. Use upward strokes.

BATHING

Bathing cleans the skin. It also cleans the mucous membranes of the genital and anal areas. Microbes, dead skin, perspiration, and excess oils are removed. A bath is refreshing and relaxing. Circulation is stimulated and body parts exercised. Observations are made, and you have time to talk to the person.

Complete or partial bed baths, tub baths, or showers are given. The method depends on the person's condition, self-care abilities, and personal choice. Bathing is common after breakfast. However, the person's choice of bath time is respected whenever possible.

Bathing frequency is a personal matter. Some people bathe daily. Others bathe twice a week. Personal choice, weather, activity, and illness affect bathing frequency. Ill persons may have fevers and perspire heavily. They need frequent bathing. Other illnesses and dry skin may limit bathing to every 2 or 3 days. The care plan tells you when to bathe the person.

The rules for bathing are in Box 13-1. *See Persons With Dementia: Bathing.*

Persons With Dementia

Bathing

Bathing may scare or frighten persons with dementia. They do not understand what is happening or why. They may fear harm or danger. Therefore they may resist care and become agitated and combative. They may shout at the caregiver and cry out for help.

The rules in Box 13-1 apply when bathing persons with dementia. The care plan includes measures to help the person through the bathing procedure. Such measures include:

- Complete pre-procedure activities—ready supplies and linens, increase room temperature, and so on.
- Do not rush the person.
- Use a calm, pleasant voice.
- Divert the person's attention.
- Be gentle.
- Calm the person.
- Try the bath later if the person continues to resist care.

Towel Baths

Persons with dementia often respond well to towel baths. They are quick, soothing, and relaxing. An over-sized towel is used. It covers the body from the neck to the feet. The towel is completely wet with a cleansing solution—water, cleaning agent, and skin-softening agent. It also has a drying agent so the person's body dries quickly. The nurse and care plan tell you when to use a towel bath. To give a towel bath, follow the agency's procedures.

BOX 13-1 Rules For Bathing

- Follow the care plan for bathing method and skin care products.
- Allow personal choice whenever possible.
- Follow Standard Precautions and the Bloodborne Pathogen Standard.
- Collect needed items before starting the procedure.
- Provide for privacy. Screen the person. Close doors, shades, or drapes.
- Assist with elimination. Bathing stimulates the need to urinate. Comfort and relaxation increase if urination needs are met.
- Cover the person for warmth and privacy.
- Reduce drafts. Close doors and windows.
- Protect the person from falling.
- Use good body mechanics at all times.

- Know what water temperature to use. See *Delegation Guidelines: Bathing*, p. 214.
- Keep bar soap in the soap dish between latherings. This prevents soapy water.
- Wash from the cleanest to the dirtiest areas.
- Encourage the person to help as much as is safely possible.
- Rinse the skin thoroughly. You must remove all soap.
- Pat the skin dry to avoid irritating or breaking the skin. Do not rub the skin.
- Dry under the breasts, between skin folds, in the perineal area, and between the toes.
- Bathe the skin whenever feces or urine is present. This prevents skin breakdown and odors.

DELEGATION GUIDELINES
Bathing

To assist with bathing, you need this information from the nurse and the care plan:

- What bath to give—complete bed bath, partial bath, tub bath, or shower.
- How much help the person needs.
- The person's activity or position limits.
- What water temperature to use. Bath water cools rapidly. Therefore water temperature for a complete bed bath is usually between 110° and 115° F (43.3° and 46.1° C) for adults.
- What skin care products to use and what the person prefers.
- What observations to report and record:
    - The color of the skin, lips, nail beds, and sclera (whites of the eyes)
    - The location and description of rashes
    - Dry skin
    - Bruises or open skin areas
    - Pale or reddened areas, particularly over bony parts
    - Drainage or bleeding from wounds or body openings
    - Swelling of the feet and legs
    - Corns or calluses on the feet
    - Skin temperature
    - Complaints of pain or discomfort

The Complete Bed Bath

The *complete bed bath* involves washing the person's entire body in bed. Persons who are unconscious, paralyzed, in a cast or traction, or weak from illness or surgery may need bed baths.

A bed bath is new to some people. Some are embarrassed to have others see their bodies. Some fear exposure. Explain how the bed bath is given. Also explain how you cover the body for privacy.

Text continued on p. 220

PROMOTING SAFETY AND COMFORT
Bathing

Safety

Hot water can burn delicate and fragile skin. Older persons are at risk. Measure water temperature according to agency policy. If unsure if the water is too hot, ask the nurse to check it.

Protect the person from falls. Practice the measures presented in Chapter 8.

Use caution when applying powder. Do not use powders near persons with respiratory disorders. Inhaling powder can irritate the airway and lungs. Before applying powder, check with the nurse and the care plan. Do not shake or sprinkle powder onto the person. To safely apply powder:

- Turn away from the person.
- Sprinkle a small amount of powder onto your hands or a cloth.
- Apply the powder in a thin layer.

Beds are made after baths. After making the bed, lower the bed to its lowest position. Then lock the bed wheels. For an occupied bed, raise or lower bed rails according to the care plan.

Protect the person and yourself from infection. When giving baths and making beds, contact with blood, body fluids, secretions, and excretions is likely. Follow Standard Precautions and the Bloodborne Pathogen Standard.

Comfort

Before bathing, allow the person to use the bathroom, commode, bedpan, or urinal. Bathing tends to stimulate the need to urinate. The person is more comfortable if his or her bladder is empty. Also bathing is not interrupted.

Provide for warmth. Cover the person with a bath blanket. Make sure the water is warm enough for the person. Cool water causes chilling.

Remove the person's gown or pajamas after washing the face, ears, and neck. Waiting to remove the gown at this time helps the person feel less exposed and more comfortable with the bath. However, it is acceptable to remove the gown before washing the face, ears, and neck.

Giving a Complete Bed Bath

Quality of Life

Remember to:

- Knock before entering the person's room
- Address the person by name
- Introduce yourself by name and title

- Explain the procedure to the person before beginning and during the procedure
- Protect the person's rights during the procedure
- Handle the person gently during the procedure

Pre-Procedure

1 Follow *Delegation Guidelines: Bathing.* See *Promoting Safety and Comfort: Bathing.*
2 Practice hand hygiene.
3 Identify the person. Check the ID bracelet against the assignment sheet. Call the person by name.
4 Collect clean linen for a closed bed. (See procedure: *Making a Closed Bed* in Chapter 12.) Place linen on a clean surface.
5 Collect the following:
- Wash basin
- Soap
- Bath thermometer
- Orange stick or nail file
- Washcloth
- Two bath towels and two hand towels

- Bath blanket
- Clothing, gown, or pajamas
- Lotion
- Powder
- Deodorant or antiperspirant
- Brush and comb
- Other grooming items if requested
- Paper towels
- Gloves

6 Cover the overbed table with paper towels. Arrange items on the overbed table. Adjust the height as needed.
7 Provide for privacy.
8 Raise the bed for body mechanics. Bed rails are up if used.

Procedure

9 Remove the signal light.
10 Decontaminate your hands. Put on gloves.
11 Cover the person with a bath blanket. Remove top linens (see procedure: *Making an Occupied Bed* in Chapter 12).
12 Lower the head of the bed. It is as flat as possible. The person has at least one pillow.
13 Fill the wash basin (two-thirds) full with water. Water temperature is usually 110° to 115° F (43.3° to 46.1° C) for adults. Measure water temperature. Use a bath thermometer. Or test the water by dipping your elbow or inner wrist into the basin.
14 Place the basin on the overbed table.
15 Lower the bed rail near you if up.
16 Place a hand towel over the person's chest.
17 Make a mitt with the washcloth (Fig. 13-8, p. 217). Use a mitt for the entire bath.
18 Wash around the person's eyes with water. Do not use soap. Gently wipe from the inner to the outer aspect of the eye with a corner of the mitt (Fig. 13-9, p. 217). Clean around the far eye

first. Repeat this step for the near eye. Use a clean part of the washcloth for each stroke.
19 Ask the person if you should use soap to wash the face.
20 Wash the face, ears, and neck. Rinse and pat dry with the towel on the chest.
21 Help the person move to the side of the bed near you.
22 Remove the gown. Do not expose the person.
23 Place a bath towel lengthwise under the far arm.
24 Support the arm with your palm under the person's elbow. His or her forearm rests on your forearm.
25 Wash the arm, shoulder, and underarm. Use long, firm strokes (Fig. 13-10, p. 218). Rinse and pat dry.
26 Place the basin on the towel. Put the person's hand into the water (Fig. 13-11. p. 218). Wash it well. Clean under fingernails with an orange stick or nail file.
27 Have the person exercise the hand and fingers.
28 Remove the basin. Dry the hand well. Cover the arm with the bath blanket.

Continued

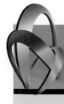
Procedure—cont'd

29 Repeat steps 23 to 28 for the near arm.

30 Place a bath towel over the chest crosswise. Hold the towel in place. Pull the bath blanket from under the towel to the waist.

31 Lift the towel slightly, and wash the chest (Fig. 13-12, p. 218). Do not expose the person. Rinse and pat dry, especially under breasts.

32 Move the towel lengthwise over the chest and abdomen. Do not expose the person. Pull the bath blanket down to the pubic area.

33 Lift the towel slightly, and wash the abdomen (Fig. 13-13, p. 219). Rinse and pat dry.

34 Pull the bath blanket up to the shoulders, covering both arms. Remove the towel.

35 Change soapy or cool water. Measure bath water as in step 13. If bed rails are used, raise the bed rail near you before leaving the bedside. Lower it when you return.

36 Uncover the far leg. Do not expose the genital area. Place a towel lengthwise under the foot and leg.

37 Bend the knee, and support the leg with your arm. Wash it with long, firm strokes. Rinse and pat dry.

38 Place the basin on the towel near the foot.

39 Lift the leg slightly. Slide the basin under the foot.

40 Place the foot in the basin (Fig. 13-14, p. 219). Use an orange stick or nail file to clean under toenails if necessary. If the person cannot bend the knees:

   a Wash the foot. Carefully separate the toes. Rinse and pat dry.

   b Clean under the toenails with an orange stick or nail file if necessary.

41 Remove the basin. Dry the leg and foot. Apply lotion to the foot if directed by the nurse and care plan. Cover the leg with the bath blanket. Remove the towel.

42 Repeat steps 36 to 41 for the near leg.

43 Change the water. Measure water temperature as in step 13. If bed rails are used, raise the bed rail near you before leaving the bedside. Lower it when you return.

44 Turn the person onto the side away from you. The person is covered with the bath blanket.

45 Uncover the back and buttocks. Do not expose the person. Place a towel lengthwise on the bed along the back.

46 Wash the back. Work from the back of the neck to the lower end of the buttocks. Use long, firm, continuous strokes (Fig. 13-15, p. 219). Rinse and dry well.

47 Give a back massage (p. 225). The person may want the back massage after the bath.

48 Turn the person onto his or her back.

49 Change the water for perineal care. Measure water temperature as in step 13. (Some state competency tests also require changing gloves and hand hygiene at this time.) If bed rails are used, raise the bed rail near you before leaving the bedside. Lower it when you return.

50 Let the person wash the genital area. Adjust the overbed table so he or she can reach the wash basin, soap, and towels with ease. Place the signal light within reach. Ask the person to signal when finished. Make sure the person understands what to do.

51 Remove the gloves. Decontaminate your hands.

52 Answer the signal light promptly. Provide perineal care if the person cannot do so (p. 228). (Decontaminate your hands and wear gloves for perineal care.)

53 Give a back massage if you have not already done so.

54 Apply deodorant or antiperspirant. Apply lotion and powder as requested. See *Promoting Safety and Comfort: Bathing.*

55 Put clean garments on the person.

56 Comb and brush the hair (Chapter 14).

57 Make the bed.

Post-Procedure

58 Provide for comfort. (See the inside of the front book cover.)

59 Place the signal light within reach.

60 Lower the bed to its lowest position.

61 Raise or lower bed rails. Follow the care plan.

62 Empty and clean the wash basin. Return it and other supplies to their proper place.

63 Wipe off the overbed table with the paper towels. Discard the paper towels.

64 Unscreen the person.

65 Complete a safety check of the room. (See the inside of the front book cover.)

66 Follow agency policy for dirty linen.

67 Decontaminate your hands.

68 Report and record your observations.

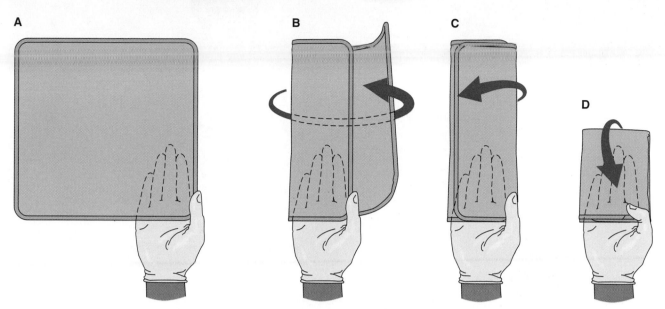

FIG. **13-8** Making a mitted washcloth. **A,** Grasp the near side of the washcloth with your thumb. **B,** Bring the washcloth around and behind your hand. **C,** Fold the side of the washcloth over your palm as you grasp it with your thumb. **D,** Fold the top of the washcloth down and tuck it under next to your palm.

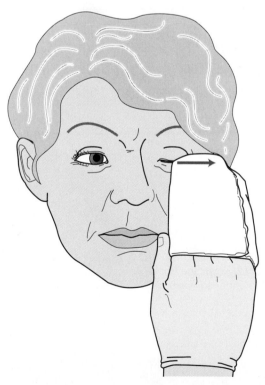

FIG. **13-9** Wash around the person's eyes with a mitted washcloth. Wipe from the inner to the outer aspect of the eye.

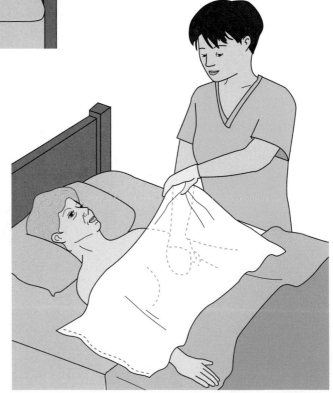

FIG. **13-10** The person's arm is washed with firm, long strokes using a mitted washcloth.

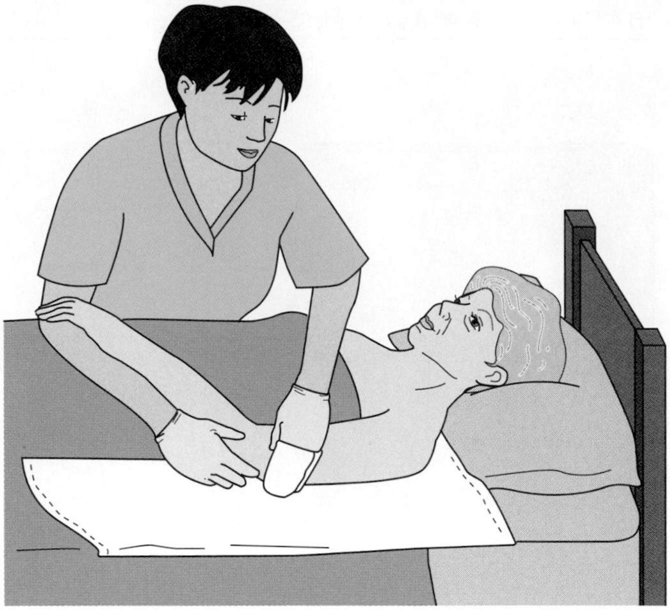

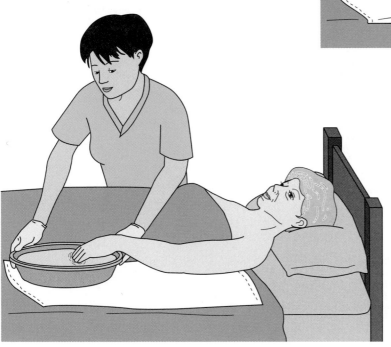

FIG. **13-11** The person's hand is washed by placing the wash basin on the bed.

FIG. **13-12** The person's breasts are not exposed during the bath. A bath towel is placed horizontally over the chest area. The towel is lifted slightly to reach under to wash the breasts and chest.

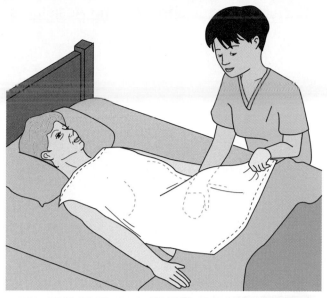

FIG. **13-13** The bath towel is turned so that it is vertical to cover the breasts and abdomen. The towel is lifted slightly to bathe the abdomen. The bath blanket covers the pubic area.

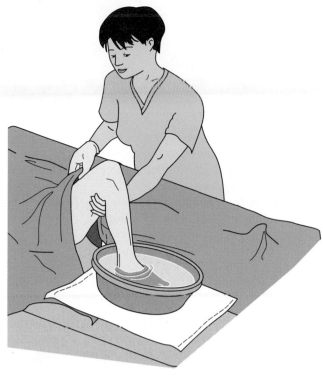

FIG. **13-14** The foot is washed by placing it in the wash basin on the bed.

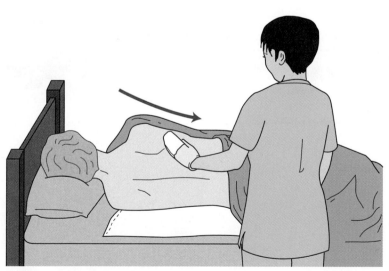

FIG. **13-15** The back is washed with long, firm, continuous strokes. Note that the person is in a side-lying position. A towel is placed lengthwise on the bed to protect the linens from water.

The Partial Bath

The *partial bath* involves bathing the face, hands, axillae (underarms), back, buttocks, and perineal area. Odors or discomfort occurs if these areas are not clean. Some persons bathe themselves in bed or at the sink. You assist as needed. Most need help washing the back. You give partial baths to persons who cannot bathe themselves.

The rules for bathing apply (see Box 13-1). So do the complete bed bath considerations.

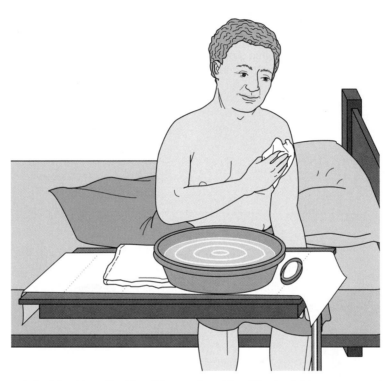

FIG. **13-16** The person is bathing himself while sitting on the side of the bed. Necessary equipment is within his reach.

Giving a Partial Bath

Quality of Life

Remember to:

- Knock before entering the person's room
- Address the person by name
- Introduce yourself by name and title
- Explain the procedure to the person before beginning and during the procedure
- Protect the person's rights during the procedure
- Handle the person gently during the procedure

Pre-Procedure

1. Follow *Delegation Guidelines: Bathing*, p. 214. See *Promoting Safety and Comfort: Bathing*, p. 214.

2. Follow steps 2 through 7 in *Giving a Complete Bed Bath*, p. 215.

Procedure

3. Make sure the bed is in the lowest position.
4. Remove top linen. Cover the person with a bath blanket.
5. Fill the wash basin with water. Water temperature is 110° to 115° F (43.3° to 46.1° C) or as directed by the nurse. Measure water temperature with the bath thermometer. Or test bath water by dipping your elbow or inner wrist into the basin.
6. Place the basin on the overbed table.
7. Position the person in the Fowler's position. Or assist him or her to sit at the bedside.
8. Adjust the overbed table so the person can reach the basin and supplies.
9. Help the person undress. Provide for privacy and warmth with the bath blanket.
10. Ask the person to wash easy to reach body parts (Fig. 13-16). Explain that you will wash the back and areas the person cannot reach.
11. Place the signal light within reach. Ask him or her to signal when help is needed or bathing is complete.
12. Leave the room after decontaminating your hands.

13. Return when the signal light is on. Knock before entering. Decontaminate your hands.
14. Change the bath water. Measure bath water temperature as in step 5.
15. Raise the bed for body mechanics. The far bed rail is up if used.
16. Ask what was washed. Put on gloves. Wash and dry areas the person could not reach. The face, hands, underarms, back, buttocks, and perineal area are washed for the partial bath.
17. Remove the gloves. Decontaminate your hands.
18. Give a back massage.
19. Apply lotion, powder, and deodorant or antiperspirant as requested.
20. Help the person put on clean garments.
21. Assist with hair care and other grooming needs.
22. Assist the person to a chair. (Lower the bed if the person transfers to a chair.) Otherwise, turn the person onto the side away from you.
23. Make the bed. (Raise the bed for body mechanics.)

Post-Procedure

24. Provide for comfort. (See the inside of the front book cover.)
25. Place the signal light within reach.
26. Lower the bed to its lowest position.
27. Raise or lower bed rails. Follow the care plan.
28. Empty and clean the basin. Return the basin and supplies to their proper place.
29. Wipe off the overbed table with the paper towels. Discard the paper towels.
30. Unscreen the person.
31. Complete a safety check of the room. (See the inside of the front book cover.)
32. Follow agency policy for dirty linen.
33. Decontaminate your hands.
34. Report and record your observations.

Tub Baths and Showers

Many people like tub baths or showers. Falls, chilling, and burns from hot water are risks. Safety is important (Box 13-2). The measures in Box 13-1 also apply.

BOX 13-2   Safety Measures For Tub Baths and Showers

- Know what water temperature to use. See *Delegation Guidelines: Tub Baths and Showers.*
- Clean and disinfect the tub or shower before and after use.
- Dry the tub or shower room floor.
- Check hand rails, grab bars, hydraulic lifts, and other safety aids. They must be in working order.
- Place a bath mat in the tub or on the shower floor. This is not needed if there are non-skid strips or a non-skid surface.
- Cover the person for warmth and privacy. This includes during transport to and from the shower room or tub room.
- Place needed items within the person's reach.
- Place the signal light within the person's reach.
- Show the person how to use the signal light in the shower or tub room.
- Have the person use grab bars when getting in and out of the tub. The person must not use towel bars for support.
- Turn cold water on first, then hot water. Turn hot water off first, then the cold water.
- Adjust water temperature and pressure to prevent chilling or burns. Do this before the person gets into the shower. If a shower chair is used, position it first.
- Direct water away from the person while adjusting water temperature and pressure.
- Fill the tub before the person gets into it.
- Measure water temperature. For showers and tub baths, use the digital display. Or you can use a bath thermometer for a tub bath.
- Keep the water spray directed toward the person during the shower. This helps keep him or her warm.
- Keep bar soap in the soap dish between latherings. This prevents soapy water. It reduces the risk of slipping and falls in showers and tubs.
- Avoid using bath oils. They make tub and shower surfaces slippery.
- Do not leave weak or unsteady persons unattended.
- Stay within hearing distance if the person can be left alone. Wait outside the shower curtain or door. You will be nearby if the person calls for you or has an accident.
- Turn the shower off before the person gets out of the shower. Drain the tub before the person gets out of the tub. Cover him or her to protect from exposure and chilling.

Tub Baths

A tub bath can cause a person to feel faint, weak, or tired. These are greater risks for persons who were on bedrest. A tub bath lasts no longer than 20 minutes.

Some agencies have portable tubs (Fig. 13-17). The person is transferred to the tub and transported to the tub room.

Whirlpool tubs have special lifts. A chair or stretcher and person are lifted into the tub (Fig. 13-18). The tub has a whirlpool action that cleanses. You wash the upper body. Carefully wash under breasts, between skin folds, and in the perineal area. Dry the person after the bath.

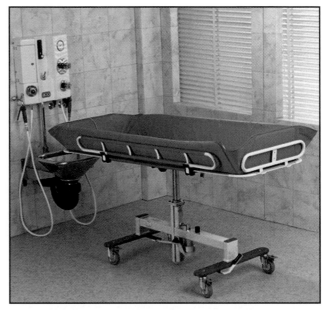

FIG. **13-17** Portable tub. (Courtesy Arjo, Inc, Morton Grove, Ill.)

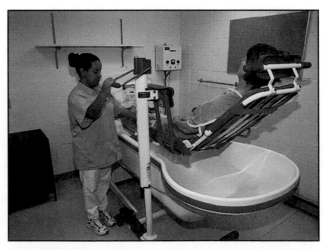

FIG. **13-18** The stretcher and person are lowered into the tub.

Showers

Some patients and residents use shower chairs (Fig. 13-19). Water drains through an opening in the seat. The chair is used to transport the person to and from the shower. The wheels are locked during the shower to prevent the chair from moving.

People who can stand in the shower should use the grab bars for support. Like tubs, showers have non-skid surfaces. If not, provide a bath mat. Never let weak or unsteady persons stand in the shower. They need to use a shower chair.

Some shower rooms have two or more stalls. Protect the person's privacy. The person has the right not to have his or her body seen by others. Properly screen and cover the person. Also, close doors and the shower curtain.

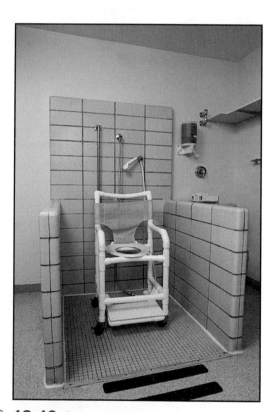

FIG. **13-19** Shower chair in a shower stall. An open area on the seat lets water drain off the chair.

DELEGATION GUIDELINES
Tub Baths and Showers

Before assisting with a tub bath or shower, you need this information from the nurse and the care plan:

- If the person takes a tub bath or shower
- What water temperature to use (usually 105° F; 40.5° C)
- If any special equipment is needed
- How much help the person needs
- If the person can bathe unattended
- What observations to report and record:
  - Dizziness
  - Light-headedness
  - See *Delegation Guidelines: Bathing* (p. 214)

PROMOTING SAFETY AND COMFORT
Tub Baths and Showers

Safety

Some persons are very weak or large. Two staff members are needed to safely assist them with tub baths and showers.

You may use portable tubs, whirlpool equipment, and shower chairs. Always follow the manufacturer's instructions. Also, protect the person from falls, chilling, and burns. Follow the safety measures in Chapter 8. Remember to measure water temperature.

Clean and disinfect the tub or shower before and after use. This prevents the spread of microbes and infection.

Comfort

Warmth and privacy promote comfort during tub baths and showers. You need to:

- Make sure the tub or shower room is warm.
- Provide for privacy. Close the room door, screen the person, and close shades, blinds, or curtains.
- Make sure water temperature is warm enough for the person.
- Have the person remove his or her robe and remove footwear just before getting into the tub or shower. Do not let the person remain exposed longer than necessary.
- Leave the room if the person can bathe alone.

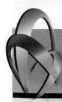

Assisting With a Tub Bath or Shower

Quality of Life

Remember to:

- Knock before entering the person's room
- Address the person by name
- Introduce yourself by name and title

- Explain the procedure to the person before beginning and during the procedure
- Protect the person's rights during the procedure
- Handle the person gently during the procedure

Pre-Procedure

1. Follow *Delegation Guidelines:*
   - *Bathing,* p. 214
   - *Tub Baths and Showers,* p. 223
   See *Promoting Safety and Comfort:*
   - *Bathing,* p. 214
   - *Tub Baths and Showers,* p. 223
2. Reserve the bathtub or shower.
3. Practice hand hygiene.
4. Identify the person. Check the ID bracelet against the assignment sheet. Call the person by name.

5. Collect the following:
   - Washcloth and two bath towels
   - Soap
   - Bath thermometer (for a tub bath)
   - Clothing, gown, or pajamas
   - Grooming items as requested
   - Robe and non-skid footwear
   - Rubber bath mat if needed
   - Disposable bath mat
   - Gloves
   - Wheelchair or shower chair

Procedure

6. Place items in the tub or shower room. Use the space provided or a chair.
7. Clean and disinfect the tub or shower.
8. Place a rubber bath mat in the tub or on the shower floor. Do not block the drain.
9. Place the disposable bath mat on the floor in front of the tub or shower.
10. Put the OCCUPIED sign on the door.
11. Return to the person's room. Provide for privacy. Decontaminate your hands.
12. Help the person sit on the side of the bed.
13. Help the person put on a robe and non-skid footwear.
14. Assist or transport the person to the tub or shower room.
15. Have the person sit on a chair if he or she walked into the tub room or shower.
16. Provide for privacy.
17. *For a tub bath:*
    a. Fill the tub halfway with warm water (105° F; 40.5° C).
    b. Measure water temperature with the bath thermometer. Or check the digital display.
18. *For a shower:*
    a. Turn on the shower.
    b. Adjust water temperature and pressure. Check the digital temperature display.
19. Help the person undress and remove footwear.
20. Help the person into the tub or shower. Position the shower chair, and lock the wheels.

21. Assist with washing if necessary. Wear gloves.
22. Ask the person to use the signal light when done or when help is needed. Remind the person that a tub bath lasts no longer than 20 minutes.
23. Place a towel across the chair.
24. Leave the room if the person can bathe alone. If not, stay in the room or remain nearby. Remove the gloves and decontaminate your hands if you will leave the room.
25. Check the person every 5 minutes.
26. Return when he or she signals for you. Knock before entering.
27. Turn off the shower or drain the tub. Cover the person while the tub drains.
28. Help the person out of the tub or shower and onto the chair.
29. Help the person dry off. Pat gently. Dry under breasts, between skin folds, in the perineal area, and between the toes.
30. Assist with lotion and other grooming items as needed.
31. Help the person dress and put on footwear.
32. Help the person return to the room. Provide for privacy.
33. Assist the person to a chair or into bed.
34. Provide a back massage if the person returns to bed.
35. Assist with hair care and other grooming needs.

Assisting With a Tub Bath or Shower—cont'd

Post-Procedure

36 Provide for comfort. (See the inside of the front book cover.)

37 Place the signal light within reach.

38 Raise or lower bed rails. Follow the care plan.

39 Unscreen the person.

40 Complete a safety check of the room. (See the inside of the front book cover.)

41 Clean and disinfect the tub or shower. Remove soiled linen. Wear gloves for this step.

42 Discard disposable items. Put the UNOCCUPIED sign on the door. Return supplies to their proper place.

43 Follow agency policy for dirty linen.

44 Decontaminate your hands.

45 Report and record your observations.

THE BACK MASSAGE

The back massage (back rub) relaxes muscles and stimulates circulation. Massages are given after the bath and with evening care. You can also give back massages at other times. Examples include after repositioning or helping the person to relax.

Back massages last 3 to 5 minutes. Observe the skin before the massage. Look for breaks in the skin, bruises, reddened areas, and other signs of skin breakdown.

Lotion reduces friction during the massage. It is warmed before being applied. To warm lotion, do one of the following.

- Rub some lotion between your hands.
- Place the bottle in the bath water.
- Hold the bottle under warm water.

Use firm strokes. Always keep your hands in contact with the person's skin. After the massage, apply some lotion to the elbows, knees, and heels. This keeps the skin soft. These bony areas are at risk for skin breakdown.

Text continued on p. 228

DELEGATION GUIDELINES
Back Massage

Before giving a back massage, you need this information from the nurse and the care plan:

- Can the person have a back massage (see *Promoting Safety and Comfort: Back Massage*)
- How to position the person
- Does the person have position limits
- When should the person receive a back massage
- Does the person need frequent back massages for comfort and to relax
- What observations to report and record:
  - Breaks in the skin
  - Bruising
  - Reddened areas
  - Signs of skin breakdown

PROMOTING SAFETY AND COMFORT
Back Massage

Safety

Back massages are dangerous for persons with certain heart diseases, back injuries, back surgeries, skin diseases, and some lung disorders. Check with the nurse and care plan before giving back massages to persons with these conditions.

Do not massage bony areas that are reddened. Reddened areas signal skin breakdown and pressure ulcers. Massage can lead to further tissue damage.

Wear gloves if the person's skin is not intact. Always follow Standard Precautions and the Bloodborne Pathogen Standard.

Comfort

The prone position is best for a massage. The side-lying position is often used. Older and disabled persons usually find the side-lying position more comfortable.

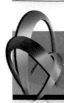

Giving a Back Massage

Quality of Life

Remember to:

- Knock before entering the person's room
- Address the person by name
- Introduce yourself by name and title
- Explain the procedure to the person before beginning and during the procedure
- Protect the person's rights during the procedure
- Handle the person gently during the procedure

Pre-Procedure

1 Follow *Delegation Guidelines: Back Massage*, p. 225. See *Promoting Safety and Comfort: Back Massage*, p. 225.
2 Practice hand hygiene.
3 Identify the person. Check the ID bracelet against the assignment sheet. Call the person by name.
4 Collect the following:
 • Bath blanket
 • Bath towel
 • Lotion
5 Provide for privacy.
6 Raise the bed for body mechanics. Bed rails are up if used.

Procedure

7 Lower the bed rail near you if up.
8 Position the person in the prone or side-lying position. The back is toward you.
9 Expose the back, shoulders, upper arms, and buttocks. Cover the rest of the body with the bath blanket.
10 Lay the towel on the bed along the back. (This step is done if the person is in a side-lying position.)
11 Warm the lotion.
12 Explain that the lotion may feel cool and wet.
13 Apply lotion to the lower back area.
14 Stroke up from the buttocks to the shoulders. Then stroke down over the upper arms. Stroke up the upper arms, across the shoulders, and down the back to the buttocks (Fig. 13-20). Use firm strokes. Keep your hands in contact with the person's skin.
15 Repeat step 14 for at least 3 minutes.
16 Knead by grasping skin between your thumb and fingers (Fig. 13-21). Knead half of the back. Start at the buttocks and move up to the shoulder. Then knead down from the shoulder to the buttocks. Repeat on the other half of the back.
17 Apply lotion to bony areas. Use circular motions with the tips of your index and middle fingers. (Do not massage reddened bony areas.)
18 Use fast movements to stimulate. Use slow movements to relax the person.
19 Stroke with long, firm movements to end the massage. Tell the person you are finishing.
20 Straighten and secure the gown. Cover the person. Remove the towel and bath blanket.

Post-Procedure

21 Provide for comfort. (See the inside of the front book cover.)
22 Place the signal light within reach.
23 Lower the bed to its lowest position.
24 Raise or lower bed rails. Follow the care plan.
25 Return lotion to its proper place.
26 Unscreen the person.
27 Complete a safety check of the room. (See the inside of the front book cover.)
28 Follow agency policy for dirty linen.
29 Decontaminate your hands.
30 Report and record your observations.

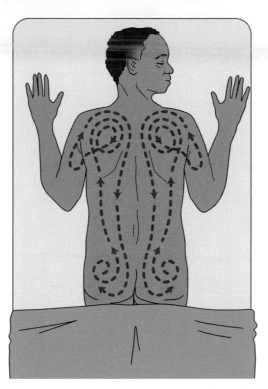

FIG. **13-20** The person lies in the prone position for a back massage. Stroke upward from the buttocks to the shoulders, down over the upper arms, back up the upper arms, across the shoulders, and down the back to the buttocks.

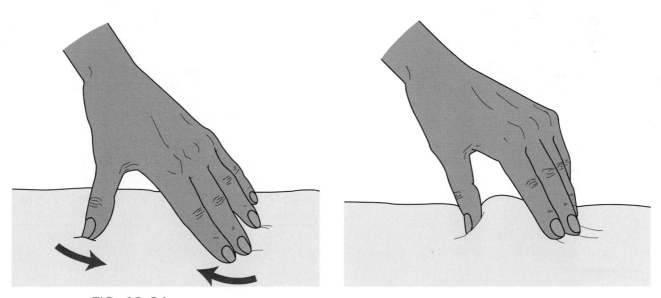

FIG. **13-21** Kneading is done by picking up tissue between the thumb and fingers.

PERINEAL CARE

Perineal care (*pericare*) involves cleaning the genital and anal areas. It prevents infection and odors, and it promotes comfort. Perineal care is done daily during the bath. It also is done whenever the area is soiled with urine or feces.

The person does perineal care if able. Otherwise, it is given by nursing staff. The procedure embarrasses many people and nursing staff, especially when it involves the other sex. *Perineum* and *perineal* are not common terms. Most people understand *privates*, *private parts*, *crotch*, *genitals*, or the *area between your legs*. Use terms the person understands. The term must also be in good taste professionally.

Standard Precautions, medical asepsis, and the Bloodborne Pathogen Standard are followed. Work from the cleanest area to the dirtiest. This is commonly called cleaning from "front to back." The urethral area (the front) is the cleanest. The anal area (the back) is the dirtiest. Therefore clean from the urethra to the anal area.

The perineal area is delicate and easily injured. Use warm water, not hot. Use washcloths, towelettes, cotton balls, or swabs according to agency policy. Rinse thoroughly. Pat dry after rinsing. This reduces moisture and promotes comfort.

DELEGATION GUIDELINES
Perineal Care

Before giving perineal care, you need this information from the nurse and the care plan:

- When perineal care needs to be done
- What terms the person understands—perineum, privates, private parts, crotch, genitals, area between the legs, and so on
- How much help the person needs
- What water temperature to use—usually 105° to 109° F (40.5° to 42.7° C)
- What cleaning agent to use
- Any position restrictions or limits
- What observations to report and record:
  - Odors
  - Redness, swelling, discharge, or irritation
  - Complaints of pain, burning, or other discomfort
  - Signs of urinary or fecal incontinence (Chapters 15 and 16)

PROMOTING SAFETY AND COMFORT
Perineal Care

Safety

Hot water can burn delicate perineal tissues. To prevent burns, measure water temperature according to agency policy. If the water seems too hot, ask the nurse to check it.

Protect yourself and the person from infection. Contact with blood, body fluids, secretions, and excretions is likely during perineal care. Follow Standard Precautions and the Bloodborne Pathogen Standard.

Persons who are incontinent need perineal care. You must protect the person and dry garments and linens from the wet incontinence product. After cleaning and drying the perineal area, remove the wet incontinence products, garments, and linen. Then apply clean, dry ones. (See Chapter 15.)

Comfort

To avoid embarrassment, it is best if the person does perineal care. If you need to provide this care, explain how you will provide for the person's privacy. Act in a professional manner at all times.

Giving Female Perineal Care

Quality of Life

Remember to:

- Knock before entering the person's room
- Address the person by name
- Introduce yourself by name and title

- Explain the procedure to the person before beginning and during the procedure
- Protect the person's rights during the procedure
- Handle the person gently during the procedure

Pre-Procedure

1 Follow *Delegation Guidelines: Perineal Care*. See *Promoting Safety and Comfort: Perineal Care*.
2 Practice hand hygiene.
3 Collect the following:
 - Soap or other cleaning agent as directed
 - At least 4 washcloths
 - Bath towel
 - Bath blanket
 - Bath thermometer
 - Wash basin
 - Waterproof pad
 - Gloves
 - Paper towels
4 Cover the overbed table with paper towels. Arrange items on top of them.
5 Identify the person. Check the ID bracelet against the assignment sheet. Call her by name.
6 Provide for privacy.
7 Raise the bed for body mechanics. Bed rails are up if used.

Procedure

8 Lower the bed rail near you if up.
9 Decontaminate your hands. Put on gloves.
10 Cover the person with a bath blanket. Move top linens to the foot of the bed.
11 Position the person on her back.
12 Drape her as in Figure 13-22, p. 230.
13 Raise the bed rail if used.
14 Fill the wash basin. Water temperature is about 105° to 109° F (40.5° to 42.7° C). Measure water temperature according to agency policy.
15 Place the basin on the overbed table.
16 Lower the bed rail if up.
17 Help the person flex her knees and spread her legs. Or help her spread her legs as much as possible with her knees straight.
18 Place a waterproof pad under her buttocks.
19 Fold the corner of the bath blanket between her legs onto her abdomen.
20 Wet the washcloths.
21 Squeeze out excess water from a washcloth. Make a mitted washcloth. Apply soap.
22 Separate the labia. Clean downward from front to back with one stroke (Fig. 13-23, p. 230).
23 Repeat steps 21 and 22 until the area is clean. Use a clean part of the washcloth for each stroke. Use more than one washcloth if needed.

24 Rinse the perineum with a clean washcloth. Separate the labia. Stroke downward from front to back. Repeat as necessary. Use a clean part of the washcloth for each stroke. Use more than one washcloth if needed.
25 Pat the area dry with the towel. Dry from front to back.
26 Fold the blanket back between her legs.
27 Help the person lower her legs and turn onto her side away from you.
28 Apply soap to a mitted washcloth.
29 Clean the rectal area. Clean from the vagina to the anus with one stroke (Fig. 13-24, p. 230).
30 Repeat steps 28 and 29 until the area is clean. Use a clean part of the washcloth for each stroke. Use more than one washcloth if needed.
31 Rinse the rectal area with a washcloth. Stroke from the vagina to the anus. Repeat as necessary. Use a clean part of the washcloth for each stroke. Use more than one washcloth if needed.
32 Pat the area dry with the towel. Dry from front to back.
33 Remove the waterproof pad.
34 Provide clean and dry linens and incontinence products as needed.
35 Remove and discard the gloves. Decontaminate your hands.

Continued

Post-Procedure

36 Cover the person. Remove the bath blanket.
37 Provide for comfort. (See the inside of the front book cover.)
38 Place the signal light within reach.
39 Lower the bed to its lowest position.
40 Raise or lower bed rails. Follow the care plan.
41 Empty and clean the wash basin. Wear gloves.
42 Return the basin and supplies to their proper place.

43 Wipe off the overbed table with the paper towels. Discard the paper towels.
44 Remove the gloves. Decontaminate your hands.
45 Unscreen the person.
46 Complete a safety check of the room. (See the inside of the front book cover.)
47 Follow agency policy for dirty linen.
48 Decontaminate your hands.
49 Report and record your observations.

A
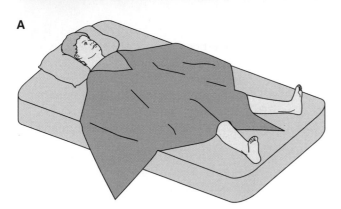

B
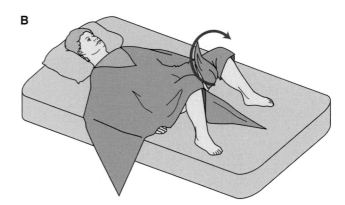

FIG. **13-22** Draping for perineal care. **A,** Position the bath blanket like a diamond: one corner is at the neck, there is a corner at each side, and one corner is between the person's legs. **B,** Wrap the blanket around the leg by bringing the corner around under the leg and over the top. Tuck the corner under the hip.

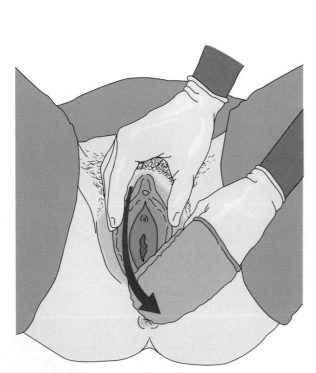

FIG. **13-23** Separate the labia with one hand. Use a mitted washcloth to cleanse between the labia with downward strokes.

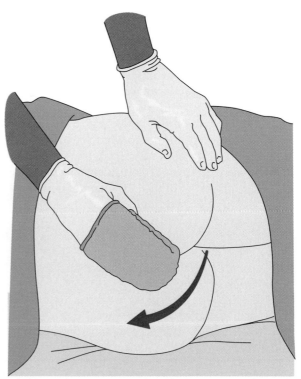

FIG. **13-24** The rectal area is cleaned by wiping from the vagina to the anus. The side-lying position allows the anal area to be cleaned more thoroughly.

Quality of Life

Remember to:

- Knock before entering the person's room
- Address the person by name
- Introduce yourself by name and title

- Explain the procedure to the person before beginning and during the procedure
- Protect the person's rights during the procedure
- Handle the person gently during the procedure

Procedure

1. Follow steps 1 through 16 in procedure: *Giving Female Perineal Care*, p. 229. Drape the person as in Figure 13-25.
2. Retract the foreskin if the person is uncircumcised (see Fig. 13-25).
3. Grasp the penis.
4. Clean the tip. Use a circular motion. Start at the meatus of the urethra, and work outward (Fig. 13-26). Repeat as needed. Use a clean part of the washcloth each time.
5. Rinse the area with another washcloth.
6. Return the foreskin to its natural position.
7. Clean the shaft of the penis. Use firm downward strokes. Rinse the area.
8. Help the person flex his knees and spread his legs. Or help him spread his legs as much as possible with his knees straight.
9. Clean the scrotum. Rinse well. Observe for redness and irritation in the skin folds.
10. Pat dry the penis and scrotum. Use the towel.
11. Fold the bath blanket back between his legs.
12. Help him lower his legs and turn onto his side away from you.
13. Clean the rectal area (see procedure: *Giving Female Perineal Care*). Rinse and dry well.
14. Remove the waterproof pad.
15. Provide clean and dry linens and incontinence products as needed.
16. Remove and discard the gloves. Decontaminate your hands.

Post-Procedure

17. Follow steps 37 through 49 in procedure: *Giving Female Perineal Care*.

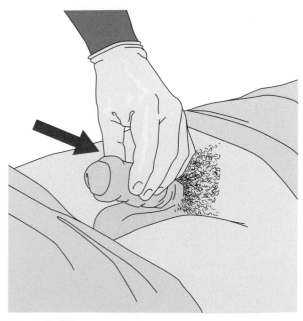

FIG. **13-25** The foreskin of the uncircumcised male is pulled back for perineal care. It is returned to the normal position immediately after cleaning.

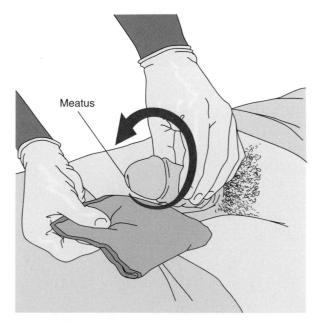

FIG. **13-26** The penis is cleaned with circular motions starting at the meatus of the urethra.

FOCUS ON THE PERSON

You must provide hygiene in a way that maintains or improves the person's quality of life, health, and safety. See *Focus on the Person: Assisting With Hygiene.*

Focus on the PERSON

Assisting With Hygiene

Providing comfort—Privacy is important for the person's mental comfort. Protect the right to privacy by:
- Not exposing the person.
- Asking visitors to leave the room before you give care.
- Closing doors, privacy curtains, shades, and drapes before giving care.
- Exposing only the body part involved in the procedure.
- Covering persons who are taken to and from tubs or shower rooms.

Ethical behavior—Water gets soapy during a complete bed bath. It also cools. You must change the water when it is soapy or cool. It takes time to safely leave the bedside and change water. However, it is the right thing to do. Not changing the water is the wrong thing.

Remaining independent—Personal choice helps the person remain independent. Hygiene is a very personal matter. Personal choice is allowed in such matters as bath time, products used, what to wear, and hair-styling. Encourage the person to do as much self-care as safely possible.

Speaking up—During hygiene procedures, you must make sure that the person is warm enough. You can ask:
- "Is the water warm enough?" "Is it too hot?" "Is it too cold?"
- "Do you need another bath blanket?"
- "Is the water starting to cool?"
- "Is the room warm enough?"

OBRA and other laws—OBRA requires that nursing center residents appear clean and neat. Survey teams observe how care is given and the person's appearance.

Nursing teamwork—Many agencies do not have tubs, portable tubs, showers, and shower chairs for each person. You need to reserve the room and needed equipment for the person. Other nursing team members need to do the same for their patients or residents. Consider the needs of others. For example, you reserve the shower room from 0945 to 1030. Do your very best to follow the schedule. Make sure the shower room is clean and ready for the next person. Or you and a co-worker schedule something for the same time. Discuss the matter with your co-worker to work out a new schedule.

Circle **T** if the answer is true or **F** if the answer is false.

1 **T F** Hygiene is needed for comfort, safety, and health.

2 **T F** After lunch, a person asks for a back massage. You can give a back massage then.

3 **T F** A hard-bristled toothbrush is good for oral hygiene.

4 **T F** Unconscious persons are supine for mouth care.

5 **T F** A person is unconscious. You use your fingers to keep the mouth open for oral hygiene.

6 **T F** Dentures are washed over the bathroom counter.

7 **T F** A tub bath lasts 30 minutes.

8 **T F** You can give permission for showers.

9 **T F** Weak persons are left alone in the shower if they are sitting.

10 **T F** A back massage relaxes muscles and stimulates circulation.

11 **T F** Perineal care helps prevent infection.

12 **T F** Foreskin is returned to its normal position immediately after cleaning.

Circle the **BEST** answer.

13 You note the following when giving oral hygiene. Which is *not* reported to the nurse?
   a Bleeding, swelling, or redness of the gums
   b Irritations, sores, or white patches in the mouth or on the tongue
   c Lips that are dry, cracked, swollen, or blistered
   d Food between the teeth

14 Which is *not* a purpose of bathing?
   a Increasing circulation
   b Promoting drying of the skin
   c Exercising body parts
   d Refreshing and relaxing the person

15 Which action is *wrong* when bathing Mrs. Bell?
   a Covering her for warmth and privacy
   b Rinsing her skin thoroughly to remove all soap
   c Washing from the dirtiest to cleanest area
   d Patting her skin dry

16 What is a safe water temperature for a complete bed bath?
   a 95° F
   b 100° F
   c 110° F
   d 120° F

17 You are going to give a back massage. Which is *false*?
   a It should last 3 to 5 minutes.
   b Lotion is warmed before being applied.
   c Your hands are always in contact with the skin.
   d The side-lying position is best.

Answers to these questions are on p. 468.

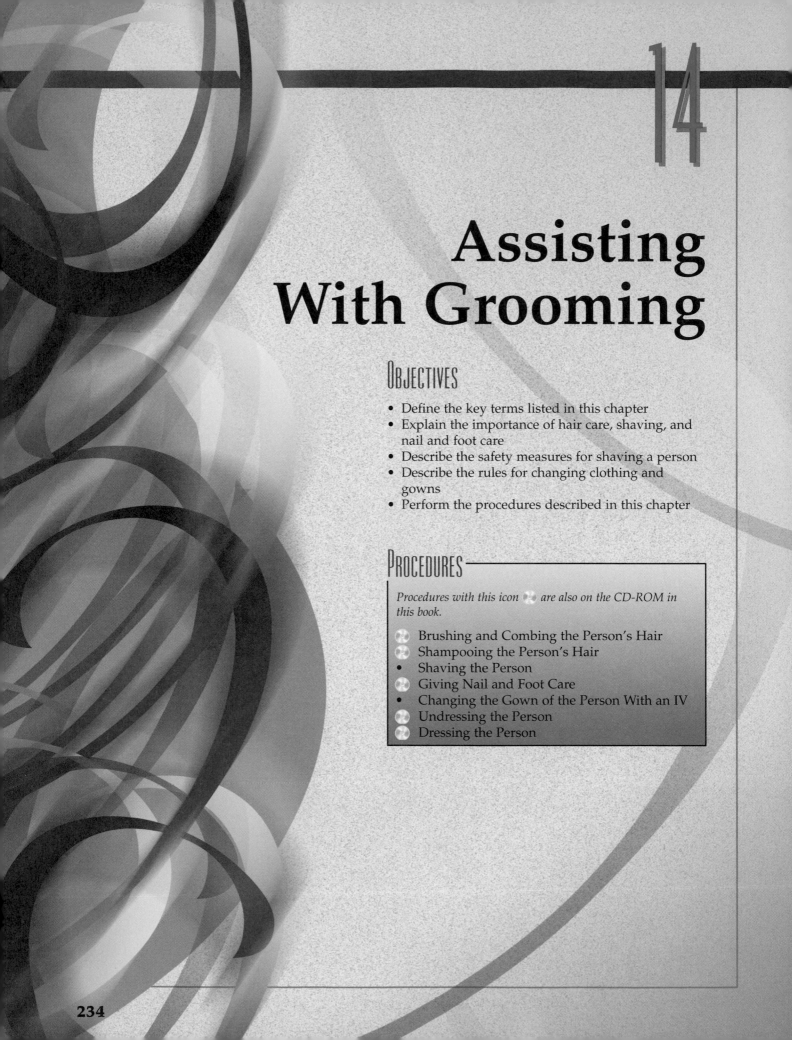

Assisting With Grooming

OBJECTIVES

- Define the key terms listed in this chapter
- Explain the importance of hair care, shaving, and nail and foot care
- Describe the safety measures for shaving a person
- Describe the rules for changing clothing and gowns
- Perform the procedures described in this chapter

PROCEDURES

Procedures with this icon ✿ *are also on the CD-ROM in this book.*

✿ Brushing and Combing the Person's Hair
✿ Shampooing the Person's Hair
• Shaving the Person
✿ Giving Nail and Foot Care
• Changing the Gown of the Person With an IV
✿ Undressing the Person
✿ Dressing the Person

KEY TERMS

alopecia Hair loss
dandruff Excessive amount of dry, white flakes from the scalp
hirsutism Excessive body hair in women and children
pediculosis (lice) Infestation with lice

Hair care, shaving, nail and foot care, and fresh garments are important to many people. Like hygiene, such measures prevent infection. They also promote comfort, well-being, and quality of life.

HAIR CARE

Many nursing centers have beauty and barber shops for residents. However, you assist patients and residents with daily hair care. The nursing process reflects the person's culture, personal choice, skin and scalp condition, health history, and self-care ability. These terms are common in care plans.

- **Alopecia** means hair loss. Hair loss may be complete or partial. Male pattern baldness occurs with aging and is the result of heredity. Hair also thins in some women with aging. Cancer treatments often cause alopecia in males and females.
- **Hirsutism** is excessive body hair in women and children. It results from heredity and abnormal amounts of male hormones.
- **Dandruff** is the excessive amount of dry, white flakes from the scalp. Itching often occurs. Sometimes eyebrows and ear canals are involved.
- **Pediculosis (lice)** is the infestation with lice. (*Infestation* means being in or on a host.) Lice bites cause severe itching in the affected area. Lice easily spreads to others through clothing, furniture, bed linen, and sexual contact. They also are spread by sharing combs and brushes. Medicated shampoos, lotions, and creams are used to treat lice. Thorough bathing is needed. So is washing clothing and linen in hot water.
  - □ *Pediculosis capitis* is the infestation of the scalp (*capitis*) with lice.
  - □ *Pediculosis pubis* is the infestation of the pubic (*pubis*) hair with lice.
  - □ *Pediculosis corporis* is the infestation of the body (*corporis*) with lice.

 ## Brushing and Combing Hair

Brushing and combing hair are part of early morning care, morning care, and afternoon care. They also are done whenever needed. Encourage patients and residents to do their own hair care. Assist as needed. The person chooses how to brush, comb, and style hair.

Long hair easily mats and tangles. Daily brushing and combing prevent the problem. So does braiding. Do not braid hair without the person's consent. *Never cut the person's hair for any reason.*

When brushing and combing hair, start at the scalp. Then brush and comb to the hair ends. You may need to comb or brush through the matting and tangling. To do this:

- Take a small section of hair near the ends.
- Comb or brush through to the hair ends.
- Working up to the scalp, add small sections of hair.
- Comb or brush through each longer section to the hair ends.
- Brush or comb from the scalp to the hair ends.

Special measures are needed for curly, coarse, and dry hair. The person may have certain practices or hair care products. They are part of the care plan. Also the person can guide you when giving hair care. *(See Caring About Culture: Braiding Hair.)*

Caring About Culture

Braiding Hair

Styling hair in in small braids is a common practice of some cultural groups. The braids are left intact for shampooing. To undo these braids, the nurse obtains the person's consent.

DELEGATION GUIDELINES
Brushing and Combing Hair

You need this information from the nurse and care plan before brushing and combing hair:
- How much help the person needs
- What to do if hair is matted or tangled
- What measures are needed for curly, coarse, or dry hair
- What hair care products to use
- The person's preferences and routine hair care measures
- What observations to report and record:
  - Scalp sores
  - Flaking
  - Itching
  - Presence of lice
  - Patches of hair loss
  - Very dry or very oily hair
  - Matted or tangled hair

PROMOTING SAFETY AND COMFORT
Brushing and Combing Hair

Safety

Sharp brush bristles can injure the scalp. So can a comb with sharp or broken teeth. Tell the nurse if you have concerns about the person's brush or comb.

Comfort

When giving hair care, place a towel across the person's back and shoulders to protect the person's garments. If the person is in bed, give hair care before changing the pillowcase. If done after a linen change, place a towel across the pillow to collect falling hair.

Brushing and Combing the Person's Hair

Quality of Life

Remember to:

- Knock before entering the person's room
- Address the person by name
- Introduce yourself by name and title

- Explain the procedure to the person before beginning and during the procedure
- Protect the person's rights during the procedure
- Handle the person gently during the procedure

Pre-Procedure

1 Follow *Delegation Guidelines: Brushing and Combing Hair.* See *Promoting Safety and Comfort: Brushing and Combing Hair.*
2 Practice hand hygiene.
3 Identify the person. Check the ID bracelet against the assignment sheet. Call the person by name.

4 Ask the person how to style hair.
5 Collect the following:
   - Comb and brush
   - Bath towel
   - Hair care items as requested
6 Arrange items on the bedside stand.
7 Provide for privacy.

Procedure

8 Lower the bed rail if used.
9 Help the person to the chair. The person puts on a robe and non-skid footwear when up. (If the person is in bed, raise the bed for body mechanics. Bed rails are up if used. Lower the near bed rail. Assist the person to a semi-Fowler's position if allowed.)
10 Place a towel across the back and shoulders or across the pillow.
11 Ask the person to remove eyeglasses. Put them in the eyeglass case. Put the case inside the bedside stand.

12 Use the comb to part the hair.
   a Part hair down the middle into 2 sides (Fig. 14-1, *A*).
   b Divide one side into 2 smaller sections (Fig. 14-1, *B*). Use the comb for this step.
13 Brush one of the small sections of hair. Start at the scalp, and brush toward the hair ends (Fig. 14-2). Do the same for the other small section of hair.
14 Repeat steps 12b and 13 for the other side.
15 Style the hair as the person prefers.
16 Remove the towel.
17 Let the person put on the eyeglasses.

Post-Procedure

18 Provide for comfort. (See the inside of the front book cover.)

19 Place the signal light within reach.

20 Lower the bed to its lowest position.

21 Raise or lower bed rails. Follow the care plan.

22 Clean and return items to their proper place.

23 Unscreen the person.

24 Complete a safety check of the room. (See the inside of the front book cover.)

25 Follow agency policy for dirty linen.

26 Decontaminate your hands.

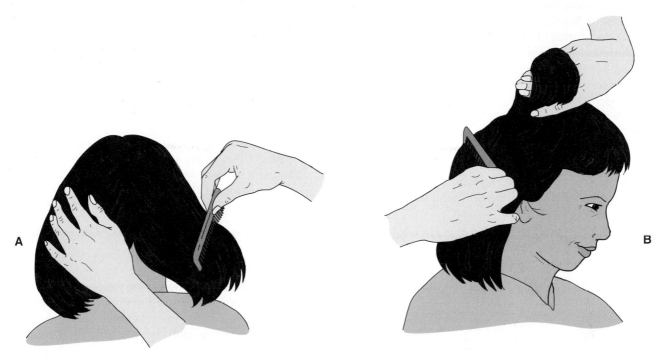

FIG. **14-1** Parting hair. **A,** Part hair down the middle. Divide it into two sides. **B,** Then part the one side into two smaller sections.

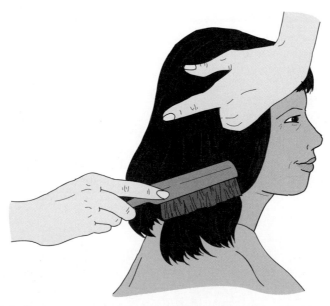

FIG. **14-2** Brush hair by starting at the scalp. Brush down to the hair ends.

Shampooing

Most people shampoo 1, 2, or 3 times a week. Others shampoo every day. In nursing centers, shampooing is usually done weekly on the person's bath or shower day. If a person's hair is done in the beauty shop, do not shampoo hair. Provide a shower cap for the bath or shower.

After shampooing, dry and style hair as quickly as possible. Women may want hair curled or rolled up before drying. Check with the nurse before doing so.

The shampooing method used depends on the person's condition, safety factors, and personal choice. The nurse tells you what method to use.

- *Shampoo during the shower or tub bath.* The person shampoos in the shower. A hand-held nozzle is used for those using shower chairs or taking tub baths. A spray of water is directed to the hair.
- *Shampoo at the sink.* The person sits facing away from the sink. A folded towel is placed over the sink edge to protect the neck. The head is tilted back over the edge of the sink. A water pitcher or hand-held nozzle is used to wet and rinse the hair.
- *Shampoo on a stretcher.* The stretcher is in front of the sink. A towel is placed under the neck. The head is tilted over the edge of the sink (Fig. 14-3). A water pitcher or hand-held nozzle is used to wet and rinse the hair.
- *Shampoo in bed.* The person's head and shoulders are moved to the edge of the bed if possible. A shampoo tray placed under the head drains water into a basin placed on a chair by the bed (Fig. 14-4). Use a water pitcher to wet and rinse the hair.

DELEGATION GUIDELINES
Shampooing

Before shampooing hair, you need this information from the nurse and the care plan:
- When to shampoo the persons' hair
- What method to use
- What shampoo and conditioner to use
- The person's position restrictions or limits
- What water temperature to use—usually 105° F (40.5° C)
- If hair is curled or rolled up before drying
- What observations to report and record:
  - Scalp sores
  - Hair falling out in patches
  - The presence of lice
  - How the person tolerated the procedure

PROMOTING SAFETY AND COMFORT
Shampooing

Safety

Keep shampoo out of the eyes. Have the person hold a washcloth over the eyes. Do not let shampoo get near the eyes. When rinsing, cup your hand at the person's forehead. This keeps soapy water from running down the person's forehead and into the eyes.

Return medicated shampoo or conditioner to the nurse. Never leave it at the bedside unless instructed to do so.

Wear gloves if the person has scalp sores. Follow Standard Precautions and the Bloodborne Pathogen Standard.

When shampooing on a stretcher, follow the rules for stretcher use (Chapter 8). Lock the stretcher wheels and use the safety straps and side rails. The far side rail is raised during the procedure.

Some people can shampoo themselves during a bath or shower. Place an extra towel, shampoo, and hair conditioner within the person's reach. Assist as needed.

Comfort

When shampooing during the tub bath or shower, the person tips his or her head back to keep shampoo and water out of the eyes. Support the back of the head with one hand as you shampoo with the other. Some older people cannot tip their heads back. They lean forward and hold a washcloth over the eyes. Support the forehead with one hand as you shampoo with the other. Make sure the person can breathe easily.

Many older people have limited range of motion in their necks. They are not shampooed at the sink or on a stretcher.

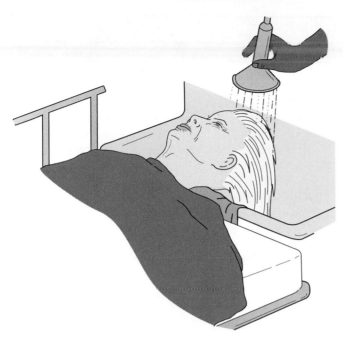

FIG. **14-3** Shampooing while the person is on a stretcher. The stretcher is in front of the sink.

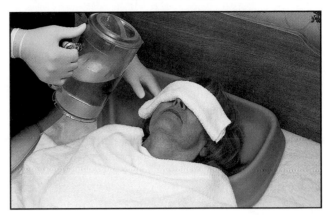

FIG. **14-4** A shampoo tray is used to shampoo a person in bed. The tray is directed to the side of the bed so water drains into a collecting basin.

Shampooing the Person's Hair

NNAAP™

Quality of Life

Remember to:

- Knock before entering the person's room
- Address the person by name
- Introduce yourself by name and title

- Explain the procedure to the person before beginning and during the procedure
- Protect the person's rights during the procedure
- Handle the person gently during the procedure

Pre-Procedure

1 Follow *Delegation Guidelines: Shampooing,* p. 238. See *Promoting Safety and Comfort: Shampooing,* p. 238.
2 Practice hand hygiene.
3 Collect the following:
   - Two bath towels
   - Washcloth
   - Shampoo
   - Hair conditioner (if requested)
   - Bath thermometer
   - Pitcher or nozzle (if needed)
   - Shampoo tray (if needed)
   - Basin or pan (if needed)
   - Waterproof pad (if needed)
   - Gloves (if needed)
   - Comb and brush
   - Hair dryer
4 Arrange items nearby.
5 Identify the person. Check the ID bracelet against the assignment sheet. Call the person by name.
6 Provide for privacy.
7 Raise the bed for body mechanics for a shampoo in bed. Bed rails are up if used.
8 Decontaminate your hands.

Continued

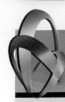

Shampooing the Person's Hair—cont'd

NNAAP™

Procedure

9 Lower the bed rail near you if up.

10 Cover the person's chest with a towel.

11 Brush and comb the hair to remove snarls and tangles.

12 Position the person for the method you will use. To shampoo the person in bed:
 a Lower the head of the bed and remove the pillow.
 b Place the waterproof pad and shampoo tray under the head and shoulders.
 c Support the head and neck with a folded towel if necessary.

13 Raise the bed rail if up.

14 Obtain water. Water temperature should be about 105° F (40.5° C). Test water temperature according to agency policy.

15 Lower the bed rail near you if up.

16 Put on gloves (if needed).

17 Ask the person to hold a washcloth over the eyes. It should not cover the nose and mouth. (A damp washcloth is easier to hold. It will not slip. However, some state competency tests require a dry washcloth.)

18 Use the pitcher or nozzle to wet the hair.

19 Apply a small amount of shampoo.

20 Work up a lather with both hands. Start at the hairline. Work toward the back of the head.

21 Massage the scalp with your fingertips. Do not scratch the scalp.

22 Rinse the hair until the water runs clear.

23 Repeat steps 19 through 22.

24 Apply conditioner. Follow directions on the container.

25 Squeeze water from the person's hair.

26 Cover hair with a bath towel.

27 Remove the shampoo tray and the waterproof pad.

28 Dry the person's face with the towel. Use the towel on the person's chest.

29 Help the person raise the head if appropriate. For the person in bed, raise the head of the bed.

30 Rub the hair and scalp with the towel. Use the second towel if the first one is wet.

31 Comb the hair to remove snarls and tangles.

32 Dry and style hair as quickly as possible.

33 Remove and discard the gloves (if used). Decontaminate your hands.

Post-Procedure

34 Provide for comfort. (See the inside of the front cover.)

35 Place the signal light within reach.

36 Lower the bed to its lowest position.

37 Raise or lower bed rails. Follow the care plan.

38 Unscreen the person.

39 Complete a safety check of the room. (See the inside of the front book cover.)

40 Clean and return equipment to its proper place. Remember to clean the brush and comb. Discard disposable items.

41 Follow agency policy for dirty linen.

42 Decontaminate your hands.

43 Report and record your observations.

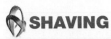 **SHAVING**

Many men shave for comfort and mental well-being. Many women shave their legs and underarms. Women with coarse facial hair may shave. Or they may use other hair removal methods. See Box 14-1 for shaving rules.

Safety and electric shavers are used. If the agency's electric shaver is used, clean it between each use. Follow agency policy.

Safety razors (blade razors) involve razor blades. They can cause nicks or cuts. Do not use them for persons taking anticoagulant drugs. An *anticoagulant* prevents or slows down *(anti)* blood clotting *(coagulant)*. Bleeding occurs easily. A nick or cut can cause serious bleeding.

Soften the beard and skin before using a safety razor. Apply a warm washcloth or towel to the face for a few minutes. Then lather the face with soap and water or a shaving cream.

Legs and underarms are shaved after the bath when the skin is soft. Soap and water, shaving cream, or lotion is used for lather. Collect shaving items with bath items. Use the kidney basin to rinse the razor. Do not use the bath water.

See Persons With Dementia: Shaving.

Caring for Mustaches and Beards

Beards and mustaches need daily care. Food can collect in hair. So can mouth and nose drainage. Daily washing and combing are needed. Ask the person how to groom his beard or mustache. *Never trim or shave a beard or mustache without the person's consent.*

BOX 14-1	**Rules For Shaving**

- Use electric shavers for persons taking anticoagulant drugs. Never use safety razors.
- Protect bed linens. Place a towel under the part being shaved. Or place a towel across the shoulders to protect clothing.
- Soften the skin before shaving.
- Encourage the person to do as much as safely possible.
- Hold the skin taut as needed.
- Shave in the direction of hair growth when shaving the face and underarms.
- Shave up from the ankles when shaving legs. This is against hair growth.
- Do not cut, nick, or irritate the skin.
- Rinse the body part thoroughly.
- Apply direct pressure to nicks or cuts.

Persons With Dementia

Shaving

Some older persons have dementia. Do not use safety razors to shave them. They may not understand what you are doing. They may resist care and move quickly. Serious nicks and cuts can occur. Use electric shavers.

DELEGATION GUIDELINES
Shaving

You need this information from the nurse and care plan when delegated shaving tasks:

- What shaver to use—electric or safety
- If the person takes anticoagulant drugs
- When to shave the person
- What observations to report and record:
  - Nicks (report at once)
  - Cuts (report at once)
  - Bleeding (report at once)
  - Irritation

PROMOTING SAFETY AND COMFORT
Shaving

Safety

Safety razors are very sharp. Protect the person and yourself from nicks or cuts. Prevent contact with blood. If using an electric shaver, follow safety measures for electrical equipment (Chapter 8).

Rinse the safety razor often during the shaving procedure. Then wipe the razor with tissues or paper towels. To protect yourself from cuts, place the tissues or paper towels on the overbed table. Do not hold them in your hand.

Follow Standard Precautions and the Bloodborne Pathogen Standard. Discard used razor blades and disposable shavers in the sharps container.

Comfort

Some people apply lotion or after-shave to the skin after shaving. Lotion softens the skin. After-shave closes skin pores. Heat is applied before shaving to soften the skin. It also opens pores.

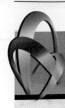

Shaving the Person

Quality of Life

Remember to:

- Knock before entering the person's room
- Address the person by name
- Introduce yourself by name and title

- Explain the procedure to the person before beginning and during the procedure
- Protect the person's rights during the procedure
- Handle the person gently during the procedure

Pre-Procedure

1 Follow *Delegation Guidelines: Shaving*, p. 241. See *Promoting Safety and Comfort: Shaving*, p. 241.
2 Practice hand hygiene.
3 Collect the following:
 - Wash basin
 - Bath towel
 - Hand towel
 - Washcloth
 - Safety razor
 - Mirror
 - Shaving cream, soap, or lotion
 - Shaving brush

- After-shave or lotion
- Tissues or paper towels
- Paper towels
- Gloves

4 Arrange paper towels and supplies on the overbed table.
5 Identify the person. Check the ID bracelet against the assignment sheet. Call the person by name.
6 Provide for privacy.
7 Raise the bed for body mechanics. Bed rails are up if used.

Procedure

8 Fill the basin with warm water.
9 Place the basin on the overbed table.
10 Lower the bed rail near you if up.
11 Decontaminate your hands. Put on gloves.
12 Assist the person to the semi-Fowler's position if allowed or to the supine position.
13 Adjust lighting to clearly see the person's face.
14 Place the bath towel over the chest.
15 Adjust the overbed table for easy reach.
16 Tighten the razor blade to the shaver.
17 Wash the person's face. Do not dry.
18 Wet the washcloth or hand towel. Wring it out.
19 Apply the washcloth or hand towel to the face for a few minutes.

20 Apply shaving cream with your hands. Or use a shaving brush to apply lather.
21 Hold the skin taut with one hand.
22 Shave in the direction of hair growth. Use shorter strokes around the chin and lips (Fig. 14-5).
23 Rinse the razor often. Wipe it with tissues or paper towels.
24 Apply direct pressure to any bleeding areas.
25 Wash off any remaining shaving cream or soap. Pat with a towel.
26 Apply after-shave or lotion if requested.
27 Remove the towel and gloves. Decontaminate your hands.

Post-Procedure

28 Provide for comfort. (See the inside of the front book cover.)
29 Place the signal light within reach.
30 Lower the bed to its lowest position.
31 Raise or lower bed rails. Follow the care plan.
32 Clean and return equipment and supplies to their proper place. Discard disposable items. Wear gloves.
33 Wipe off the overbed table with the paper towels. Discard the paper towels.

34 Remove the gloves. Decontaminate your hands.
35 Unscreen the person.
36 Complete a safety check of the room. (See the inside of the front book cover.)
37 Follow agency policy for dirty linen.
38 Decontaminate your hands.
39 Report nicks, cuts, irritation, or bleeding to the nurse. Also report and record other observations.

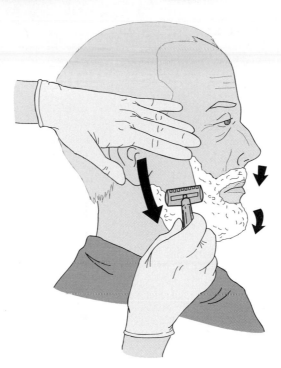

FIG. **14-5** Shave in the direction of hair growth. Use longer strokes on the larger areas of the face. Use short strokes around the chin and lips.

NAIL AND FOOT CARE

Nail and foot care prevents infection, injury, and odors. Hangnails, ingrown nails (nails that grow in at the side), and nails torn away from the skin cause skin breaks. Long or broken nails can scratch skin or snag clothing. Dirty feet, socks, or stockings harbor microbes and cause odors.

Nails are easier to trim and clean after soaking or bathing. Use nail clippers to cut fingernails. *Never use scissors.* Use extreme caution to prevent damage to nearby tissues.

Some agencies do not let nursing assistants cut or trim toenails. Follow agency policy.

DELEGATION GUIDELINES
Nail and Foot Care

Before giving nail and foot care, you need this information from the nurse and the care plan:
■ What water temperature to use
■ How long to soak fingernails (usually 5 to 10 minutes)
■ How long to soak the feet (usually 15 to 20 minutes)
■ What observations to report and record:
  ■ Reddened, irritated, or callused areas
  ■ Breaks in the skin
  ■ Corns on top of and between the toes
  ■ Very thick nails
  ■ Loose nails

PROMOTING SAFETY AND COMFORT
Nail and Foot Care

Safety

You do not cut or trim toenails if a person:

- Has diabetes
- Has poor circulation to the legs and feet
- Takes drugs that affect blood clotting
- Has very thick nails or ingrown toenails

The RN or podiatrist (foot *[pod]* doctor) cuts toenails and provides foot care for these persons.

Check between the toes for cracks and sores. These areas often are overlooked. If left untreated, a serious infection could occur.

The feet are easily burned. Persons with decreased sensation or circulatory problems may not feel hot temperatures.

After soaking, apply lotion or petrolatum jelly to the feet. This can cause slippery feet. Help the person put on non-skid footwear before you transfer the person or let the person walk.

Breaks in the skin and bleeding can occur. Follow Standard Precautions and the Bloodborne Pathogen Standard.

Comfort

Sometimes just the fingernails are trimmed. Sometimes just foot care is given. Sometimes both are done. When both are done, the person sits at the overbed table (Fig. 14-6). Make sure the person is warm and comfortable. Remember to support the foot and ankle when giving foot care.

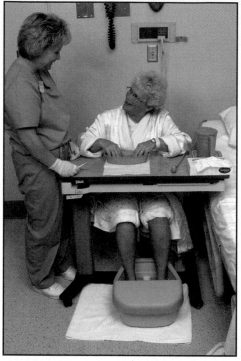

FIG. **14-6** Nail and foot care. The feet soak in a whirlpool foot bath, and the fingers soak in a kidney basin.

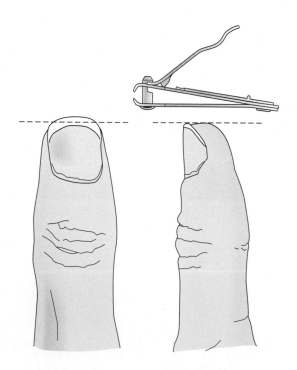

FIG. **14-7** Clip fingernails straight across. Use a nail clipper.

Giving Nail and Foot Care

Quality of Life

Remember to:

- Knock before entering the person's room
- Address the person by name
- Introduce yourself by name and title

- Explain the procedure to the person before beginning and during the procedure
- Protect the person's rights during the procedure
- Handle the person gently during the procedure

Pre-Procedure

1 Follow *Delegation Guidelines: Nail and Foot Care,* p. 243. See *Promoting Safety and Comfort: Nail and Foot Care.*
2 Practice hand hygiene.
3 Collect the following:
 - Wash basin or whirlpool foot bath
 - Soap
 - Bath thermometer
 - Bath towel
 - Hand towel
 - Washcloth
 - Kidney basin
 - Nail clippers
 - Orange stick

 - Emery board or nail file
 - Lotion for hands
 - Lotion or petrolatum jelly for feet
 - Paper towels
 - Bath mat
 - Gloves
4 Arrange paper towels and other items on the overbed table.
5 Identify the person. Check the ID bracelet against the assignment sheet. Call the person by name.
6 Provide for privacy.
7 Assist the person to the bedside chair. Place the signal light within reach.

Procedure

8 Place the bath mat under the feet.
9 Fill the wash basin or whirlpool foot bath 2/3 (two-thirds) full with water. The nurse tells you what water temperature to use. (Measure water temperature with a bath thermometer. Or test it by dipping your elbow or inner wrist into the basin. Follow agency policy.)
10 Place the basin or foot bath on the bath mat.
11 Help the person put the feet into the basin or foot bath. Make sure both feet are completely covered by water.
12 Adjust the overbed table in front of the person.
13 Fill the kidney basin 2/3 (two-thirds) full with water. See step 9 for water temperature.
14 Place the kidney basin on the overbed table.
15 Place the person's fingers into the basin. Position the arms for comfort (see Fig. 14-6).
16 Let the fingers soak for 5 to 10 minutes. Let the feet soak for 15 to 20 minutes. Rewarm water as needed.
17 Decontaminate your hands. Put on gloves.
18 Remove the kidney basin.
19 Clean under the fingernails with the orange stick. Use a towel to wipe the orange stick after each nail.

20 Dry the hands and between the fingers.
21 Clip fingernails straight across with the nail clippers (Fig. 14-7).
22 Shape nails with an emery board or nail file. Nails are smooth with no rough edges.
23 Push cuticles back with the orange stick or a washcloth (Fig. 14-8, p. 246).
24 Apply lotion to the hands. Warm lotion before applying it.
25 Move the overbed table to the side.
26 Wash the feet and between the toes with soap and a washcloth. Rinse the feet and between the toes.
27 Remove the feet from the basin or foot bath. Dry thoroughly, especially between the toes.
28 Apply lotion or petrolatum jelly to the tops and soles of the feet. Do not apply between the toes. Warm lotion before applying it. Remove excess lotion with a towel.
29 Remove and discard the gloves. Decontaminate your hands.
30 Help the person put on non-skid footwear.

Continued

Giving Nail and Foot Care—cont'd

NNAAP™

Post-Procedure

31 Provide for comfort. (See the inside of the front book cover.)
32 Place the signal light within reach.
33 Raise or lower bed rails. Follow the care plan.
34 Clean and return equipment and supplies to their proper place. Discard disposable items. Wear gloves for this step.

35 Remove the gloves. Decontaminate your hands.
36 Unscreen the person.
37 Complete a safety check of the room. (See the inside of the front book cover.)
38 Follow agency policy for dirty linen.
39 Decontaminate your hands.
40 Report and record your observations.

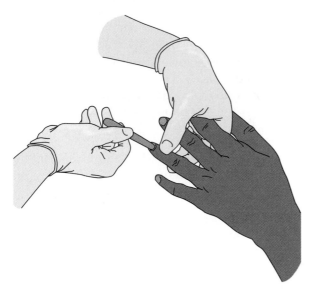

FIG. **14-8** Push the cuticle back with an orange stick.

CHANGING GOWNS AND CLOTHING

Patients and residents need to change clothes and sleepwear in the morning and at bedtime. Garments are changed whenever wet or soiled. When changing gowns or clothing, follow these rules.

- Provide for privacy. Do not expose the person.
- Encourage the person to do as much as possible.
- Let the person choose what to wear. Make sure the right undergarments are chosen.
- Remove clothing from the strong or "good" side first. This is often called the "unaffected" side.
- Put clothing on the weak side first. This is often called the "affected" side.
- Support the arm or leg when removing or putting on a garment.

DELEGATION GUIDELINES
Changing Gowns

Before changing a gown, you need this information from the nurse and the care plan:
- Which arm has the IV
- If the person has an IV pump (see *Promoting Safety and Comfort: Changing gowns.*)

PROMOTING SAFETY AND COMFORT
Changing Gowns

Safety

IV pumps control how fast fluid enters a vein. This is called the *flow rate*. If the person has an IV pump and a standard gown, do not use the following procedure. The arm with the IV is not put through the sleeve.

Changing an IV gown can cause the flow rate to change. Always ask the nurse to check the flow rate after you change a gown.

Do not disconnect or remove any part of the IV set-up. See Chapter 17.

Comfort

Some patient gowns are secured with ties at the upper back. The back and buttocks are exposed when the person stands. Other gowns overlap in the back and tie at the side. These gowns provide more privacy. Because they tie at the side, uncomfortable bows and knots at the back are avoided.

Changing Gowns

Many patients wear gowns. So do some residents. If there is injury or paralysis, the gown is removed from the strong arm first. Support the weak arm while removing the gown. Put the clean gown on the weak arm first and then on the strong arm.

Some agencies have special gowns for IV therapy. They open along the sleeve and close with ties, snaps, or Velcro. Sometimes standard gowns are used.

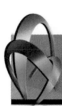

Changing the Gown of the Person With an IV

Quality of Life

Remember to:

- Knock before entering the person's room
- Address the person by name
- Introduce yourself by name and title
- Explain the procedure to the person before beginning and during the procedure
- Protect the person's rights during the procedure
- Handle the person gently during the procedure

Pre-Procedure

1 Follow *Delegation Guidelines: Changing Gowns.* See *Promoting Safety and Comfort: Changing Gowns.*
2 Practice hand hygiene.
3 Get a clean gown and a bath blanket.

4 Identify the person. Check the ID bracelet against the assignment sheet. Call the person by name.
5 Provide for privacy.
6 Raise the bed for body mechanics. Bed rails are up if used.

Procedure

7 Lower the bed rail near you (if up).
8 Cover the person with a bath blanket. Fan-fold linens to the foot of the bed.
9 Untie the gown. Free parts that the person is lying on.
10 Remove the gown from the arm with *no IV.*
11 Gather up the sleeve of the arm *with the IV.* Slide it over the IV site and tubing. Remove the arm and hand from the sleeve (Fig. 14-9, *A,* p. 248).
12 Keep the sleeve gathered. Slide your arm along the tubing to the bag (Fig. 14-9, *B,* p. 248).
13 Remove the bag from the pole. Slide the bag and tubing through the sleeve (Fig. 14-9, *C,* p. 248).

Do not pull on the tubing. Keep the bag above the person.
14 Hang the IV bag on the pole.
15 Gather the sleeve of the clean gown that will go on the arm with the IV infusion.
16 Remove the bag from the pole. Slip the sleeve over the bag at the shoulder part of the gown (Fig. 14-9, *D,* p. 248). Hang the bag.
17 Slide the gathered sleeve over the tubing, hand, arm, and IV site. Then slide it onto the shoulder.
18 Put the other side of the gown on the person. Fasten the gown.
19 Cover the person. Remove the bath blanket.

Post-Procedure

20 Provide for comfort. (See the inside of the front book cover.)
21 Place the signal light within reach.
22 Lower the bed to its lowest position.
23 Raise or lower bed rails. Follow the care plan.
24 Unscreen the person.

25 Complete a safety check of the room. (See the inside of the front book cover.)
26 Follow agency policy for dirty linen.
27 Decontaminate your hands.
28 Ask the nurse to check the flow rate.
29 Report and record your observations.

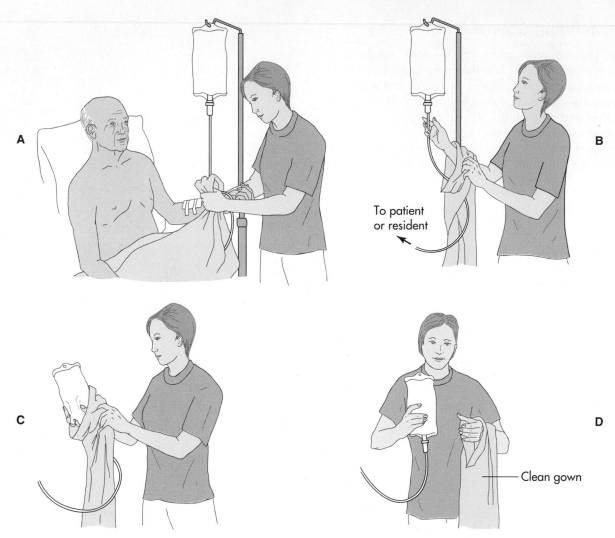

FIG. **14-9** Changing a gown. **A,** The gown is removed from the arm with no IV. The sleeve on the arm with the IV is gathered up, slipped over the IV site and tubing, and removed from the arm and hand. **B,** The gathered sleeve is slipped along the IV tubing to the bag. **C,** The IV bag is removed from the pole and passed through the sleeve. **D,** The gathered sleeve of the clean gown is slipped over the IV bag at the shoulder part of the gown.

Dressing and Undressing

Clothing changes are often necessary on admission and discharge. Some people enter and leave the agency in a gown or pajamas. Most wear street clothes. Most residents wear street clothes during the day. Some dress and undress themselves. Others need help. Personal choice is a resident right. Let the person choose what to wear. Follow the rules on p. 246 for dressing and undressing.

Text continued on p. 255

DELEGATION GUIDELINES
Dressing and Undressing

Before changing clothing, you need this information from the nurse and the care plan:
- How much help the person needs
- Which side is the person's strong side
- If the person needs to wear certain garments
- What observations to report and record:
  - How much help was given
  - How the person tolerated the procedure
  - Any complaints by the person

Undressing the Person

Quality of Life

Remember to:

- Knock before entering the person's room
- Address the person by name
- Introduce yourself by name and title

- Explain the procedure to the person before beginning and during the procedure
- Protect the person's rights during the procedure
- Handle the person gently during the procedure

Pre-Procedure

1 Follow *Delegation Guidelines: Dressing and Undressing.*
2 Practice hand hygiene.
3 Collect a bath blanket and clothing requested by the person.
4 Identify the person. Check the ID bracelet against the assignment sheet. Call the person by name.

5 Provide for privacy.
6 Raise the bed for body mechanics. Bed rails are up if used.
7 Lower the bed rail on the person's weak side.
8 Position him or her supine.
9 Cover the person with the bath blanket. Fan-fold linens to the foot of the bed.

Procedure

10 Remove garments that open in the back.
  a Raise the head and shoulders. Or turn him or her onto the side away from you.
  b Undo buttons, zippers, ties, or snaps.
  c Bring the sides of the garment to the sides of the person (Fig. 14-10, p. 250). If he or she is in a side-lying position, tuck the far side under the person. Fold the near side onto the chest (Fig. 14-11, p. 250).
  d Position the person supine.
  e Slide the garment off the shoulder on the strong side. Remove it from the arm (Fig. 14-12, p. 250).
  f Repeat step 10e for the weak side.
11 Remove garments that open in the front.
  a Undo buttons, zippers, ties, or snaps.
  b Slide the garment off the shoulder and arm on the strong side.
  c Assist the person to sit up or raise the head and shoulders. Bring the garment over to the weak side (Fig. 14-13, p. 251).
  d Lower the head and shoulders. Remove the garment from the weak side.
  e If you cannot raise the head and shoulders:
    (1) Turn the person toward you. Tuck the removed part under the person.
    (2) Turn him or her onto the side away from you.
    (3) Pull the side of the garment out from under the person. Make sure he or she will not lie on it when supine.
    (4) Return the person to the supine position.
    (5) Remove the garment from the weak side.

12 Remove pullover garments.
  a Undo any buttons, zippers, ties, or snaps.
  b Remove the garment from the strong side.
  c Raise the head and shoulders. Or turn the person onto the side away from you. Bring the garment up to the person's neck (Fig. 14-14, p. 251).
  d Remove the garment from the weak side.
  e Bring the garment over the person's head.
  f Position him or her in the supine position.
13 Remove pants or slacks.
  a Remove footwear.
  b Position the person supine.
  c Undo buttons, zippers, ties, snaps, or buckles.
  d Remove the belt.
  e Ask the person to lift the buttocks off the bed. Slide the pants down over the hips and buttocks (Fig. 14-15, p. 251). Have the person lower the hips and buttocks.
  f If the person cannot raise the hips off the bed:
    (1) Turn the person toward you.
    (2) Slide the pants off the hip and buttock on the strong side (Fig. 14-16, p. 252).
    (3) Turn the person away from you.
    (4) Slide the pants off the hip and buttock on the weak side (Fig. 14-17, p. 252).
  g Slide the pants down the legs and over the feet.
14 Dress the person. See procedure: *Dressing the Person,* p. 253.

Continued

Undressing the Person—cont'd

Post-Procedure

15 Provide for comfort. (See the inside of the front book cover.)
16 Place the signal light within reach.
17 Lower the bed to its lowest position.
18 Raise or lower bed rails. Follow the care plan.
19 Unscreen the person.

20 Complete a safety check of the room. (See the inside of the front book cover.)
21 Follow agency policy for soiled clothing.
22 Decontaminate your hands.
23 Report and record your observations.

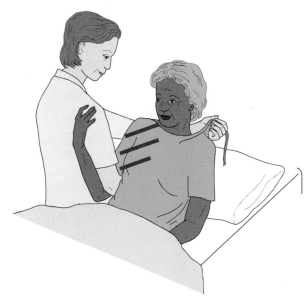

FIG. **14-10** The sides of the garment are brought from the back to the sides of the person. (Note: The "weak" side is *indicated by slash marks*.)

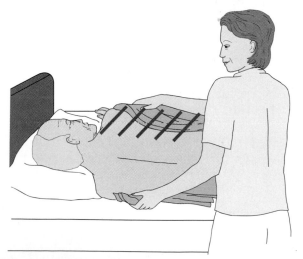

FIG. **14-11** A garment that opens in back is removed from the person in the side-lying position. The far side of the garment is tucked under the person. The near side is folded onto the person's chest. (Note: The "weak" side is *indicated by slash marks*.)

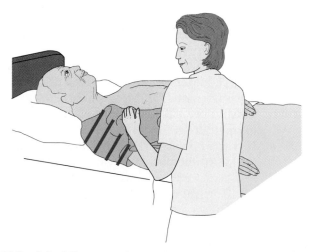

FIG. **14-12** The garment is removed from the strong side first.

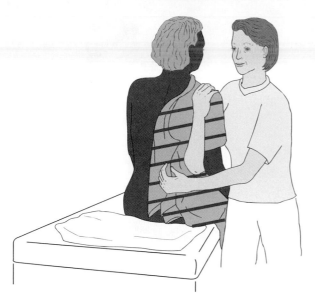

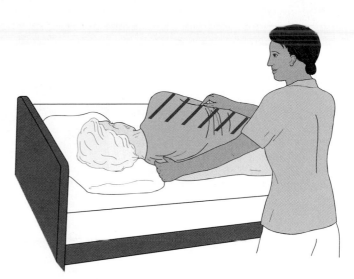

FIG. **14-13** A front-opening garment is removed with the person's head and shoulders raised. The garment is removed from the strong side first. Then it is brought around the back to the weak side. (Note: The "weak" side is *indicated by slash marks*.)

FIG. **14-14** A pullover garment is removed from the strong side first. Then the garment is brought up to the person's neck so that it can be removed from the weak side. (Note: The "weak" side is *indicated by slash marks*.)

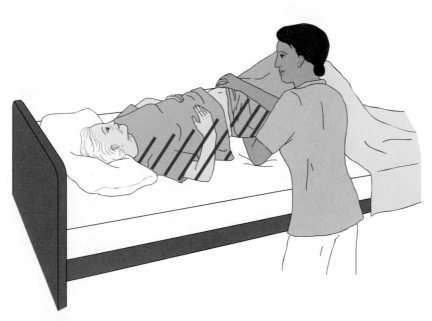

FIG. **14-15** The person lifts the hips and buttocks for removing the pants. The pants are slid down over the hips and buttocks. (Note: The "weak" side is *indicated by slash marks*.)

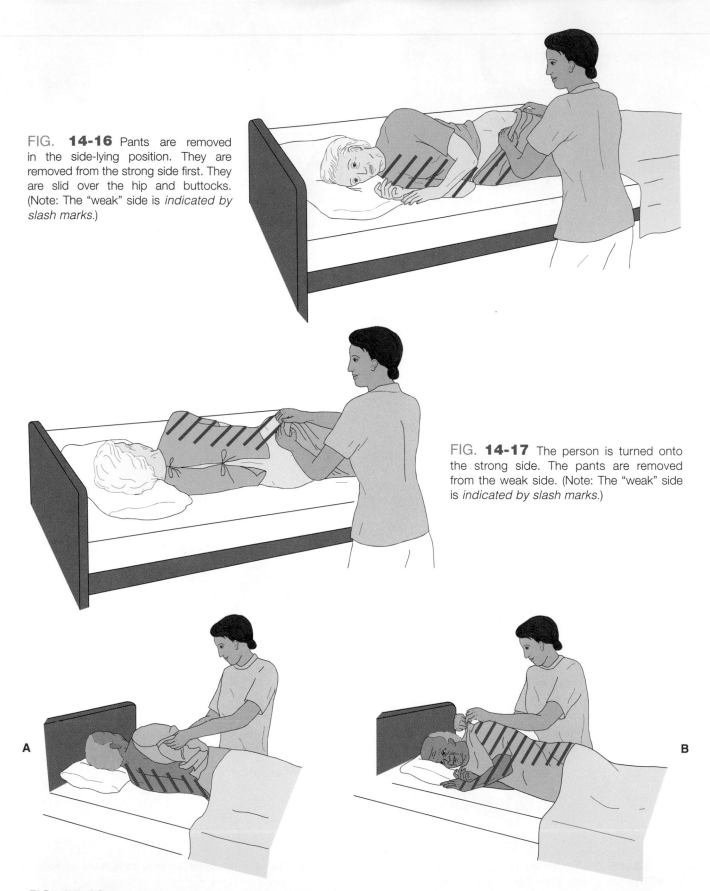

FIG. **14-16** Pants are removed in the side-lying position. They are removed from the strong side first. They are slid over the hip and buttocks. (Note: The "weak" side is *indicated by slash marks*.)

FIG. **14-17** The person is turned onto the strong side. The pants are removed from the weak side. (Note: The "weak" side is *indicated by slash marks*.)

FIG. **14-18** Dressing a person. **A,** The side-lying position can be used to put on garments that open in the back. Turn the person toward you after the garment is put on the arms. The side of the garment is brought to the person's back. **B,** Then turn the person away from you. The other side of the garment is brought to the back and fastened. (Note: The "weak" side is *indicated by slash marks*.)

Dressing the Person

Quality of Life

Remember to:

- Knock before entering the person's room
- Address the person by name
- Introduce yourself by name and title
- Explain the procedure to the person before beginning and during the procedure
- Protect the person's rights during the procedure
- Handle the person gently during the procedure

Pre-Procedure

1 Follow *Delegation Guidelines: Dressing and Undressing,* p. 248.
2 Practice hand hygiene.
3 Ask the person what he or she would like to wear.
4 Get a bath blanket and clothing requested by the person.
5 Identify the person. Check the ID bracelet against the assignment sheet. Call the person by name.
6 Provide for privacy.
7 Raise the bed for body mechanics. Bed rails are up if used.
8 Lower the bed rail (if up) on the person's strong side.
9 Position the person supine.
10 Cover the person with the bath blanket. Fan-fold linens to the foot of the bed.
11 Undress the person. (See procedure: *Undressing the Person,* p. 249).

Procedure

12 Put on garments that open in the back.
  a Slide the garment onto the arm and shoulder of the weak side.
  b Slide the garment onto the arm and shoulder of the strong side.
  c Raise the person's head and shoulders.
  d Bring the sides to the back.
  e If the person cannot raise the head and shoulders:
    (1) Turn the person toward you.
    (2) Bring one side of the garment to the person's back (Fig. 14-18, *A*).
    (3) Turn the person away from you.
    (4) Bring the other side to the person's back (Fig. 14-18, *B*).
  f Fasten buttons, ties, snaps, or zippers.
  g Position the person supine.
13 Put on garments that open in the front.
  a Slide the garment onto the arm and shoulder on the weak side.
  b Raise the head and shoulders. Bring the side of the garment around to the back. Lower the person down. Slide the garment onto the arm and shoulder of the strong arm.
  c If the person cannot raise the head and shoulders:
    (1) Turn the person away from you.
    (2) Tuck the garment under him or her.
    (3) Turn the person toward you.
    (4) Pull the garment out from under him or her.
    (5) Turn the person back to the supine position.
    (6) Slide the garment over the arm and shoulder of the strong arm.
  d Fasten buttons, ties, snaps, or zippers.
14 Put on pullover garments.
  a Position the person supine.
  b Bring the neck of the garment over the head.
  c Slide the arm and shoulder of the garment onto the weak side.
  d Raise the person's head and shoulders.
  e Bring the garment down.
  f Slide the arm and shoulder of the garment onto the strong side.
  g If the person cannot assume a semi-sitting position:
    (1) Turn the person away from you.
    (2) Tuck the garment under the person.
    (3) Turn the person toward you.
    (4) Pull the garment out from under him or her.
    (5) Position the person supine.
    (6) Slide the arm and shoulder of the garment onto the strong side.
  h Fasten buttons, ties, snaps, or zippers.
15 Put on pants or slacks.
  a Slide the pants over the feet and up the legs.
  b Ask the person to raise the hips and buttocks off the bed.

Continued

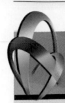

Dressing the Person—cont'd

Procedure—cont'd

c Bring the pants up over the hips and buttocks.

d Ask the person to lower the hips and buttocks.

e If the person cannot raise the hips and buttocks:

(1) Turn the person onto the strong side (away from you).

(2) Pull the pants over the hips and buttock on the weak side.

(3) Turn the person onto the weak side (toward you).

(4) Pull the pants over the hips and buttock on the strong side.

(5) Position the person supine.

f Fasten buttons, ties, snaps, the zipper, and the belt buckle.

16 Put socks and non-skid footwear on the person.

17 Help the person get out of bed. If the person will stay in bed. Cover the person. Remove the bath blanket.

Post-Procedure

18 Provide for comfort. (See the inside of the front book cover.)

19 Place the signal light within reach.

20 Lower the bed to its lowest position.

21 Raise or lower bed rails. Follow the care plan.

22 Unscreen the person.

23 Complete a safety check of the room. (See the inside of the front book cover.)

24 Follow agency policy for soiled clothing.

25 Decontaminate your hands.

26 Report and record your observations.

Focus on the PERSON

Assisting With Grooming

Providing comfort—Grooming measures promote physical comfort. They also promote mental comfort. Self-esteem and body image improve when the person likes how he or she looks. Therefore, follow the person's grooming routines. For example, style hair as the person prefers.

Ethical behavior—You may not like the person's hairstyle or clothing choices. Or you may not agree with the person's choice in personal care products. Do not judge the person by your own standards. Do not impose your choices, standards, or values on the person.

Remaining independent—Promote personal choice whenever possible. This lets the person have some control over grooming measures and clothing choices. As with hygiene, encourage the person to do as much for himself or herself as safely possible.

Speaking up—Make sure that you follow the person's grooming choices. Also make sure that you meet the person's grooming needs. You can ask:

■ "Do you want your hair brushed or combed?"

■ "Do you use hair conditioner?"

■ "Is this hair dryer too hot?"

■ "How does the whirlpool bath feel?" "Is the water too hot or too cool?"

■ "What would you like to wear today?"

■ "Would you like me to help you with those buttons?"

■ "Can I help you with that zipper?"

OBRA and other laws—OBRA requires that the person receive courteous and dignified care. You need to:

■ Groom hair, beards, and nails as the person wishes

■ Assist with dressing in the right clothing for the time of day

■ Assist with grooming measures for:

  ■ A neat and clean appearance

  ■ A clean-shaven face or a groomed beard

  ■ Clean and trimmed nails

  ■ Properly fastened clothing and shoes

Nursing teamwork—Shampoo trays, electric shavers, and whirlpool foot baths are shared among patients and residents. Let other team members know when you need to use an item. After the procedure, clean and promptly return the item to its proper place. A co-worker should not have to clean or look for an item after you use it.

FOCUS ON THE PERSON

People want to look good to others. Clean hair, nails, and clothes help mental well-being. So does a clean-shaven face or a well-groomed beard or mustache. *See Focus on the Person: Assisting With Grooming.*

REVIEW QUESTIONS

Circle the **BEST** answer.

1 A person has *alopecia*. This is
   a Excessive body hair
   b Dry, white flakes from the scalp
   c An infestation of lice
   d Hair loss

2 Which prevents hair from matting and tangling?
   a Bedrest
   b Daily brushing and combing
   c Daily shampooing
   d Cutting hair

3 A person's hair is *not* matted or tangled. When brushing the hair, start at
   a The forehead
   b The hair ends
   c The scalp
   d The back of the neck

4 Brushing keeps the hair
   a Soft and shiny
   b Clean
   c Free of lice
   d Long

5 Mr. Lee wants his hair washed. You should
   a Wash his hair during his shower
   b Wash his hair at the sink
   c Shampoo him in bed
   d Follow the care plan

6 When shaving Mr. Lee, do the following *except*
   a Practice Standard Precautions
   b Follow the Bloodborne Pathogen Standard
   c Shave in the direction of hair growth
   d Shave when the skin is dry

7 Mr. Lee is nicked during shaving. Your first action is to
   a Wash your hands
   b Apply direct pressure
   c Tell the nurse
   d Use an electric razor

8 Fingernails are cut with
   a An emery board
   b Scissors
   c A nail file
   d Nail clippers

9 Fingernails are trimmed
   a Before soaking
   b After soaking
   c Before trimming toenails
   d After trimming toenails

Circle **T** if the statement is true and **F** if it is false.

10 **T F** Mr. Lee has a mustache and beard. You think he would be more comfortable without facial hair. You can shave his beard and mustache.
11 **T F** Mr. Lee has poor circulation in his legs and feet. You can cut and trim his toenails.
12 **T F** Clothing is removed from the strong side first.
13 **T F** The person chooses what to wear.
14 **T F** You can cut matted hair.

The answers to these questions are on p. 468.

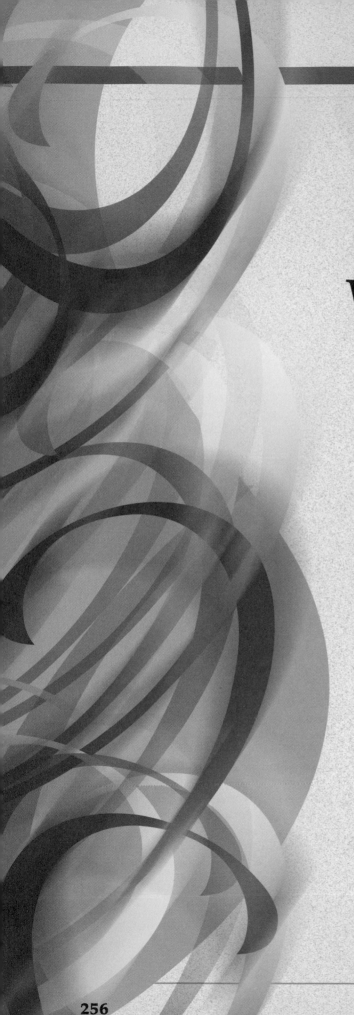

15

Assisting With Urinary Elimination

Objectives

- Define the key terms listed in this chapter
- Describe normal urine
- Describe the rules for normal urination
- Describe urinary incontinence and the care required
- Explain why catheters are used
- Explain how to care for persons with catheters
- Describe two methods of bladder training
- Perform the procedures described in this chapter

Procedures

Procedures with this icon ❀ *are also on the CD-ROM in this book.*

❀ Giving the Bedpan
- Giving the Urinal
- Helping the Person to the Commode
❀ Giving Catheter Care
- Emptying a Urinary Drainage Bag
- Applying a Condom Catheter

KEY TERMS

catheter A tube used to drain or inject fluid through a body opening

dysuria Painful or difficult *(dys)* urination *(uria)*

functional incontinence The person has bladder control but cannot use the toilet in time

hematuria Blood *(hemat)* in the urine *(uria)*

nocturia Frequent urination *(uria)* at night *(noct)*

oliguria Scant amount *(olig)* of urine *(uria)*; less than 500 ml in 24 hours

overflow incontinence Urine leaks when the bladder is too full

polyuria Abnormally large amounts *(poly)* of urine *(uria)*

reflex incontinence The loss of urine at predictable intervals when the bladder is full

stress incontinence When urine leaks during exercise and certain movements

urge incontinence Urine is lost in response to a sudden, urgent need to void; the person cannot get to a toilet in time

urinary frequency Voiding at frequent intervals

urinary incontinence The loss of bladder control

urinary urgency The need to void at once

urination The process of emptying urine from the bladder; voiding

voiding Urination

Eliminating waste is a physical need. The urinary system removes waste products from the blood. It also maintains the body's water balance.

NORMAL URINATION

The healthy adult produces about 1500 ml (milliliters) (3 pints) of urine a day. Many factors affect urine production. They include age, disease, the amount and kinds of fluid ingested, dietary salt, and drugs. Some substances increase urine production: coffee, tea, alcohol, and some drugs. A diet high in salt causes the body to retain water. When water is retained, less urine is produced.

Urination (voiding) mean the process of emptying urine from the bladder. The amount of fluid intake, habits, and available toilet facilities affect frequency. So do activity, work, and illness. People usually void at bedtime, after getting up, and before meals. Some people void every 2 to 3 hours.

Some persons need help getting to the bathroom. Others use bedpans, urinals, or commodes. Follow the rules in Box 15-1 and the person's care plan.

BOX 15-1	Rules For Normal Elimination

- Practice medical asepsis.
- Follow Standard Precautions and the Bloodborne Pathogen Standard.
- Provide fluids as the nurse and care plan direct.
- Follow the person's voiding routines and habits. Check with the nurse and the care plan.
- Help the person to the bathroom when the request is made. Or provide the commode, bedpan, or urinal. The need to void may be urgent.
- Help the person assume a normal position for voiding if possible. Women sit or squat. Men stand.
- Warm the bedpan or urinal.
- Cover the person for warmth and privacy.
- Provide for privacy. Pull the curtain around the bed and close room and bathroom doors. Also close drapes, blinds, or window shades. Leave the room if the person can be alone.
- Tell the person that running water, flushing the toilet, or playing music can mask voiding sounds. Voiding with others close by embarrasses some people.
- Stay nearby if the person is weak or unsteady.
- Place the signal light and toilet tissue within reach.
- Allow enough time to void. Do not rush the person.
- Promote relaxation. Some people like to read.
- Run water in a sink if the person cannot start the stream. Or place the person's fingers in warm water.
- Provide perineal care as needed (Chapter 13).
- Assist with hand washing after voiding. Provide a wash basin, soap, washcloth, and towel.
- Assist the person to the bathroom or offer the bedpan, urinal, or commode at regular times. Some people are embarrassed or are too weak to ask for help.

Observations

Normal urine is pale yellow, straw-colored, or amber. It is clear with no particles. A faint odor is normal. Observe urine for color, clarity, odor, amount, and particles.

Ask the nurse to observe urine that looks or smells abnormal. Report these problems:

- **Dysuria**—painful or difficult *(dys)* urination *(uria)*
- **Hematuria**—blood *(hemat)* in the urine *(uria)*
- **Nocturia**—frequent urination *(uria)* at night *(noct)*
- **Oliguria**—scant amount *(olig)* of urine *(uria)*, less than 500 ml in 24 hours
- **Polyuria**—abnormally large amounts *(poly)* of urine *(uria)*
- **Urinary frequency**—voiding at frequent intervals
- **Urinary incontinence**—the loss of bladder control
- **Urinary urgency**—the need to void at once

Bedpans

Bedpans are used by persons who cannot be out of bed. Women use bedpans for voiding and bowel movements. Men use them only for bowel movements.

A *fracture pan* has a thin rim. It is only about ½-inch deep at one end (Fig. 15-1). The smaller end is placed under the buttocks (Fig. 15-2). Fracture pans are used:

- By persons with casts or in traction
- By persons with limited back motion
- After spinal cord injury or surgery
- After a hip fracture or hip replacement surgery

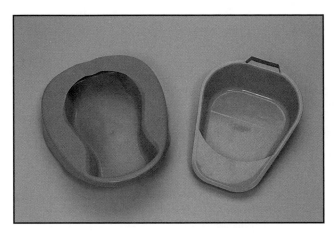

FIG. **15-1** Standard bedpan *(left)* and the fracture pan *(right)*.

DELEGATION GUIDELINES
Bedpans

Before assisting with a bedpan, you need this information from the nurse and care plan:

- What bedpan to use—standard bedpan or fracture pan
- Position or activity limits
- If the person can be left alone.
- If the nurse needs to observe the results before disposing of the contents
- What observations to report and record:
  - Urine color, clarity, and odor
  - Amount
  - Presence of particles
  - Complaints of urgency, burning, dysuria, or other problems
  - For bowel movements, see Chapter 16

PROMOTING SAFETY AND COMFORT
Bedpans

Safety

Urine and bowel movements may contain blood and microbes. Microbes can live and grow in dirty bedpans. Follow Standard Precautions and the Bloodborne Pathogen Standard when handling bedpans and their contents. Thoroughly clean and disinfect bedpans after use.

Comfort

Some older persons have fragile bones from osteoporosis or painful joints from arthritis (Chapter 24). Fracture pans provide more comfort for them than standard bedpans.

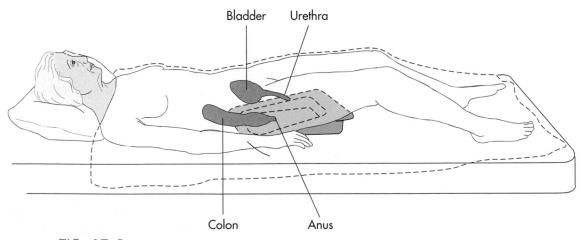

Bladder   Urethra

Colon   Anus

FIG. **15-2** A person positioned on a fracture pan. The small end is under the buttocks.

Giving the Bedpan

Quality of Life

Remember to:

- Knock before entering the person's room
- Address the person by name
- Introduce yourself by name and title

- Explain the procedure to the person before beginning and during the procedure
- Protect the person's rights during the procedure
- Handle the person gently during the procedure

Pre-Procedure

1 Follow *Delegation Guidelines: Bedpans.* See *Promoting Safety and Comfort: Bedpans.*
2 Provide for privacy.
3 Practice hand hygiene.
4 Put on gloves.

5 Collect the following:
  - Bedpan
  - Bedpan cover
  - Toilet tissue
  - Waterproof pad (if required by the agency)
6 Arrange equipment on the chair or bed.

Procedure

7 Warm and dry the bedpan if necessary.
8 Lower the bed rail near you if up.
9 Position the person supine. Raise the head of the bed slightly.
10 Fold the top linens and gown out of the way. Keep the lower body covered.
11 Ask the person to flex the knees and raise the buttocks by pushing against the mattress with his or her feet.
12 Slide your hand under the lower back. Help raise the buttocks. If using a waterproof pad, place it under the buttocks.
13 Slide the bedpan under the person (Fig. 15-3, p. 260).
14 If the person cannot assist in getting on the bedpan:
  a Place the waterproof pad under the buttocks if using one.
  b Turn the person onto the side away from you.
  c Place the bedpan firmly against the buttocks (Fig. 15-4, *A*, p. 261).
  d Push the bedpan down and toward the person (Fig. 15-4, *B*, p. 261).
  e Hold the bedpan securely. Turn the person onto the back.
  f Make sure the bedpan is centered under the person.
15 Cover the person.
16 Raise the head of the bed so the person is in a sitting position.
17 Make sure the person is correctly positioned on the bedpan (Fig. 15-5, p. 261).
18 Raise the bed rail if used.
19 Place the toilet tissue and signal light within reach.

20 Ask the person to signal when done or when help is needed.
21 Remove the gloves. Decontaminate your hands.
22 Leave the room, and close the door.
23 Return when the person signals. Or check on the person every 5 minutes. Knock before entering.
24 Decontaminate your hands. Put on gloves.
25 Raise the bed for body mechanics. Lower the bed rail (if used) and the head of the bed.
26 Ask the person to raise the buttocks. Remove the bedpan. Or hold the bedpan and turn him or her onto the side away from you.
27 Clean the genital area if the person cannot do so. Clean from front (urethra) to back (anus) with toilet tissue. Use fresh tissue for each wipe. Provide perineal care if needed. Remove and discard the waterproof pad if using one.
28 Cover the bedpan. Take it to the bathroom. Raise the bed rail (if used) before leaving the bedside.
29 Note the color, amount, and character of urine or feces.
30 Empty the bedpan contents into the toilet and flush.
31 Rinse the bedpan. Pour the rinse into the toilet and flush.
32 Clean the bedpan with a disinfectant.
33 Remove soiled gloves. Practice hand hygiene, and put on clean gloves.
34 Return the bedpan and clean cover to the bedside stand.
35 Help the person with hand washing.
36 Remove the gloves. Decontaminate your hands.

Continued

NNAAP™

Giving the Bedpan—cont'd

Post-Procedure

37 Provide for comfort. (See the inside of the front book cover.)

38 Place the signal light within reach.

39 Lower the bed to its lowest position.

40 Raise or lower bed rails. Follow the care plan.

41 Unscreen the person.

42 Complete a safety check of the room. (See the inside of the front book cover.)

43 Follow agency policy for soiled linen.

44 Decontaminate your hands.

45 Report and record your observations.

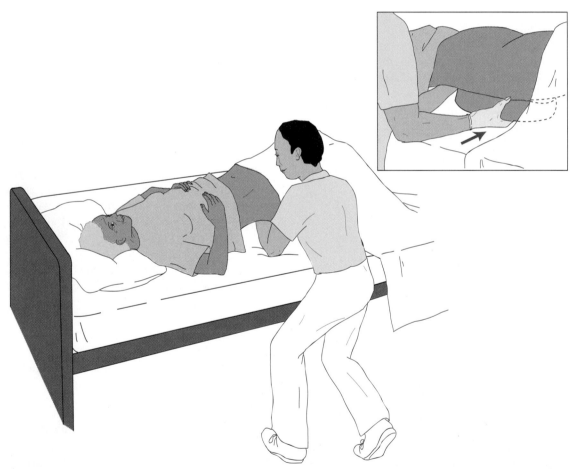

FIG. **15-3** The person raises the buttocks off the bed with help. The bedpan is slid under the person.

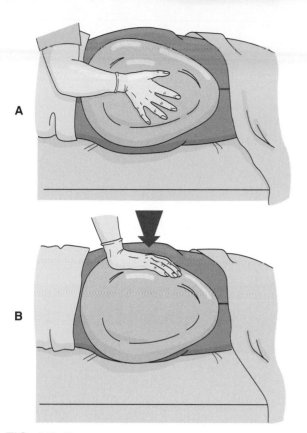

FIG. **15-4** Giving a bedpan. **A,** Position the person on one side. Place the bedpan firmly against the buttocks. **B,** Push downward on the bedpan and toward the person.

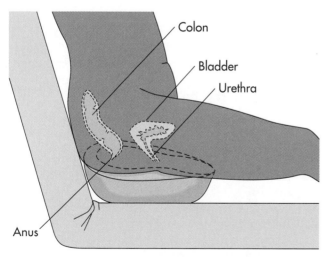

FIG. **15-5** The person is positioned on the bedpan so the urethra and anus are directly over the opening.

Urinals

Men use urinals to void (Fig. 15-6). Urinals have caps and hook-type handles. The urinal hooks to the bed rail within the man's reach. He stands to use the urinal if possible. Or he sits on the side of the bed or lies in bed to use it. Some men need support when standing. You may have to place and hold the urinal for some men.

After voiding, the cap is closed. This prevents urine spills. Remind men to hang urinals on bed rails and to signal after using them. Remind them not to place urinals on overbed tables and bedside stands. Some agencies do not use bed rails. Follow agency policy for where to place urinals.

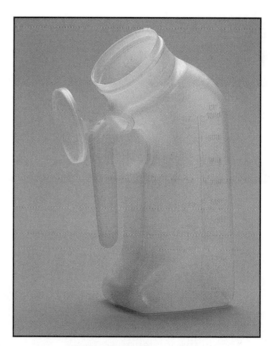

FIG. **15-6** Male urinal.

DELEGATION GUIDELINES
Urinals

Before assisting with urinals, you need this information from the nurse and care plan:
- How the urinal is used—standing, sitting, or lying in bed
- If help is needed with placing or holding the urinal
- If the man needs support to stand (If yes, how many staff members are needed.)
- If you can leave the room or if you need to stay with the person.
- If the nurse needs to observe the urine before its disposal
- What observations to report and record (see *Delegation Guidelines: Bedpans,* p. 258)

Safety

Follow Standard Precautions and the Bloodborne Pathogen Standard when handling urinals and their contents. Empty them promptly to prevent odors and the spread of microbes. A filled urinal spills easily causing safety hazards. Also, it is an unpleasant site and a source of odor. Urinals are cleaned and disinfected like bedpans.

Comfort

You may have to place the urinal for some men. This means that you need to place the penis in the urinal. This may embarrass both you and the person. Act in a professional manner at all times.

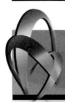

Giving the Urinal

Quality of Life

Remember to:

- Knock before entering the person's room
- Address the person by name
- Introduce yourself by name and title

- Explain the procedure to the person before beginning and during the procedure
- Protect the person's rights during the procedure
- Handle the person gently during the procedure

Pre-Procedure

1 Follow *Delegation Guidelines: Urinals*, p. 261. See *Promoting Safety and Comfort: Urinals*.
2 Provide for privacy.
3 Determine if the man will stand, sit, or lie in bed.
4 Practice hand hygiene.
5 Put on gloves.

Procedure

6 Give him the urinal if he is in bed. Remind him to tilt the bottom down to prevent spills.
7 If he is going to stand:
  a Help him sit on the side of the bed.
  b Put non-skid footwear on him.
  c Help him stand. Provide support if he is unsteady.
  d Give him the urinal.
8 Position the urinal if necessary. Position his penis in the urinal if he cannot do so.
9 Place the signal light within reach. Or check on him every 5 minutes. Ask him to signal when done or when he needs help.
10 Provide for privacy.
11 Remove the gloves. Decontaminate your hands.
12 Leave the room, and close the door.

13 Return when he signals for you. Or check on the person every 5 minutes. Knock before entering.
14 Decontaminate your hands. Put on gloves.
15 Close the cap on the urinal. Take it to the bathroom.
16 Note the color, amount, and character of the urine.
17 Empty the urinal into the toilet and flush.
18 Rinse the urinal with cold water. Pour the rinse into the toilet and flush.
19 Clean the urinal with a disinfectant.
20 Return the urinal to its proper place.
21 Remove soiled gloves. Practice hand hygiene, and put on clean gloves.
22 Assist with hand washing.
23 Remove the gloves. Decontaminate your hands.

Post-Procedure

24 Provide for comfort. (See the inside of the front book cover.)
25 Place the signal light within reach.
26 Raise or lower bed rails. Follow the care plan.
27 Unscreen him.

28 Complete a safety check of the room. (See the inside of the front book cover.)
29 Follow agency policy for soiled linen.
30 Decontaminate your hands.
31 Report and record your observations.

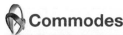 Commodes

A commode is a chair or wheelchair with an opening for a bedpan or container (Fig. 15-7). Persons unable to walk to the bathroom often use commodes. The commode allows a normal position for elimination. Some commodes are wheeled into bathrooms and placed over toilets. The container is removed if the commode is used with the toilet.

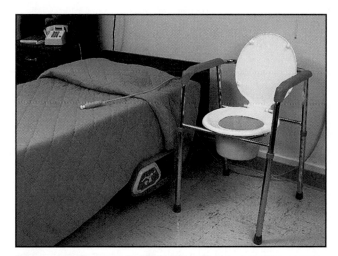

FIG. **15-7** The commode has a toilet seat with a container. The container slides out from under the seat for emptying.

DELEGATION GUIDELINES
Commodes

You need this information from the nurse and care plan when assisting with commodes:

- Is the commode used at the bedside or over the toilet
- How much help the person needs
- If the person can be left alone
- If the nurse needs to observe urine or bowel movements
- What observations to report and record (see *Delegation Guidelines: Bedpans*, p. 258)

PROMOTING SAFETY AND COMFORT
Commodes

Safety

For commode use, transfer the person to or from bed or a chair or wheelchair. Practice safe transfer procedures (Chapter 11). Use the transfer belt.

Urine and feces may contain blood and microbes. Follow Standard Precautions and the Bloodborne Pathogen Standard. Thoroughly clean and disinfect the commode container after use.

Comfort

After the person transfers to the commode, cover his or her lap and legs with a bath blanket. This provides warmth and promotes privacy.

Helping the Person to the Commode

Quality of Life

Remember to:

- Knock before entering the person's room
- Address the person by name
- Introduce yourself by name and title

- Explain the procedure to the person before beginning and during the procedure
- Protect the person's rights during the procedure
- Handle the person gently during the procedure

Pre-Procedure

1 Follow *Delegation Guidelines: Commodes*. See *Promoting Safety and Comfort: Commodes*.
2 Provide for privacy.
3 Practice hand hygiene.
4 Put on gloves.

5 Collect the following:
- Commode
- Toilet tissue
- Bath blanket
- Transfer belt

Continued

Helping the Person to the Commode—cont'd

Procedure

6   Bring the commode next to the bed. Remove the chair seat and container lid.

7   Help the person sit on the side of the bed. Lower the bed rail if used,

8   Help him or her put on a robe and non-skid footwear.

9   Assist the person to the commode. Use the transfer belt.

10   Cover the person with a bath blanket for warmth.

11   Place the toilet tissue and signal light within reach.

12   Ask him or her to signal when done or when help is needed. (Stay with the person if necessary. Be respectful. Provide as much privacy as possible.)

13   Remove the gloves. Decontaminate your hands.

14   Leave the room. Close the door.

15   Return when the person signals. Or check on the person every 5 minutes. Knock before entering.

16   Decontaminate your hands. Put on the gloves.

17   Help the person clean the genital area as needed. Remove the gloves, and practice hand hygiene.

18   Help the person back to bed using the transfer belt. Remove the robe, transfer belt, and footwear. Raise the bed rail if used.

19   Put on clean gloves. Remove and cover the commode container. Clean the commode.

20   Take the container to the bathroom.

21   Observe urine and feces for color, amount, and character.

22   Empty the container contents into toilet and flush.

23   Rinse the container. Pour the rinse into the toilet and flush.

24   Clean and disinfect the container.

25   Return the container to the commode. Return other supplies to their proper place.

26   Return the commode to its proper place.

27   Remove soiled gloves. Practice hand hygiene, and put on clean gloves.

28   Assist with hand washing.

29   Remove the gloves. Decontaminate your hands.

Post-Procedure

30   Provide for comfort. (See the inside of the front book cover.)

31   Place the signal light within reach.

32   Raise or lower bed rails. Follow the care plan.

33   Unscreen the person.

34   Complete a safety check of the room. (See the inside of the front book cover.)

35   Follow agency policy for soiled linen.

36   Decontaminate your hands.

37   Report and record your observations.

URINARY INCONTINENCE

Urinary incontinence is the loss of bladder control. It may be temporary or permanent. There are basic types of incontinence.

- **Stress incontinence.** Urine leaks during exercise and certain movements. Urine loss is small (less than 50 ml). Often called *dribbling*, it occurs with laughing, sneezing, coughing, lifting, or other activities.
- **Urge incontinence.** Urine is lost in response to a sudden, urgent need to void. The person cannot get to a toilet in time. Urinary frequency, urinary urgency, and night-time voidings are common.

- **Overflow incontinence.** Urine leaks when the bladder is too full. The person feels like the bladder is not empty. The person only dribbles or has a weak urine stream.
- **Functional incontinence.** The person has bladder control but cannot use the toilet in time. Immobility, restraints, unanswered signal lights, no signal light within reach, and not knowing where to find the bathroom are causes. So is difficulty removing clothing. Confusion and disorientation are other causes.
- **Reflex incontinence.** Urine is lost at predictable intervals when the bladder is full. The person does not feel the need to void. Nervous system disorders and injuries are common causes.

BOX 15-2 Nursing Measures For Persons With Urinary Incontinence

- Record the person's voidings. This includes incontinent times and successful use of the toilet, commode, bedpan, or urinal.
- Answer signal lights promptly. The need to void may be urgent.
- Promote normal urinary elimination (see Box 15-1).
- Promote normal bowel elimination (Chapter 16).
- Encourage voiding at scheduled intervals.
- Follow the person's bladder training program (p. 274).
- Have the person wear easy-to-remove clothing. Incontinence can occur while trying to deal with buttons, zippers, and undergarments.
- Encourage the person to do pelvic muscle exercises as instructed by the nurse.
- Help prevent urinary tract infections.
  - Promote fluid intake as the nurse directs.
  - Have the person wear cotton underwear.
  - Keep the perineal area clean and dry.
- Decrease fluid intake before bedtime.
- Provide good skin care.
- Provide dry garments and linens.
- Observe for signs of skin breakdown (Chapter 21).
- Use incontinence products as the nurse directs. Follow the manufacturer's instructions.
- Provide perineal care as needed (Chapter 13). Remember to:
  - Use a safe and comfortable water temperature.
  - Follow Standard Precautions and the Bloodborne Pathogen Standard.
  - Protect the person and dry garments and linen from the wet incontinence product.
  - Expose only the perineal area.
  - Wash, rinse, and dry the perineal area and buttocks.
  - Remove wet incontinence products, garments, and linen. Apply clean, dry ones.

Sometimes incontinence results from intestinal, rectal, and reproductive system surgeries. More than one type of incontinence can be present. This is called *mixed incontinence.*

Incontinence is embarrassing. Garments get wet, and odors develop. The person is uncomfortable. Skin irritation, infection, and pressure ulcers are risks. Falling is a risk when trying to get to the bathroom quickly. The person's pride, dignity, and self-esteem are affected. Loss of independence, social isolation, and depression are common.

The person's care plan may include some of the measures in Box 15-2. *Good skin care and dry garments and linens are essential.* Following the rules for normal urinary elimination prevents incontinence in some people. Others need bladder training (p. 274). Sometimes catheters are ordered (p. 266).

Incontinence products help keep the person dry (Fig. 15-8). They have two layers and a waterproof back. Fluid passes through the first layer. It is absorbed by the lower layer. The nurse selects products that best meet the person's needs.

Incontinence is beyond the person's control. It is not something the person chooses to do. The person may wet again right after skin care and changing wet garments and linens. The person's needs are great. If you find yourself becoming short-tempered and impatient, talk to the nurse at once. Kindness, empathy, understanding, and patience are needed.

See Persons With Dementia: Urinary Incontinence.

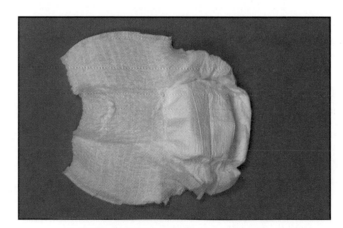

FIG. **15-8** Incontinence product.

Persons With Dementia

Urinary Incontinence

Persons with dementia may void in the wrong places. Trash cans, planters, heating vents, and closets are examples. Some persons remove incontinence products and throw them on the floor or in the toilet. Other persons resist staff efforts to keep them clean and dry. Check with the nurse and the care plan for measures to help the person. Remember, everyone has the right to safe care and to be treated with respect.

CATHETERS

A **catheter** is a tube used to drain or inject fluid through a body opening. Inserted through the urethra into the bladder, a urinary catheter drains urine. An *indwelling catheter* (*retention* or *Foley catheter*) is left in the bladder (Fig. 15-9). Tubing connects the catheter to the drainage bag. A doctor or nurse inserts the catheter (*catheterization*).

Some people are too weak or disabled to use the bedpan, commode, or toilet. For them, catheters can promote comfort and prevent incontinence. Catheters can protect wounds and pressure ulcers from contact with urine. They also allow hourly urinary output measurements. However, they are a last resort for incontinence. Catheters do not treat the cause of incontinence.

Persons with catheters are at high risk for infection. Follow the rules in Box 15-3.

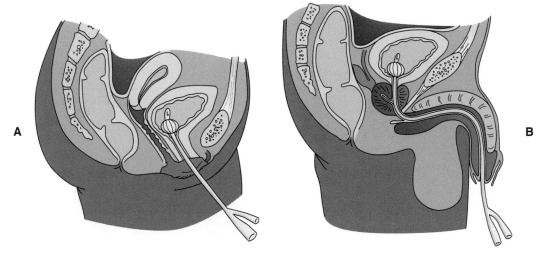

FIG. **15-9** Indwelling catheter. **A,** Indwelling catheter in the female bladder. The inflated balloon at the tip prevents the catheter from slipping out through the urethra. **B,** Indwelling catheter with the balloon inflated in the male bladder.

BOX 15-3   Caring For Persons With Indwelling Catheters

- Follow the rules of medical asepsis.
- Follow Standard Precautions and the Bloodborne Pathogen Standard.
- Allow urine to flow freely through the catheter or tubing. Tubing should not have kinks. The person should not lie on the tubing.
- Keep the catheter connected to the drainage tubing. Follow the measures on p. 269 if the catheter and drainage tube are disconnected.
- Keep the drainage bag below the bladder. This prevents urine from flowing backward into the bladder.
- Attach the drainage bag to the bed frame, back of the chair, or lower part of an IV pole. *Never attach the drainage bag to the bed rail.*
- Do not let the drainage bag rest on the floor.
- Coil the drainage tubing on the bed. Secure it to the bottom linen (Fig. 15-10). Follow agency policy. Use a clip, bed sheet clamp, tape, safety pin with rubber band, or other device as directed by the nurse. Tubing must not loop below the drainage bag.

- Secure the catheter to the inner thigh (see Fig. 15-10). Or secure it to the man's abdomen. This prevents excess catheter movement and friction at the insertion site. Secure the catheter with a tube holder, tape, or other device as the nurse directs.
- Check for leaks. Report any leaks to the nurse at once.
- Provide catheter care daily or twice a day (see procedure: *Giving Catheter Care*, p. 268). Follow the care plan.
- Provide perineal care daily, after bowel movements, and when there is vaginal drainage. Follow the care plan.
- Empty the drainage bag at the end of the shift or as the nurse directs. Measure and record the amount of urine (see procedure: *Emptying a Urinary Drainage Bag*, p. 271). Report increases or decreases in the amount of urine.
- Use a separate measuring container for each person. This prevents the spread of microbes from one person to another.
- Do not let the drain on the drainage bag touch any surface.
- Encourage fluid intake as instructed by the nurse.

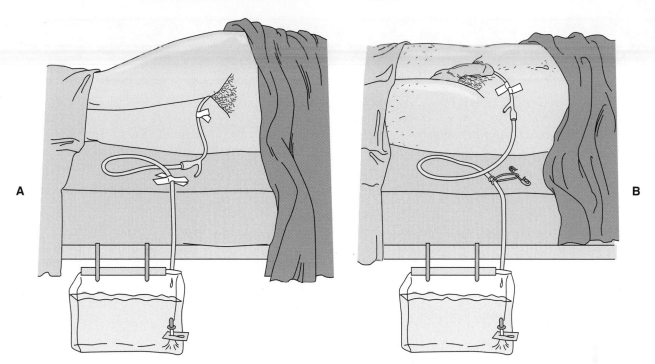

FIG. **15-10** Securing catheters. **A,** The drainage tube is coiled on the bed and secured to the bottom linens. The catheter is taped to the inner thigh. Enough slack is left on the catheter to prevent friction at the urethra. **B,** The catheter is secured to the man's abdomen.

DELEGATION GUIDELINES
Catheters

The nurse may delegate catheter care to you. If so, you need this information from the nurse and the care plan:

- When to give catheter care—daily, twice a day, after bowel movements, or when vaginal discharge is present
- Where to secure the catheter—thigh or abdomen
- What device to use to secure the catheter—tube holder, tape, or other device.
- How to secure drainage tubing—clip, bed sheet clamp, tape, safety pin and rubber band, or other device
- What observations to report and record:
  - Complaints of pain, burning, irritation, or the need to void (report at once)
  - Crusting, abnormal drainage, or secretions
  - The color, clarity, and odor of urine
  - Particles in the urine
  - Drainage system leaks

PROMOTING SAFETY AND COMFORT
Catheters

Safety

Urine may contain microbes and blood. Follow Standard Precautions and the Bloodborne Pathogen Standard.

Comfort

The catheter must not pull at the insertion site. This causes discomfort and irritation. Hold the catheter securely during catheter care. Then properly secure the catheter. Also make sure the tubing is not under the person. Besides obstructing urine flow, laying on the tubing is uncomfortable. To promote comfort, follow the rules in Box 15-3.

Giving Catheter Care

NNAAP™

Quality of Life

Remember to:

- Knock before entering the person's room
- Address the person by name
- Introduce yourself by name and title

- Explain the procedure to the person before beginning and during the procedure
- Protect the person's rights during the procedure
- Handle the person gently during the procedure

Pre-Procedure

1 Follow *Delegation Guidelines: Catheters*, p. 267. See *Promoting Safety and Comfort: Catheters*, p. 267.
2 Practice hand hygiene.
3 Collect the following:
   - Items for perineal care (Chapter 13)
   - Gloves
   - Bath blanket

4 Identify the person. Check the ID bracelet against the assignment sheet. Call the person by name.
5 Provide for privacy.
6 Raise the bed for body mechanics. Bed rails are up if used.

Procedure

7 Lower the bed rail near you if up.
8 Decontaminate your hands. Put on the gloves.
9 Cover the person with a bath blanket. Fan-fold top linens to the foot of the bed.
10 Drape the person for perineal care. (See procedure: *Giving Female Perineal Care* in Chapter 13).
11 Fold back the bath blanket to expose the genital area.
12 Place the waterproof pad under the buttocks. Ask the person to flex the knees and raise the buttocks off the bed.
13 Separate the labia (female). In an uncircumcised male, retract the foreskin (Fig. 15-11). Check for crusts, abnormal drainage, or secretions.
14 Give perineal care. (See procedure: *Giving Female Perineal Care* or *Giving Male Perineal Care* in Chapter 13.)
15 Apply soap to a clean, wet washcloth.
16 Hold the catheter near the meatus.

17 Clean the catheter from the meatus down the catheter about 4 inches (Fig. 15-12). Clean downward, away from the meatus with 1 stroke. Do not tug or pull on the catheter. Repeat as needed with a clean area of the washcloth. Use a clean washcloth if needed.
18 Rinse the catheter with a clean washcloth. Rinse from the meatus down the catheter about 4 inches. Rinse downward, away from the meatus with 1 stroke. Do not tug or pull on the catheter. Repeat as needed with a clean area of the washcloth. Use a clean washcloth if needed.
19 Pat dry the perineal area. Dry from front to back.
20 Return foreskin to its natural position.
21 Secure the catheter. Coil and secure tubing (see Fig. 15-10).
22 Remove the waterproof pad.
23 Cover the person. Remove the bath blanket.
24 Remove the gloves. Decontaminate your hands.

Post-Procedure

25 Provide for comfort. (See the inside of the front book cover.)
26 Place the signal light within reach.
27 Lower the bed to its lowest position.
28 Raise or lower bed rails. Follow the care plan.
29 Clean and return equipment to its proper place. Discard disposable items. (Wear gloves for this step.)

30 Remove the gloves. Decontaminate your hands.
31 Unscreen the person.
32 Complete a safety check of the room. (See the inside of the front book cover.)
33 Follow agency policy for soiled linen.
34 Decontaminate your hands.
35 Report and record your observations.

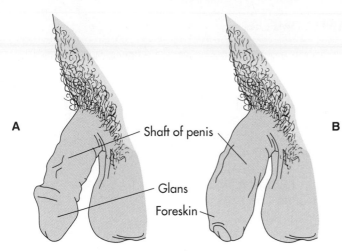

FIG. **15-11 A,** Circumcised male. **B,** Uncircumcised male.

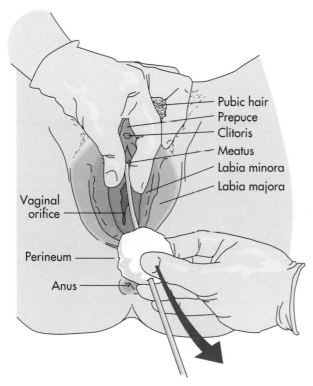

FIG. **15-12** The catheter is cleaned starting at the meatus. About 4 inches of the catheter is cleaned.

 Drainage Systems

A closed drainage system is used for indwelling catheters. Nothing can enter the system from the catheter to the drainage bag. The urinary system is sterile. Infection can occur if microbes enter the drainage system. The microbes travel up the tubing or catheter into the bladder and kidneys. A urinary tract infection can threaten health and life.

The drainage system has tubing and a drainage bag. Tubing attaches at one end to the catheter. At the other end, it attaches to the drainage bag.

The bag hangs from the bed frame, chair, or wheelchair. It must not touch the floor. The bag is always kept lower than the person's bladder (see Fig. 15-10). Microbes can grow in urine. If the drainage bag is higher than the bladder, urine can flow back into the bladder. An infection can occur. Therefore, do not hang the drainage bag on a bed rail. When the bed rail is raised, the bag is higher than bladder level. When the person walks, the bag is held lower than the bladder.

Sometimes drainage systems are disconnected accidentally. If that happens, tell the nurse at once. Do not touch the ends of the catheter or tubing. Do the following:

- Practice hand hygiene. Put on gloves.
- Wipe the end of the tube with an antiseptic wipe.
- Wipe the end of the catheter with another antiseptic wipe.
- Do not put the ends down. Do not touch the ends after you clean them.
- Connect the tubing to the catheter.
- Discard the wipes into a biohazard bag.
- Remove the gloves. Practice hand hygiene.

DELEGATION GUIDELINES
Drainage Systems

Before emptying a urinary drainage bag, you need this information from the nurse and the care plan:
- When to empty the drainage bag
- If the person uses a leg bag
- When to switch drainage bags and leg bags
- If you should clean or discard the drainage bag
- What observations to report and record:
  - The amount of urine measured
  - The color, clarity, and odor of urine
  - Particles in the urine
  - Complaints of pain, burning, irritation, or the need to urinate
  - Drainage system leaks

PROMOTING SAFETY AND COMFORT
Drainage Systems

Safety

Urine may contain microbes and blood. Follow Standard Precautions and the Bloodborne Pathogen Standard.

Some drainage bags are secured to a leg. Called "leg bags," they hold less than 1000 ml of urine (p. 272). Most drainage bags hold at least 2000 ml of urine. Therefore, leg bags fill faster than drainage bags. Check leg bags often. Empty and measure urine when the bag is half full.

Comfort

Having urine in a drainage bag is embarrassing to some people. Visitors can see the urine when they are with the person. To promote mental comfort, have visitors sit on the side away from the drainage bag. Sometimes you can empty the bag before visitors arrive.

Some agencies provide drainage bag holders. The drainage bag is placed inside the holder. Urine cannot be seen.

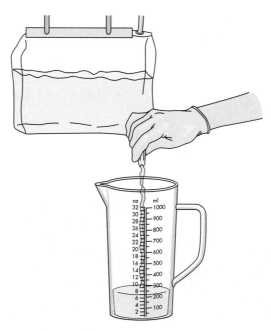

FIG. **15-13** The clamp on the drainage bag is opened. The drain is directed into the graduate. The drain must not touch the inside of the graduate.

Emptying a Urinary Drainage Bag

Quality of Life

Remember to:

- Knock before entering the person's room
- Address the person by name
- Introduce yourself by name and title

- Explain the procedure to the person before beginning and during the procedure
- Protect the person's rights during the procedure
- Handle the person gently during the procedure

Pre-Procedure

1 Follow *Delegation Guidelines: Drainage Systems*, p. 269. See *Promoting Safety and Comfort: Drainage Systems.*
2 Collect equipment:
   - Graduate (measuring container)
   - Gloves
   - Paper towels

3 Practice hand hygiene.
4 Identify the person. Check the ID bracelet against the assignment sheet. Call the person by name.
5 Provide for privacy.

Procedure

6 Put on the gloves.
7 Place a paper towel on the floor. Place the graduate on top of it.
8 Position the graduate under the collection bag.
9 Open the clamp on the drain.
10 Let all urine drain into the graduate. Do not let the drain touch the graduate (Fig. 15-13).
11 Close and position the clamp (see Fig. 15-10).
12 Measure urine.
13 Remove and discard the paper towel.

14 Empty the contents of the graduate into the toilet and flush.
15 Rinse the graduate. Empty the rinse into the toilet and flush.
16 Clean and disinfect the graduate.
17 Return the graduate to its proper place.
18 Remove the gloves. Practice hand hygiene.
19 Record the time and amount on the intake and output (I&O) record (Chapter 17).

Post-Procedure

20 Provide for comfort. (See the inside of the front book cover.)
21 Place the signal light within reach.
22 Unscreen the person.

23 Complete a safety check of the room. (See the inside of the front book cover.)
24 Report and record the amount and other observations.

The Condom Catheter

Condom catheters are often used for incontinent men. They also are called *external catheters, Texas catheters*, and *urinary sheaths*. A condom catheter is a soft sheath that slides over the penis. Tubing connects the condom catheter and drainage bag. Many men prefer leg bags (Fig. 15-14, p. 272).

Condom catheters are usually changed daily after perineal care. To apply a condom catheter, follow the manufacturer's instructions. Thoroughly wash the penis with soap and water. Then dry it before applying the catheter.

Some condom catheters are self-adhering. Adhesive inside the catheter adheres to the penis. Other catheters are secured in place with elastic tape. Use the elastic tape packaged with the catheter. Elastic tape expands when the penis changes size. This allows blood flow to the penis. *Never use adhesive tape to secure catheters. It does not expand. Blood flow to the penis is cut off, injuring the penis.*

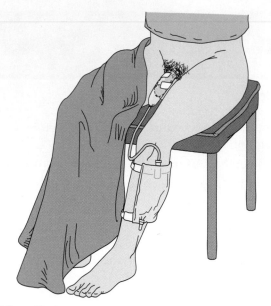

FIG. **15-14** Condom catheter attached to a leg bag.

DELEGATION GUIDELINES
Condom Catheters

Before removing or applying a condom catheter, you need this information from the nurse and the care plan:

- What size to use—small, medium, or large
- When to remove the catheter and apply a new one
- If a leg bag or standard drainage system is used
- What observations to report and record:
  - Reddened or open areas on the penis
  - Swelling of the penis
  - Color, clarity, and odor of urine
  - Particles in the urine

FIG. **15-15** A condom catheter applied to the penis. There is a 1-inch space between the penis and the end of the catheter. Elastic tape is applied in a spiral fashion to secure the condom catheter to the penis.

PROMOTING SAFETY AND COMFORT
Condom Catheters

Safety

Do not apply a condom catheter if the penis is red, irritated, or shows signs of skin breakdown. Report your observations to the nurse at once.

If you do not know how to use the condom catheters used at the agency, ask the nurse to show the correct application to you. Then ask the nurse to observe you applying the catheter.

Blood must flow to the penis. If tape is needed, use elastic tape. Apply it in a spiral.

Urine may contain microbes and blood. Follow Standard Precautions and the Bloodborne Pathogen Standard.

Comfort

To apply a condom catheter, you need to touch and handle the penis. This can embarrass the man. Some men become aroused. Always act in a professional manner. If necessary, allow the man some privacy. Provide for his safety and place the urinal within reach. Tell him when you will return, and leave the room. Remember to knock before entering the room.

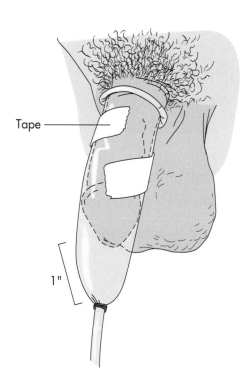

Tape

1"

Applying a Condom Catheter

Quality of Life

Remember to:

- Knock before entering the person's room
- Address the person by name
- Introduce yourself by name and title

- Explain the procedure to the person before beginning and during the procedure
- Protect the person's rights during the procedure
- Handle the person gently during the procedure

Pre-Procedure

1 Follow *Delegation Guidelines: Condom Catheters.* See *Promoting Safety and Comfort: Condom Catheters.*
2 Practice hand hygiene.
3 Collect the following:
   - Condom catheter
   - Elastic tape
   - Drainage bag or leg bag
   - Cap for the drainage bag
   - Basin of warm water
   - Soap
   - Towel and washcloths
   - Bath blanket
   - Gloves
   - Waterproof pad
   - Paper towels
4 Arrange paper towels and equipment on the overbed table.
5 Identify the person. Check the ID bracelet against the assignment sheet. Call the person by name.
6 Provide for privacy.
7 Raise the bed for body mechanics. Bed rails are up if used.

Procedure

8 Lower the bed rail near you if up.
9 Decontaminate your hands. Put on the gloves.
10 Cover the person with a bath blanket. Lower top linens to the knees.
11 Ask the person to raise his buttocks off the bed. Or turn him onto his side away from you.
12 Slide the waterproof pad under his buttocks.
13 Have the person lower his buttocks. Or turn him onto his back.
14 Secure the drainage bag to the bed frame. Or have a leg bag ready. Close the drain.
15 Expose the genital area.
16 Remove the condom catheter.
   a Remove the tape. Roll the sheath off the penis.
   b Disconnect the drainage tubing from the condom. Cap the drainage tube.
   c Discard the tape and condom.
17 Provide perineal care (see procedure: *Giving Male Perineal Care,* Chapter 13). Observe the penis for reddened areas and skin breakdown or irritation.

18 Remove the protective backing from the condom. This exposes the adhesive strip.
19 Hold the penis firmly. Roll the condom onto the penis. Leave a 1-inch space between the penis and the end of the catheter (Fig. 15-15).
20 Secure the condom.
   a For a self-adhering condom: Press the condom to the penis.
   b For a condom secured with elastic tape: Apply elastic tape in a spiral (see Fig. 15-15). Do not apply tape completely around the penis.
21 Make sure the penis tip does not touch the condom. Make sure the condom is not twisted.
22 Connect the condom to the drainage tubing. Coil and secure excess tubing on the bed. Or attach a leg bag.
23 Remove the waterproof pad and gloves. Discard them. Practice hand hygiene.
24 Cover the person. Remove the bath blanket.

Post-Procedure

25 Provide for comfort. (See the inside of the front book cover.)
26 Place the signal light within reach.
27 Lower the bed to its lowest position.
28 Raise or lower bed rails. Follow the care plan.
29 Unscreen the person.
30 Decontaminate your hands. Put on clean gloves.

31 Measure and record the amount of urine in the bag. Clean or discard the collection bag.
32 Clean and return the wash basin and other equipment. Return items to their proper place.
33 Remove the gloves. Decontaminate your hands.
34 Complete a safety check of the room. (See the inside of the front book cover.)
35 Report and record your observations.

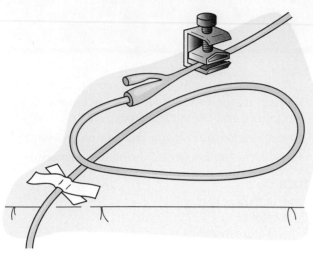

FIG. **15-16** The clamped catheter prevents urine from draining out of the bladder. The clamp is applied directly to the catheter—not to the drainage tubing.

BLADDER TRAINING

Bladder training programs help some persons with urinary incontinence. Some persons need bladder training after indwelling catheter removal. Control of urination is the goal. Bladder control promotes comfort and quality of life. You assist with bladder training as directed by the nurse and the care plan.

There are two basic methods for bladder training:

- The person uses the toilet, commode, bedpan, or urinal at certain times. Every 2 or 3 hours is common. The person is given 15 or 20 minutes to start voiding. The rules for normal urination are followed.
- The person has a catheter. The catheter is clamped to prevent urine flow from the bladder (Fig. 15-16). It is usually clamped for 1 or 2 hours at first. Over time, it is clamped for 3 to 4 hours. Urine drains when the catheter is unclamped. When the catheter is removed, voiding is encouraged every 3 to 4 hours or as directed by the nurse and the care plan.

FOCUS ON THE PERSON

People usually void in private. Illness, disease, and aging can affect this very private act. *See Focus on the Person: Assisting With Urinary Elimination.*

Focus on the PERSON

Assisting With Urinary Elimination

Providing comfort—Voiding in private promotes mental comfort. Allow as much privacy as safely possible. Follow the nurse's directions and the care plan.

Remove bedpans promptly. Do not leave the person sitting on the bedpan. Discomfort, odors, and skin breakdown are likely.

Ethical behavior—The person's elimination habits and routines may be different from yours. Do not react to things that seem odd to you. Act in a professional manner at all times. Remember, laughing at, making fun of, or ridiculing a person is abuse under OBRA.

Remaining independent—Some people can place bedpans and urinals themselves. Others can get on and off bedside commodes themselves. To promote independence, make sure these devices are kept within their reach.

Speaking up—Patients and residents may not use "voiding" and "urinating" terms. The person may not understand what you are saying. Do not ask: "Do you need to void?" Instead, ask these questions:

- "Do you need to use the bathroom?"
- "Do you need to use the bedpan."

- "Do you need to pass urine?"
- "Do you need to pee?"

OBRA and other laws—Each state has a nurse practice act. It regulates nursing practice in that state. Serving to protect the public's welfare and safety, it is used to decide what nursing assistants can do in that state. Some states allow nursing assistants to do urinary catheterizations (inserting a catheter into the bladder). If your state and agency allow you to do catheterizations:

- The procedure must be in your job description.
- You must have the necessary education and training.
- You must know how to use the agency's supplies and equipment.
- A nurse must be available to answer questions and supervise you.

Nursing teamwork—A person's need to void may be urgent. Answer signal lights promptly. Also answer signal lights for co-workers. Otherwise incontinence may result. The person is wet and embarrassed. He or she is at risk for skin breakdown and infection. Your co-worker has extra work—changing linens and garments. You like help when you are busy. So do your co-workers.

REVIEW QUESTIONS

Circle the **BEST** answer.

1 Which is *false*?
   a Urine is normally clear and yellow or amber in color.
   b Urine normally has an ammonia odor.
   c People usually void before bedtime and on rising.
   d A person normally voids about 1500 ml a day.

2 Which is *not* a rule for normal urinary elimination?
   a Help the person assume a normal position for voiding.
   b Provide for privacy.
   c Help the person to the bathroom or commode. Or provide the bedpan or urinal as soon as requested.
   d Always stay with the person who is on a bedpan.

3 The best position for using a bedpan is
   a Fowler's position
   b The supine position
   c The prone position
   d The side-lying position

4 After using the urinal, the man should
   a Put it on the bedside stand
   b Use the signal light
   c Put it on the overbed table
   d Empty it

5 Urinary incontinence
   a Is always permanent
   b Requires good skin care
   c Is treated with a catheter
   d Requires bladder training

6 A person has a catheter. Which action is *wrong*?
   a Keep the drainage bag above the level of the bladder.
   b Keep drainage tubing free of kinks.
   c Coil the drainage tubing on the bed.
   d Secure the catheter according to agency policy.

7 A person has a catheter. Which action is *wrong*?
   a Tape any leaks at the connection site.
   b Follow Standard Precautions and the Bloodborne Pathogen Standard.
   c Empty the drainage bag at the end of each shift.
   d Report complaints of pain, burning, the need to urinate, or irritation at once.

8 Mr. Powers has a condom catheter. You apply elastic tape
   a Completely around the penis
   b To the inner thigh
   c To the abdomen
   d In a spiral fashion

9 The goal of bladder training is to
   a Remove the catheter
   b Allow the person to walk to the bathroom
   c Gain control of urination
   d Void every 3 or 4 hours

10 Which is *not* a cause of functional incontinence?
   a Unanswered signal lights
   b No signal light within reach
   c Problems removing clothing
   d Laughing, sneezing, or coughing

Answers to these questions are on p. 469.

275

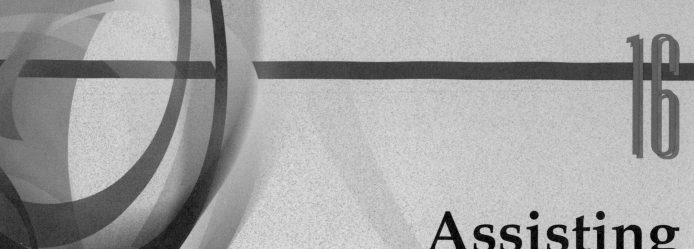

Assisting With Bowel Elimination

OBJECTIVES

- Define the key terms listed in this chapter
- Describe normal defecation and the observations to report
- Identify the factors that affect bowel elimination
- Describe common bowel elimination problems
- Explain how to promote comfort and safety during defecation
- Describe bowel training
- Explain why enemas are given
- Describe the common enema solutions
- Describe the rules for giving enemas
- Describe how to care for a person with an ostomy
- Perform the procedures described in this chapter

PROCEDURES

Procedures with this icon 🌸 are also on the CD-ROM in this book.

- Giving a Cleansing Enema
- Giving a Small-Volume Enema

KEY TERMS

colostomy A surgically created opening (*stomy*) between the colon (*colo*) and abdominal wall

constipation The passage of a hard, dry stool

defecation The process of excreting feces from the rectum through the anus; bowel movement

diarrhea The frequent passage of liquid stools

enema The introduction of fluid into the rectum and lower colon

fecal impaction The prolonged retention and buildup of feces in the rectum

fecal incontinence The inability to control the passage of feces and gas through the anus

feces The semi-solid mass of waste products in the colon that are expelled through the anus

flatulence The excessive formation of gas in the stomach and intestines

flatus Gas or air passed through the anus

ileostomy A surgically created opening (*stomy*) between the ileum (small intestine [*ileo*]) and the abdominal wall

ostomy A surgically created opening

stoma An opening; see colostomy and ileostomy

stool Excreted feces

suppository A cone-shaped, solid drug that is inserted into a body opening; it melts at body temperature

Bowel elimination is a basic physical need. Wastes are excreted from the gastrointestinal tract. You assist patients and residents in meeting their elimination needs.

NORMAL BOWEL MOVEMENTS

Some people have a bowel movement every day. Others have one every 2 to 3 days. Some people have two or three bowel movements a day. Many people have a bowel movement after breakfast. Others do so in the evening. To assist with bowel elimination, you need to know these terms:

- **Defecation**—the process of excreting feces from the rectum through the anus (a bowel movement)
- **Feces**—the semi-solid mass of waste products in the colon that are expelled through the anus
- **Stool**—excreted feces

Stools are normally brown. Bleeding in the stomach and small intestine causes black or tarry stools. Bleeding in the lower colon and rectum causes red-colored stools. Diseases and infection can cause clay-colored or white, pale, orange-colored, or green-colored stools.

Stools are normally soft, formed, moist, and shaped like the rectum. They have a normal odor.

Observations

Carefully observe stools before disposing of them. Observe and report the following to the nurse: color, amount, consistency, odor, shape, size, frequency of defecation, and complaints of pain. Ask the nurse to observe abnormal stools.

FACTORS AFFECTING BOWEL ELIMINATION

These factors affect stool frequency, consistency, color, and odor. The nurse considers them when using the nursing process to meet the person's elimination needs. Normal, regular elimination is the goal.

- *Privacy.* Lack of privacy can prevent defecation despite having the urge. Odors and sounds are embarrassing. Some people ignore the urge when others are present.
- *Habits.* Many people have a bowel movement after breakfast. Some drink a hot beverage, read, or take a walk to relax. Defecation is easier when a person is relaxed, not tense.
- *Diet.* A well-balanced diet and bulk are needed. High-fiber foods leave a residue for needed bulk and help prevent constipation. Fruits, vegetables, and whole grain cereals and breads are high in fiber. So is bran. In nursing centers, bran is often added to cereal, prunes, or prune juice. Spicy foods can irritate the intestines. Frequent stools or diarrhea can result. Gas-forming foods stimulate peristalsis, which aids defecation. They include onions, beans, cabbage, cauliflower, radishes, and cucumbers. Older persons often avoid gas-forming foods to prevent "stomach-aches" or "bloating."
- *Fluids.* Feces contain water. Stool consistency depends on the amount of water absorbed in the colon. Feces harden and dry when large amounts of water are absorbed or when fluid intake is poor. Hard, dry feces move slowly through the colon. Constipation can occur. Drinking 6 to 8 glasses of water daily promotes normal bowel elimination. Warm fluids—coffee, tea, hot cider, and warm water—increase peristalsis.
- *Activity.* Exercise and activity maintain muscle tone and stimulate peristalsis.
- *Drugs.* Drugs can prevent constipation or control diarrhea. Other drugs have diarrhea or constipation as side effects.
- *Disability.* Some people cannot control bowel movements. They defecate whenever feces enter the rectum. A bowel training program is needed (p. 279).

BOX 16-1	Comfort and Safety During Bowel Elimination

- Help the person to the toilet or commode. Or provide the bedpan as soon as requested.
- Wheel the person into the bathroom on the commode if possible. Place the commode over the toilet. This provides privacy.
- Provide for privacy. Ask visitors to leave the room. Close doors and pull privacy curtains. Also close window curtains, blinds, or shades.
- Make sure the bedpan is warm.
- Position the person in a normal sitting or squatting position.
- Cover the person for warmth and privacy.
- Allow enough time for defecation. Do not rush the person.
- Place the signal light and toilet tissue within reach.
- Leave the room if the person can be alone.
- Stay nearby if the person is weak or unsteady.
- Provide perineal care.
- Dispose of feces promptly. This reduces odors and prevents the spread of microbes.
- Assist the person with hand washing after elimination.
- Follow the care plan if the person has fecal incontinence. The care plan tells you when to assist with elimination.
- Follow Standard Precautions and the Bloodborne Pathogen Standard.

- *Age.* Aging slows down the passage of feces through the intestines. This results in constipation. For some people, the changes from aging cause loss of bowel control. (See Fecal Incontinence.)

Safety and Comfort

The care plan includes measures to meet the person's elimination needs. It may involve diet, fluids, and exercise. Follow the measures in Box 16-1 to promote comfort and safety.

COMMON PROBLEMS

Common problems include constipation, fecal impaction, diarrhea, fecal incontinence, and flatulence.

Constipation

Constipation is the passage of a hard, dry stool. The person usually strains to have a bowel movement. Stools are large or marble-sized. Large stools cause pain as they pass through the anus. Constipation occurs when feces move slowly through the bowel. This allows more time for water absorption. Common causes include a low-fiber diet, ignoring the urge to defecate, decreased fluid intake, inactivity,

drugs, aging, and certain diseases. Dietary changes, fluids, and activity prevent or relieve constipation. So do drugs and enemas.

Fecal Impaction

A **fecal impaction** is the prolonged retention and buildup of feces in the rectum. Feces are hard or putty-like. Fecal impaction results if constipation is not relieved. The person cannot defecate. More water is absorbed from already hard feces. Liquid feces pass around the hardened fecal mass in the rectum. The liquid feces seep from the anus.

The person tries many times to have a bowel movement. Abdominal discomfort, nausea, loss of appetite, cramping, and rectal pain are common. Report these signs and symptoms to the nurse.

Diarrhea

Diarrhea is the frequent passage of liquid stools. Feces move through the intestines rapidly. This reduces the time for fluid absorption. The need to defecate is urgent. Some people cannot get to a bathroom in time. Abdominal cramping, nausea, and vomiting may occur.

Causes of diarrhea include infections, some drugs, irritating foods, and microbes in food and water. Diet and drugs reduce peristalsis. You need to:

- Assist with elimination needs promptly.
- Dispose of stools promptly. This prevents odors and the spread of microbes.
- Give good skin care. Liquid feces irritate the skin. So does frequent wiping with toilet tissue. Skin breakdown and pressure ulcers are risks.

The amount of body water decreases with aging. Report signs of diarrhea at once. Ask the nurse to observe the stool.

Fecal Incontinence

Fecal incontinence is the inability to control the passage of feces and gas through the anus. Causes include intestinal diseases and nervous system diseases and injuries. Fecal impaction, diarrhea, some drugs, and aging are other causes. Unanswered signal lights is another cause.

Fecal incontinence is frustrating and embarrassing. Anger and humiliation are common. The person may need:

- Bowel training
- Help with elimination after meals and every 2 to 3 hours
- Incontinence products to keep garments and linens clean
- Good skin care
  See Persons With Dementia: Fecal Incontinence.

Flatulence

Gas and air are normally in the stomach and intestines. They are expelled through the mouth (belching, eructating) and anus. Gas and air passed through the anus is called **flatus. Flatulence** is the excessive formation of gas or air in the stomach and intestines. Causes include:

- Swallowing air while eating and drinking
- Bacterial action in the intestines
- Gas-forming foods (onions, beans, cabbage, cauliflower, radishes, and cucumbers)
- Constipation
- Bowel and abdominal surgeries
- Drugs that decrease peristalsis

If flatus is not expelled, the intestines distend. That is, they swell or enlarge from the pressure of the gases. Abdominal cramping or pain, shortness of breath, and a swollen abdomen occur. "Bloating" is a common complaint. Walking, moving in bed, and the left-side lying position often produce flatus. Doctors may order enemas or drugs to relieve flatulence.

BOWEL TRAINING

Bowel training has two goals.

- To gain control of bowel movements.
- To develop a regular pattern of elimination. Fecal impaction, constipation, and fecal incontinence are prevented.

Meals, especially breakfast, stimulate the urge to defecate. The person's usual time of day for defecation is noted on the care plan. Toilet, commode, or bedpan use is offered at this time. Factors that promote elimination are part of the care plan and bowel training program.

The doctor may order a suppository to stimulate defecation. A **suppository** is a cone-shaped, solid drug that is inserted into a body opening. It melts at body temperature. A nurse inserts a rectal suppository into the rectum (Fig. 16-1). A bowel movement occurs about 30 minutes later.

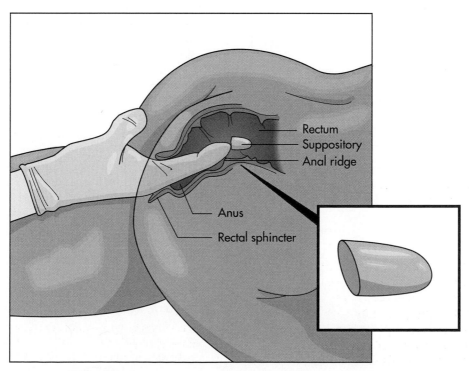

FIG. **16-1** The suppository (inset) is inserted into the rectum.

ENEMAS

An **enema** is the introduction of fluid into the rectum and lower colon. Doctors order enemas to remove feces and relieve constipation, fecal impaction, or flatulence.

Comfort and safety measures for bowel elimination are practiced when giving enemas (see Box 16-1). Also follow the rules in Box 16-2.

The doctor orders the enema solution. The solution depends on the enema's purpose.

- *Tap-water enema*—obtained from a faucet.
- *Soapsuds enema (SSE)*—add 3 to 5 ml of castile soap to 500 to 1000 ml of tap water.
- *Saline enema*—a solution of salt and water. Add 1 to 2 teaspoons of table salt to 500 to 1000 ml of tap water.
- *Oil-retention enema*—mineral, olive, or cotton-seed oil.
- *Small-volume enema*—contains about 120 ml (4 ounces) of solution.

BOX 16-2 Comfort and Safety Measures For Giving Enemas

- Have the person void first. This increases the person's comfort during the enema procedure.
- Measure solution temperature with a bath thermometer. See *Delegation Guidelines: Enemas.*
- Give the amount of solution ordered.
- Position the person as the nurse directs. The Sims' position or the left side-lying position is preferred.
- Ask the nurse and check the procedure manual to see how far to insert the enema tubing. It is usually inserted 3 to 4 inches in adults.
- Lubricate the enema tip before inserting it.
- Stop tube insertion if you feel resistance, the person complains of pain, or bleeding occurs.
- Ask the nurse how high to raise the enema bag. For adults, it is usually held 12 inches above the anus.
- Give the solution slowly. Usually it takes 10 to 15 minutes to give 750 to 1000 ml.
- Hold the enema tube in place while giving the solution.
- Ask the nurse how long the person should retain the solution. The length of time depends on the amount and type of solution.
- Make sure the bathroom will be vacant when the person needs to defecate. Make sure that another person will not use the bathroom.
- Have the bedpan or commode ready if the person will not use the bathroom.
- Ask the nurse to observe the enema results.
- Do not give enemas that contain drugs. Nurses give these enemas.

DELEGATION GUIDELINES
Enemas

Some states and agencies let nursing assistants give enemas. Others do not. Before giving an enema, make sure that:

- Your state allows you to perform the procedure
- The procedure is in your job description
- You have the necessary education and training
- You review the procedure with a nurse
- A nurse is available to answer questions and to supervise you

If the above conditions are met, you need this information from the nurse:

- What type of enema to give—cleansing, small-volume, or oil-retention
- When to give the enema
- What size enema tube to use
- How many times to repeat the enema
- The amount of solution ordered by the doctor—usually 500 to 1000 ml for a cleansing enema
- How much castile soap to use for an SSE
- How much salt to use for a saline enema
- What the solution temperature should be—usually 105° F (40.5° C) for adults
- How to position the person—Sims' or the left side-lying position
- How far to insert the enema tubing—usually 3 to 4 inches for adults
- How high to hold the solution container
- How fast to give the solution—750 to 1000 ml are usually given over 10 to 15 minutes
- How long the person should try to retain the solution
- What to report and record:
  - The amount of solution given
  - If bleeding or resistance was noted when inserting the tube
  - How long the person retained the solution
  - Color, amount, consistency, shape, and odor of stools
  - Complaints of cramping, pain, or discomfort
  - How the person tolerated the procedure

PROMOTING SAFETY AND COMFORT
Enemas

Safety

Enemas are usually safe procedures. Many people give themselves enemas at home. However, enemas are dangerous for older persons and those with certain heart and kidney diseases.

Contact with stools is likely when giving enemas. They may contain microbes and blood. Follow Standard Precautions and the Bloodborne Pathogen Standard.

Comfort

Before starting the procedure, make sure that the bathroom will be available for the person's use. If the person will use the commode or bedpan, make sure the device is ready. Always keep a bedpan nearby in case the person starts to expel the enema solution and feces. Mental comfort is promoted when the person knows that the bathroom, commode, or bedpan is ready for his or her use.

Make sure the person is comfortable in the Sims' or left side-lying position. When comfortable, it is easier for the person to tolerate the procedure.

Prevent cramping by:
- Using the correct water temperature. Cool water causes cramping.
- Giving the solution slowly.

The Cleansing Enema

Cleansing enemas clean the bowel of feces and flatus. They relieve constipation and fecal impaction. They are needed before certain surgeries and diagnostic procedures.

The doctor orders a soapsuds, tap-water, or saline enema. The doctor may order *enemas until clear*. This means that enemas are given until the return solution is clear and free of feces. Ask the nurse how many enemas to give. Agency policy may allow repeating them 2 or 3 times.

Text continued on p. 284

 # Giving a Cleansing Enema

Quality of Life

Remember to:
- Knock before entering the person's room
- Address the person by name
- Introduce yourself by name and title

- Explain the procedure to the person before beginning and during the procedure
- Protect the person's rights during the procedure
- Handle the person gently during the procedure

Continued

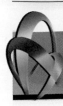 **Giving a Cleansing Enema—cont'd**

Pre-Procedure

1 Follow *Delegation Guidelines: Enemas,* p. 280. See *Promoting Safety and Comfort: Enemas,* p. 281.
2 Practice hand hygiene.
3 Collect the following:
   • Bedpan or commode
   • Disposable enema kit as directed by the nurse (enema bag, tube, clamp, and waterproof pad)
   • Bath thermometer
   • Waterproof pad (if not in the enema kit)
   • Water-soluble lubricant
   • Gloves
   • 3 to 5 ml (1 teaspoon) castile soap or 1 to 2 teaspoons of salt
   • Toilet tissue
   • Bath blanket
   • IV pole
   • Robe and non-skid footwear
   • Paper towels
4 Identify the person. Check the ID bracelet with the assignment sheet. Call the person by name.
5 Provide for privacy.
6 Raise the bed for body mechanics. Bed rails are up if used.

Procedure

7 Lower the bed rail near you if up.
8 Decontaminate your hands. Put on gloves.
9 Cover the person with a bath blanket. Fanfold top linens to the foot of the bed.
10 Position the IV pole so the enema bag is 12 inches above the anus. Or it is at a height directed by the nurse.
11 Raise the bed rail if used.
12 Prepare the enema:
   a Close the clamp on the tube.
   b Adjust water flow until it is lukewarm.
   c Fill the enema bag for the amount ordered.
   d Measure water temperature with the bath thermometer. It is usually 105° F (40.5° C) for adults.
   e Prepare the enema solution as directed by the nurse (p. 280):
      (1) Saline enema: add salt as directed
      (2) Soapsuds enema: add castile soap as directed
      (3) Tap-water enema: add nothing
   f Stir the solution with the bath thermometer. Scoop off any suds (SSE).
   g Seal the bag.
   h Hang the bag on the IV pole.
13 Lower the bed rail near you if up.
14 Position the person in Sims' position or in a left side-lying position.
15 Place a waterproof pad under the buttocks.
16 Expose the anal area.
17 Place the bedpan behind the person.
18 Position the enema tube in the bedpan. Remove the cap from the tubing.

19 Open the clamp. Let solution flow through the tube to remove air. Clamp the tube.
20 Lubricate the tube 3 to 4 inches from the tip.
21 Separate the buttocks to see the anus.
22 Ask the person to take a deep breath through the mouth.
23 Insert the tube gently 3 to 4 inches into the adult's rectum (Fig. 16-2). Do this when the person is exhaling. Stop if the person complains of pain, you feel resistance, or bleeding occurs.
24 Check the amount of solution in the bag.
25 Unclamp the tube. Give the solution slowly (Fig. 16-3).
26 Ask the person to take slow deep breaths. This helps the person relax.
27 Clamp the tube if the person needs to defecate, has cramping, or starts to expel solution. Unclamp when symptoms subside.
28 Give the amount of solution ordered. Stop if the person cannot tolerate the procedure.
29 Clamp the tube before it is empty. This prevents air from entering the bowel.
30 Hold toilet tissue around the tube and against the anus. Remove the tube.
31 Discard the toilet tissue into the bedpan.
32 Wrap the tubing tip with paper towels. Place it inside the enema bag.
33 Help the person onto the bedpan. Raise the head of the bed, and raise the bed rail if used. Or assist the person to the bathroom or commode. The person wears a robe and non-skid footwear when up. The bed is in the lowest position.

Giving a Cleansing Enema—cont'd

Procedure—cont'd

34 Place the signal light and toilet tissue within reach. Remind the person not to flush the toilet.
35 Discard disposable items.
36 Remove the gloves. Decontaminate your hands.
37 Leave the room if the person can be left alone.
38 Return when the person signals. Or check on the person every 5 minutes. Knock before entering.
39 Decontaminate your hands, and put on gloves. Lower the bed rail if up.
40 Observe enema results for amount, color, consistency, and odor. Call for the nurse to observe the results.

41 Provide perineal care as needed.
42 Remove the waterproof pad.
43 Empty, clean, and disinfect the bedpan or commode. Flush the toilet after the nurse observes the results. Return items to their proper place.
44 Remove the gloves. Practice hand hygiene.
45 Assist with hand washing. Wear gloves if needed.
46 Cover the person. Remove the bath blanket.

Post-Procedure

47 Provide for comfort. (See the inside of the front book cover.)
48 Place the signal light within reach.
49 Lower the bed to its lowest position.
50 Raise or lower bed rails. Follow the care plan.
51 Unscreen the person.

52 Complete a safety check of the room. (See the inside of the front book cover.)
53 Follow agency policy for soiled linen and used supplies.
54 Decontaminate your hands.
55 Report and record your observations.

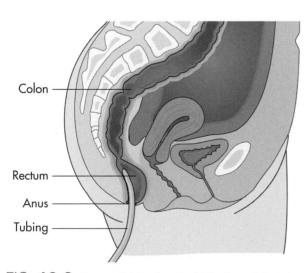

FIG. **16-2** Enema tubing inserted into the adult rectum.

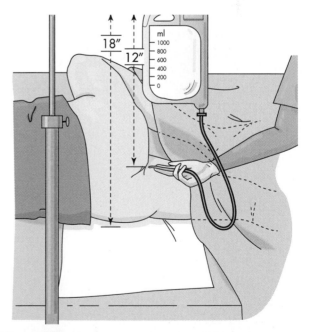

FIG. **16-3** Giving an enema. The person is in Sims' position. The enema bag hangs from an IV pole. The bag is 12 inches above the anus and 18 inches above the mattress.

The Small-Volume Enema

Small-volume enemas irritate and distend the rectum. This causes defecation. They are often ordered for constipation or when the bowel does not need complete cleansing.

These enemas are ready to give. The solution is usually given at room temperature. To give the enema, squeeze and roll up the plastic bottle from the bottom. Do not release pressure on the bottle. Otherwise, solution is drawn from the rectum back into the bottle.

Urge the person to retain the solution until there is a need to defecate. This usually takes about 5 to 10 minutes. Staying in the Sims' or left side-lying position helps to retain the enema.

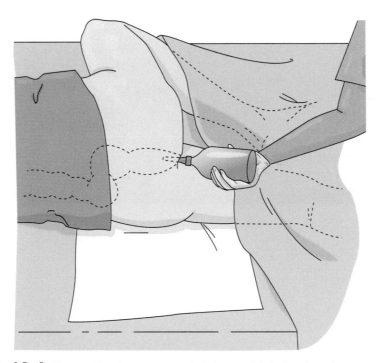

FIG. **16-4** The small-volume enema tip is inserted 2 inches into the rectum.

Giving a Small-Volume Enema

Quality of Life

Remember to:

■ Knock before entering the person's room

■ Address the person by name

■ Introduce yourself by name and title

■ Explain the procedure to the person before beginning and during the procedure

■ Protect the person's rights during the procedure

■ Handle the person gently during the procedure

Pre-Procedure

1   Follow *Delegation Guidelines: Enemas*, p. 280. See *Promoting Safety and Comfort: Enemas*, p. 281.

2   Practice hand hygiene.

3   Collect the following:
   • Small volume enema
   • Bedpan or commode
   • Waterproof pad
   • Toilet tissue
   • Gloves
   • Robe and non-skid footwear
   • Bath blanket

4   Identify the person. Check the ID bracelet against the assignment sheet. Call the person by name.

5   Provide for privacy.

6   Raise the bed for body mechanics. Bed rails are up if used.

Procedure

7   Lower the bed rail near you if up.

8   Decontaminate your hands. Put on the gloves.

9   Cover the person with a bath blanket. Fan-fold top linens to the foot of the bed.

10 Position the person in Sims' or a left side-lying position.

11 Place the waterproof pad under the buttocks.

12 Expose the anal area.

13 Position the bedpan near the person.

14 Remove the cap from the enema tip.

15 Separate the buttocks to see the anus.

16 Ask the person to take a deep breath through the mouth.

17 Insert the enema tip 2 inches into the rectum (Fig. 16-4). Do this when the person is exhaling. Insert the tip gently. Stop if the person complains of pain, you feel resistance, or bleeding occurs.

18 Squeeze and roll the bottle gently. Release pressure on the bottle after you remove the tip from the rectum.

19 Put the bottle into the box, tip first.

20 Help the person onto the bedpan; raise the head of the bed. Raise or lower bed rails according to the care plan. Or assist the person to the bathroom or commode. The person wears a robe and non-skid footwear when up. The bed is in the lowest position.

21 Place the signal light and toilet tissue within reach. Remind the person not to flush the toilet.

22 Discard disposable items.

23 Remove the gloves. Decontaminate your hands.

24 Leave the room if the person can be left alone.

25 Return when the person signals. Or check on the person every 5 minutes. Knock before entering.

26 Decontaminate your hands. Put on gloves.

27 Lower the bed rail if up.

28 Observe enema results for amount, color, consistency, shape, and odor.

29 Help the person with perineal care.

30 Remove the waterproof pad.

31 Empty, clean, and disinfect the bedpan or commode. Flush the toilet after the nurse observes the results.

32 Return equipment to its proper place.

33 Remove the gloves. Practice hand hygiene.

34 Assist with hand washing. Wear gloves if necessary.

35 Return top linens. Remove the bath blanket.

Post-Procedure

36 Follow steps 47 through 55 in procedure: *Giving a Cleansing Enema*, p. 283.

The Oil-Retention Enema

Oil-retention enemas relieve constipation and fecal impactions. The oil is retained for 30 to 60 minutes or longer (1 to 3 hours). Retaining oil softens feces and lubricates the rectum. This lets feces pass with ease. Most oil-retention enemas are commercially prepared.

Giving an oil-retention enema is like giving a small-volume enema. After giving an oil-retention enema:

- Leave the person in the Sims' or left side-lying position. Cover the person for warmth.
- Urge the person to retain the enema for the time ordered.
- Place extra waterproof pads on the bed if needed.
- Check the person often while the person retains the enema.

THE PERSON WITH AN OSTOMY

Sometimes part of the intestines are removed surgically. Cancer, bowel disease, and trauma (stab or bullet wounds) are common reasons. An ostomy is sometimes necessary. An **ostomy** is a surgically created opening. The opening is called a **stoma.** The person wears a pouch over the stoma to collect feces and flatus.

Colostomy

A **colostomy** is a surgically created opening *(stomy)* between the colon *(colo)* and abdominal wall. Part of the colon is brought out onto the abdominal wall and a stoma made. Feces and flatus pass through the stoma instead of through the anus. With a permanent colostomy, the diseased part of the colon is removed. A temporary colostomy gives the diseased or injured bowel time to heal. After healing, surgery is done to reconnect the bowel.

The colostomy site depends on the site of disease or injury (Fig. 16-5). Stool consistency depends on the colostomy site. Consistency ranges from liquid to formed. The more colon remaining to absorb water, the more solid and formed the stool. If the colostomy is near the start of the colon, stools are liquid. A colostomy near the end of the colon results in formed stools.

Feces irritate the skin. Skin care prevents skin breakdown around the stoma. The skin is washed and dried. Then a skin barrier is applied around the stoma. It prevents feces from having contact with the skin. The skin barrier is part of the pouch or a separate device.

Ileostomy

An **ileostomy** is a surgically created opening *(stomy)* between the ileum (small intestine *[ileo]*) and the abdominal wall. Part of the ileum is brought out onto the

abdominal wall, and a stoma is made. The entire colon is removed (Fig. 16-6). Liquid feces drain constantly from an ileostomy. Water is not absorbed because the colon was removed. Feces in the small intestine contain digestive juices that are very irritating to the skin. The ileostomy pouch must fit well. Feces must not touch the skin. Good skin care is required.

Ostomy Pouches

The pouch has an adhesive backing that is applied to the skin. Sometimes pouches are secured to ostomy belts (Fig. 16-7). Many pouches have a drain at the bottom that closes with clips, clamps, or wire closures. The drain is opened to empty the pouch. The pouch is emptied when feces are present. It is opened when it balloons or bulges with flatus. The drain is wiped with toilet tissue before it is closed.

The pouch is changed every 3 to 7 days and when it leaks. Frequent pouch changes can damage the skin.

Odors are prevented. Good hygiene is needed. The pouch is emptied when feces are present. A deodorant is put in the pouch as directed by the nurse. The person is advised to avoid gas-forming foods.

The person can wear normal clothes. However, tight garments can prevent feces from entering the pouch. Also, bulging from feces and flatus can be seen with tight clothes.

Peristalsis increases after eating. Therefore stomas are usually quiet before breakfast. Expelling feces is less likely at this time. If the person showers or bathes with the pouch off, it is best done before breakfast. Delay a shower or bath for 1 or 2 hours after a new pouch is applied. This gives adhesive time to stick to the skin.

Do not flush pouches down the toilet. Follow agency policy for disposing of them.

PROMOTING SAFETY AND COMFORT
Ostomy Pouches

Safety

When emptying an ostomy pouch, contact with feces is likely. They may contain microbes or blood. Follow Standard Precautions and the Bloodborne Pathogen Standard.

Report signs of skin breakdown to the nurse.

Comfort

Stomas do not have nerve endings. Therefore, they are not painful. You will not hurt the person when touching the stoma.

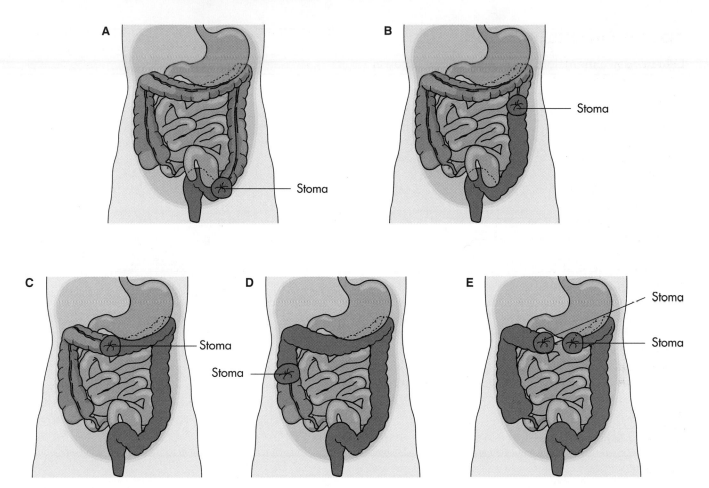

FIG. **16-5** Colostomy sites. *Shading* shows the part of the bowel surgically removed. **A,** Sigmoid colostomy. **B,** Descending colostomy. **C,** Transverse colostomy. **D,** Ascending colostomy. **E,** Double-barrel colostomy has two stomas. One allows for the excretion of feces. The other is for the introduction of drugs to help the bowel heal. This type of colostomy is usually temporary.

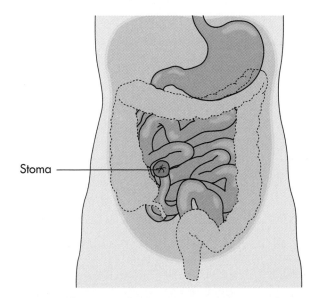

FIG. **16-6** An ileostomy. The entire large intestine is surgically removed.

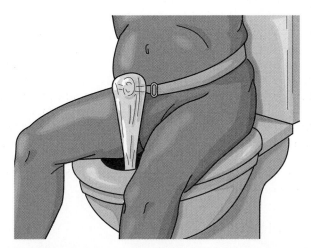

FIG. **16-7** The ostomy pouch is secured to an ostomy belt. The pouch is emptied by directing it into the toilet and unclamping the end.

FOCUS ON THE PERSON

Like urinary elimination, people usually have bowel movements in private. Illness, disease, surgery, and aging can affect this very private act.

See Focus on the Person: Assisting With Bowel Elimination.

Focus on the **PERSON**

Assisting With Bowel Elimination

Providing comfort—Physical and mental comfort promotes bowel elimination. The person must be in a comfortable position. Privacy is important. So is having enough time to defecate. The person should not feel rushed.

Ethical behavior—Odors and sounds often occur with bowel elimination. You must control your verbal and nonverbal responses. Do not comment about odors or sounds.

Remaining independent—Persons with ostomies manage their own care if able. Some have had ostomies for a long time. They may have special routines or care measures. Their choices in ostomy care are followed.

Speaking up—Many patients and residents tend to their own bowel elimination needs. However, information is still needed for the person's record and the nursing process. You may need to ask some of these questions:

- "Did you have a bowel movement today?"

- "Please tell me about your bowel movement. When did you have it? What was the amount? Were the stools formed or loose? Did you have any bleeding, pain, or problems having a bowel movement?"
- "Did you pass any gas?"
- "How much gas did you pass?"
- "Do you need help cleaning yourself?"

OBRA and other laws—Leaving a person sitting or lying in his or her urine or feces is neglect. It is a form of physical abuse. State laws and OBRA require the reporting and investigating of abuse. If found guilty of abuse, neglect, or mistreatment of a resident, you will lose your job. The offense is noted on your registry information. You cannot work in a nursing center or on a skilled care nursing unit in a hospital.

Nursing teamwork—The need to have a bowel movement may be urgent. Answer signal lights promptly. Also help co-workers answer signal lights. Patients and residents must not be left sitting on toilets, bedpans, or commodes. They must not be left sitting or lying in feces.

REVIEW QUESTIONS

Circle the **BEST** answer.

1 Which is *false?*
   a A person must have a bowel movement every day.
   b Stools are normally brown, soft, and formed.
   c Diarrhea occurs when feces move rapidly through the bowels.
   d Constipation results when feces move slowly through the colon.

2 The prolonged retention and accumulation of feces in the rectum is called
   a Constipation
   b Fecal impaction
   c Diarrhea
   d Fecal incontinence

3 Which will *not* promote comfort and safety for bowel elimination?
   a Asking visitors to leave the room
   b Helping the person to a sitting position
   c Offering the bedpan after meals
   d Telling the person that you will return in a few minutes

4 Bowel training is aimed at
   a Gaining control of bowel movements and developing a regular elimination pattern
   b Ostomy control
   c Preventing fecal impaction, constipation, and anal incontinence
   d Preventing bleeding

5 Which is *not* used for a cleansing enema?
   a Soap suds
   b Saline
   c Oil
   d Tap water

6 Which is *false?*
   a Enema solutions should be 105° F (40.5° C).
   b The Sims' position is used for an enema.
   c The enema bag is held 12 inches above the anus.
   d The enema solution is given rapidly.

7 In adults, the enema tube is inserted
   a 2 inches
   b 4 inches
   c 6 inches
   d 8 inches

8 The oil-retention enema is usually retained for
   a 10 to 15 minutes
   b 15 to 30 minutes
   c 30 to 60 minutes
   d 60 to 90 minutes

9 Which statement about ostomies is *false?*
   a Good skin care around the stoma is essential.
   b Deodorants can control odors.
   c The person wears a pouch.
   d Feces are always liquid.

10 An ostomy pouch is usually emptied
   a Every morning
   b At bedtime
   c When feces are present
   d Every 3 days

Answers to these questions are on p. 469.

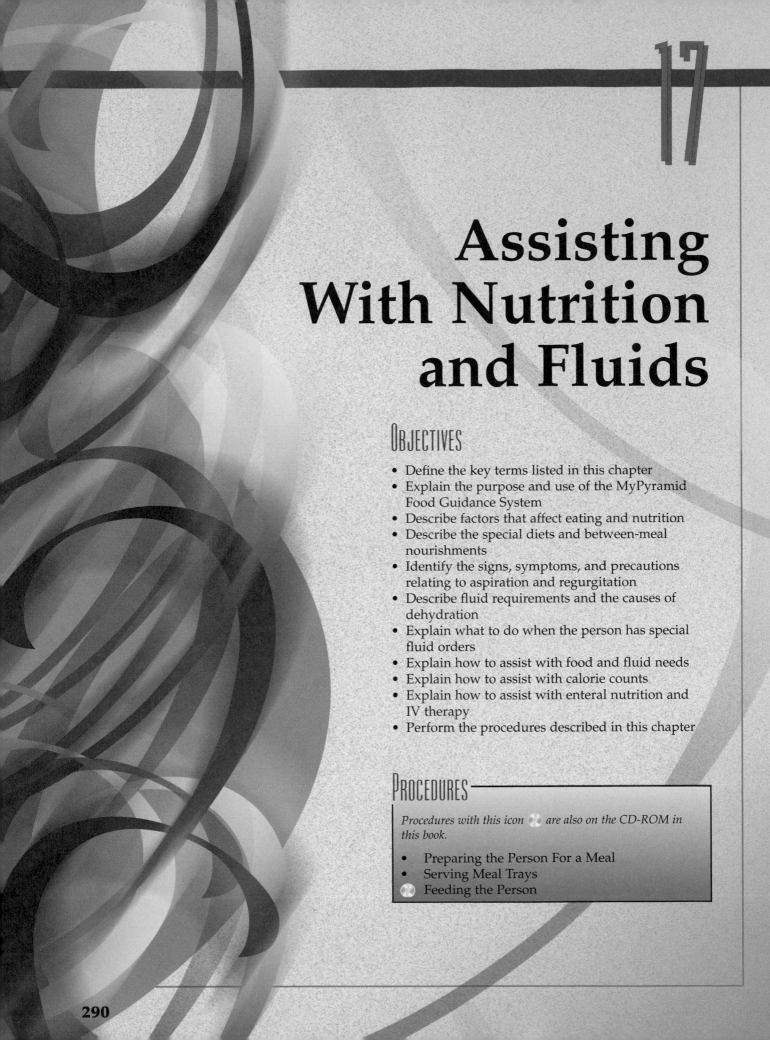

Assisting With Nutrition and Fluids

OBJECTIVES

- Define the key terms listed in this chapter
- Explain the purpose and use of the MyPyramid Food Guidance System
- Describe factors that affect eating and nutrition
- Describe the special diets and between-meal nourishments
- Identify the signs, symptoms, and precautions relating to aspiration and regurgitation
- Describe fluid requirements and the causes of dehydration
- Explain what to do when the person has special fluid orders
- Explain how to assist with food and fluid needs
- Explain how to assist with calorie counts
- Explain how to assist with enteral nutrition and IV therapy
- Perform the procedures described in this chapter

PROCEDURES

Procedures with this icon are also on the CD-ROM in this book.

- Preparing the Person For a Meal
- Serving Meal Trays
- Feeding the Person

Key Terms

anorexia The loss of appetite

aspiration Breathing fluid or an object into the lungs

calorie The amount of energy produced when the body burns food

dehydration A decrease in the amount of water in body tissues

dysphagia Difficulty (*dys*) swallowing (*phagia*)

edema The swelling of body tissues with water

enteral nutrition Giving nutrients through the gastrointestinal tract (*enteral*)

flow rate The number of drops per minute (*gtt/min*)

gavage Tube feeding

intravenous (IV) therapy Giving fluids through a needle or catheter inserted into a vein; IV and IV infusion

nutrient A substance that is ingested, digested, absorbed, and used by the body

nutrition The processes involved in the ingestion, digestion, absorption, and use of foods and fluids by the body

regurgitation The backward flow of food from the stomach into the mouth

Food and water are physical needs. They are necessary for life. The amount and quality of food affects physical and mental well-being. A poor diet and poor eating habits increase the risk for infection and disease. Chronic illnesses become worse. Healing problems occur. Physical and mental function is affected, increasing the risk for accidents and injuries.

BASIC NUTRITION

Nutrition is the processes involved in the ingestion, digestion, absorption, and use of foods and fluids by the body. Good nutrition is needed for growth, healing, and body functions. Foods and fluids contain nutrients. A **nutrient** is a substance that is ingested, digested, absorbed, and used by the body. Nutrients are grouped into fats, proteins, carbohydrates, vitamins, minerals, and water.

Fats, proteins, and carbohydrates give the body fuel for energy. A **calorie** is the amount of energy produced when the body burns food.

- 1 gram of fat—9 calories
- 1 gram of protein—4 calories
- 1 gram of carbohydrate—4 calories

MyPyramid

Released in April 2005, the *MyPryamid Food Guidance System* (Fig. 17-1, p. 292) replaces the 1992 *Food Guide Pyramid*. Smart and healthy food choices and daily activity are encouraged.

The MyPyramid symbol shows the "Steps To a Healthier You."

- *The kind and amounts of food to eat daily.* This depends on the person's age, gender (male or female), and activity level. (See the MyPyramid.gov website.)
- *Gradual improvement.* People can take small steps each day to improve their diet and life-style.
- *Physical activity.* This is shown by the steps and the person climbing them. They are a reminder of the importance of physical activity. For health benefits, at least 30 minutes of physical activity are needed on most days of the week. It is best to do so every day. Activity should be moderate or vigorous (Box 17-1, p. 293). The activity can be done in one 30-minute period. Or it can be done in 2 or 3 parts as long as the total time is at least 30 minutes a day.
- *Variety.* The six color bands stand for the 5 food groups and oils. Food from the 5 groups are needed each day for good health.
- *Moderation.* This means to avoid extremes. The bands narrow as they go from the bottom to the top of the pyramid. Foods near the base have the most nutritional value and the fewest calories. They have little or no solid fats, added sugars, or caloric sweeteners. Foods lower in the band should be chosen more often than those higher in the band.
- *The right amount from each food group band.* The bands differ in width. The widths suggest how much food to choose from each group. The wider the band, the more foods the person should choose from that group.

Grains

The orange band is for grains. Any food made from wheat, rice, oats, cornmeal, barley, or other cereal grain is a grain product. Bread, pasta, oatmeal, breakfast cereals, tortillas, and grits are examples. There are two types of grains:

- *Whole grains* contain the entire grain kernel. Whole-wheat flour, bulgur (cracked wheat), oatmeal, whole cornmeal, and brown rice are examples.
- *Refined grains* have been processed to remove the grain kernel. These grains have a finer texture. White flour, white bread, and white rice are examples. They have less dietary fiber than whole grains.

A person needs at least 3 ounces of whole-grain cereals, breads, crackers, rice, or pasta every day. For a 2000-calorie diet, 6 ounces are needed daily. See Figure 17-1 and Table 17-1.

Grains have the following health benefits:

■ Reduce the risk of coronary artery disease.

■ May prevent constipation.
■ May help with weight management.
■ May prevent certain birth defects.
■ Contain these nutrients—dietary fiber, and several B vitamins (thiamin, riboflavin, niacin, folate), and minerals (iron, magnesium, and selenium).

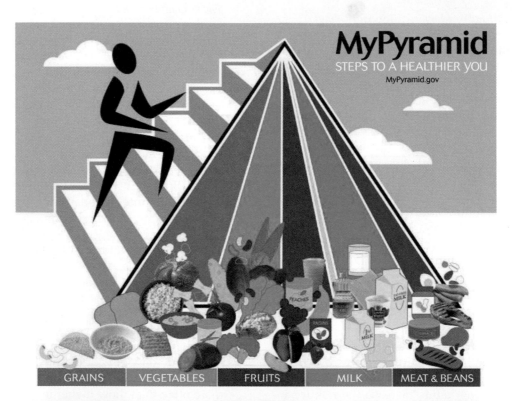

FIG. **17-1** MyPyramid: Steps to a healthier you. (Courtesy U.S. Department of Agriculture, Center for Nutrition and Policy Promotion, April 2005, CNPP-15).

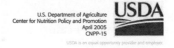

BOX 17-1	MyPyramid: Physical Activity

Moderate Physical Activities	**Vigorous Physical Activities**
• Walking briskly (about 3½ miles per hour) • Hiking • Gardening/yard work • Dancing • Golf (walking and carrying clubs) • Bicycling (less than 10 miles per hour) • Weight training (general light workout)	• Running/jogging (5 miles per hour) • Bicycling (more than 10 miles per hour) • Swimming (freestyle laps) • Aerobics • Walking very fast (4½ miles per hour) • Heavy yard work (chopping wood) • Weight lifting (vigorous effort) • Basketball (competitive)

TABLE 17-1	MyPyramid Serving Sizes For a 2000-Calorie Diet	
Group (color band)	**Servings**	**Serving Sizes**
Grains (orange band)	At least 6 ounces (6 oz) of whole-grain cereals, breads, crackers, rice, or pasta daily	1 ounce = 1 slice of bread 1 ounce = 1 cup of breakfast cereal 1 ounce = ½ cup of cooked rice, cereal, or pasta
Vegetables (green band)	At least 2½ cups per day Vegetable subgroups amounts per week: Dark green—3 cups Orange—2 cups Dry beans and peas—3 cups Starchy—3 cups Other—6½ cups	1 cup = 1 cup of raw or cooked vegetables or vegetable juice 1 cup = 2 cups of raw leafy greens
Fruits (red band)	At least 2 cups per day	1 cup = 1 cup fruit 1 cup = 1 cup fruit juice 1 cup = ½ cup dried fruit
Milk (blue band)	At least 3 cups per day	1 cup = 1 cup milk or yogurt 1 cup = 1½ ounces natural cheese 1 cup = 2 ounces processed cheese
Meat and beans (purple band)	At least 5½ ounces per day	1 ounce = 1 ounce of lean meat, poultry, or fish 1 ounce = 1 egg 1 ounce = 1 tablespoon peanut butter 1 ounce = ¼ cup cooked dry beans 1 ounce = ½ ounce of nuts or seeds
Oils (yellow band)	At least 6 teaspoons daily	1 teaspoon = 1 teaspoon

Modified from MyPyramid: Food Intake Patterns, US Department of Agriculture, Center for Nutrition and Policy Promotion, April 2005.

Vegetables

The green band is for vegetables. A person should vary the kinds of vegetables eaten. Most should come from the dark green, orange, and dry peas and beans subgroups.

- *Dark green vegetables*—bok choy, collard greens, dark green leafy lettuce, kale, mesclun, mustard greens, romaine lettuce, spinach, turnips, watercress
- *Orange vegetables*—acorn squash, butternut squash, carrots, hubbard squash, pumpkin, sweet potatoes
- *Dry beans and peas (legumes)*—black beans, black-eyed peas, garbanzo peas (chickpeas), kidney beans, lentils, lima beans (mature), navy beans, pinto beans, soy beans, split peas, tofu, white beans
- *Starchy vegetables*—corn, green peas, lima beans (green), potatoes
- *Other vegetables*—artichokes, asparagus, bean sprouts, beets, Brussels sprouts, cabbage, cauliflower, celery, cucumbers, eggplant, green beans, green or red peppers, iceberg (head) lettuce, mushrooms, okra, onions, parsnips, tomatoes, tomato juice, vegetable juice, turnips, wax beans, zucchini

A least 1 cup of vegetables is needed daily on a 1000-calorie diet. For a 2000 calorie diet, 2½ cups are needed daily. See Figure 17-1 and Table 17-1. A person can choose fresh, frozen, canned, and dried vegetables as well as vegetable juices.

Vegetables have these health benefits:

- May reduce the risk for stroke, coronary artery disease, other cardiovascular diseases, and type 2 diabetes.
- Protect against certain cancers. Cancers of the mouth, stomach, and colon-rectum are examples.
- May reduce the risk of developing kidney stones.
- May reduce the risk of bone loss.
- May help lower calorie intake. Most vegetables are naturally low in fat and calories.
- Contain no cholesterol.
- Contain these nutrients—potassium, dietary fiber, folate (folic acid), vitamin A, vitamin E, and vitamin C.

Fruits

The red band is for fruits. Any fruit or 100% fruit juice counts as part of the fruit group. Fruit choices should vary. Fresh, frozen, canned, or dried fruits are best. Avoid fruits canned in syrup. Syrup contains added sugar. Choose fruits canned in 100% fruit juice or water.

For a 1000-calorie diet, at least 1 cup of fruit is needed daily. For a 2000-calorie diet, 2 cups are needed daily. See Figure 17-1 and Table 17-1.

Fruits have these health benefits:

- May reduce the risk for stroke, coronary artery disease, other cardiovascular diseases, and type 2 diabetes.
- Protect against certain cancers. Cancers of the mouth, stomach, and colon-rectum are examples.
- May reduce the risk of developing kidney stones.
- May reduce the risk of bone loss.
- May help lower calorie intake. Most fruits are naturally low in fat and calories.
- Contain no cholesterol.
- Are naturally low in sodium.
- Contain these nutrients—potassium, dietary fiber, vitamin C, and folate (folic acid).

Milk

The blue band is for milk and milk products. Low-fat or fat-free choices are best. The milk group includes all fluid milk. It also includes yogurt and cheese. (Cream, cream cheese, and butter are not part of the group.)

On a 1000-calorie diet, 2 cups are needed daily. A 2000-calorie diet requires 3 cups daily. See Figure 17-1 and Table 17-1.

Milk has these health benefits:

- Helps build and maintain bone mass throughout the lifespan. This may reduce the risk of osteoporosis.
- Improves the overall quality of the diet.
- Contains these nutrients—calcium, potassium, and vitamin D.

Meat and Beans

The purple band is for meats and beans. This group includes all foods made from meat, poultry, fish, dry beans or peas, eggs, nuts, and seeds. Most meat and poultry choices should be lean or low-fat. Fish, nuts, and seeds contain healthy oils. They should be chosen often instead of meat or poultry.

Remember the following when selecting foods from this group:

- Choose lean or low-fat meat and poultry. Higher fat choices include regular ground beef (75% to 80% lean) and chicken with skin.
- Using fat for cooking increases the caloric value of the food. Fried chicken and eggs fried in butter are examples.
- Salmon, trout, and herring are rich in substances that may reduce the risk of heart disease.
- Liver and other organ meats are high in cholesterol.
- Egg yolks are high in cholesterol. Egg whites are cholesterol-free.
- Processed meats have added sodium (salt). They include ham, sausage, frankfurters, and luncheon and deli meats.
- Sunflower seeds, almonds, and hazelnuts are rich sources of vitamin E.

A 1000-calorie diet allows 2 ounces daily from the meat and beans group. A 2000-calorie diet allows 5½ ounces daily. See Figure 17-1 and Table 17-1.

Foods in this group are high in fat and cholesterol. Heart disease is a major risk. However, the meat and beans group provides these nutrients needed for health and body maintenance:

- Protein
- B vitamins (niacin, thiamin, riboflavin, and B6) and vitamin E
- Iron, zinc, and magnesium

Oils

The yellow band is for oils. Oils are fats that are liquid at room temperature. Vegetable oils used in cooking are examples. They include canola oil, corn oil, and olive oil. Some foods are naturally high in oil—nuts, olives, some fish, and avocados.

Remember the following when making oil choices:

- Oils are high in calories.
- The best oil choices come from fish, nuts, and vegetable oils.
- Some foods are mainly oil. Mayonnaise, certain salad dressings, and soft margarine (tub or squeeze) are examples.
- Oils from plant sources do not contain cholesterol.
- Solid fats are those that are solid at room temperature. Common solid fats include butter, beef fat (tallow, suet), chicken fat, pork fat (lard), stick margarine, and shortening.

Oils contain some fatty acids that are essential for health. Oils also are a major source of vitamin E.

Enough oil is usually consumed daily from nuts, fish, cooking oil, and salad dressings. On a 1000-calorie diet, 3 teaspoons of oils are allowed. On a 2000-calorie diet, 6 teaspoons of oils are allowed. See Figure 17-1 and Table 17-1.

Nutrients

No food or food group has every essential nutrient. A well-balanced diet has servings from the five food groups in MyPyramid. It ensures an adequate intake of essential nutrients.

- *Protein* is the most important nutrient. It is needed for tissue growth and repair. Sources include meat, fish, poultry, eggs, milk and milk products, cereals, beans, peas, and nuts.
- *Carbohydrates* provide energy and fiber for bowel elimination. They are found in fruits, vegetables, breads, cereals, and sugar. Fiber is not digested. It provides the bulky part of chyme for elimination.

- *Fats* provide energy. They add flavor to food and help the body use certain vitamins. Sources include meats, lard, butter, shortening, oils, milk, cheese, egg yolks, and nuts. Dietary fat not needed by the body is stored as body fat (adipose tissue).
- *Vitamins* are needed for certain body functions. They do not provide calories. The body stores vitamins A, D, E, and K. Vitamin C and the B complex vitamins are not stored. They must be ingested daily. The lack of a certain vitamin results in signs and symptoms of an illness.
- *Minerals* are needed for bone and tooth formation, nerve and muscle function, fluid balance, and other body processes.
- *Water* is needed for all body processes. See p. 299.

FACTORS AFFECTING EATING AND NUTRITION

Many factors affect nutrition and eating habits. Some begin during infancy and continue throughout life. Others develop later.

- *Age.* Many changes occur in the digestive system. See Chapter 7.
- *Culture.* Culture influences food choices and food preparation. Frying, baking, smoking, or roasting food or eating raw food are cultural practices. So is the use of sauces and spices. (*See Caring About Culture: Food Practices*, p. 296.)
- *Religion.* Selecting, preparing, and eating food often involve religious practices. A person may follow all, some, or none of the dietary practices of his or her faith. You must respect the person's religious practices.
- *Appetite.* Appetite relates to the desire for food. A hungry person seeks food and eats until satisfied. However, loss of appetite (**anorexia**) can occur. Causes include illness, drugs, anxiety, pain, and depression. Unpleasant sights, thoughts, and smells are other causes. Older persons may have loss of appetite from decreased senses of taste and smell.
- *Personal choice.* Food likes and dislikes are personal. They are influenced by food served in the home. Body reactions affect food choices. People usually avoid foods that cause allergic reactions, nausea, vomiting, diarrhea, indigestion, or headaches.
- *Illness.* Appetite usually decreases during illness and recovery from injuries and surgery. However, nutritional needs are increased. The body must fight infection, heal tissue, and replace lost blood cells. Nutrients lost through vomiting and diarrhea need replacement. Some diseases and drugs cause a sore mouth. This makes eating painful.

Caring About Culture

Food Practices

Food practices vary among cultural groups. Rice and beans are protein sources in *Mexico*. In the *Philippines*, rice is preferred with every meal. A diet high in starch and fat is common in *Poland*. Potatoes, rye, and wheat are common. The diet in *China* is low in fat but high in sodium. The sodium content is from the use of soy sauce and dried and preserved foods.

Eating beef is common in the *United States*. Beef is not eaten in *India*.

(Modified from D'Avanzo CE, Geissler EM: *Pocket guide to cultural health assessment*, ed 3, St Louis, 2003, Mosby.)

OBRA DIETARY REQUIREMENTS

OBRA has these requirements for food served in nursing centers:

- The person's nutritional and dietary needs are met.
- The person's diet is well-balanced. It is nourishing and tastes good. Food is well seasoned. It is not too salty or too sweet.
- Food is appetizing. It has an appealing aroma and is attractive.
- Hot food is served hot. Cold food is served cold.
- Food is served promptly.
- Food is prepared to meet each person's needs. Some people need food cut, ground, or chopped. Others have special diets ordered by the doctor.
- Each person receives at least three meals a day. A bedtime snack is offered.
- The center provides any special eating equipment and utensils (Fig. 17-2). Called adaptive equipment, such devices promote independence in eating. Make sure needed equipment is available for the person.

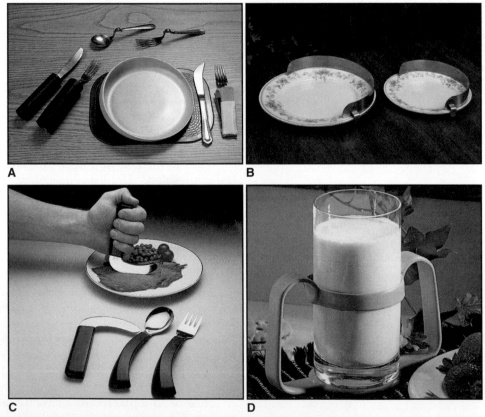

FIG. **17-2** Eating utensils for persons with special needs. **A,** The curved fork fits over the hand. The rounded plate helps keep food on the plate. Special grips and swivel handles are helpful for some persons. **B,** Plate guards help keep food on the plate. **C,** Knives with rounded blades are rocked back and forth to cut food. The person does not need a fork in one hand and a knife in the other. **D,** Glass or cup holder. (Courtesy Sammons Preston Roylan: an AbilityOne Co., Bolingbrook, Ill.)

SPECIAL DIETS

Doctors may order special diets for a nutritional deficiency or a disease. They also order them to remove or decrease certain substances in the diet. The health team works together to meet the person's nutritional needs.

Regular diet, general diet, and *house diet* mean no dietary limits or restrictions. Table 17-2 describes common diets.

TABLE **17-2**	Special Diets	
Diet	**Use**	**Foods Allowed**
Clear-liquid—foods liquid at body temperature and which leave small amounts of residue; nonirritating and nongas-forming	Postoperatively, acute illness, infection, nausea and vomiting, and before gastrointestinal exams	Water, tea, and coffee (without milk or cream); carbonated beverages; gelatin; clear fruit juices (apple, grape, and cranberry); fat-free clear broth; hard candy, sugar, and Popsicles
Full-liquid—foods liquid at room temperature or melt at body temperature	Advance from clear-liquid diet postoperatively; for stomach irritation, fever, nausea, and vomiting; and for persons unable to chew, swallow, or digest solid foods	Foods on the clear-liquid diet; custard; eggnog; strained soups; strained fruit and vegetable juices; milk and milk shakes; strained, cooked cereals; plain ice cream and sherbet; pudding; yogurt
Mechanical soft—semi-solid foods that are easily digested	Advance from full-liquid diet, chewing problems, gastrointestinal disorders, and infections	All liquids; eggs (not fried); broiled, baked, or roasted meat, fish, or poultry that is chopped or shredded; mild cheeses (American, Swiss, cheddar, cream, and cottage); strained fruit juices; refined bread (no crust) and crackers; cooked cereal; cooked or pureed vegetables; cooked or canned fruit without skin or seeds; pudding; plain cakes and soft cookies without fruit or nuts
Fiber- and residue-restricted—food that leaves a small amount of residue in the colon	Diseases of the colon and diarrhea	Coffee, tea, milk, carbonated beverages, strained fruit juices; refined bread and crackers; creamed and refined cereal; rice; cottage and cream cheese; eggs (not fried); plain puddings and cakes; gelatin; custard; sherbet and ice cream; strained vegetable juices; canned or cooked fruit without skin or seeds; potatoes (not fried); strained cooked vegetables; plain pasta; and no raw fruits and vegetables
High-fiber—foods that increase the amount of residue and fiber in the colon to stimulate peristalsis	Constipation and GI disorders	All fruits and vegetables; whole wheat bread; whole grain cereals; fried foods; whole grain rice; milk, cream, butter, and cheese; and meats
Bland—foods that are mechanically and chemically nonirritating and low in roughage; foods served at moderate temperatures; and no strong spices or condiments	Ulcers, gallbladder disorders, and some intestinal disorders; after abdominal surgery	Lean meats; white bread; creamed and refined cereals; cream or cottage cheese; gelatin; plain puddings, cakes, and cookies; eggs (not fried); butter and cream; canned fruits and vegetables without skin and seeds; strained fruit juices; potatoes (not fried); pastas and rice; strained or soft cooked carrots, peas, beets, spinach, squash, and asparagus tips; creamed soups from allowed vegetables; no fried foods
High-calorie—calorie intake is increased to about 3000 to 4000; includes 3 full meals and between-meal snacks	Weight gain and some thyroid imbalances	Dietary increases in all foods; large portions of a regular diet with 3 between-meal snacks
Calorie-controlled—provides adequate nutrients while controlling calories to promote weight loss and reduction of body fat	Weight reduction	Foods low in fats and carbohydrates and lean meats; avoid butter, cream, rice, gravies, salad oils, noodles, cakes, pastries, carbonated and alcoholic beverages, candy, potato chips, and similar foods

continued

TABLE 17-2 Special Diets—cont'd

Diet	Use	Foods Allowed
High-iron—foods that are high in iron	Anemia; following blood loss; for women during the reproductive years	Liver and other organ meats; lean meats; egg yolks; shellfish; dried fruits; dried beans; green leafy vegetables; lima beans; peanut butter; enriched breads and cereals
Fat-controlled (low-cholesterol)—foods low in fat and foods prepared without adding fat	Heart disease, gallbladder disease, disorders of fat digestion, liver disease, diseases of the pancreas	Skim milk or buttermilk; cottage cheese (no other cheeses allowed); gelatin; sherbet; fruit; lean meat, poultry, and fish (baked, broiled, or roasted); fat-free broth; soups made with skim milk; margarine; rice, pasta, breads, and cereals; vegetables; potatoes
High-protein—aids and promotes tissue healing	For burns, high fever, infection, and some liver diseases	Meat, milk, eggs, cheese, fish, poultry; breads and cereals; green leafy vegetables
Sodium-controlled—a certain amount of sodium is allowed	Heart disease, fluid retention, liver disease, and some kidney diseases	Fruits and vegetables and unsalted butter are allowed; adding salt at the table is not allowed; highly salted foods and foods high in sodium are not allowed; the use of salt during cooking may be restricted
Diabetes meal planning—the same amount of carbohydrates, protein, and fat are eaten at the same time each day	Diabetes	Depends on nutritional and energy requirements

The Sodium-Controlled Diet

The average amount of sodium in the daily diet is 3000 to 5000 mg. The body needs no more than 2400 mg. Healthy people excrete excess sodium in the urine.

Heart, liver, and kidney diseases, and certain drugs cause the body to retain extra sodium. Sodium causes the body to retain water. If there is too much sodium, the body retains more water. Tissues swell with water. There is excess fluid in the blood vessels. The heart has to work harder. The sodium-controlled diet decreases the amount of sodium in the body. The body retains less water. Less water in the tissues and blood vessels reduces the heart's workload.

The doctor orders the amount of sodium restriction.

Diabetes Meal Planning

Diabetes is a chronic disease from a lack of insulin (Chapter 24). The pancreas produces and secretes insulin. Insulin lets the body use sugar. Without enough insulin, sugar builds up in the bloodstream. It is not used by cells for energy. Diabetes is usually treated with insulin or other drugs, diet, and exercise.

The dietitian and person develop a meal plan. Consistency is key. It involves:
- Food preferences (likes and dislikes), eating habits, mealtimes, culture, and life-style. Food amounts and preparation may be restricted.
- Calories needed. The same amount of carbohydrates, protein, and fat are eaten each day.
- Eating meals and snacks at regular times. The person eats at the same time every day. This is done to maintain a certain blood sugar level.

Serve the person's meals and snacks on time. Then check the tray to see what was eaten. Tell the nurse what the person did and did not eat. If all food was not eaten, a between-meal nourishment is needed (p. 306). The nurse tells you what to give. The between-meal nourishment makes up for food not eaten at the meal.

The Dysphagia Diet

Dysphagia means difficulty (*dys*) swallowing (*phagia*). In severe cases, food enters the airway (aspiration). **Aspiration** is breathing fluid or an object into the lungs (p. 307). To prevent aspiration, food thickness is changed to meet the person's needs (Box 17-2).

Promote safety when feeding a person with dysphagia. You must:
- Know the signs and symptoms of dysphagia (Box 17-3).
- Position the person's head and neck correctly. Follow the care plan.
- Feed the person according to the care plan.
- Follow aspiration precautions (Box 17-4).
- Report changes in how the person eats.
- Report choking, coughing, or difficulty breathing during or after meals. Also report abnormal breathing or respiratory sounds. Report these observations at once.

BOX 17-2 Dysphagia Diet

Consistency	Description
Thickened liquid	No lumps. Pureed with milk, gravy, or broth to thickness of baby food. Thickener is added to some pureed foods as needed. Does not mound on a plate. May be called creamy or sauce. Stir before serving if the food settles. Use a spoon.
Medium thick	The thickness of nectar or V-8 juice (does not hold its shape). Stir right before serving.
Extra thick	Thick like honey. Mounds a bit on a spoon. Drinkable from a cup. Stir before serving.
Yogurt like consistency	Thick like yogurt. Holds its shape. Served with a spoon.
Puree	No lumps; mounds on plate. May be thick like mashed potatoes.

BOX 17-3 Signs and Symptoms of Dysphagia

- The person avoids foods that need chewing.
- The person avoids foods with certain textures and temperatures.
- The person tires during a meal.
- Food spills out of the person's mouth while eating.
- Food "pockets" or is "squirreled" in the person's cheeks.
- The person eats slowly, especially solid foods.
- The person complains that food will not go down or the food is stuck.
- The person frequently coughs or chokes before, during, or after swallowing.
- The person regurgitates food after eating (p. 307).
- The person spits out food suddenly and almost violently.
- Food comes up through the person's nose.
- The person is hoarse—especially after eating.
- After swallowing, the person makes gargling sounds while talking or breathing.
- The person has a runny nose, sneezes, or has excessive drooling of saliva.
- The person complains of frequent heartburn.
- Appetite is decreased.

FLUID BALANCE

Water is needed to live. Death can result from too much or too little water. Water is ingested through fluids and foods. It is lost through urine, feces, vomit, the skin (perspiration), and the lungs (expiration).

The amount of fluid taken in (intake) and the amount of fluid lost (output) must be equal. If fluid intake exceeds fluid output, tissues swell with water. This is called **edema.** Edema is common in people with heart and kidney diseases. **Dehydration** is a decrease in the amount of water in body tissues. Fluid output exceeds intake. Common causes are poor fluid intake, vomiting, diarrhea, bleeding, excess sweating, and increased urine production.

Normal Fluid Requirements

An adult needs 1500 ml of water daily to survive. About 2000 to 2500 ml of fluid per day are needed for normal fluid balance. Water requirements increase with hot weather, exercise, fever, illness, and excess fluid losses.

Body water decreases with age. So does the thirst sensation. Older persons may not feel thirsty even when their bodies need water. Offer fluids according to the care plan.

BOX 17-4 Aspiration Precautions

- Help the person with meals and snacks. Follow the care plan.
- Position the person in Fowler's position or upright in a chair for meals and snacks.
- Support the upper back, shoulders, and neck with a pillow. Follow the care plan.
- Observe for signs and symptoms of aspiration during meals and snacks.
- Check the person's mouth after each meal and snack for pocketing. Check inside the cheeks, under the tongue, and on the roof of the mouth. Remove any food present.
- Position the person in a chair or in semi-Fowler's position after each meal or snack. The person maintains this position for at least 1 hour after eating. Follow the care plan.
- Provide mouth care after each meal or snack.
- Report and record your observations.

MEETING FOOD AND FLUID NEEDS

Weakness, illness, and confusion can affect appetite and ability to eat. So can unpleasant odors, sights, and sounds. An uncomfortable position, the need for oral hygiene, the need to eliminate, and pain also affect appetite.

Special Orders

The doctor may order the amount of fluid a person can have in 24 hours. This is done to maintain fluid balance. Found on the care plan, common orders are:

- *Encourage fluids.* The person drinks an increased amount of fluid. The order is general or states the amount to ingest. Intake records are kept (Chapter 18). A variety of fluids are offered and kept within reach. Serve them at the correct temperature. Offer fluids often to persons who cannot feed themselves.
- *Restrict fluids.* Fluids are limited to a certain amount. They are offered in small amounts and in small containers. The water pitcher is removed from the room or kept out of sight. Intake records are kept. Provide frequent oral hygiene to keep the mouth moist.
- *Nothing by mouth.* The person cannot eat or drink anything. *NPO* stands for *non per os.* It means nothing *(non)* by *(per)* mouth *(os).* NPO is ordered before and after surgery, before some diagnostic tests and procedures, and to treat certain illnesses. An NPO sign is posted in the room. The water pitcher and glass are removed. Frequent oral hygiene is needed, but the person must not swallow any fluid. The person is NPO for 6 to 8 hours before surgery and before certain diagnostic tests and procedures.

DELEGATION GUIDELINES
Preparing For Meals

To prepare a person for a meal, you need this information from the nurse and the care plan:

- How much help the person needs
- Where the person will eat—room or dining room
- What the person uses for elimination—bathroom, commode, bedpan, urinal, or specimen pan
- What type of oral hygiene the person needs
- If the person wears dentures
- How to position the person—in bed or in a chair or wheelchair
- If the person wears eyeglasses or hearing aids
- How the person gets to the dining room—by self or with help
- If the person uses a wheelchair, walker, or cane

PROMOTING SAFETY AND COMFORT
Preparing For Meals

Safety

Before meals, the person needs to eliminate and have oral hygiene. Follow Standard Precautions and the Bloodborne Pathogen Standard. Also follow them when cleaning equipment and the room.

Comfort

The meal setting must be free of unpleasant sights, sounds, and odors. Remove unpleasant equipment from the room.

 Preparing for Meals

You need to prepare patients and residents for meals. If they are ready to eat, you can serve meals promptly. They need to eliminate and have oral care. They need dentures, eyeglasses, and hearing aids in place. If incontinent, they need to be clean and dry. Hand washing and a comfortable position for eating are important.

Preparing the Person For a Meal

Quality of Life

Remember to:

- Knock before entering the person's room
- Address the person by name
- Introduce yourself by name and title

- Explain the procedure to the person before beginning and during the procedure
- Protect the person's rights during the procedure
- Handle the person gently during the procedure

Pre-Procedure

1 Follow *Delegation Guidelines: Preparing For Meals.* See *Promoting Safety and Comfort: Preparing For Meals.*
2 Practice hand hygiene.
3 Collect the following:
   - Equipment for oral hygiene
   - Bedpan, urinal, commode, or specimen pan and toilet tissue

   - Wash basin
   - Soap
   - Washcloth
   - Towel
   - Gloves
4 Provide for privacy.

Procedure

5 Make sure eyeglasses and hearing aids are in place.
6 Assist with oral hygiene. Make sure dentures are in place. Wear gloves, and practice hand hygiene after removing them.
7 Assist with elimination. Make sure the incontinent person is clean and dry. Wear gloves and practice hand hygiene after removing them.
8 Assist with hand washing. Wear gloves and practice hand hygiene after removing them.
9 Do the following if the person will eat in bed:
   a Raise the head of the bed to a comfortable position.
   b Clean the overbed table. Adjust it in front of the person.

   c Place the signal light within reach.
   d Unscreen the person.
10 Do the following if the person will sit in a chair:
   a Position the person in a chair or wheelchair.
   b Remove items from the overbed table. Clean the table.
   c Adjust the overbed table in front of the person.
   d Place the signal light within reach.
   e Unscreen the person.
11 Assist the person to the dining area. (This is for the person who eats in a dining area.)

Post-Procedure

12 Provide for comfort. (See the inside of the front book cover.)
13 Clean and return equipment to its proper place. Wear gloves for this step.
14 Straighten the room. Eliminate unpleasant noise, odors, or equipment.

15 Complete a safety check of the room. (See the inside of the front book cover.)
16 Remove the gloves. Decontaminate your hands.

Dining Programs

Some residents are alert and enjoy eating with others. Some prefer to eat in their rooms. Others are confused and noisy at mealtime. Incontinence or odors are other problems. Weak or very ill persons cannot leave their rooms. To meet these varying needs, nursing centers have dining programs:

- *Social dining.* Residents eat at a dining room table with 4 to 6 others. Tables have tablecloths or placemats. Food is served as in a restaurant. Residents are oriented and feed themselves.
- *Family dining.* Food is served in bowls and on platters. Residents serve themselves like at home. They are oriented and feed themselves.
- *Assistive dining.* The dining room has horseshoe-shaped tables. Residents need help eating. You sit at the center and feed up to 4 people (Fig. 17-3).
- *Low-stimulation dining.* Distractions are prevented during meals. The health team decides on the best place for each person to sit.

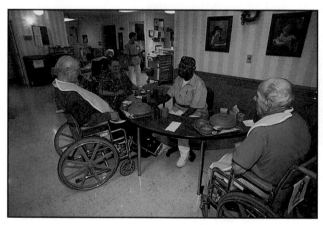

FIG. **17-3** A horseshoe-shaped table is used for assistive dining. The nursing assistant feeds three residents at one time. Residents are in the company of others.

Serving Meal Trays

Food is served in containers that keep foods at the correct temperature. Hot food is kept hot. Cold food is kept cold. You serve meal trays after preparing persons for meals. You can serve trays promptly if patients and residents are ready to eat. Prompt serving keeps food at the right temperature.

If a meal tray is not served within 15 minutes, recheck food temperature. To check the temperature, follow agency policy. If not at the right temperature, get another tray. Some agencies allow reheating in microwave ovens.

DELEGATION GUIDELINES
Serving Meal Trays

Before serving meal trays, you need this information from the nurse and the care plan:
- What adaptive equipment the person uses
- How much help the person needs opening cartons, cutting food, buttering bread, and so on
- If the person's intake and output (I&O) are measured (Chapter 18)
- If calorie counts are done (p. 306)

PROMOTING SAFETY AND COMFORT
Serving Meal Trays

Safety

Always check food temperature after reheating. Food that is too hot can burn the person.

Comfort

Check the person's position when serving meal trays. The position may have changed after the person was prepared to eat. Provide other comfort measures as needed. See the inside of the front book cover.

Serving Meal Trays

Quality of Life

Remember to:

- Knock before entering the person's room
- Address the person by name
- Introduce yourself by name and title

- Explain the procedure to the person before beginning and during the procedure
- Protect the person's rights during the procedure
- Handle the person gently during the procedure

Pre-Procedure

1 Follow *Delegation Guidelines: Serving Meal Trays.* See *Promoting Safety and Comfort: Serving Meal Trays.*

2 Practice hand hygiene.

Procedure

3 Make sure the tray is complete. Check items on the tray with the dietary card. Make sure adaptive equipment is included.
4 Identify the person. Check the ID bracelet against the dietary card. Call the person by name.
5 Place the tray within the person's reach. Adjust the overbed table as needed.
6 Remove food covers. Open cartons, cut meat, and butter bread as needed.
7 Place the napkin, clothes protector, adaptive equipment, and eating utensils within reach.

8 Measure and record intake if ordered (Chapter 18). Note the amount and type of foods eaten (p. 306).
9 Check for and remove any food in the mouth (pocketing). Wear gloves. Decontaminate your hands after removing the gloves.
10 Remove the tray.
11 Clean spills. Change soiled linen and clothing.
12 Help the person return to bed if needed.

Post-Procedure

13 Assist with oral hygiene and hand washing. Wear gloves.
14 Remove the gloves. Decontaminate your hands.
15 Provide for comfort. (See the inside of the front book cover.)
16 Place the signal light within reach.

17 Raise or lower bed rails. Follow the care plan.
18 Complete a safety check of the room. (See the inside of the front book cover.)
19 Follow agency policy for soiled linen.
20 Decontaminate your hands.
21 Report and record your observations.

Feeding the Person

Weakness, paralysis, casts, confusion, and other limits may make self-feeding impossible. These persons are fed.

Serve food and fluids in the order the person prefers. Offer fluids during the meal. Fluids help the person chew and swallow.

Use spoons to feed the person. They are less likely to cause injury than forks. The spoon should only be one-third full. This portion is chewed and swallowed easily. Some people need smaller portions. Follow the care plan.

Persons who need to be fed are often angry, humiliated, and embarrassed. Some refuse to eat. Let

them do as much as possible. Some can manage "finger foods" (bread, cookies, crackers). If strong enough, let them hold cold drinks (never hot drinks). Do not exceed activity limits ordered by the doctor. Provide support. Encourage them to try even if food is spilled.

Visually impaired persons are often very aware of food aromas. They may know the food served. Always tell the person what is on the tray. When feeding a visually impaired person, describe what you are offering. For persons who feed themselves, describe foods and fluids and their place on the tray. Use the numbers on a clock for the location of foods (Fig. 17-4, p. 304).

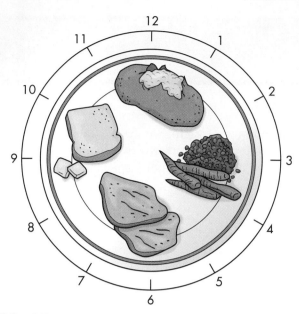

FIG. **17-4** The numbers on a clock are used to help a visually impaired person locate food.

Many people pray before eating. Allow time and privacy for prayer. This shows respect and care about the person.

Meals provide social contact with others. Engage the person in pleasant conversation. However, allow time for chewing and swallowing. Also, sit facing the person. By facing the person, you can see how well the person is eating. You can also see if the person has problems swallowing.

See Persons With Dementia: Feeding the Person.

DELEGATION GUIDELINES
Feeding the Person

Before feeding a person, you need this information from the nurse and the care plan:
- Why the person needs help
- How much help the person needs
- If the person can manage finger foods
- What the person's activity limits are
- What the person's dietary restrictions are
- What size portion to feed the person—⅓ spoonful or less
- What safety measures are needed if the person has dysphagia
- If the person can use a straw
- What observations to report and record:
  - The amount and kind of food eaten
  - Complaints of nausea or dysphagia
  - Signs and symptoms of dysphagia (p. 299)
  - Signs and symptoms of aspiration (p. 307)

Persons With Dementia

Feeding the Person

Persons with dementia may become distracted during meals. Some cannot sit long enough to finish a meal. Others forget how to use eating utensils. Some persons resist your efforts to help them eat. Confused persons may throw or spit food.

A quiet and calm setting is often helpful. So are special mealtimes. The person may eat small meals 4 or 5 times a day. Follow the care plan. Talk to the nurse if you feel upset or impatient. You must treat the person with dignity and respect.

PROMOTING SAFETY AND COMFORT
Feeding the Person

Safety

Check food temperature. Very hot foods can burn the person.

Prevent aspiration. Check the person's mouth before offering more food or fluids. The person's mouth must be empty between bites and swallows.

Comfort

The person will eat better if not rushed. Show the person that you have time for him or her. Do this by sitting to feed the person. Standing communicates that you are in a hurry.

Wipe the person's hands, face, and mouth as needed during the meal. Use the napkin. If necessary, use a wet wash cloth. Then dry the person with a towel.

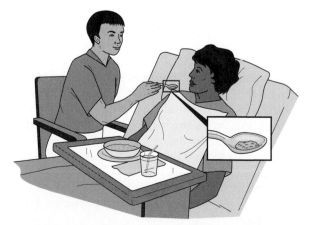

FIG. **17-5** A spoon is used to feed the person. The spoon is no more than one-third full.

Feeding the Person

NNAAP™

Quality of Life

Remember to:

- Knock before entering the person's room
- Address the person by name
- Introduce yourself by name and title

- Explain the procedure to the person before beginning and during the procedure
- Protect the person's rights during the procedure
- Handle the person gently during the procedure

Pre-Procedure

1 Follow *Delegation Guidelines: Feeding the Person.* See *Promoting Safety and Comfort: Feeding the Person.*
2 Practice hand hygiene.

3 Position the person in a comfortable position for eating—usually sitting or Fowler's.
4 Get the tray. Place it on the overbed table or dining table.

Procedure

5 Identify the person. Check the ID bracelet with the dietary card. Call the person by name.
6 Drape a napkin across the person's chest and underneath the chin.
7 Tell the person what foods and fluids are on the tray.
8 Prepare food for eating. Season food as the person prefers and is allowed on the care plan.
9 Serve foods in the order the person prefers. Identify foods as you serve them. Alternate between solid and liquid foods. Use a spoon for safety (Fig. 17-5). Allow enough time for chewing and swallowing. Do not rush the person.
10 Check the person's mouth before offering more food or fluids. Make sure the person's mouth is empty between bites and swallows.
11 Use straws for liquids if the person cannot drink out of a glass or cup. Have one straw for each liquid. Provide short straws for weak persons.

12 Wipe the person's hands, face, and mouth as needed during the meal. Use the napkin.
13 Follow the care plan if the person has dysphagia. (Some persons with dysphagia do not use straws.) Give thickened liquid with a spoon.
14 Converse with the person in a pleasant manner.
15 Encourage him or her to eat as much as possible.
16 Wipe the person's mouth with a napkin. Discard the napkin.
17 Note how much and which foods were eaten. See "calorie counts" on p. 306.
18 Measure and record intake if ordered (Chapter 18).
19 Remove the tray.
20 Take the person back to his or her room (if in a dining area).
21 Assist with oral hygiene and hand washing. Provide for privacy, and put on gloves. Decontaminate your hands after removing the gloves.

Post-Procedure

22 Provide for comfort. (See the inside of the front book cover.)
23 Place the signal light within reach.
24 Raise or lower bed rails. Follow the care plan.

25 Complete a safety check of the room. (See the inside of the front book cover.)
26 Return the food tray to the food cart.
27 Decontaminate your hands.
28 Report and record your observations.

Between-Meal Nourishments

Many special diets involve between-meal nourishments. Common nourishments are crackers, milk, juice, a milkshake, cake, wafers, a sandwich, gelatin, and custard. They are served upon arrival on the nursing unit. Provide needed utensils, a straw, and a napkin. Follow the same considerations and procedures for serving meal trays and feeding persons.

Providing Drinking Water

Patients and residents need fresh drinking water each shift. They also need water whenever the pitcher is empty. Before providing water, ask the nurse about the person's fluid orders (p. 300). Some persons cannot have ice.

Follow the agency's procedure for providing fresh drinking water. Also practice medical asepsis. Water glasses and pitchers can spread microbes. To prevent the spread of microbes:

- Make sure the water pitcher is labeled with the person's name and room and bed number.
- Do not touch the rim or inside of the water glass or pitcher.
- Do not let the ice scoop touch the rim or inside of the water glass or pitcher.
- Do not put the ice scoop in the ice container or dispenser. Place it in the scoop holder or on a towel for the scoop.

Calorie Counts

Calorie records are kept for some people. On a flow sheet, you note what the person ate and how much. For example, a person is served a chicken breast, rice, beans, a roll, pudding, and two pats of butter. The person ate all the chicken, half the rice, and the roll. One pat of butter was used. The beans and pudding were not eaten. Note these on the flow sheet. A nurse or dietitian will convert these portions into calories. The nurse tells you which persons need calorie counts.

MEETING SPECIAL NEEDS

Many persons cannot eat or drink because of illness, surgery, or injury. The doctor orders other methods to meet their food and fluid needs.

Enteral Nutrition

Persons who cannot chew or swallow often require enteral nutrition. **Enteral nutrition** is giving nutrients through the gastrointestinal tract *(enteral)*. A nurse gives formula through a feeding tube (Fig. 17-6). (**Gavage** means tube feeding.)

- A *nasogastric (NG) tube* is inserted through the nose *(naso)* and esophagus into the stomach *(gastro)* (Fig. 17-7). A doctor or an RN inserts the tube.
- A *gastrostomy tube (stomach tube)* is inserted into the stomach. A surgically created opening *(stomy)* in the stomach *(gastro)* is needed (Fig. 17-8).

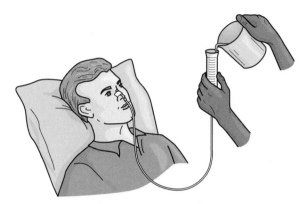

FIG. **17-6** A tube feeding is given.

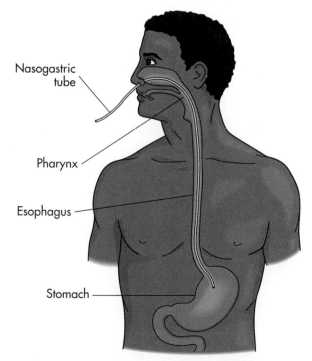

Nasogastric tube

Pharynx

Esophagus

Stomach

FIG. **17-7** A nasogastric tube is inserted through the nose and esophagus into the stomach.

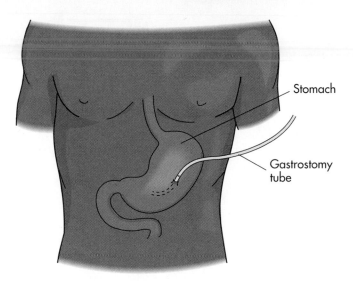

FIG. **17-8** A gastrostomy tube.

Stomach

Gastrostomy
tube

Preventing Aspiration

Aspiration is a major risk with feeding tubes. Remember, *aspiration* is the breathing of fluid or an object into the lungs. It can cause pneumonia and death.

The NG tube is passed through the esophagus then into the stomach. During insertion, the tube can slip into the airway. After insertion, the tube can move out of place from coughing, sneezing, vomiting, suctioning, and poor positioning. The tube can move from the stomach into the esophagus and then into the airway. *The RN checks tube placement before a tube feeding. Checking tube placement is never your responsibility.*

Aspiration also occurs from regurgitation. **Regurgitation** is the backward flow of food from the stomach into the mouth. Delayed stomach emptying and overfeeding are common causes. To prevent regurgitation, follow the care plan. Usually the person is in semi-Fowler's position for 1 or 2 hours or at all times. Semi-Fowler's position allows formula to move through the gastrointestinal system and prevents aspiration. The left side-lying position is avoided. It prevents the stomach from emptying.

Observations

Aspiration is a major risk. Other risks include diarrhea, constipation, and delayed stomach emptying. Report the following to the nurse at once:

■ Nausea
■ Discomfort during the tube feeding
■ Vomiting
■ Diarrhea
■ Distended (enlarged and swollen) abdomen
■ Coughing
■ Complaints of indigestion or heartburn
■ Redness, swelling, drainage, odor, or pain at the ostomy site
■ Elevated temperature
■ Signs and symptoms of respiratory distress (Chapter 22)
■ Increased pulse rate
■ Complaints of flatulence (Chapter 16)

Comfort Measures

The person with a feeding tube is usually NPO. Dry mouth, dry lips, and sore throat cause discomfort. Some persons can have hard candy or gum. Oral hygiene, lubricant to the lips, and mouth rinses are done every 2 hours while the person is awake. The nose and nostrils are cleaned every 4 to 8 hours. Give care as directed by the nurse and care plan.

NG tubes can irritate and cause pressure on the nose. They can alter the shape of the nostrils or cause pressure ulcers. Securing the tube helps prevent these problems. Tape or a tube holder secures the tube to the nose (Fig. 17-9, p. 308). Follow agency policy for securing the tube to the gown.

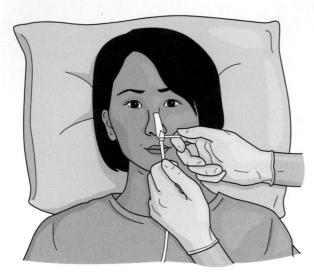

FIG. **17-9** The feeding tube is secured to the nose.

Intravenous Therapy

Intravenous (IV) therapy is giving fluids through a needle or catheter inserted into a vein. *IV* and *IV infusion* also refer to IV therapy. The basic equipment used is shown in Figure 17-10.

- The fluid is in a plastic *IV bag*.
- A *catheter* or *needle* is inserted into a vein.
- The infusion tubing *(IV tube)* connects the IV bag to the catheter or needle.
- Fluid drips from the bag into the *drip chamber*.
- The *clamp* is used to regulate the flow rate.
- The IV bag hangs from an IV pole or ceiling hook. *IV standard* is another name for an IV pole.

Flow Rate

The doctor orders the amount of fluid to give (infuse) and the amount of time to give it in. With this information, the RN calculates the flow rate. The **flow rate** is the number of drops per minute (gtt/min). The abbreviation *gtt* means drops. The Latin word *guttae* means drops.

The RN sets the clamp for the flow rate. Or an electronic pump controls the flow rate. An alarm sounds if something is wrong. Tell the nurse at once if you hear an alarm. *Never change the position of the clamp or adjust any controls on IV pumps.*

You can check the flow rate. The RN tells you the number of drops per minute. To check the flow rate, count the number of drops in 1 full minute (Fig. 17-11). Tell the RN at once:

- If no fluid is dripping
- If the rate is too fast
- If the rate is too slow

A rate that is too fast or too slow can be harmful. Changes in flow rate can occur from position changes. Kinked tubes and lying on the tubing also are common problems.

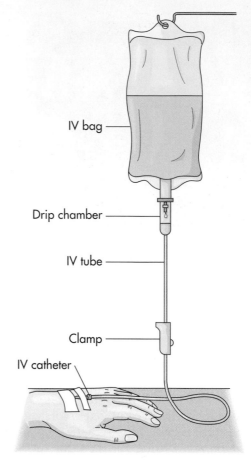

FIG. **17-10** Equipment for IV therapy.

IV bag

Drip chamber

IV tube

Clamp

IV catheter

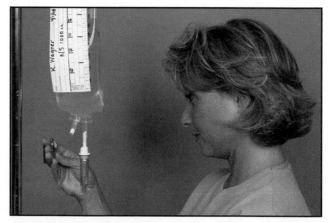

FIG. **17-11** The flow rate is checked by counting the number of drops per minute.

Assisting With IV therapy

You help meet the safety, hygiene, and activity needs of persons with IVs. *You are never responsible for starting or maintaining IV therapy. Nor do you regulate the flow rate or change IV bags. You never give blood or IV drugs.* Follow the nurse's directions and the care plan. Complications can occur from IV therapy. Report any of the signs and symptoms listed in Box 17-5 at once.

BOX 17-5	**Signs and Symptoms of IV Therapy Complications**

At the IV Site

- Bleeding
- Puffiness or swelling
- Pale or reddened skin
- Complaints of pain at or above the IV site
- Hot or cold skin near the site

Involving the Whole Body

- Fever
- Itching
- Drop in blood pressure

- Pulse rate greater than 100 beats per minute
- Irregular pulse
- Cyanosis
- Changes in mental function
- Loss of consciousness
- Difficulty breathing
- Shortness of breath
- Decreasing or no urine output
- Chest pain
- Nausea
- Confusion

FOCUS ON THE PERSON

Good nutrition promotes health and prevents disease. It is needed for healing and to gain strength. Meeting food and fluid needs is part of your job.

See *Focus on the Person: Nutrition and Fluids.*

Focus on the PERSON

Nutrition and Fluids

Providing comfort—Some nursing centers have areas where the resident can dine with a partner, family, or friends. They can enjoy holidays, birthdays, anniversaries, and other special events together. The dietary department provides the meal or it is brought by the family.

Food complaints are common. Food tastes bad. Food is cold. Food is not appealing, and so on. Many hospitals are serving food in new ways. For example:

- *24-hour catering.* Meals and snacks are provided 24 hours a day. This is for persons who cannot or do not want to eat at the usual mealtimes. The person can order food directly from the food service department.
- *Mobile food carts.* Food service staff bring a food cart to the nursing unit. The patient selects food and a tray is prepared.

Ethical behavior—The person may offer you some food on the meal tray. The person may say that he or she is not that hungry, does not plan to eat it all, or does not like the food served. The person is given food that he or she selected off of a menu. The amount provided is what the person needs to heal and gain strength. Eating the person's food is unethical.

Remaining independent—Disease or injury can affect the hands, wrists, and arms. Adaptive equipment lets the person eat independently. Make sure the person has the needed equipment.

Speaking up—You may have to assist some patients and residents with filling out their menus. Speak clearly and slowly as you read from the menu.

The person may not eat all the food served. You need to find out why and tell the nurse. You can ask these questions. Then ask the person to explain his or her answer.

- "Please tell me why you didn't eat everything."
- "Was there something wrong with your food?"
- "Did your food taste okay?"
- "Was your food too hot or too cold?"
- "Would you prefer something else?"
- "Weren't you hungry?"

OBRA and other laws—Patients and residents must receive proper nutrition. Survey teams make sure that:

- Needed help is provided
- Assistive devices are provided
- Medical asepsis is practiced when serving food and fluids
- Meals, snacks, and between-meal nourishments are served promptly
- Other food is offered if the person refuses the food served

Nursing teamwork—Meal trays arrive on the nursing unit in a meal cart. Each tray is in a slot. Trays are served in the order that they appear in the cart. The entire nursing team serves trays. You may serve trays to patients or residents of other staff members. They do the same for you. The goal is to serve food promptly and at the correct temperature.

REVIEW QUESTIONS

Circle the **BEST** answer.

1 The MyPyramid Food Guidance System encourages the following *except*
   a The same diet for everyone
   b Smart food choices
   c Physical activity
   d Small steps to improve diet and life-style

2 On a 2000-calorie a day diet, how many daily servings of grains are needed?
   a 6 ounces   c 3 to 4 ounces
   b 4 to 5 ounces   d 2 ounces

3 On a 2000-calorie a day diet, how many daily servings of the meat group are needed?
   a 2½ ounces   c 4 to 5 ounces
   b 3 to 4 ounces   d 5½ ounces

4 Which food group contains the *most* fat?
   a Grains   c Milk
   b Vegetables   d Meat and beans

5 These statements are about oils. Which is *false?*
   a Oils are high in calories.
   b The best oil choices come from fish, nuts, and vegetable oils.
   c Oils from plant sources contain cholesterol.
   d Mayonnaise, certain salad dressings, and soft margarine are mainly oil.

6 Protein is needed for
   a Tissue growth and repair
   b Energy and the fiber for bowel elimination
   c Body heat and the protection of organs from injury
   d Improving the taste of food

7 Which foods provide the *most* protein?
   a Butter and cream
   b Tomatoes and potatoes
   c Meats and fish
   d Corn and lettuce

8 Diabetes meal planning involves the following *except*
   a The person's food preferences
   b Eating the same amount of carbohydrates, protein, and fat each day
   c Eating at regular times
   d Sodium control

9 Which is *not* a sign of a swallowing problem?
   a Drooling
   b Coughing while eating
   c Pocketing
   d Dysphagia

10 These statements are about OBRA requirements. Which *is false?*
   a 24-hour meal service is required.
   b Hot food must be served hot. Cold food must be served cold.
   c Food must smell and taste good.
   d Special eating equipment must be provided.

11 Adult fluid requirements for normal fluid balance are about
   a 1000 to 1500 ml daily   c 2000 to 2500 ml daily
   b 1500 to 2000 ml daily   d 2500 to 3000 ml daily

12 A person is NPO. You should
   a Provide a variety of fluids
   b Offer fluids in small amounts and small containers
   c Remove the water pitcher and glass
   d Prevent the person from having oral hygiene

13 Which statement about feeding a person is *not correct?*
   a Ask if he or she wants to pray before eating.
   b Use a fork to feed the person.
   c Ask the person the order in which to serve foods.
   d Engage the person in a pleasant conversation.

14 To prevent regurgitation, the person is positioned in
   a Semi-Fowler's position
   b The prone position
   c The left side-lying position
   d The right side-lying position

15 A person with a feeding tube is usually
   a Allowed a regular diet
   b On bedrest
   c NPO
   d In a coma

16 You note that the IV flow rate is too slow. You must
   a Tell the RN at once
   b Adjust the flow rate
   c Reposition the person
   d Clamp the tubing

The answers to these questions are on p. 469.

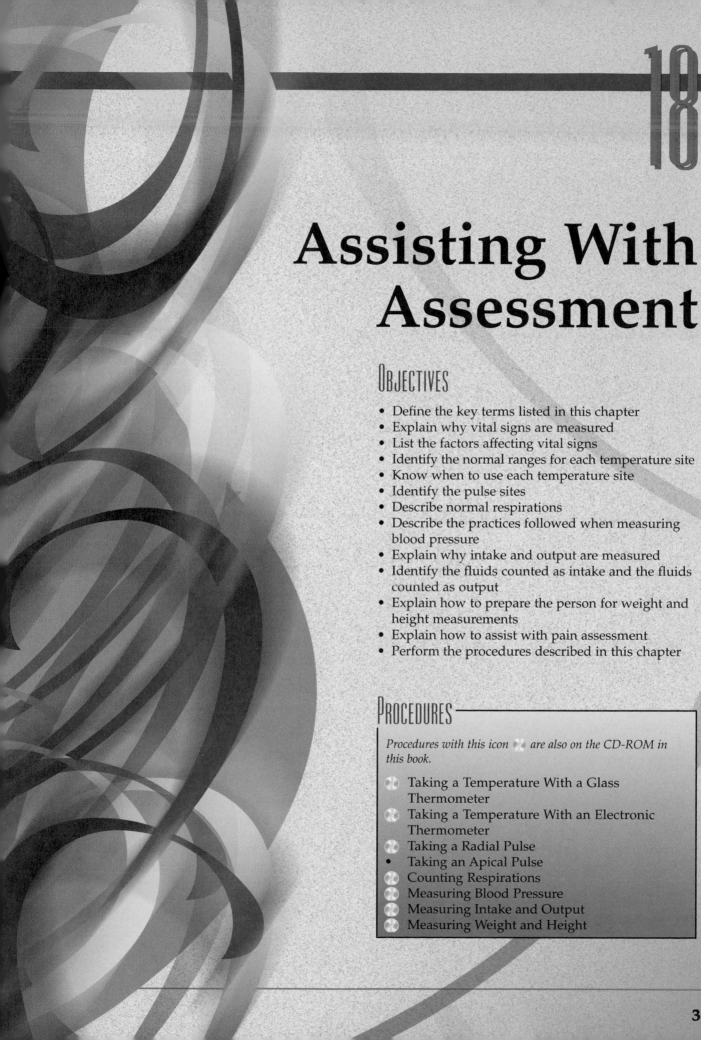

Assisting With Assessment

OBJECTIVES

- Define the key terms listed in this chapter
- Explain why vital signs are measured
- List the factors affecting vital signs
- Identify the normal ranges for each temperature site
- Know when to use each temperature site
- Identify the pulse sites
- Describe normal respirations
- Describe the practices followed when measuring blood pressure
- Explain why intake and output are measured
- Identify the fluids counted as intake and the fluids counted as output
- Explain how to prepare the person for weight and height measurements
- Explain how to assist with pain assessment
- Perform the procedures described in this chapter

PROCEDURES

Procedures with this icon 🔆 are also on the CD-ROM in this book.

- 🔆 Taking a Temperature With a Glass Thermometer
- 🔆 Taking a Temperature With an Electronic Thermometer
- 🔆 Taking a Radial Pulse
- Taking an Apical Pulse
- 🔆 Counting Respirations
- 🔆 Measuring Blood Pressure
- 🔆 Measuring Intake and Output
- 🔆 Measuring Weight and Height

KEY TERMS

blood pressure The amount of force exerted against the walls of an artery by the blood

body temperature The amount of heat in the body that is a balance between the amount of heat produced and the amount lost by the body

diastolic pressure The pressure in the arteries when the heart is at rest

fever Elevated body temperature

hypertension Blood pressure measurements that remain above (hyper) a systolic pressure of 140 mm Hg or a diastolic pressure of 90 mm Hg

hypotension When the systolic blood pressure is below (hypo) 90 mm Hg and the diastolic pressure is below 60 mm Hg

pulse The beat of the heart felt at an artery as a wave of blood passes through the artery

pulse rate The number of heartbeats or pulses felt in 1 minute

respiration Breathing air into (inhalation) and out of (exhalation) the lungs

systolic pressure The amount of force needed to pump blood out of the heart into the arterial circulation

vital signs Temperature, pulse, respirations, and blood pressure

You assist the nurse with the assessment step of the nursing process. Some observations involve measurements. You measure **vital signs**—temperature, pulse, respirations, and blood pressure. You also measure intake and output and weight and height. The nurse and care plan tell you when to take these measurements.

The nurse also assesses the person's pain. You report observations about pain to the nurse.

VITAL SIGNS

Vital signs reflect three body processes: regulation of body temperature, breathing, and heart function. A person's vital signs vary within certain limits. They are affected by sleep, activity, eating, weather, noise, exercise, drugs, anger, fear, anxiety, pain, and illness.

Vital signs show even minor changes in a person's condition. They tell about a person's response to treatment. They often signal life-threatening events.

Accuracy is essential when you measure, record, and report vital signs. If unsure of your measurements, promptly ask the nurse to take them again. Unless otherwise ordered, take vital signs with the person at rest in a lying or sitting position. Report the following at once:

- Any vital sign that is changed from a prior measurement
- Vital signs above or below the normal range

Body Temperature

Body temperature is the amount of heat in the body. It is a balance between the amount of heat produced and the amount lost by the body. Heat is produced as cells use food for energy. It is lost through the skin, breathing, urine, and feces. Body temperature stays fairly stable. It is lower in the morning and higher in the afternoon and evening. Body temperature is affected by age, weather, exercise, emotions, stress, and illness.

Thermometers are used to measure temperature. It is measured using the Fahrenheit (F) and centigrade or Celsius (C) scale. Temperature sites are the mouth, rectum, tympanic membrane (ear), and axilla (underarm) (Box 18-1). Each site has a normal range (Table 18-1).

Older persons have lower body temperatures than younger adults. An oral temperature of 98.6° F may signal **fever** (elevated body temperature) in an older person.

Glass Thermometers

The glass thermometer is a hollow glass tube (Fig. 18-1). The tube is filled with a substance—mercury or a mercury-free mixture. When heated, the substance expands and rises in the tube. When cooled, the substance contracts and moves down the tube.

Long- or slender-tip thermometers are used for oral and axillary temperatures. So are thermometers with stubby and pear-shaped tips. Rectal thermometers have stubby tips and are color-coded in red.

Glass thermometers are reusable. However, the following are problems:

- They take a long time to register.
- They break easily. Broken rectal thermometers can injure the rectum and colon.
- The person may bite down on and break an oral thermometer. Cuts in the mouth are risks. Swallowed mercury can cause mercury poisoning.

Reading a Glass Thermometer. Fahrenheit thermometers have long and short lines. Every other long line is marked in an even degree from 94° to 108° F. The short lines mean 0.2 (two tenths) of a degree (Fig. 18-2, A).

PROMOTING SAFETY AND COMFORT
Glass Thermometers

Safety

If a mercury–glass thermometer breaks, tell the nurse at once. Mercury is a hazardous substance. Do not touch the mercury. Do not let the person do so. The agency must follow special procedures for handling all hazardous materials. See Chapter 8.

BOX **18-1**	**Temperature Sites**

Oral Site

Oral temperatures are *not* taken if the person:
- Is an infant or a child under 6 years of age
- Is unconscious
- Has had surgery or an injury to the face, neck, nose, or mouth
- Is receiving oxygen
- Breathes through the mouth
- Has a nasogastric tube
- Is delirious, restless, confused, or disoriented
- Is paralyzed on one side of the body
- Has a sore mouth
- Has a convulsive (seizure) disorder

Rectal Site

Rectal temperatures are taken when the oral route cannot be used. Rectal temperatures are *not* taken if the person:
- Has diarrhea
- Has a rectal disorder or injury

- Has heart disease
- Had rectal surgery
- Is confused or agitated

Tympanic Membrane Site

This site has fewer microbes than the mouth or rectum. Therefore the risk of spreading infection is reduced. This site is *not* used if the person has:
- An ear disorder
- Ear drainage

Axillary Site

Less reliable than the other sites. It is used when the other sites cannot be used.

TABLE **18-1**	**Normal Body Temperatures**	
Site	**Baseline**	**Normal Range**
Rectal	99.6° F (37.5° C)	98.6° to 100.6° F (37.0° to 38.1° C)
Oral	98.6° F (37° C)	97.6° to 99.6° F (36.5° to 37.5° C)
Tympanic membrane	98.6° F (37° C)	98.6° F (37° C)
Axillary	97.6° F (36.5° C)	96.6° to 98.6° F (35.9° to 37.0° C)

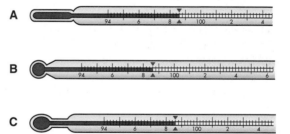

FIG. **18-1** Types of glass thermometers. **A,** The long or slender tip. **B,** The stubby tip (rectal thermometer). **C,** The pear-shaped tip.

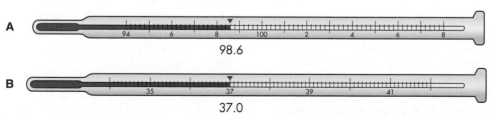

FIG. **18-2 A,** A Fahrenheit thermometer. The temperature measurement is 98.6° F. **B,** Centigrade thermometer. The temperature measurement is 37.0° C.

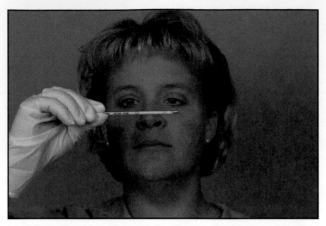

FIG. **18-3** The thermometer is held at the stem. It is read at eye level.

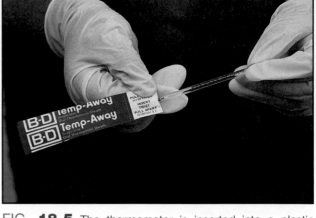

FIG. **18-5** The thermometer is inserted into a plastic cover.

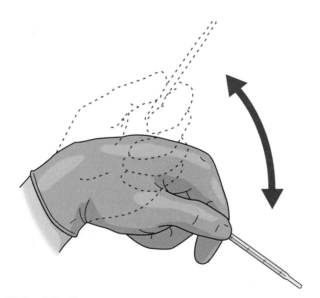

FIG. **18-4** The wrist is snapped to shake down the thermometer.

On a centigrade thermometer, each long line means 1 degree. Degrees range from 34° to 42° C. Each short line means 0.1 (one tenth) of a degree (Fig. 18-2, *B*).

To read a glass thermometer:

- Hold it at the stem (Fig. 18-3). Bring it to eye level.
- Turn it until you can see the numbers and the long and short lines.
- Turn it back and forth slowly until you see the silver or red line.
- Read the nearest degree (long line).
- Read the nearest tenth of a degree (short line).

Using a Glass Thermometer. Do the following to prevent infection, promote safety, and obtain an accurate measurement.

- Use only the person's thermometer.
- Use a rectal thermometer only for rectal temperatures.
- Rinse the thermometer under cold running water if it was soaking in a disinfectant. Dry it from the stem to the bulb end with tissues.
- Check the thermometer for breaks, cracks, and chips. Discard it according to agency policy if it is broken, cracked, or chipped.
- Shake down the thermometer to move the substance down in the tube. Hold it at the stem. Stand away from walls, tables, or other hard surfaces. Flex and snap your wrist until the substance is below 94° F or 34° C. See Figure 18-4.
- Clean and store the thermometer following agency policy. Wipe it with tissues first to remove mucus, feces, or sweat. Do not use hot water. It causes the mercury or mercury-free mixture to expand so much that the thermometer could break. After cleaning, rinse the thermometer under cold running water. Then store it in a container with disinfectant solution.
- Use plastic covers following agency policy (Fig. 18-5). To take a temperature, insert the thermometer into a cover. Remove the cover to read the thermometer. Discard the cover after use.
- Practice medical asepsis. Follow Standard Precautions and the Bloodborne Pathogen Standard.

Taking Temperatures

Glass thermometers are used for oral, rectal, and axillary temperatures. Special measures are needed for each site.

- *The oral site.* The glass thermometer remains in place 2 to 3 minutes or as required by agency policy.
- *The rectal site.* Lubricate the rectal thermometer for easy insertion and to prevent tissue injury. Hold it in place so it is not lost into the rectum or broken. A glass thermometer remains in the rectum for 2 minutes or as required by agency policy. Privacy is important. The buttocks and anus are exposed. The procedure embarrasses many people.
- *The axillary site.* The axilla (underarm) must be dry. Do not use this site right after bathing. Hold the glass thermometer in place for 5 to 10 minutes or as required by agency policy.

DELEGATION GUIDELINES
Taking Temperatures

The nurse may ask you to take temperatures. If so, you need this information from the nurse and the care plan:

- What site to use—oral, rectal, axillary, or tympanic membrane
- What thermometer to use—glass, electronic, or other type
- How long to leave a glass thermometer in place
- When to take temperatures
- Which persons are at risk for elevated temperatures
- What observations to report and record:
  - A temperature that is changed from a prior measurement
  - A temperature above or below the normal range

PROMOTING SAFETY AND COMFORT
Taking Temperatures

Safety

Thermometers are inserted into the mouth, rectum, and axilla. Each area has many microbes. The area may contain blood. Therefore each person has his or her own glass thermometer. This prevents the spread of microbes and infection. Follow Standard Precautions and the Bloodborne Pathogen Standard when taking temperatures.

When taking a rectal temperature, your gloved hands may come in contact with feces. If so, remove the gloves and decontaminate your hands. Then note the temperature on your notepad or assignment sheet. Put on clean gloves to complete the procedure.

Comfort

Remove the thermometer in a timely manner. Do not leave the thermometer in place longer than needed. This affects the person's comfort. For example, an oral thermometer is left in place for 2 to 3 minutes. Do not leave it in place longer than that.

Taking a Temperature With a Glass Thermometer

NNAAP™

Quality of Life

Remember to:

- Knock before entering the person's room
- Address the person by name
- Introduce yourself by name and title

- Explain the procedure to the person before beginning and during the procedure
- Protect the person's rights during the procedure
- Handle the person gently during the procedure

Continued

Pre-Procedure

1 Follow *Delegation Guidelines: Taking Temperatures*, p. 315. See *Promoting Safety and Comfort:*
   • *Glass Thermometers*, p. 313.
   • *Taking Temperatures*, p. 315.
2 For an *oral temperature*, ask the person not to eat, drink, smoke, or chew gum for at least 15 to 20 minutes or as required by agency policy.
3 Practice hand hygiene.
4 Collect the following:
   • Oral or rectal thermometer and holder

• Tissues
• Plastic covers if used
• Gloves
• Toilet tissue (rectal temperature)
• Water-soluble lubricant (rectal temperature)
• Towel (axillary temperature)

5 Identify the person. Check the ID bracelet against the assignment sheet. Call the person by name.
6 Provide for privacy.

Procedure

7 Put on the gloves.
8 Rinse the thermometer in cold water if it was soaking in a disinfectant. Dry it with tissues.
9 Check for breaks, cracks, or chips.
10 Shake down the thermometer below the lowest number. Hold the thermometer by the stem.
11 Insert it into a plastic cover if used.
12 For an *oral temperature*:
   a Ask the person to moisten his or her lips.
   b Place the bulb end of the thermometer under the tongue and to one side (Fig. 18-6).
   c Ask the person to close the lips around the thermometer to hold it in place.
   d Ask the person not to talk. Remind the person not to bite down on the thermometer.
   e Leave it in place for 2 to 3 minutes or as required by agency policy. (Note: Some state competency tests require leaving the thermometer in place for 3 minutes.)
13 For a *rectal temperature*:
   a Position the person in Sims' position.
   b Put a small amount of lubricant on a tissue. Lubricate the bulb end of the thermometer.
   c Fold back top linens to expose the anal area.
   d Raise the upper buttock to expose the anus (Fig. 18-7).
   e Insert the thermometer 1 inch into the rectum. Do not force the thermometer. Remember, glass thermometers can break.
   f Hold the thermometer in place for 2 minutes or as required by agency policy. Do not let go of it while it is in the rectum.
14 For an *axillary temperature*:
   a Help the person remove an arm from the gown. Do not expose the person.

   b Dry the axilla with the towel.
   c Place the bulb end of the thermometer in the center of the axilla.
   d Ask the person to place the arm over the chest to hold the thermometer in place (Fig. 18-8). Hold it and the arm in place if he or she cannot help.
   e Leave the thermometer in place for 5 to 10 minutes or as required by agency policy.
15 Remove the thermometer.
16 Use tissues to remove the plastic cover. Discard the cover and tissues. Wipe the thermometer with a tissue if no cover was used. Wipe from the stem to the bulb end. Discard the tissue.
17 Read the thermometer.
18 Note the person's name and temperature on your notepad or assignment sheet. Write *R* for a rectal temperature. Write *A* for an axillary temperature.
19 For a *rectal temperature*:
   a Place used toilet tissue on several thicknesses of toilet tissue.
   b Place the thermometer on clean toilet tissue.
   c Wipe the anal area to remove excess lubricant and any feces.
   d Cover the person.
20 For an *axillary temperature:* Help the person put the gown back on.
21 Shake down the thermometer.
22 Clean the thermometer according to agency policy. Return it to the holder.
23 Discard tissue and dispose of toilet tissue.
24 Remove the gloves. Decontaminate your hands.

Post-Procedure

25 Provide for comfort. (See the inside of the front book cover.)
26 Place the signal light within reach.
27 Unscreen the person.
28 Complete a safety check of the room. (See the inside of the front book cover.)

29 Decontaminate your hands.
30 Report and record the temperature. Note the temperature site when reporting and recording. Report any abnormal temperature at once.

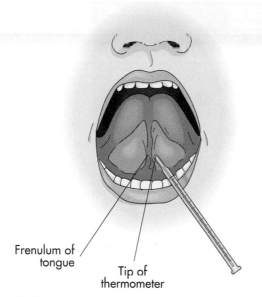

Frenulum of
tongue
　　　Tip of
　　　thermometer

FIG. **18-6** The thermometer is placed at the base of the tongue and to one side.

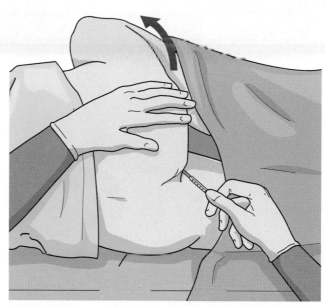

FIG. **18-7** The rectal temperature is taken with the person in the Sims' position. The buttock is raised to expose the anus.

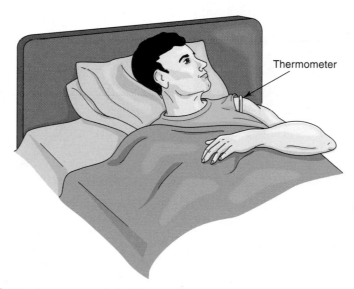

Thermometer

FIG. **18-8** The thermometer is held in place in the axilla by bringing the person's arm over the chest.

Electronic Thermometers

Electronic thermometers are battery operated (Fig. 18-9, p. 318). They measure temperature in a few seconds. The temperature is shown on the front of the device. The hand-held unit is kept in a battery charger when not in use.

Electronic thermometers have oral and rectal probes. A disposable cover (sheath) covers the probe and is discarded after use. This helps prevent the spread of infection.

Tympanic Membrane Thermometers. Tympanic membrane thermometers measure temperature at the tympanic membrane in the ear (Fig. 18-10, p. 318). The covered probe is gently inserted into the ear. The temperature is measured in 1 to 3 seconds.

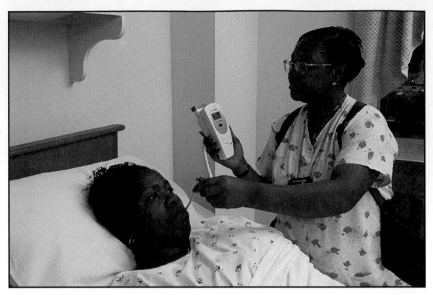

FIG. **18-9** The covered probe of the electronic thermometer is inserted under the tongue.

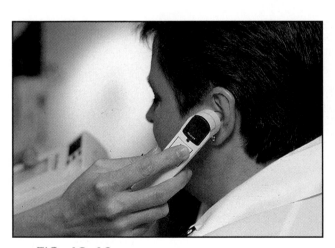

FIG. **18-10** Tympanic membrane thermometer.

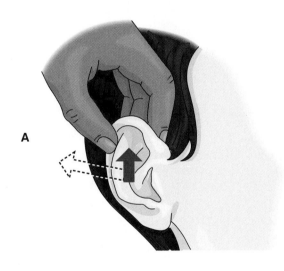

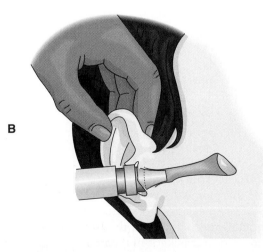

FIG. **18-11** Using a tympanic membrane thermometer. **A,** The ear is pulled up and back. **B,** The probe is inserted into the ear canal.

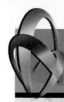

Taking a Temperature With an Electronic Thermometer

Pre-Procedure

1. Follow *Delegation Guidelines: Taking Temperatures*, p. 315. See *Promoting Safety and Comfort: Taking Temperatures*, p. 315.
2. For an *oral temperature*, ask him or her not to eat, drink, smoke, or chew gum for at least 15 to 20 minutes.
3. Collect the following:
   - Thermometer—electronic or tympanic membrane
   - Probe (Blue for an oral or axillary temperature. Red for a rectal temperature.)
   - Probe covers
   - Toilet tissue (rectal temperature)
   - Water-soluble lubricant (rectal temperature)
   - Gloves
   - Towel (axillary temperature)
4. Plug the probe into the thermometer. (This is not done for a tympanic membrane thermometer.)
5. Practice hand hygiene.
6. Identify the person. Check the ID bracelet against the assignment sheet. Call the person by name.

Procedure

7. Provide for privacy. Position the person for an oral, rectal, axillary, or tympanic membrane temperature.
8. Put on gloves if contact with blood, body fluids, secretions, or excretions is likely.
9. Insert the probe into a probe cover.
10. For an *oral temperature*:
    - a Ask the person to open the mouth and raise the tongue.
    - b Place the covered probe at the base of the tongue and to one side (see Fig. 18-9).
    - c Ask the person to lower the tongue and close the mouth.
11. For a *rectal temperature*:
    - a Place some lubricant on toilet tissue.
    - b Lubricate the end of the covered probe.
    - c Expose the anal area.
    - d Raise the upper buttock.
    - e Insert the probe ½ inch into the rectum.
    - f Hold the probe in place.
12. For an *axillary temperature*:
    - a Help the person remove an arm from the gown. Do not expose the person.
    - b Dry the axilla with the towel.
    - c Place the covered probe in the axilla.
    - d Place the person's arm over the chest.
    - e Hold the probe in place.
13. For a *tympanic membrane temperature*:
    - a Ask the person to turn his or her head so the ear is in front of you.
    - b Pull up and back on the ear to straighten the ear canal (Fig. 18-11).
    - c Insert the covered probe gently.
14. Start the thermometer.
15. Hold the probe in place until you hear a tone or see a flashing or steady light.
16. Read the temperature on the display.
17. Remove the probe. Press the eject button to discard the cover.
18. Note the person's name and temperature on your notepad or assignment sheet. Note the temperature site.
19. Return the probe to the holder.
20. Help the person put the gown back on (axillary temperature). For a rectal temperature:
    - a Wipe the anal area with toilet tissue to remove lubricant.
    - b Cover the person.
    - c Dispose of used toilet tissue.
    - d Remove the gloves. Decontaminate your hands.

Post-Procedure

21. Provide for comfort. (See the inside of the front book cover.)
22. Place the signal light within reach.
23. Unscreen the person.
24. Complete a safety check of the room. (See the inside of the front book cover.)
25. Return the thermometer to the charging unit.
26. Decontaminate your hands.
27. Report and record the temperature. Note the temperature site when reporting and recording. Report any abnormal temperature at once.

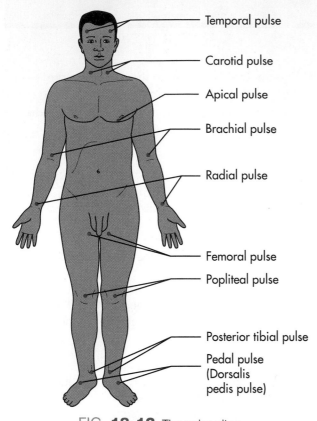

FIG. **18-12** The pulse sites.

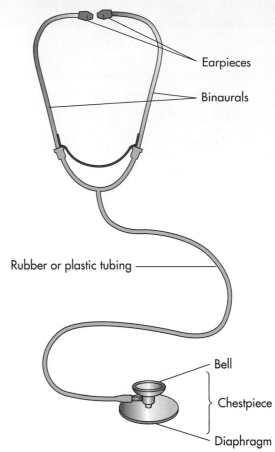

FIG. **18-13** Parts of a stethoscope.

Pulse

The **pulse** is the beat of the heart felt at an artery as a wave of blood passes through the artery. A pulse is felt every time the heart beats.

The temporal, carotid, brachial, radial, femoral, popliteal, posterior tibial, and dorsalis pedis (pedal) pulses are on each side of the body (Fig. 18-12). The radial site is used most often. It is easy to reach and find. You can take a radial pulse without disturbing or exposing the person.

The apical pulse is felt over the apex of the heart. It is taken with a stethoscope.

Using a Stethoscope

A *stethoscope* is an instrument used to listen to the sounds produced by the heart, lungs, and other body organs (Fig. 18-13). It is used to take apical pulses and blood pressures. Follow these rules when using a stethoscope.

- Wipe the earpieces and diaphragm with antiseptic wipes before and after use.
- Place the earpiece tips in your ears. The bend of the tips points forward. Earpieces should fit snugly to block out noises. They should not cause pain or ear discomfort.
- Place the diaphragm over the artery. Hold it in place as in Figure 18-14.
- Prevent noise. Do not let anything touch the tubing. Ask the person to be silent.

PROMOTING SAFETY AND COMFORT
Using a Stethoscope

Safety

Stethoscopes are in contact with many persons and staff. Therefore you must prevent infection. Wipe the earpieces and diaphragm with antiseptic wipes before and after use.

Comfort

Stethoscope diaphragms tend to be cold. Warm the diaphragm in your hand before applying it to the person (Fig. 18-15). Cold diaphragms can startle the person.

Pulse Rate

The **pulse rate** is the number of heartbeats or pulses felt in 1 minute. The pulse rate is affected by many factors—age, fever, exercise, fear, anger, anxiety, excitement, heat, position, and pain. These and other factors cause the heart to beat faster. Some drugs also increase the pulse rate. Other drugs slow down the pulse.

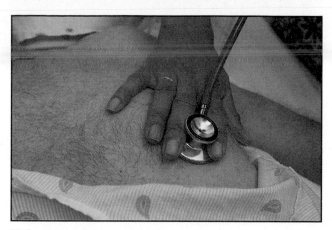

FIG. **18-14** The stethoscope is held in place with the fingertips of the index and middle fingers.

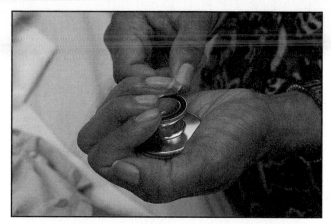

FIG. **18-15** The diaphragm of the stethoscope is warmed in the palm of the hand.

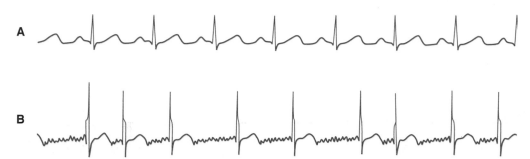

FIG. **18-16** **A,** The electrocardiogram shows a regular pulse. The beats occur at regular intervals. **B,** These beats occur at irregular intervals.

The adult pulse rate is between 60 and 100 beats per minute. A rate of less than 60 or greater than 100 is considered abnormal. Report abnormal rates to the nurse at once.

Rhythm and Force of the Pulse

The rhythm of the pulse should be regular. That is, pulses are felt in a pattern. The same time interval occurs between beats. An irregular pulse occurs when the beats are not evenly spaced or beats are skipped (Fig. 18-16).

Force relates to pulse strength. A forceful pulse is easy to feel. It is described as *strong, full,* or *bounding.* Hard-to-feel pulses are described as *weak, thready,* or *feeble.*

 Taking a Radial Pulse

The radial pulse is used for routine vital signs. Place the first 2 or 3 fingers of one hand against the radial artery. The radial artery is on the thumb side of the wrist (Fig. 18-17). Count the pulse for 30 seconds.

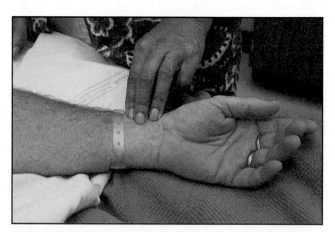

FIG. **18-17** The middle 3 fingers are used to take the radial pulse.

Then multiply the number by 2. This gives the number of beats per minute. If the pulse is irregular, count it for 1 minute.

In some agencies, all radial pulses are taken for 1 minute. Follow agency policy.

DELEGATION GUIDELINES
Taking Pulses

Before taking a pulse, you need this information from the nurse and the care plan:

- What pulse to take—radial or apical
- When to take the pulse
- What other vital signs to measure
- How long to count the pulse—30 seconds or 1 minute
- If the nurse has concerns about certain patients or residents
- What observations to report and record:
  - The pulse site
  - The pulse rate—report a pulse rate less than 60 *(bradycardia)* or more than 100 beats *(tachycardia)* per minute at once
  - If the pulse is regular or irregular
  - Pulse force—strong, full, bounding, weak, thready, or feeble

PROMOTING SAFETY AND COMFORT
Taking Pulses

Safety

Do not use your thumb to take a pulse. The thumb has a pulse. You could mistake the pulse in your thumb for the person's pulse. Reporting and recording the wrong pulse rate can harm the person.

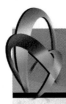

Taking a Radial Pulse

Quality of Life

Remember to:

- Knock before entering the person's room
- Address the person by name
- Introduce yourself by name and title

- Explain the procedure to the person before beginning and during the procedure
- Protect the person's rights during the procedure
- Handle the person gently during the procedure

Pre-Procedure

1 Follow *Delegation Guidelines: Taking Pulses.* See *Promoting Safety and Comfort: Taking Pulses.*
2 Practice hand hygiene.

3 Identify the person. Check the ID bracelet against the assignment sheet. Call the person by name.
4 Provide for privacy.

Procedure

5 Have the person sit or lie down.
6 Locate the radial pulse. Use your first 2 or 3 middle fingers (see Fig. 18-17).
7 Note if the pulse is strong or weak, and regular or irregular.
8 Count the pulse for 30 seconds. Multiply the number of beats by 2. Or count the pulse for

1 minute as directed by the nurse or if required by agency policy. (Note: Some state competency tests require counting the pulse for 1 minute.)
9 Count the pulse for 1 minute if it is irregular.
10 Note the person's name and pulse on your notepad or assignment sheet. Note the strength of the pulse. Note if it was regular or irregular.

Post-Procedure

11 Provide for comfort. (See the inside of the front book cover.)
12 Place the signal light within reach.
13 Unscreen the person.

14 Complete a safety check of the room. (See the inside of the front book cover.)
15 Decontaminate your hands.
16 Report and record the pulse rate and your observations. Report an abnormal pulse at once.

Taking an Apical Pulse

The apical pulse is taken with a stethoscope. Apical pulses are taken on persons who have heart disease, have irregular heart rhythms, or who take drugs that affect the heart. The apical pulse is on the left side of the chest slightly below the nipple (Fig. 18-18).

Count the apical pulse for 1 minute. The heartbeat normally sounds like a *lub-dub*. Count each *lub-dub* as 1 beat. Do not count the *lub* as 1 beat and the *dub* as another.

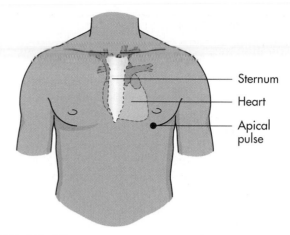

FIG. **18-18** The apical pulse is located 2 to 3 inches to the left of the sternum (breastbone) and below the left nipple.

Taking an Apical Pulse

Quality of Life

Remember to:

- Knock before entering the person's room
- Address the person by name
- Introduce yourself by name and title

- Explain the procedure to the person before beginning and during the procedure
- Protect the person's rights during the procedure
- Handle the person gently during the procedure

Pre-Procedure

1 Follow *Delegation Guidelines: Taking Pulses.* See *Promoting Safety and Comfort: Using a Stethoscope,* p. 320.
2 Collect a stethoscope and antiseptic wipes.
3 Practice hand hygiene.

4 Identify the person. Check the ID bracelet against the assignment sheet. Call the person by name.
5 Provide for privacy.

Procedure

6 Clean the earpieces and diaphragm with the wipes.
7 Have the person sit or lie down.
8 Expose the nipple area of the left chest. Do not expose a woman's breasts.
9 Warm the diaphragm in your palm.
10 Place the earpieces in your ears.

11 Find the apical pulse. Place the diaphragm 2 to 3 inches to the left of the breastbone and below the left nipple (see Fig. 18-18).
12 Count the pulse for 1 minute. Note if it is regular or irregular.
13 Cover the person. Remove the earpieces.
14 Note the person's name and pulse on your notepad or assignment sheet. Note if the pulse was regular or irregular.

Post-Procedure

15 Provide for comfort. (See the inside of the front book cover.)
16 Place the signal light within reach.
17 Unscreen the person.
18 Complete a safety check of the room. (See the inside of the front book cover.)

19 Clean the earpieces and diaphragm with the wipes.
20 Return the stethoscope to its proper place.
21 Decontaminate your hands.
22 Report and record your observations. Record the pulse rate with *Ap* for apical pulse. Report an abnormal pulse at once.

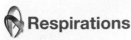

Respirations

Respiration means breathing air into (inhalation) and out of (exhalation) the lungs. Each respiration involves 1 inhalation and 1 exhalation. Respirations are normally quiet, effortless, and regular. Both sides of the chest rise (inhalation) and fall (exhalation) equally.

The healthy adult has 12 to 20 respirations per minute. The respiratory rate is affected by the factors that affect temperature and pulse. Heart and respiratory diseases usually increase the respiratory rate.

People tend to change breathing patterns when they know their respirations are being counted. Therefore the person should not know that you are counting them.

Count respirations right after taking a pulse. Keep your fingers or stethoscope over the pulse site. (The person assumes you are taking the pulse.) To count respirations, watch the chest rise and fall. Count them for 30 seconds. Multiply the number by 2 for the number of respirations in 1 minute. If an abnormal pattern is noted, count the respirations for 1 minute.

In some agencies, respirations are counted for 1 minute. Follow agency policy.

DELEGATION GUIDELINES
Respirations

Before counting respirations, you need this information from the nurse and the care plan:

- How long to count respirations—30 seconds or 1 minute
- When to count respirations
- What other vital signs to measure
- What observations to report and record:
  - The respiratory rate
  - Equality and depth of respirations
  - If the respirations were regular or irregular
  - If the person has pain or difficulty in breathing
  - Any respiratory noises
  - Any abnormal respiratory patterns (Chapter 22)

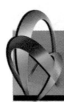

Counting Respirations

Procedure

1 Follow *Delegation Guidelines: Respirations*.
2 Keep your fingers or the stethoscope over the pulse site.
3 Do not tell the person you are counting respirations.
4 Begin counting when the chest rises. Count each rise and fall of the chest as 1 respiration.
5 Note the following:
- If respirations are regular
- If both sides of the chest rise equally
- The depth of respirations
- If the person has any pain or difficulty breathing

6 Count respirations for 30 seconds. Multiply the number by 2. (Note: Some state competency tests require counting respirations for 1 minute.) Or count respirations for 1 minute as directed by the nurse or if required by agency policy.
7 Count respirations for 1 minute if they are abnormal or irregular.
8 Note the person's name, respiratory rate, and other observations on your notepad or assignment sheet.

Post-Procedure

9 Provide for comfort. (See the inside of the front book cover.)
10 Place the signal light within reach.
11 Unscreen the person.
12 Complete a safety check of the room. (See the inside of the front book cover.)
13 Decontaminate your hands.
14 Report and record the respiratory rate and your observations. Report abnormal respirations at once.

Blood Pressure

Blood pressure is the amount of force exerted against the walls of an artery by the blood. The period of heart muscle contraction is called *systole*. The period of heart muscle relaxation is called *diastole*.

Systolic and diastolic pressures are measured. The **systolic pressure** is the amount of force needed to pump blood out of the heart into the arterial circulation. It is the higher pressure. The **diastolic pressure** is the pressure in the arteries when the heart is at rest. It is the lower pressure.

Blood pressure is measured in millimeters (mm) of mercury (Hg). The systolic pressure is recorded over the diastolic pressure. A systolic pressure of 120 mm Hg and a diastolic pressure of 80 mm Hg is written as 120/80 mm Hg.

Normal and Abnormal Blood Pressures

Blood pressure can change from minute to minute. Because it can vary so easily, blood pressure has normal ranges.

- *Systolic pressure*—less than 120 mm Hg
- *Diastolic pressure*—less than 80 mm Hg

Treatment is indicated for measurements that remain above *(hyper)* a systolic pressure of 140 mm Hg or a diastolic pressure of 90 mm Hg. This condition is known as **hypertension.** Report any systolic pressure above 120 mm Hg. A diastolic pressure above 80 mm Hg also is reported. Likewise, systolic pressures below *(hypo)* 90 mm Hg and diastolic pressures below 60 mm Hg are reported. This is called **hypotension.**

PROMOTING SAFETY AND COMFORT
Equipment

Safety

Mercury is a hazardous substance. Handle mercury manometers carefully. If one breaks, call for the nurse at once. Do not touch the mercury. Do not let the person touch it. The agency must follow special procedures for handling all hazardous substances. See Chapter 8.

Comfort

Inflate the cuff only to the extent necessary (see procedure: *Measuring Blood Pressure,* p. 327). The inflated cuff causes discomfort. The higher the inflation, the greater the discomfort.

Equipment

A stethoscope and a sphygmomanometer are used to measure blood pressure. The *sphygmomanometer* has a cuff and a measuring device.

- The *aneroid* type has a round dial and a needle that points to the numbers (Fig. 18-19, *A*).
- The *mercury* type has a column of mercury within a calibrated tube (Fig. 18-19, *B*).
- The *electronic* type shows the systolic and diastolic blood pressures on the front of the device (Fig. 18-19, *C*). Follow the manufacturer's instructions.

A

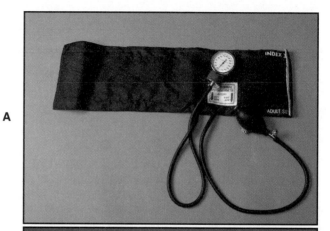

B

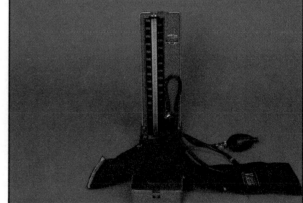

C

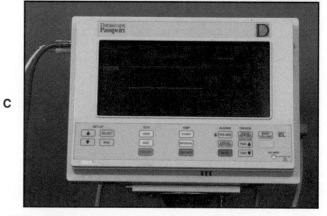

FIG. **18-19** Blood pressure equipment. **A,** Aneroid manometer and cuff. **B,** Mercury manometer and cuff. **C,** Electronic sphygmomanometer.

The blood pressure cuff is wrapped around the upper arm. Tubing connects the cuff to the manometer. Another tube connects the cuff to a small, hand-held bulb. A valve on the bulb is turned so the cuff inflates as the bulb is squeezed. The inflated cuff causes pressure over the brachial artery. The valve is turned the other way to deflate the cuff. Blood pressure is measured as the cuff is deflated.

Sounds are produced as blood flows through the arteries. The stethoscope is used to listen to the sounds in the brachial artery as the cuff is deflated. Stethoscopes are not needed with electronic manometers.

 Measuring Blood Pressure

Blood pressure is normally measured in the brachial artery. Box 18-2 lists the guidelines for measuring blood pressure.

DELEGATION GUIDELINES
Measuring Blood Pressure

Before measuring blood pressure, you need this information from the nurse and the care plan:

- When to measure blood pressure
- If the person has an arm IV infusion, a cast, or dialysis access site
- If the person had breast surgery, on what side was the surgery done
- If the person needs to be lying down, sitting, or standing
- What size cuff to use—regular, child-size, or extra-large
- What observations to report and record

BOX 18-2   Guidelines for Measuring Blood Pressure

- Do not take blood pressure on an arm with an IV infusion, a cast, or a dialysis access site. If a person had breast surgery, do not take blood pressure on that side. Avoid taking blood pressure on an injured arm.
- Let the person rest for 10 to 20 minutes before measuring blood pressure.
- Measure blood pressure with the person sitting or lying. Sometimes the doctor orders blood pressure measured in the standing position.
- Apply the cuff to the bare upper arm. Clothing can affect the measurement.
- Make sure the cuff is snug. Loose cuffs can cause inaccurate readings.
- Use a larger cuff if the person is obese or has a large arm. Ask the nurse what size to use.
- Place the diaphragm of the stethoscope firmly over the brachial artery. The entire diaphragm must have contact with the skin.
- Make sure the room is quiet. Talking, TV, radio, and sounds from the hallway can affect an accurate measurement.
- Have the sphygmomanometer where you can clearly see it.
- Measure the systolic and diastolic pressures. Expect to hear the first blood pressure sound at the point where you last felt the radial or brachial pulse. The first sound is the systolic pressure. The point where the sound disappears is the diastolic pressure.
- Take the blood pressure again if you are not sure of an accurate measurement. Wait 30 to 60 seconds before repeating the measurement.
- Tell the nurse at once if you cannot hear the blood pressure.

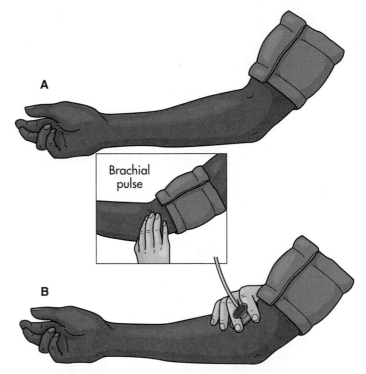

FIG. **18-20** Measuring blood pressure. **A,** The cuff is over the brachial artery. **B,** The diaphragm of the stethoscope is over the brachial artery.

Measuring Blood Pressure

Quality of Life

Remember to:

- Knock before entering the person's room
- Address the person by name
- Introduce yourself by name and title

- Explain the procedure to the person before beginning and during the procedure
- Protect the person's rights during the procedure
- Handle the person gently during the procedure

Pre-Procedure

1 Follow *Delegation Guidelines: Measuring Blood Pressure.* See *Promoting Safety and Comfort:*
   - *Using a Stethoscopes*, p. 320.
   - *Equipment*, p. 325.
2 Collect the following:
   - Sphygmomanometer
   - Stethoscope
   - Antiseptic wipes
3 Practice hand hygiene.
4 Identify the person. Check the ID bracelet against the assignment sheet. Call the person by name.
5 Provide for privacy.

Procedure

6 Wipe the stethoscope earpieces and diaphragm with the wipes.
7 Have the person sit or lie down.
8 Position the person's arm level with the heart. The palm is up.
9 Stand no more than 3 feet away from the manometer. A mercury model is vertical, on a flat surface, and at eye level. The aneroid type is directly in front of you.
10 Expose the upper arm.
11 Squeeze the cuff to expel any remaining air. Close the valve on the bulb.
12 Find the brachial artery at the inner aspect of the elbow. Use your fingertips.
13 Place the arrow on the cuff over the brachial artery (Fig. 18-20, *A*). Wrap the cuff around the upper arm at least 1 inch above the elbow. It is even and snug.
14 *One-step method:*
   a Place the stethoscope earpieces in your ears.
   b Find the radial or brachial artery.
   c Inflate the cuff until you can no longer feel the pulse. Note this point.
   d Inflate the cuff 30 mm Hg beyond the point where you last felt the pulse.
15 *Two-step method:*
   a Find the radial or brachial artery.

b Inflate the cuff until you can no longer feel the pulse. Note this point.
c Inflate the cuff 30 mm Hg beyond the point where you last felt the pulse.
d Deflate the cuff slowly. Note the point when you feel the pulse.
e Wait 30 seconds.
f Place the stethoscope earpieces in your ears.
g Inflate the cuff 30 mm Hg beyond the point where you felt the pulse return.
16 Place the diaphragm over the brachial artery (Fig. 18-20, *B*). Do not place it under the cuff.
17 Deflate the cuff at an even rate of 2 to 4 millimeters per second. Turn the valve counterclockwise to deflate the cuff.
18 Note the point where you hear the first sound. This is the systolic reading. It is near the point where the radial pulse disappeared.
19 Continue to deflate the cuff. Note the point where the sound disappears. This is the diastolic reading.
20 Deflate the cuff completely. Remove it from the person's arm. Remove the stethoscope earpieces from your ears.
21 Note the person's name and blood pressure on your notepad or assignment sheet.
22 Return the cuff to the case or wall holder.

Post-Procedure

23 Provide for comfort. (See the inside of the front book cover.)
24 Place the signal light within reach.
25 Unscreen the person.
26 Complete a safety check of the room. (See the inside of the front book cover.)

27 Clean the earpieces and diaphragm with the wipes.
28 Return the equipment to its proper place.
29 Decontaminate your hands.
30 Report and record the blood pressure. Report an abnormal blood pressure at once.

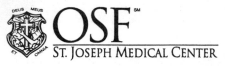

FLUID BALANCE CHART

Water Glass	250ml		Ice Cream	120ml
Styrofoam Cup	180ml		Ice Chips	1/2 amt. of
Cup (coffee)	250ml			ml's in cup
Milk Carton	240ml			
Pop (1 can)	360ml		Pitcher	
Broth-Soup	175ml		(Yellow)	1000ml
Juice Carton	120ml			
Juice Glass	120ml			
Jello	120ml			

DATE ___6/15___

		INTAKE			OUTPUT					
		Parenteral		Amt. ml Absbd.	URINE		OTHER		CONT. IRRIGATION	
TIME	ORAL				Method Collected	Amt. (ml)	Method Collected	Amt. (ml)	In	Out
2400-0100		ml from previous shift			V	150				
0100-0200							Vom.	150		
0200-0300										
0300-0400										
0400-0500										
0500-0600	125				V	200				
0600-0700										
0700-0800										
	125	8 - hour Sub-total			8-hr T	350	8-hr T	150		
0800-0900	400	ml from previous shift			V	250				
0900-1000	100									
1000-1100										
1100-1200										
1200-1300	400				V	250				
1300-1400										
1400-1500	200									
1500-1600										
	1100	8 - hour Sub-total			8-hr T	500	8-hr T			
1600-1700		ml from previous shift			V	270				
1700-1800	350									
1800-1900	50									
1900-2000	200									
2000-2100					V	400				
2100-2200										
2200-2300										
2300-2400										
	600	8 - hour Sub-total			8-hr T	670	8-hr T			
	1825	24 - hour Sub-total			24-hr T	1520	24-hr T	150		

Source Key:

  URINE

V	- Voided
C	- Catheter
INC	- Incontinent
U.C.	- Ureteral Catheter

Source Key:

  OTHER

G.I.T.	- Gastric Intestinal Tube
T.T.	- T. Tube
Vom.	- Vomitus
Liq S.	- Liquid Stool
H.V.	- Hemovac

310'   Marie Mills

Form No. MF36722 (Rev. 5/97)   MFI

FIG. **18-21** An intake and output record. (Modified from OSF St. Joseph Medical Center, Bloomington, Ill.)

INTAKE AND OUTPUT

The doctor or nurse may order intake and output (I&O) measurements. I&O records are kept by the nursing team. They are used to evaluate fluid balance and kidney function. They also are kept when the person has special fluid orders (Chapter 17).

All fluids taken by mouth are measured and recorded—water, milk, coffee, tea, juices, soups, and soft drinks. So are foods that melt at room temperature—ice cream, sherbet, custard, pudding, gelatin, and Popsicles. The nurse measures and records IV fluids and tube feedings. Output includes urine, vomitus, diarrhea, and wound drainage.

 ## Measuring Intake and Output

Intake and output are measured in milliliters (ml). You need to know these amounts.
- 1 ounce (oz) equals 30 ml
- A pint is about 500 ml
- A quart is about 1000 ml

You need to know the serving sizes of bowls, dishes, cups, pitchers, glasses, and other containers. The information may be on the I&O record (Fig. 18-21).

A *graduate* is used to measure leftover fluids, urine, vomitus, and drainage from suction. Like a measuring cup, the graduate is marked in ounces and in milliliters (Fig. 18-22). Plastic urinals and kidney basins often have amounts marked.

An I&O record is kept at the bedside. When intake or output is measured, the amount is recorded in the correct column (see Fig. 18-21). Amounts are totaled at the end of the shift. The totals are recorded in the person's record.

The urinal, commode, bedpan, or specimen pan is used for voiding. Remind the person not to void in the toilet. Also remind the person not to put toilet tissue into the receptacle.

DELEGATION GUIDELINES
Intake and Output

When measuring I&O, you need this information from the nurse and the care plan:
- Does the person have a special fluid order—encourage fluids, restrict fluids, or NPO
- When to report measurements—hourly or end-of-shift
- What the person uses for voiding—urinal, bedpan, commode, or specimen pan
- If the person has a catheter

PROMOTING SAFETY AND COMFORT
Intake and Output

Safety

Urine may contain microbes or blood. Microbes can grow in urinals, commodes, bedpans, specimen pans, and drainage systems. Follow Standard Precautions and the Bloodborne Pathogen Standard when handling such equipment. Thoroughly clean the item after it is used. Use a disinfectant for cleaning.

Comfort

Promptly measure the contents of urinals, commodes, bedpans, and specimen pans. This helps prevent or reduce odors. Odors can disturb the person.

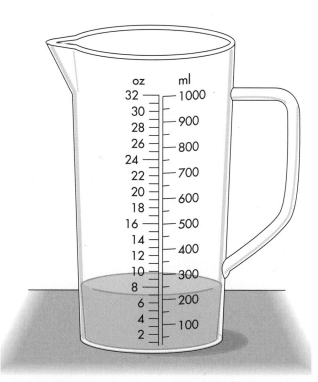

FIG. **18-22** A graduate marked in ounces and milliliters.

Measuring Intake and Output

NNAAP™

Quality of Life

Remember to:

- Knock before entering the person's room
- Address the person by name
- Introduce yourself by name and title

- Explain the procedure to the person before beginning and during the procedure
- Protect the person's rights during the procedure
- Handle the person gently during the procedure

Pre-Procedure

1 Follow *Delegation Guidelines: Intake and Output*, p. 329. See *Promoting Safety and Comfort: Intake and Output*, p. 329.
2 Practice hand hygiene.

3 Collect the following:
  • Intake and output (I&O) record
  • Graduates
  • Gloves

Procedure

4 Put on gloves.
5 Measure intake as follows:
  a Pour liquid remaining in a container into the graduate.
  b Measure the amount at eye level. Keep the container level.
  c Check the serving amount on the I&O record.
  d Subtract the remaining amount from the full serving amount. Record the amount.
  e Pour the fluid in the graduate back into the container.
  f Repeat steps 5a through 5e for each liquid.
  g Add the amounts from each liquid together.
  h Record the time and amount on the I&O record.

6 Measure output as follows:
  a Pour the fluid into the graduate used to measure output.
  b Measure the amount at eye level. Keep the container level.
7 Dispose of fluid in the toilet. Avoid splashes.
8 Clean and rinse the graduates. Dispose of rinse into the toilet. Return the graduates to their proper place.
9 Clean and rinse the bedpan, urinal, kidney basin, or other drainage container. Discard the rinse into the toilet. Return the item to its proper place.
10 Remove the gloves. Decontaminate your hands.
11 Record the amount on the I&O record.

Post-Procedure

12 Provide for comfort. (See the inside of the front book cover.)
13 Make sure the signal light is within reach.

14 Complete a safety check of the room. (See the inside of the front book cover.)
15 Report and record your observations.

MEASURING WEIGHT AND HEIGHT

Weight and height are measured on admission to the agency. The person is weighed daily, weekly, or monthly. This is done to measure weight gain or loss.

Standing, chair, and lift scales are used. Chair and lift scales are used for persons who cannot stand. Follow the manufacturer's instructions and agency procedures.

When measuring weight and height, follow these guidelines:

- The person only wears a gown or pajamas. Clothes add weight. No footwear is worn. Footwear adds to the weight and height measurements.
- The person voids before being weighed. A full bladder adds weight.
- Weigh the person at the same time of day. Before breakfast is the best time. Food and fluids add weight.
- Use the same scale for daily, weekly, and monthly weights. Scales weigh differently.
- Balance the scale at zero before weighing the person. For balance scales, move the weights to zero. A digital scale should read at zero.

DELEGATION GUIDELINES
Measuring Weight and Height

Before measuring weight and height, you need this information from the nurse and the care plan:
- When to measure weight and height
- What scale to use

PROMOTING SAFETY AND COMFORT
Measuring Weight and Height

Safety

Follow the manufacturer's instructions when using chair or lift scales. Also follow the agency's procedures. Practice safety measures to prevent falls.

Comfort

The person wears only a gown or pajamas for the weight measurement. Prevent chilling and drafts (Chapter 12).

Measuring Weight and Height

Quality of Life

Remember to:

- Knock before entering the person's room
- Address the person by name
- Introduce yourself by name and title

- Explain the procedure to the person before beginning and during the procedure
- Protect the person's rights during the procedure
- Handle the person gently during the procedure

Pre-Procedure

1 Follow *Delegation Guidelines: Measuring Weight and Height*. See *Promoting Safety and Comfort: Measuring Weight and Height.*
2 Ask the person to void.
3 Practice hand hygiene.
4 Bring the scale and paper towels to the person's room.

5 Decontaminate your hands.
6 Identify the person. Check the ID bracelet against the assignment sheet. Call the person by name.
7 Provide for privacy.

Continued

Measuring Weight and Height—cont'd

NNAAP™

Procedure

8 Place the paper towels on the scale platform.
9 Raise the height rod.
10 Move the weights to zero (0). The pointer is in the middle.
11 Have the person remove the robe and footwear. Assist as needed.
12 Help the person stand on the scale. The person stands in the center of the scale. Arms are at the sides.
13 Move the weights until the balance pointer is in the middle (Fig. 18-23).
14 Note the weight on your notepad or assignment sheet.

15 Ask the person to stand very straight.
16 Lower the height rod until it rests on the person's head (Fig. 18-24).
17 Note the height on your notepad or assignment sheet.
18 Raise the height rod. Help the person step off of the scale.
19 Help the person put on a robe and non-skid footwear if he or she will be up. Or help the person back to bed.
20 Lower the height rod. Adjust the weight rods to zero (0) if this is your agency policy.

Post-Procedure

21 Provide for comfort. (See the inside of the front book cover.)
22 Place the signal light within reach.
23 Raise or lower bed rails. Follow the care plan.
24 Unscreen the person.

25 Complete a safety check of the room. (See the inside of the front book cover.)
26 Discard the paper towels.
27 Return the scale to its proper place.
28 Decontaminate your hands.
29 Report and record the measurements.

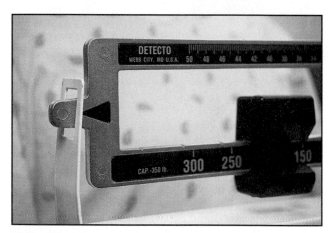

FIG. **18-23** The weight is read when the balance pointer is in the middle.

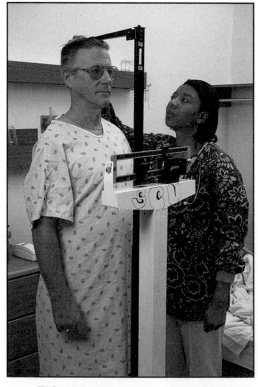

FIG. **18-24** Height is measured.

PAIN

Pain means to ache, hurt, or be sore. Pain is a warning from the body. It means there is tissue damage.

Pain is personal. It differs for each person. What *hurts* to one person may *ache* to another. What one person calls *sore*, another may call *aching*. If a person complains of pain, the person *has* pain. You must believe the person.

There are different types of pain.

- *Acute pain* is felt suddenly from injury, disease, trauma, or surgery. There is tissue damage. Acute pain lasts a short time, usually less than 6 months. It lessens with healing.
- *Chronic pain* lasts longer than 6 months. Pain is constant or occurs off and on. There is no longer tissue damage. Chronic pain remains long after healing. Arthritis and cancer are common causes.
- *Radiating pain* is felt at the site of tissue damage and in nearby areas. Pain from a heart attack is often felt in the left chest, left jaw, left shoulder, and left arm. Gallbladder disease can cause pain in the right upper abdomen, the back, and right shoulder (Fig. 18-25).
- *Phantom pain* is felt in a body part that is no longer there. A person with an amputated leg may still sense leg pain.

Signs and Symptoms

You cannot see, hear, feel, or smell a person's pain. You must rely on what the person tells you. Promptly report any information you collect about pain. Use the person's exact words when reporting and recording. The nurse needs this information:

- *Location.* Where is the pain? Ask the person to point to the area of pain. Pain can radiate. Ask the person if the pain is anywhere else and to point to those areas.
- *Onset and duration.* When did the pain start? How long has it lasted?
- *Intensity.* Does the person complain of mild, moderate, or severe pain? Ask the person to rate the pain on a scale of 1 to 10, with 10 as the most severe (Fig. 18-26).
- *Description.* Ask the person to describe the pain.
- *Factors causing pain.* These are called *precipitating* factors. To precipitate means to cause. Such factors include moving or turning in bed, coughing or deep breathing, and exercise. Ask what the person was doing before the pain started and when it started.
- *Vital signs.* Measure the person's pulse, respirations, and blood pressure. Increases in these vital signs often occur with acute pain. Vital signs may be normal with chronic pain.
- *Other signs and symptoms.* Does the person have other symptoms—dizziness, nausea, vomiting, weakness, numbness or tingling, or others? Box 18-3, p. 334 lists the signs and symptoms that often occur with pain.

PAIN: Ask person to rate pain on scale of 1-10										
No pain										Worst pain imaginable
0	1	2	3	4	5	6	7	8	9	10

FIG. **18-26** Pain rating scale. (Modified from DeWit, SC: *Fundamental concepts and skills for nursing*, Philadelphia, 2001, Saunders.)

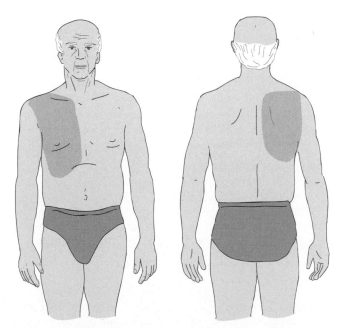

FIG. **18-25** Gallbladder pain radiates to the right upper abdomen, the back, and the right shoulder.

BOX 18-3   Signs and Symptoms of Pain

Body Responses

- Increased pulse, respirations, and blood pressure
- Nausea
- Pale skin (pallor)
- Sweating (diaphoresis)
- Vomiting

Behaviors

- Changes in speech: slow or rapid; loud or quiet
- Crying
- Gasping
- Grimacing
- Groaning
- Grunting
- Holding the affected body part (splinting)
- Irritability
- Maintaining one position; refusing to move
- Moaning
- Quietness
- Restlessness
- Rubbing
- Screaming

FOCUS ON THE PERSON

Vital signs, other measurements, and observations about the person's pain are important for the nursing process. They help the nurse plan for and evaluate the person's care. *See Focus on the Person: Assisting With Assessment.*

Focus on the PERSON

Assisting With Assessment

Providing comfort—Vital signs, intake and output, and weight and height measurements cause little physical discomfort. However, rectal temperatures can embarrass the person. You must provide for the person's privacy. Also act in a professional manner at all times.

The nurse uses your observations to assess the person's pain. Then the nurse plans measures to promote comfort and relieve pain. Follow the person's care plan.

Ethical behavior—Your measurements must be accurate. Tell the nurse if you cannot feel a pulse or hear a blood pressure. Do not make up a measurement. That could harm the person.

Remaining independent—Personal choices help the person remain independent. The person may prefer that you use the right or left arm for pulses and blood pressures. If safe to do so, use the arm the person prefers.

Speaking up—Patients and residents like to know their measurements. If agency policy allows, you can tell the person the measurements. Remember, this information is private and confidential. Roommates and visitors must not hear what you are saying.

A measurement may be abnormal. Or you may not be able to feel a pulse or hear a blood pressure. Do not alarm the person. You can say:

- "I'm not sure that I counted your pulse correctly. I want the nurse to take it too."
- "I'm not sure that I heard your blood pressure correctly. I'll ask the nurse to take it again."
- "Your pulse is a little slow (or fast). I'll ask the nurse to check it."
- "Your temperature is higher than normal. I'm going to check it with another thermometer. I'll also ask the nurse to check you."

OBRA and other laws—OBRA requires that residents be weighed on admission. They are weighed daily, weekly, or monthly to check for weight loss or gain.

The nurse must complete a pain assessment whenever the person's behavior or level of function changes. You must report changes and complaints of pain to the nurse at once.

Nursing teamwork—Electronic and tympanic membrane thermometers are shared with other nursing team members. When using these devices, tell your co-workers what thermometer you have. Work quickly, but carefully. Return the device to the charging unit in a timely manner.

REVIEW QUESTIONS

Circle the **BEST** answer.

1 Which should you report at once?
   a   An oral temperature of 98.4° F
   b   A rectal temperature of 101.6° F
   c   An axillary temperature of 97.6° F
   d   An oral temperature of 99.0° F

2 A rectal temperature is taken when the person
   a   Is unconscious
   b   Has heart disease
   c   Is confused
   d   Has diarrhea

3 Which is usually used to take a pulse?
   a   The radial pulse
   b   The carotid pulse
   c   The apical pulse
   d   The brachial pulse

4 Which is reported to the nurse at once?
   a   A pulse of 66 beats per minute
   b   A pulse of 40 beats per minute
   c   A pulse of 80 beats per minute
   d   A pulse of 96 beats per minute

5 The following describe normal respirations *except*
   a   There are 12 to 20 per minute
   b   They are quiet and effortless
   c   Both sides of the chest rise and fall equally
   d   The person breathes through the mouth

6 Respirations are usually counted
   a   After taking the temperature
   b   After taking the pulse
   c   Before taking the pulse
   d   After taking the blood pressure

7 Which blood pressure is normal for an adult?
   a   88/54 mm Hg
   b   210/100 mm Hg
   c   112/78 mm Hg
   d   152/90 mm Hg

8 When taking a blood pressure, you should do the following *except*
   a   Take the blood pressure in the arm with an IV infusion
   b   Apply the cuff to a bare upper arm
   c   Turn off the TV and radio
   d   Locate the brachial artery

9 Which is the systolic blood pressure?
   a   The point where the pulse is no longer felt
   b   The point where the first sound is heard
   c   The point where the last sound is heard
   d   The point 30 mm Hg above where the pulse was felt

10 Which are *not* counted as liquid foods?
   a   Coffee, tea, juices, and soft drinks
   b   Sauces and melted cheese
   c   Ice cream and sherbet
   d   Popsicles and soup

11 Which is *not* measured as output?
   a   Urine
   b   Vomitus
   c   Perspiration
   d   Wound drainage

12 For an accurate weight measurement, the person
   a   Wears footwear
   b   Wears a robe and gown
   c   Voids first
   d   Chooses what scale to use

13 A person has pain in the left chest, the left jaw, and in the left shoulder and arm. This is
   a   Acute pain
   b   Chronic pain
   c   Radiating pain
   d   Phantom pain

14 Mr. Smith complains of pain. You should do the following *except*
   a   Ask him to point to where the pain is felt
   b   Ask him to rate the pain on a scale of 1 to 10
   c   Ask him to describe the pain
   d   Ask to look at the pain

Answers to these questions are on p. 469.

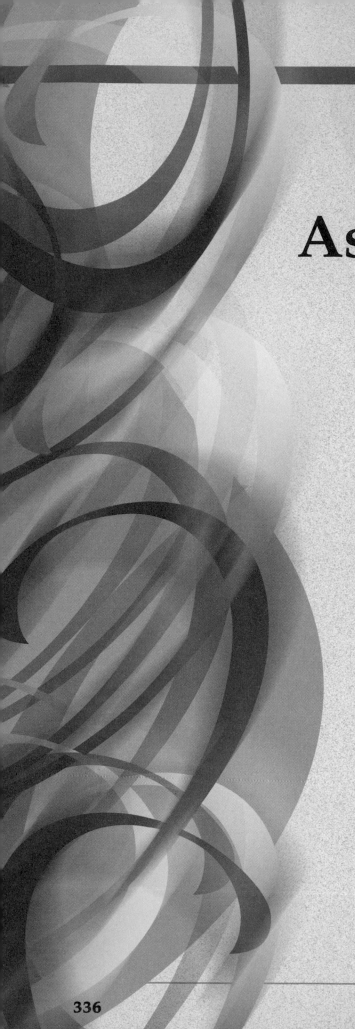

19

Assisting With Specimens

OBJECTIVES

- Define the key terms listed in this chapter
- Explain why specimens are collected
- Describe the different types of urine specimens
- Explain why urine specimens are tested
- Explain the rules for collecting specimens
- Perform the procedures described in this chapter

PROCEDURES

Procedures with this icon 💿 are also on the CD-ROM in this book.

- Collecting a Random Urine Specimen
- Collecting a Midstream Specimen
- Collecting a Double-Voided Specimen
- Testing Urine With Reagent Strips
- Collecting a Stool Specimen
- Collecting a Sputum Specimen

KEY TERMS

acetone A substance that appears in urine from the rapid breakdown of fat for energy; ketone body or ketone

glucosuria Sugar (*glucos*) in the urine (*uria*); glycosuria

glycosuria Sugar (*glycos*) in the urine (*uria*); glucosuria

hematuria Blood (*hemat*) in the urine (*uria*)

hemoptysis Bloody (*hemo*) sputum (*ptysis* means "to spit")

ketone Acetone; ketone body

ketone body Acetone; ketone

sputum Mucus from the respiratory system that is expectorated (expelled) through the mouth

Specimens (samples) are collected and tested to prevent, detect, and treat disease. The doctor orders what specimen to collect and the test needed. Most specimens are tested in the laboratory. All specimens sent to the laboratory require requisition slips. The slip has the person's identifying information and the test ordered. Some tests are done at the bedside. When collecting specimens, follow the rules in Box 19-1.

BOX 19-1	**Rules For Collecting Specimens**

- Follow the rules of medical asepsis.
- Follow Standard Precautions and the Bloodborne Pathogen Standard.
- Use a clean container for each specimen.
- Use the correct container.
- Label the container accurately.
- Do not touch the inside of the container or lid.
- Identify the person. Check the ID bracelet against the laboratory requisition slip or assignment sheet. Compare all information.
- Collect the specimen at the correct time.
- Ask the person not to have a bowel movement when collecting a urine specimen. The specimen must not contain feces.
- Ask the person to put toilet tissue in the toilet or wastebasket. Urine and stool specimens must not contain tissue.
- Place the specimen container in a plastic bag.
- Take the specimen and requisition slip to the laboratory. Or take it to the storage area.

URINE SPECIMENS

Urine specimens are collected for urine tests. Follow the rules in Box 19-1.

DELEGATION GUIDELINES
Urine Specimens

Before collecting a urine specimen, you need this information from the nurse:

- The type of specimen needed
- What time to collect the specimen
- What special measures are needed
- If you need to test the specimen (p. 341)
- What observations to report and record:
  - Problems obtaining the specimen
  - Color, clarity, and odor of urine
  - Particles in the urine
  - Complaints of pain, burning, urgency, dysuria, or other problems

PROMOTING SAFETY AND COMFORT
Urine Specimens

Safety

Microbes can grow in urine. Urine also may contain blood. Follow Standard Precautions and the Bloodborne Pathogen Standard.

Comfort

Urine specimens may embarrass some people. They do not like clear specimen containers that show urine. Placing the urine specimen container in a paper bag is often helpful.

 ## The Random Urine Specimen

The random urine specimen is collected for a routine urinalysis. No special measures are needed. It is collected at any time during a 24-hour period. Many people can collect the specimen themselves. Weak and very ill persons need help.

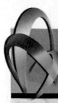

Collecting a Random Urine Specimen

Pre-Procedure

1 Follow *Delegation Guidelines: Urine Specimens,* p. 337. See *Promoting Safety and Comfort: Urine Specimens,* p. 337.
2 Practice hand hygiene. Put on gloves.
3 Collect the following:
   - Voiding receptacle—bedpan and cover, urinal, or specimen pan (Fig. 19-1)

- Specimen container and lid
- Label
- Gloves
- Plastic bag

Procedure

4 Label the container.
5 Put the container and lid in the bathroom.
6 Remove the gloves. Decontaminate your hands.
7 Identify the person. Check the ID bracelet against the requisition slip. Call the person by name.
8 Provide for privacy.
9 Put on the gloves.
10 Ask the person to void into the receptacle. Remind him or her to put toilet tissue into the wastebasket or toilet. Toilet tissue is not put in the bedpan or specimen pan.

11 Take the receptacle to the bathroom.
12 Pour about 120 ml (4 oz) of urine into the specimen container. Dispose of excess urine.
13 Place the lid on the specimen container. Put the container in the plastic bag.
14 Clean and return the receptacle to its proper place.
15 Remove the gloves, and practice hand hygiene. Put on clean gloves.
16 Assist with hand washing.
17 Remove the gloves. Decontaminate your hands.

Post-Procedure

18 Provide for comfort. (See the inside of the front book cover.)
19 Place the signal light within reach.
20 Raise or lower bed rails. Follow the care plan.
21 Unscreen the person.

22 Complete a safety check of the room. (See the inside of the front book cover.)
23 Decontaminate your hands.
24 Report and record your observations.
25 Take the specimen and the requisition slip to the storage area or laboratory.

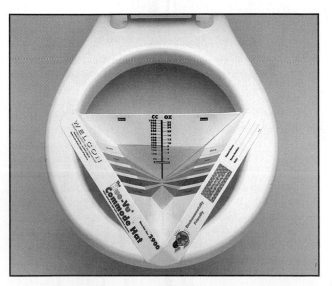

FIG. **19-1** The specimen pan is placed on the toilet rim. It has a color chart for urine. (Courtesy Welcon, Inc., Forth Worth, Tex.)

 The Midstream Specimen

The midstream specimen is also called a *clean-voided specimen* or a *clean-catch specimen.* The perineal area is cleaned before collecting the specimen. This reduces the number of microbes in the urethral area. The person starts to void into a receptacle. Then the person stops the stream of urine, and a sterile specimen container is positioned. The person voids into the container until the specimen is obtained.

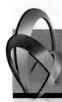

Collecting a Midstream Specimen

Quality of Life

Pre-Procedure

1 Follow *Delegation Guidelines: Urine Specimens,* p. 337. See *Promoting Safety and Comfort: Urine Specimens,* p. 337.
2 Practice hand hygiene. Put on gloves.
3 Collect the following:
   - Midstream specimen kit (with antiseptic solution)
   - Label
   - Disposable gloves
   - Sterile gloves (if not part of the kit)
   - Voiding receptacle—bedpan, urinal, or commode if needed
   - Plastic bag
   - Supplies for perineal care
4 Label the container.
5 Remove the gloves. Decontaminate your hands.
6 Identify the person. Check the ID bracelet against the requisition slip. Call the person by name.
7 Provide for privacy.

Procedure

8 Provide perineal care. (Wear gloves for this step. Decontaminate your hands after removing them).
9 Open the sterile kit.
10 Put on the sterile gloves.
11 Pour the antiseptic solution over the cotton balls.
12 Open the sterile specimen container. Do not touch the inside of the container or lid. Set the lid down so the inside is up.
13 *For a female*—clean the perineum with cotton balls.
   a Spread the labia with your thumb and index finger. Use your non-dominant hand. (This hand is now contaminated. It must not touch anything sterile.)
   b Clean down the urethral area from front to back. Use a clean cotton ball for each stroke.
   c Keep the labia separated to collect the urine specimen (steps 15 through 18).
14 *For a male*—clean the penis with cotton balls.
   a Hold the penis with your non-dominant hand.
   b Clean the penis starting at the meatus. Use a cotton ball and clean in a circular motion. Start at the center and work outward.
   c Keep holding the penis until the specimen is collected (steps 15 through 18).
15 Ask the person to void into the receptacle.
16 Pass the specimen container into the stream of urine. Keep the labia separated (Fig. 19-2, p. 340).
17 Collect about 30 to 60 ml of urine (1 to 2 oz).
18 Remove the specimen container before the person stops voiding.
19 Release the labia or penis.
20 Let the person finish voiding into the receptacle.
21 Put the lid on the specimen container. Touch only the outside of the container or lid.
22 Wipe the outside of the container.
23 Place the container in a plastic bag.
24 Provide toilet tissue after the person is done voiding.
25 Take the receptacle to the bathroom.
26 Measure urine if intake and output is ordered. Include the amount in the specimen container.
27 Clean the receptacle and other items. Return equipment to its proper place.
28 Remove the gloves. Practice hand hygiene.
29 Put on clean gloves.
30 Assist with hand washing.
31 Remove the gloves. Decontaminate your hands.

Post-Procedure

32 Follow steps 18 through 25 in *Collecting a Random Urine Specimen.*

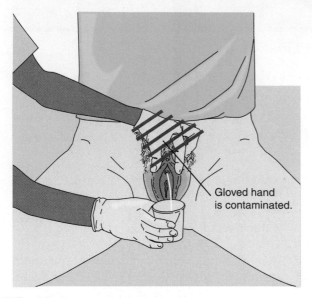

FIG. **19-2** The labia are separated to collect a midstream specimen.

Gloved hand is contaminated.

 The Double-Voided Specimen

Fresh-fractional urine specimen is another term for a double-voided specimen. The person voids twice. The first time the bladder is emptied of "stale" urine. "Fresh" urine collects in the bladder after the first voiding. In 30 minutes the person voids again. The second voiding is usually a very small or "fractional" amount of urine.

Fresh-fractional specimens are used to test urine for glucose and ketones.

 Collecting a Double-Voided Specimen

Quality of Life

Remember to:

- Knock before entering the person's room
- Address the person by name
- Introduce yourself by name and title

- Explain the procedure to the person before beginning and during the procedure
- Protect the person's rights during the procedure
- Handle the person gently during the procedure

Pre-Procedure

1 Follow *Delegation Guidelines: Urine Specimens,* p. 337. See *Promoting Safety and Comfort: Urine Specimens,* p. 337.
2 Practice hand hygiene. Put on gloves.
3 Collect the following:
  • Voiding receptacle—bedpan, urinal, commode, or specimen pan

  • Two specimen containers
  • Urine testing equipment
  • Gloves
4 Remove the gloves. Decontaminate your hands.
5 Identify the person. Check the ID bracelet against the assignment sheet. Call the person by name.
6 Provide for privacy.

Procedure

7 Put on the gloves.
8 Ask the person to void into the receptacle. Remind the person not to put toilet tissue in the receptacle.
9 Take the receptacle to the bathroom.
10 Pour some urine into the specimen container.
11 Test the specimen in case you cannot obtain a second specimen. Discard the urine. Note the result on your assignment sheet.
12 Clean the receptacle, and return the receptacle to its proper place.
13 Remove the gloves, and practice hand hygiene. Put on clean gloves.

14 Assist with hand washing.
15 Remove the gloves. Decontaminate your hands.
16 Ask the person to drink an 8-ounce glass of water.
17 Provide for comfort. (See the inside of the front book cover.) Raise the bed rails if needed. Place the signal light within reach.
18 Unscreen the person.
19 Decontaminate your hands.
20 Complete a safety check of the room. (See the inside of the front book cover.)
21 Return to the room in 20 to 30 minutes.
22 Repeat steps 6 through 15.

Collecting a Double-Voided Specimen—cont'd

Post-Procedure

23 Provide for comfort. (See the inside of the front book cover.)
24 Place the signal light within reach.
25 Raise the bed rails if needed. Follow the care plan.
26 Unscreen the person.

27 Complete a safety check of the room. (See the inside of the front book cover.)
28 Decontaminate your hands.
29 Report the results of the second test and any other observations.

 ## Testing Urine

The nurse may ask you to do simple urine tests. You can test for pH, glucose, ketones, and blood using reagent strips. The doctor orders the type and frequency of urine tests.

- *Testing for pH*—Urine pH measures if urine is acidic or alkaline. Changes in normal pH (4.6 to 8.0) occur from illness, foods, and drugs. A routine urine specimen is needed.
- *Testing for glucose and ketones*—In diabetes the pancreas does not secrete enough insulin (Chapter 24). The body needs insulin to use sugar for energy. If not used, sugar builds up in the blood. Some sugar appears in the urine. **Glucosuria** or **glycosuria** means sugar (*glucos, glycos*) in the urine (*uria*). The diabetic person may also have **acetone (ketone bodies, ketones)** in the urine. These substances appear in urine from the rapid breakdown of fat for energy. The body uses fat for energy if it cannot use sugar. Urine is also tested for ketones. These tests are usually done four times a day—30 minutes before each meal and at bedtime. The doctor uses the test to make drug and diet decisions. Double-voided specimens are best for these tests.
- *Testing for blood*—Injury and disease can cause blood (*hemat*) to appear in the urine (*uria*). This is called **hematuria.** Sometimes blood is seen in the urine. At other times it is unseen (*occult*). A routine urine specimen is needed.

DELEGATION GUIDELINES
Testing Urine

When testing urine is delegated to you, you need this information from the nurse and the care plan:
- What test is needed
- What equipment to use
- When to test urine
- Specific instructions for the test ordered
- If the nurse wants to observe the results of each test
- What observations to report and record:
  - Test results
  - Problems obtaining the specimen
  - Color, clarity, and odor of urine
  - Particles in the urine
  - Complaints of pain, burning, urgency, dysuria, or other problems

PROMOTING SAFETY AND COMFORT
Testing Urine

Safety

When using reagent strips, read and follow the manufacturer's instructions. Otherwise you could get the wrong result. The doctor uses the test results in diagnosing and treating the person. A wrong result could lead to serious harm.

You must be accurate when testing urine. Promptly report the results to the nurse. Ordered drugs may depend on the results.

Microbes can grow in urine. Urine also may contain blood. Follow Standard Precautions and the Bloodborne Pathogen Standard.

Comfort

The person may want to know the test results. If allowed by agency policy, you can tell the person the results. Remember, this information is private and confidential. Make sure only the person hears what you are saying.

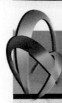

Testing Urine With Reagent Strips

Quality of Life

Remember to:

- Knock before entering the person's room
- Address the person by name
- Introduce yourself by name and title

- Explain the procedure to the person before beginning and during the procedure
- Protect the person's rights during the procedure
- Handle the person gently during the procedure

Pre-Procedure

1. Follow *Delegation Guidelines: Testing Urine,* p. 341. See *Promoting Safety and Comfort: Testing Urine,* p. 341.

2. Practice hand hygiene.
3. Identify the person. Check the ID bracelet against the assignment sheet. Call the person by name.

Procedure

4. Put on the gloves.
5. Collect the following:
   - Urine specimen (routine specimen for pH and occult blood; double-voided specimen for sugar and ketones)
   - Reagent strip as ordered
   - Gloves
6. Remove a strip from the bottle. Put the cap on the bottle at once. It must be on tight.
7. Dip the strip test areas into the urine.

8. Remove the strip after the correct amount of time. See the manufacturer's instructions.
9. Tap the strip gently against the container. This removes excess urine.
10. Wait the required amount of time. See the manufacturer's instructions.
11. Compare the strip with the color chart on the bottle (Fig. 19-3). Read the results.
12. Discard disposable items and the specimen.
13. Remove the gloves. Decontaminate your hands.

Post-Procedure

14. Provide for comfort. (See the inside of the front book cover.)
15. Place the signal light within reach.
16. Clean and return equipment to its proper place. (Wear gloves for this step.)

17. Complete a safety check of the room. (See the inside of the front book cover.)
18. Remove the gloves. Practice hand hygiene.
19. Report and record the results and other observations.

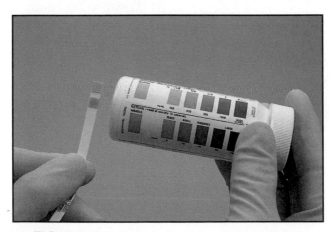

FIG. **19-3** Reagent strips for sugar and ketones.

STOOL SPECIMENS

When internal bleeding is suspected, feces are checked for blood. Stools are also studied for fat, microbes, worms, and other abnormal contents. The stool specimen must not be contaminated with urine. Some tests require a warm stool. The specimen is taken to the laboratory at once if a warm stool is needed. Remember to follow the rules in Box 19-1.

DELEGATION GUIDELINES
Stool Specimens

Before collecting a stool specimen, you need this information from the nurse:
- What time to collect the specimen
- What special measures are needed
- What observations to report and record:
  - Problems obtaining the specimen
  - Color, amount, consistency, and odor of feces
  - Complaints of pain or discomfort

PROMOTING SAFETY AND COMFORT
Stool Specimens

Safety

Stools contain microbes. And they may contain blood. Follow Standard Precautions and the Bloodborne Pathogen Standard.

Comfort

Stools normally have an odor. A person may be embarrassed that you need to collect a specimen. Complete the task quickly and carefully. Also act in a professional manner.

Collecting a Stool Specimen

Quality of Life

Remember to:
- Knock before entering the person's room
- Address the person by name
- Introduce yourself by name and title
- Explain the procedure to the person before beginning and during the procedure
- Protect the person's rights during the procedure
- Handle the person gently during the procedure

Pre-Procedure

1 Follow *Delegation Guidelines: Stool Specimens.* See *Promoting Safety and Comfort: Stool Specimens.*
2 Practice hand hygiene. Put on gloves.
3 Collect the following:
- Bedpan and cover or commode
- Urinal for voiding
- Specimen pan for the toilet or commode
- Specimen container and lid
- Tongue blade
- Disposable bag
- Gloves
- Toilet tissue
- Laboratory requisition slip
- Plastic bag

Continued

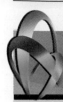

Collecting a Stool Specimen—cont'd

Procedure

4 Label the container.

5 Remove the gloves. Decontaminate your hands.

6 Identify the person. Check the ID bracelet against the requisition slip. Call the person by name.

7 Provide for privacy.

8 Put on gloves.

9 Ask the person to void. Provide the bedpan, commode, or urinal for voiding if the person does not use the bathroom. Empty and clean the device.

10 Put the specimen pan on the toilet if the person will use the bathroom. Place it at the back of the toilet (Fig. 19-4).

11 Assist the person onto the bedpan or to the toilet or commode. The person wears a robe and non-skid footwear when up.

12 Ask the person not to put toilet tissue in the bedpan, commode, or specimen pan. Provide a bag for toilet tissue.

13 Place the signal light and toilet tissue within reach. Raise or lower bed rails. Follow the care plan.

14 Remove the gloves, and decontaminate your hands. Leave the room.

15 Return when the person signals. Or check on the person every 5 minutes. Knock before entering. Decontaminate your hands.

16 Lower the bed rail near you if up.

17 Put on the gloves. Provide perineal care if needed.

18 Use a tongue blade to take about 2 tablespoons of stool to the specimen container (Fig. 19-5). Take the sample from the middle of a formed stool. If required by agency policy, take stool from 2 different places on the specimen.

19 Put the lid on the specimen container. Do not touch the inside of the lid or container. Place the container in the plastic bag.

20 Wrap the tongue blade in toilet tissue.

21 Discard the tongue blade into the bag.

22 Empty, clean, and disinfect equipment.

23 Remove the gloves. Decontaminate your hands.

24 Return equipment to its proper place.

25 Put on clean gloves.

26 Assist with hand washing.

27 Remove the gloves. Decontaminate your hands.

Post-Procedure

28 Provide for comfort. (See the inside of the front book cover.)

29 Place the signal light within reach.

30 Raise or lower bed rails. Follow the care plan.

31 Unscreen the person.

32 Complete a safety check of the room. (See the

inside of the front book cover.)

33 Take the specimen and requisition slip to the laboratory.

34 Decontaminate your hands.

35 Report and record your observations.

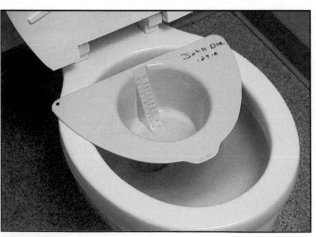

FIG. **19-4** The specimen pan is placed at the back of the toilet for a stool specimen.

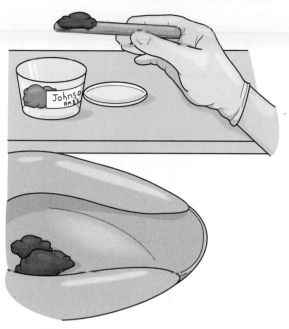

FIG. **19-5** A tongue blade is used to transfer a small amount of stool from the bedpan to the specimen container.

Before collecting a sputum specimen, you need this information from the nurse:
- When to collect the specimen
- How much sputum is needed—usually 1 to 2 tablespoons
- If the person uses the bathroom
- If the person can hold the specimen container
- What observations to report and record:
  - The time the specimen was collected
  - The amount of sputum collected
  - How easily the person raised the sputum
  - Sputum color—clear, white, yellow, green, brown, or red
  - Sputum odor—none or foul odor
  - Sputum consistency—thick, watery, or frothy (with bubbles or foam)
  - **Hemoptysis**—bloody *(hemo)* sputum *(ptysis,* meaning "to spit")
  - If the person was not able to produce a specimen
  - Any other observations

 SPUTUM SPECIMENS

Respiratory disorders cause the lungs, bronchi, and trachea to secrete mucus. Mucus from the respiratory system is called **sputum** when expectorated (expelled) through the mouth. Sputum specimens are studied for blood, microbes, and abnormal cells.

The person coughs up sputum from the bronchi and trachea. This is often painful and hard to do. It is easier to collect a specimen in the morning. Secretions are coughed up upon awakening.

The person rinses the mouth with water. Rinsing decreases saliva and removes food particles. Mouthwash is not used. It destroys some of the microbes in the mouth.

Remember to follow the rules in Box 19-1.

Safety

Follow Standard Precautions and the Bloodborne Pathogen Standard to prevent contact with mucus. It may contain blood or microbes.

The doctor may order Isolation Precautions if the person has or may have tuberculosis (TB) (Chapter 24). Protect yourself by wearing a tuberculosis respirator (Chapter 10).

Comfort

The procedure can embarrass the person. Coughing and expectorating sounds can disturb those nearby. Also, sputum is unpleasant to look at. For these reasons, privacy is important. Cover the specimen container and place it in a bag. Some sputum containers hide the contents.

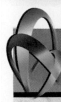

Collecting a Sputum Specimen

Quality of Life

Remember to:

- Knock before entering the person's room
- Address the person by name
- Introduce yourself by name and title

- Explain the procedure to the person before beginning and during the procedure
- Protect the person's rights during the procedure
- Handle the person gently during the procedure

Pre-Procedure

1 Follow *Delegation Guidelines: Sputum Specimens,* p. 345. See *Promoting Safety and Comfort: Sputum Specimens,* p. 345.
2 Practice hand hygiene.
3 Collect the following:
   - Sputum specimen container and label
   - Laboratory requisition slip
   - Disposable bag

   - Gloves
   - Tissues
4 Label the container.
5 Identify the person. Check the ID bracelet against the requisition slip. Call the person by name.
6 Provide for privacy. If able, the person uses the bathroom for the procedure.

Procedure

7 Put on the gloves.
8 Ask the person to rinse the mouth out with clear water.
9 Have the person hold the container. Only the outside is touched.
10 Ask the person to cover the mouth and nose with tissues when coughing.
11 Ask him or her to take 2 or 3 deep breaths and cough up the sputum.
12 Have the person expectorate directly into the container (Fig. 19-6). Sputum should not touch the outside.

13 Collect 1 to 2 tablespoons of sputum unless told to collect more.
14 Put the lid on the container.
15 Place the container in the bag. Attach the requisition slip to the bag.
16 Remove the gloves, and decontaminate your hands. Put on clean gloves.
17 Assist with hand washing.
18 Remove the gloves. Decontaminate your hands.

Post-Procedure

19 Provide for comfort. (See the inside of the front book cover.)
20 Place the signal light within reach.
21 Unscreen the person.
22 Complete a safety check of the room. (See the inside of the front book cover.)

23 Decontaminate your hands.
24 Take the bag to the laboratory or storage area.
25 Decontaminate your hands.
26 Report and record your observations.

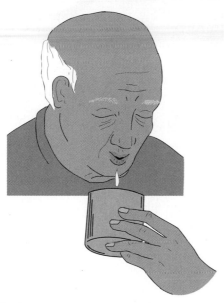

FIG. **19-6** The person expectorates into the center of the specimen container.

FOCUS ON THE PERSON

You must collect specimens correctly and carefully. Test results depend on proper specimen collection. Correct test results are needed for the doctor to detect and treat disease. *See Focus on the Person: Assisting With Specimens.*

Focus on the PERSON

Assisting With Specimens

Providing comfort—Specimen collection embarrasses many people. Promote comfort by explaining the procedure to the person. This helps the person know what to expect and what to do. For example, do not say that you need a stool specimen and leave the specimen container in the bathroom. The person may think that the specimen container is used to have a bowel movement. To do so would be most uncomfortable and embarrassing.

Ethical behavior—Ethics is concerned with right and wrong behavior. If you did not collect a specimen correctly, do not send it to the laboratory. Tell the nurse what happened. Then collect the specimen at the next opportunity. Test results must be accurate for correct diagnosis and treatment.

Remaining independent—Some people can collect their own urine and sputum specimens. Doing so promotes independence. It also helps reduce embarrassment.

Speaking up—Always explain the procedure before you begin. Explain what the person needs to do and what you will do. Also show what equipment and supplies you will use. For example: "The doctor wants your stools tested. Meaning, we need a specimen from a bowel movement. I'm going to place this specimen pan

(show the specimen pan) at the back of the toilet seat. Your stools will collect in it rather than in the toilet. Please put toilet tissue in the toilet, not in the specimen pan. After you have a bowel movement, put your signal light on right away. I'll use a tongue blade (show tongue blade) to take some stool from the specimen pan to put in this specimen container (show specimen container)."

After explaining the procedure, ask the person if he or she has any questions. If you do not know the answer, refer the question to the nurse.

Also make sure the person understands what to do. You can say: "Mrs. Clark, please help me make sure that you understand what I said. To collect a stool specimen, please tell me what you're going to do and what I need to do."

OBRA and other laws—You must correctly identify the person. Specimens must be collected and tests done on the right person. Otherwise one or both persons could suffer harm. Before collecting or testing a specimen, carefully identify the person. Check the ID bracelet against the laboratory requisition slip or assignment sheet. Compare all information, not just the person's name.

Nursing teamwork—You may need to take a specimen to the laboratory. Before you go, ask if other staff need to have specimens taken there. This saves staff time. It also prevents having too many staff members off the unit at the same time.

REVIEW QUESTIONS

Circle the **BEST** answer.

1 You are going to collect a random urine specimen. You should do the following *except*
   a Label the container as requested
   b Use the correct container
   c Collect the specimen at the right time
   d Use sterile supplies

2 The perineum is cleaned before collecting a
   a Random specimen
   b Midstream specimen
   c Stool specimen
   d Double-voided specimen

3 Urine is tested for sugar and ketones
   a At bedtime
   b 30 minutes after meals and at bedtime
   c 30 minutes before meals and at bedtime
   d Before breakfast

4 Which specimen is best for sugar and ketone testing?
   a A random specimen
   b A clean-voided specimen
   c A reagent specimen
   d A double-voided specimen

5 A stool specimen must be kept warm. After collecting the specimen, you need to
   a Put it in the oven
   b Take it to the storage area
   c Take it to the laboratory
   d Cover it with a towel

6 The best time to collect a sputum specimen is
   a On awakening
   b After meals
   c At bedtime
   d After oral hygiene

7 A sputum specimen is needed. You should ask the person to
   a Use mouthwash
   b Rinse the mouth with clear water
   c Brush the teeth
   d Remove dentures

Answers to these questions are on page 469.

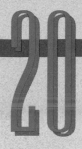

Assisting With Exercise and Activity

OBJECTIVES

- Define the key terms listed in this chapter
- Describe bedrest and how to prevent related complications
- Describe the devices used to support and maintain body alignment
- Describe range-of-motion exercises
- Explain how to help a falling person
- Describe four walking aids
- Perform the procedures described in this chapter

PROCEDURES

Procedures with this icon are also on the CD-ROM in this book.

- Performing Range-of-Motion Exercises
- Helping the Person to Walk
- Helping the Falling Person

Key Terms

abduction Moving a body part away from the midline of the body

adduction Moving a body part toward the midline of the body

ambulation The act of walking

atrophy The decrease in size or a wasting away of tissue

contracture The lack of joint mobility caused by abnormal shortening of a muscle

dorsiflexion Bending the toes and foot up at the ankle

extension Straightening a body part

external rotation Turning the joint outward

flexion Bending a body part

footdrop The foot falls down at the ankle; permanent plantar flexion

hyperextension Excessive straightening of a body part

internal rotation Turning the joint inward

orthostatic hypotension Abnormally low *(hypo)* blood pressure when the person suddenly stands up *(ortho* and *static)*; postural hypotension

plantar flexion The foot *(plantar)* is bent *(flexion)*; bending the foot down at the ankle

postural hypotension Orthostatic hypotension

pronation Turning the joint downward

range of motion (ROM) The movement of a joint to the extent possible without causing pain

rotation Turning the joint

supination Turning the joint upward

Illness, surgery, injury, pain, and aging can limit activity. Inactivity, whether mild or severe, affects every body system. It also affects mental well-being. Exercise and activity are promoted in all persons to the extent possible. The care plan and your assignment sheet include the person's activity level and needed exercises.

BEDREST

The doctor orders bedrest to treat a health problem. Sometimes it is a nursing measure if the person's condition changes. Bedrest is ordered to:

- Reduce physical activity
- Reduce pain
- Encourage rest
- Regain strength
- Promote healing

These types of bedrest are common.

- *Bedrest.* Some activities of daily living (ADL) are allowed. Self-feeding, oral hygiene, bathing, shaving, and hair care are often allowed.

- *Strict bedrest.* Everything is done for the person. No ADL are allowed.
- *Bedrest with commode privileges.* A commode is used for elimination.
- *Bedrest with bathroom privileges (bedrest with BRP).* The bathroom is used for elimination.

Complications of Bedrest

Bedrest and lack of exercise and activity can cause serious complications. Pressure ulcers, constipation, and fecal impaction can result. Urinary tract infections and renal calculi (kidney stones) can occur. So can blood clots (thrombi) and pneumonia (infection of the lung).

The musculoskeletal system is affected by the lack of exercise and activity. These complications must be prevented to maintain normal movement.

- A **contracture** is the lack of joint mobility caused by abnormal shortening of a muscle. The contracted muscle is fixed into position, is deformed, and cannot stretch (Fig. 20-1). Common sites are the fingers, wrists, elbows, toes, ankles, knees, hips, neck, and spine. The person is permanently deformed and disabled.
- **Atrophy** is the decrease in size or the wasting away of tissue. Tissues shrink in size. Muscle atrophy is a decrease in size or a wasting away of muscle (Fig. 20-2).

Orthostatic hypotension is abnormally low *(hypo)* blood pressure when the person suddenly stands up *(ortho* and *static)*. It is also called **postural hypotension.** *(Postural* relates to posture or standing.) When a person moves from lying or sitting to a standing position, the blood pressure drops. The person is dizzy and weak and has spots before the eyes. Fainting can occur. Slowly changing positions is key to preventing orthostatic hypotension.

Good nursing care prevents complications from bedrest. Good alignment, range-of-motion exercises, and frequent position changes are important. They are part of the care plan.

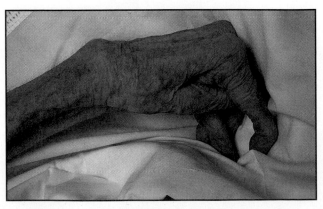

FIG. **20-1** A contracture.

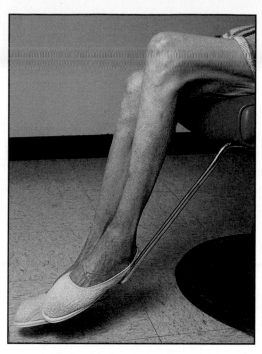

FIG. **20-2** Muscle atrophy.

Positioning

Body alignment and positioning were discussed in Chapter 11. Supportive devices are often used to support and maintain the person in a certain position.

- *Bed boards*—are placed under the mattress to prevent it from sagging (Fig. 20-3).
- *Foot boards*—prevent plantar flexion that can lead to footdrop. In **plantar flexion**, the foot *(plantar)* is bent *(flexion)*. **Footdrop** is when the foot falls down at the ankle (permanent plantar flexion). The foot board is placed so the soles of the feet are flush against it (Fig. 20-4). Foot boards also keep top linens off the feet and toes.
- *Trochanter rolls*—prevent the hips and legs from turning outward (external rotation). A bath blanket is folded to the desired length and rolled up. The loose end is placed under the person from the hip to the knee (Fig. 20-5). Then the roll is tucked alongside the body.
- *Hip abduction wedges*—keep the hips abducted (Fig. 20-6, p. 352). The wedge is placed between the person's legs. These are common after hip replacement surgery.
- *Handrolls or hand grips*—prevent contractures of the thumb, fingers, and wrist (Fig. 20-7, p. 352). Sponges, rubber balls, and finger cushions (Fig. 20-8, p. 352) also are used.
- *Splints*—keep the elbows, wrists, thumbs, fingers, ankles, and knees in normal position (Fig. 20-9, p. 353).
- *Bed cradles*—keep the weight of top linens off the feet and toes (Fig. 20-10, p. 353). The weight of top linens can cause footdrop and pressure ulcers.

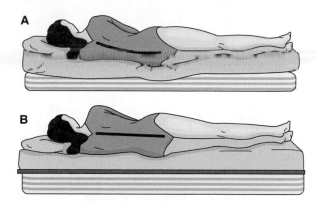

FIG. **20-3** Bed boards. **A,** Mattress sagging without bed boards. **B,** Bed boards are under the mattress. No sagging occurs.

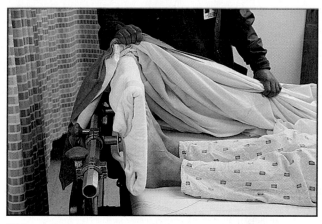

FIG. **20-4** A foot board. Feet are flush with the board to keep them in normal alignment.

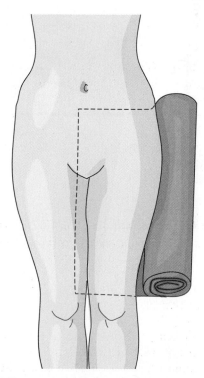

FIG. **20-5** A trochanter roll is made from a bath blanket. It extends from the hip to the knee.

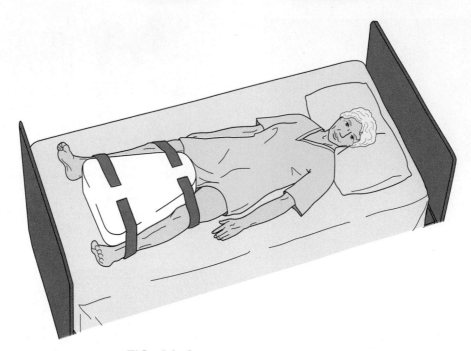

FIG. **20-6** Hip abduction wedge.

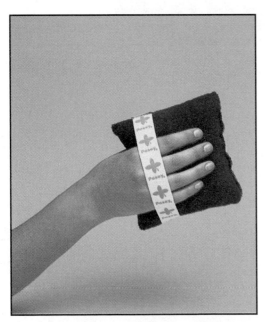

FIG. **20-7** Hand grip. (Courtesy JT Posey Co., Arcadia, Calif.)

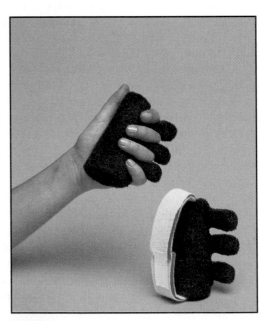

FIG. **20-8** Finger cushion. (Courtesy JT Posey Co., Arcadia, Calif.)

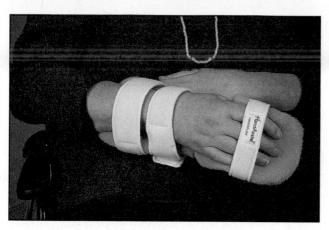

FIG. **20-9** A splint.

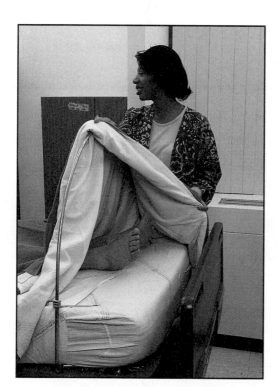

FIG. **20-10** A bed cradle.

 RANGE-OF-MOTION EXERCISES

The movement of a joint to the extent possible without causing pain is the **range of motion (ROM)** of that joint. Range-of-motion exercises involve moving the joints through their complete range of motion (Box 20-1). They are usually done at least twice a day. The doctor or nurse may order:

■ *Active* range-of-motion exercises—are done by the person.
■ *Passive* range-of-motion exercises—another person moves the joints.
■ *Active-assistive* range-of-motion exercises—the person does the exercises with some help from another person.

Text continued on p. 359

BOX 20-1	**Joint Movements**

Abduction—moving a body part away from the midline of the body
Adduction—moving a body part toward the midline of the body
Extension—straightening a body part
Flexion—bending a body part
Hyperextension—excessive straightening of a body part
Dorsiflexion—bending the toes and foot up at the ankle
Rotation—turning the joint
Internal rotation—turning the joint inward
External rotation—turning the joint outward
Plantar flexion—bending the foot down at the ankle
Pronation—turning the joint downward
Supination—turning the joint upward

DELEGATION GUIDELINES
Range-of-Motion Exercises

When delegated range-of-motion exercises, you need this information from the nurse and the care plan:

■ The kind of range-of-motion exercises ordered—active, passive, active-assistive
■ Which joints to exercise
■ How often the exercises are done
■ How many times to repeat each exercise
■ What observations to report and record:
  ■ The time the exercises were performed
  ■ The joints exercised
  ■ The number of times the exercises were performed on each joint
  ■ Complaints of pain or signs of stiffness or spasm
  ■ The degree to which the person took part in the exercises

PROMOTING SAFETY AND COMFORT
Range-of-Motion Exercises

Safety

Range-of-motion exercises can cause injury if not done properly. Muscle strain, joint injury, and pain are possible. Practice the rules in Box 20-2 when performing or assisting with range-of-motion exercises.

Range-of-motion exercises to the neck can cause serious injury if not done properly. Some agencies require that nursing assistants have special training before doing such exercises. Other agencies do not let nursing assistants do them. Know your agency's policy. Perform range-of-motion exercises to the neck only if allowed by your agency and if the nurse instructs you to do so.

Comfort

To promote physical comfort during range-of-motion exercises, follow the rules in Box 20-2. Also cover the person with a bath blanket. Expose only the part being exercised. Providing for privacy promotes mental comfort.

> **BOX 20-2**   **Performing Range-of-Motion Exercises**
>
> - Exercise only the joints the nurse tells you to exercise.
> - Expose only the body part being exercised.
> - Use good body mechanics.
> - Support the part being exercised.
> - Move the joint slowly, smoothly, and gently.
> - Do not force a joint beyond its present range of motion or to the point of pain.
> - *Perform range-of-motion exercises to the neck only if allowed by agency policy.* In some agencies, only physical or occupational therapists do neck exercises. This is because of the danger of neck injuries.

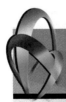

Performing Range-of-Motion Exercises

Quality of Life

Remember to:

- Knock before entering the person's room
- Address the person by name
- Introduce yourself by name and title

- Explain the procedure to the person before beginning and during the procedure
- Protect the person's rights during the procedure
- Handle the person gently during the procedure

Pre-Procedure

1. Follow *Delegation Guidelines: Range-of-Motion Exercises*, p. 353. See *Promoting Safety and Comfort: Range-of-Motion Exercises.*
2. Practice hand hygiene.
3. Identify the person. Check the ID bracelet against the assignment sheet. Call the person by name.
4. Obtain a bath blanket.
5. Provide for privacy.
6. Raise the bed for body mechanics. Bed rails are up if used.

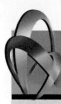
Procedure

7 Lower the bed rail near you if up.

8 Position the person supine.

9 Cover the person with a bath blanket. Fan-fold top linens to the foot of the bed.

10 Exercise the neck *if allowed by your agency and if the RN instructs you to do so* (Fig. 20-11, p. 357):
   a Place your hands over the person's ears to support the head. Support the jaws with your fingers.
   b Flexion—bring the head forward. The chin touches the chest.
   c Extension—straighten the head.
   d Hyperextension—bring the head backward until the chin points up.
   e Rotation—turn the head from side to side.
   f Lateral flexion—move the head to the right and to the left.
   g Repeat flexion, extension, hyperextension, rotation, and lateral flexion 5 times—or the number of times stated on the care plan.

11 Exercise the shoulder (Fig. 20-12, p. 357):
   a Grasp the wrist with one hand. Grasp the elbow with the other hand.
   b Flexion—raise the arm straight in front and over the head.
   c Extension—bring the arm down to the side.
   d Hyperextension—move the arm behind the body. (Do this if the person sits in a straight-backed chair or is standing.)
   e Abduction—move the straight arm away from the side of the body.
   f Adduction—move the straight arm to the side of the body.
   g Internal rotation—bend the elbow. Place it at the same level as the shoulder. Move the forearm down toward the body.
   h External rotation—move the forearm toward the head.
   i Repeat flexion, extension, hyperextension, abduction, adduction, and internal and external rotation 5 times—or the number of times stated on the care plan.

12 Exercise the elbow (Fig. 20-13, p. 357):
   a Grasp the person's wrist with one hand. Grasp the elbow with your other hand.
   b Flexion—bend the arm so the same-side shoulder is touched.
   c Extension—straighten the arm.
   d Repeat flexion and extension 5 times—or the number of times stated on the care plan.

13 Exercise the forearm (Fig. 20-14, p. 357):
   a Pronation—turn the hand so the palm is down.
   b Supination—turn the hand so the palm is up.
   c Repeat pronation and supination 5 times—or the number of times stated on the care plan.

14 Exercise the wrist (Fig. 20-15, p. 357):
   a Hold the wrist with both of your hands.
   b Flexion—bend the hand down.
   c Extension—straighten the hand.
   d Hyperextension—bend the hand back.
   e Radial flexion—turn the hand toward the thumb.
   f Ulnar flexion—turn the hand toward the little finger.
   g Repeat flexion, extension, hyperextension, and radial flexion and ulnar flexion 5 times—or the number of times stated on the care plan.

15 Exercise the thumb (Fig. 20-16, p. 357):
   a Hold the person's hand with one hand. Hold the thumb with your other hand.
   b Abduction—move the thumb out from the inner part of the index finger.
   c Adduction—move the thumb back next to the index finger.
   d Opposition—touch each fingertip with the thumb.
   e Flexion—bend the thumb into the hand.
   f Extension—move the thumb out to the side of the fingers.
   g Repeat abduction, adduction, opposition, flexion, and extension 5 times—or the number of times stated on the care plan.

16 Exercise the fingers (Fig. 20-17, p. 358):
   a Abduction—spread the fingers and the thumb apart.
   b Adduction—bring the fingers and thumb together.
   c Extension—straighten the fingers so the fingers, hand, and arm are straight.
   d Flexion—make a fist.
   e Repeat abduction, adduction, extension, and flexion 5 times—or the number of times stated on the care plan.

Continued

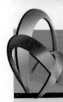

Performing Range-of-Motion Exercises—cont'd

NNAAP™

Procedure—cont'd

17 Exercise the hip (Fig. 20-18, p. 358):
  a Support the leg. Place one hand under the knee. Place your other hand under the ankle.
  b Flexion—raise the leg.
  c Extension—straighten the leg.
  d Abduction—move the leg away from the body.
  e Adduction—move the leg toward the other leg.
  f Internal rotation—turn the leg inward.
  g External rotation—turn the leg outward.
  h Repeat flexion, extension, abduction, adduction, and internal and external rotation 5 times—or the number of times stated on the care plan.

18 Exercise the knee (Fig. 20-19, p. 358):
  a Support the knee. Place one hand under the knee. Place your other hand under the ankle.
  b Flexion—bend the leg.
  c Extension—straighten the leg.
  d Repeat flexion and extension of the knee 5 times—or the number of times stated on the care plan.

19 Exercise the ankle (Fig. 20-20, p. 358):
  a Support the foot and ankle. Place one hand under the foot. Place your other hand under the ankle.
  b Dorsiflexion—pull the foot forward. Push down on the heel at the same time.

  c Plantar flexion—turn the foot down. Or point the toes.
  d Repeat dorsiflexion and plantar flexion 5 times—or the number of times stated on the care plan.

20 Exercise the foot (Fig. 20-21, p. 359):
  a Continue to support the foot and ankle.
  b Pronation—turn the outside of the foot up and the inside down.
  c Supination—turn the inside of the foot up and the outside down.
  d Repeat pronation and supination 5 times— or the number of times stated on the care plan.

21 Exercise the toes (Fig. 20-22, p. 359):
  a Flexion—curl the toes.
  b Extension—straighten the toes.
  c Abduction—spread the toes apart.
  d Adduction—pull the toes together.
  e Repeat flexion, extension, abduction, and adduction 5 times—or the number of times stated on the care plan.

22 Cover the leg. Raise the bed rail if used.
23 Go to the other side. Lower the bed rail near you if up.
24 Repeat steps 11 through 21.

Post-Procedure

25 Provide for comfort. (See the inside of the front book cover.)
26 Remove the bath blanket.
27 Place the signal light within reach.
28 Lower the bed to its lowest position.
29 Raise or lower bed rails. Follow the care plan.

30 Return the bath blanket to its proper place.
31 Unscreen the person.
32 Complete a safety check of the room. (See the inside of the front book cover.)
33 Decontaminate your hands.
34 Report and record your observations.

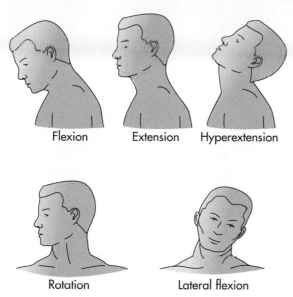

Flexion   Extension   Hyperextension

Rotation   Lateral flexion

FIG. **20-11** Range-of-motion exercises for the neck.

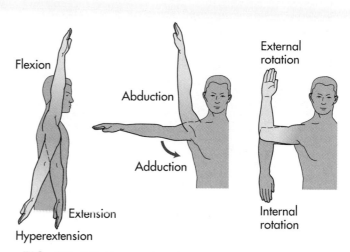

Flexion

Abduction

Adduction

Extension

Hyperextension

External rotation

Internal rotation

FIG. **20-12** Range-of-motion exercises for the shoulder.

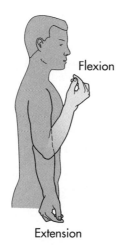

Flexion

Extension

FIG. **20-13** Range-of-motion exercises for the elbow.

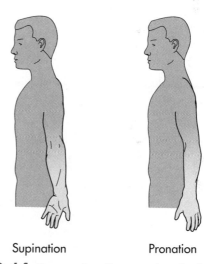

Supination   Pronation

FIG. **20-14** Range-of-motion exercises for the forearm.

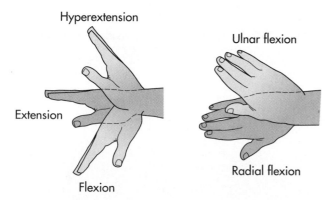

Hyperextension

Ulnar flexion

Extension

Flexion

Radial flexion

FIG. **20-15** Range-of-motion exercises for the wrist.

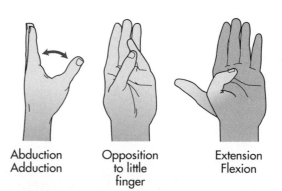

Abduction Adduction   Opposition to little finger   Extension Flexion

FIG. **20-16** Range-of-motion exercises for the thumb.

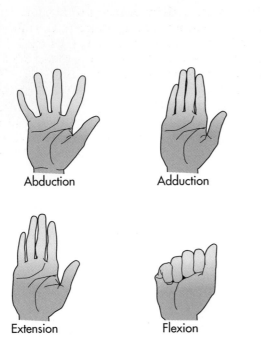

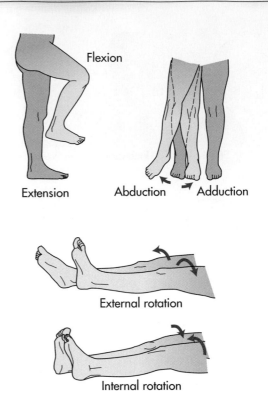

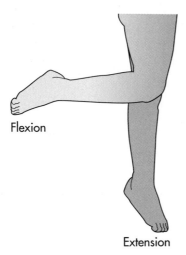

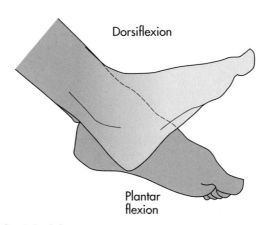

FIG. **20-17** Range-of-motion exercises for the fingers.

FIG. **20-18** Range-of-motion exercises for the hip.

FIG. **20-19** Range-of-motion exercises for the knee.

FIG. **20-20** Range-of-motion exercises for the ankle.

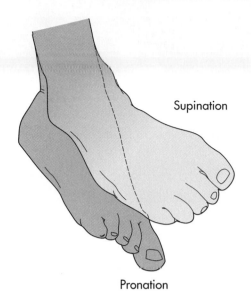

FIG. **20-21** Range-of-motion exercises for the foot.

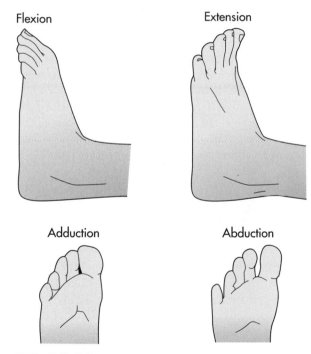

FIG. **20-22** Range-of-motion exercises for the toes.

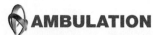 **AMBULATION**

After bedrest, activity increases slowly and in steps. The person sits up in bed, and then sits on the side of the bed (dangles). Sitting in a bedside chair follows. Next the person walks in the room and then in the hallway. **Ambulation** is the act of walking.

Some people are weak and unsteady from bedrest, illness, surgery, or injury. Help them walk according to the care plan. Use a gait (transfer) belt if the person is weak or unsteady. The person also uses hand rails along the wall. Always check the person for orthostatic hypotension (p. 350).

DELEGATION GUIDELINES
Ambulation

Before helping with ambulation, you need this information from the nurse and the care plan:
- How much help the person needs
- If the person uses a cane, walker, crutches, or a brace
- Areas of weakness—right arm or leg, left arm or leg
- How far to walk the person
- What observations to report and record:
    - How well the person tolerated the activity
    - Shuffling, sliding, limping, or walking on tip-toes
    - Complaints of pain or discomfort
    - Complaints of orthostatic hypotension—weakness, dizziness, spots before the eyes, feeling faint
    - The distance walked

PROMOTING SAFETY AND COMFORT
Ambulation

Safety

Practice the safety measures to prevent falls (Chapter 8). Use a gait belt when helping a person with ambulation. Also use it to help the person to stand.

Comfort

The fear of falling affects the person's mental comfort. Explain the purpose of the gait belt. Also explain how you will help the person if or she starts to fall (p. 361).

Helping the Person to Walk

NNAAP™

Quality of Life

Remember to:

- Knock before entering the person's room
- Address the person by name
- Introduce yourself by name and title
- Explain the procedure to the person before beginning and during the procedure
- Protect the person's rights during the procedure
- Handle the person gently during the procedure

Pre-Procedure

1 Follow *Delegation Guidelines: Ambulation*, p. 359. See *Promoting Safety and Comfort: Ambulation*, p. 359.
2 Practice hand hygiene.
3 Collect the following:
   • Robe and non-skid shoes
   • Paper or sheet to protect bottom linens
   • Gait (transfer) belt

4 Identify the person. Check the ID bracelet against the assignment sheet. Call the person by name.
5 Provide for privacy.

Procedure

6 Lower the bed to its lowest position. Lock the bed wheels. Lower the bed rail if up.
7 Fan-fold top linens to the foot of the bed.
8 Place the paper or sheet under the person's feet. Put the shoes on the person. Fasten the shoes.
9 Help the person to dangle. (See procedure: *Helping the Person to Sit on the Side of the Bed [Dangle]* in Chapter 11).
10 Help the person put on the robe.
11 Apply the gait belt. (See procedure: *Applying a Transfer Belt* in Chapter 11.)
12 Help the person stand. (See procedure: *Transferring the Person to a Chair or Wheelchair* in Chapter 11.) Grasp the gait belt at each side. If not using a gait belt, place your arms under the person's arms around to the shoulder blades.
13 Stand at the person's weak side while he or she gains balance. Hold the belt at the side and back. If not using a gait belt, have one arm around the back and the other at the elbow to support the person.

14 Encourage the person to stand erect with the head up and back straight.
15 Help the person walk. Walk to the side and slightly behind the person on the person's weak side. Provide support with the gait belt (Fig. 20-23). If not using a gait belt, have one arm around the back and the other at the elbow to support the person. Encourage the person to use the hand rail on his or her strong side.
16 Encourage the person to walk normally. The heel strikes the floor first. Discourage shuffling, sliding, or walking on tiptoes.
17 Walk the required distance if the person tolerates the activity. Do not rush the person.
18 Help the person return to bed. Remove the gait belt. (See procedure: *Transferring the Person From a Chair or Wheelchair to Bed* in Chapter 11.)
19 Lower the head of the bed. Help the person to the center of the bed.
20 Remove the shoes. Remove the paper or sheet over the bottom sheet.

Post-Procedure

21 Provide for comfort. (See the inside of the front book cover.)
22 Place the signal light within reach.
23 Raise or lower bed rails. Follow the care plan.
24 Return the robe and shoes to their proper place.

25 Unscreen the person.
26 Complete a safety check of the room. (See the inside of the front book cover.)
27 Decontaminate your hands.
28 Report and record your observations.

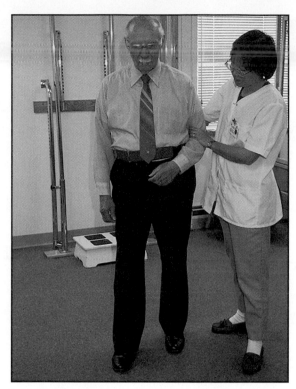

FIG. **20-23** Assist with ambulation by walking to the side and slightly behind the person. Use a gait belt for the person's safety.

The Falling Person

A person may start to fall when standing or walking. The person may be weak, light-headed, or dizzy. Fainting may occur. Falling may be caused by slipping or sliding on spills, waxed floors, throw rugs, or improper shoes (Chapter 8). Head, wrist, arm, hip, and knee injuries could occur.

Do not try to prevent the fall. You could injure yourself and the person while twisting and straining to stop the fall. If a person starts to fall, ease him or her to the floor. This lets you control the direction of the fall. You can also protect the person's head. Do not let the person move or get up before the nurse checks for injuries.

See Persons With Dementia: The Falling Person.

Persons With Dementia

The Falling Person

A confused person may not understand why you do not want him or her to move or get up after a fall. Forcing a person not to move may injure the person and you. You may need to let the person move for his or her safety and your own. Never use force or hold a person down. Stay calm, and protect the person from injury. Talk to the person in a quiet, soothing voice. Call for help.

Helping the Falling Person

Procedure

1 Stand with your feet apart. Keep your back straight.
2 Bring the person close to your body as fast as possible. Use the gait belt. Or wrap your arms around the person's waist. If necessary, you can also hold the person under the arms (Fig. 20-24, *A*, p. 362).
3 Move your leg so the person's buttocks rest on it (Fig. 20-24, *B*, p. 362). Move the leg near the person.
4 Lower the person to the floor. The person slides down your leg to the floor (Fig. 20-24, *C*, p. 362). Bend at your hips and knees as you lower the person.
5 Call a nurse to check the person. Stay with the person.
6 Help the nurse return the person to bed. Get other staff to help if needed.

Post-Procedure

7 Provide for comfort. (See the inside of the front book cover.)
8 Place the signal light within reach.
9 Raise or lower the bed rails. Follow the care plan.
10 Complete a safety check of the room. (See the inside of the front book cover.)
11 Report and record the following:

• How the fall occurred
• How far the person walked
• How activity was tolerated before the fall
• Complaints before the fall
• How much help the person needed while walking

12 Complete an incident report (Chapter 8).

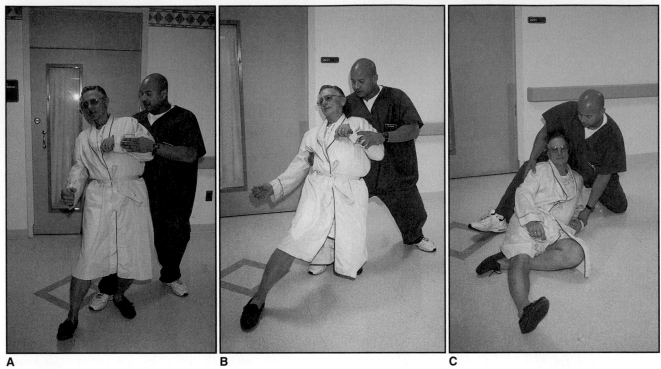

A   B   C

FIG. **20-24** A, The falling person is supported. **B,** The person's buttocks rest on the nursing assistant's leg. **C,** The person is eased to the floor on the nursing assistant's leg.

Walking Aids

Walking aids support the body. The physical therapist or nurse measures and teaches the person how to use the device.

Crutches

Crutches are used when the person cannot use one leg or when one or both legs need to gain strength. Some persons with permanent leg weakness can use crutches. Falls are a risk. Follow these safety measures:

- Check the crutch tips. They must not be worn down, torn, or wet. Replace worn or torn crutch tips. Dry wet tips with a towel or paper towels.
- Check wooden crutches for cracks and metal crutches for bends.
- Tighten all bolts.
- Street shoes are worn. They must be flat and have non-skid soles.
- Clothes must fit well. Loose clothes may get caught between the crutches and underarms. Loose clothes and long skirts can hang forward and block the person's view of the feet and crutch tips.
- Practice safety rules to prevent falls (Chapter 8).
- Keep crutches within the person's reach. Put them by the person's chair or against a wall.

Canes

Canes are used for weakness on one side of the body. They help provide balance and support (Fig. 20-25).

A cane is held on the *strong side* of the body. (If the left leg is weak, the cane is held in the right hand.) The cane tip is about 6 to 10 inches to the side of the foot. It is about 6 to 10 inches in front of the foot on the strong side. The grip is level with the hip. The person walks as follows:

- *Step A:* The cane is moved forward 6 to 10 inches (Fig. 20-26, *A*).
- *Step B:* The weak leg (opposite the cane) is moved forward even with the cane (Fig. 20-26, *B*).
- *Step C:* The strong leg is moved forward and ahead of the cane and the weak leg (Fig. 20-26, *C*).

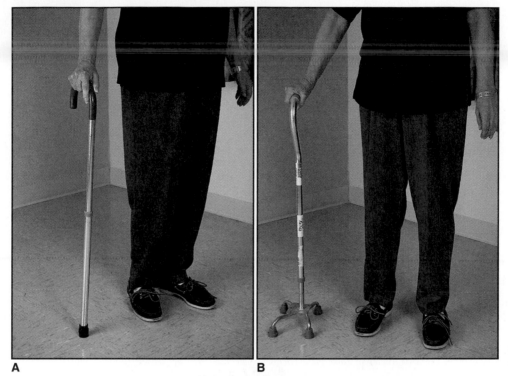

FIG. **20-25** **A,** Single-tip cane. **B,** Four-point cane.

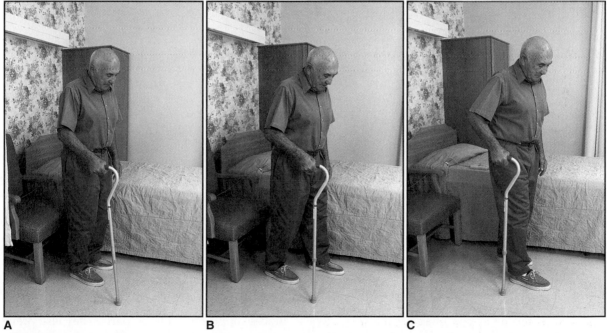

FIG. **20-26** Walking with a cane. **A,** The cane is moved forward about 6 to 10 inches. **B,** The leg opposite the cane (weak leg) is brought forward even with the cane. **C,** The leg on the cane side (strong side) is moved ahead of the cane and the weak leg.

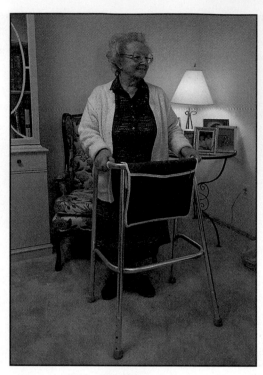

FIG. **20-27** A walker.

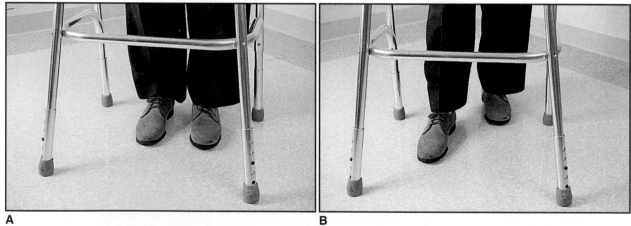

A   **B**

FIG. **20-28** Walking with a walker. **A,** The walker is moved about 6 inches in front of the person. **B,** Both feet are moved up to the walker.

Walkers

A walker gives more support than a cane (Fig. 20-27). The walker is picked up and moved about 6 to 8 inches in front of the person. The person then moves the weak leg and foot and then the strong leg and foot up to the walker (Fig. 20-28).

Baskets, pouches, and trays attach to the walker (see Fig. 20-27). They are used for needed items. This allows more independence.

Braces

Braces support weak body parts. They also prevent or correct deformities or prevent joint movement. A brace is applied over the ankle, knee, or back (Fig. 20-29).

Skin and bony points under braces are kept clean and dry. This prevents skin breakdown. Report redness or signs of skin breakdown at once (Chapter 21). Also report complaints of pain or discomfort. The nurse assesses the skin under braces every shift. The care plan tells you when to apply and remove a brace.

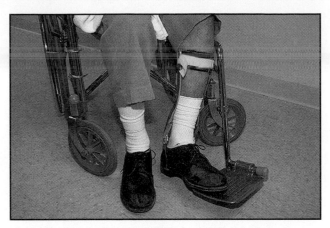

FIG. **20-29** Leg brace.

FOCUS ON THE PERSON

Exercise and activity help prevent complications from bedrest. They also promote independence.

See Focus on the Person: Assisting With Exercise and Activity.

Focus on the PERSON

Assisting with Exercise and Activity

Providing comfort—Physical and mental comfort is important during exercise and activity. To promote physical comfort, make sure the person wears the correct clothing and footwear. Footwear must fit properly to prevent falls, pain, discomfort, and blisters.

Privacy promotes mental comfort. Make sure the person's garments provide needed privacy during ambulation. The person must not walk in the room or hallway with a gown open in the back. During range-of-motion exercises, cover the person with a bath blanket. Expose only the body part being exercised.

Ethical behavior—Range-of-motion exercises are important for the person's well-being. They prevent muscle atrophy and contractures. You must follow delegation guidelines (p. 353). That is the right thing to do.

Remaining independent—Exercise and activity help maintain normal joint and muscle function. They also promote normal function of all body systems. Good conditioning has long-term effects. The more active the person is in the present, the more likely that or she will remain active in the future. Encourage the person to be as active as possible. Being active helps the person remain independent.

Speaking up—Orthostatic hypotension can occur when the person moves from lying or sitting to standing. Fainting is a risk. To check for orthostatic hypotension, ask the person these questions:
- "Do you feel weak?"
- "Do you feel dizzy?"
- "Do you see spots before your eyes?"
- "Do you feel like fainting?"

OBRA and other laws—OBRA requires activity programs for nursing center residents. They are important for physical and mental well-being. Activities must meet the interests and physical, mental, and psychosocial needs of each resident. Bingo, movies, dances, exercise groups, shopping and museum trips, concerts, and guest speakers are often arranged. Some centers have gardening activities.

Protect the right to personal choice. Well-being is promoted when the person attends activities of personal choice. Do not force the person to take part in activities that do not interest him or her.

Nursing teamwork—Some residents need help getting to activity programs. Some also need help with activities. When you can, help co-workers assist residents to and with activity programs. For example, you may have 1 or 2 residents who need help. A co-worker may have 4 or 5 persons needing help.

REVIEW QUESTIONS

Circle the **BEST** answer.

1 Ms. Porter is on bedrest. Which is *false?*
   a She has orthostatic hypotension.
   b Bedrest helps reduce pain and promotes healing.
   c Pressure ulcers, constipation, and blood clots are risks.
   d Contractures and muscle atrophy can occur.

2 Which helps to prevent plantar flexion?
   a Bed boards
   b A foot board
   c A trochanter roll
   d Handrolls

3 Which prevents the hip from turning outward?
   a Bed boards
   b A foot board
   c Trochanter roll
   d A leg brace

4 A contracture is
   a The loss of muscle strength from inactivity
   b The lack of joint mobility from shortening of a muscle
   c A decrease in the size of a muscle
   d A blood clot in the muscle

5 Passive range-of-motion exercises are performed by
   a The person
   b Someone else
   c The person with the help of another
   d The person with the use of hand grips

6 ROM exercises are ordered for a person. You do the following *except*
   a Support the part being exercised
   b Move the joint slowly, smoothly, and gently
   c Force the joint through full range of motion
   d Exercise only the joints indicated by the nurse

7 Flexion involves
   a Bending the body part
   b Straightening the body part
   c Moving the body part toward the body
   d Moving the body part away from the body

8 Which statement about ambulation is *false?*
   a A gait belt is used if the person is weak or unsteady.
   b The person can shuffle or slide when walking after bedrest.
   c Walking aids may be needed.
   d Crutches, canes, walkers, and braces are common walking aids.

9 You are getting a person ready to crutch walk. You should do the following *except*
   a Check the crutch tips
   b Have the person wear non-skid shoes
   c Get a pair of crutches from physical therapy
   d Tighten the bolts on the crutches

10 A cane is used
   a At waist level
   b On the strong side
   c On the weak side
   d On either side

Circle **T** if the statement is true and **F** if the statement is false.

11 **T F** A single-tipped cane and a four-point cane give the same support.
12 **T F** When using a cane, the feet are moved first.
13 **T F** Mr. Parker uses a walker. He moves the walker first and then his feet.
14 **T F** Mr. Parker starts to fall. You should try to prevent the fall.
15 **T F** A person has a brace. Bony areas need protection from skin breakdown.

The answers to these questions are on p. 469.

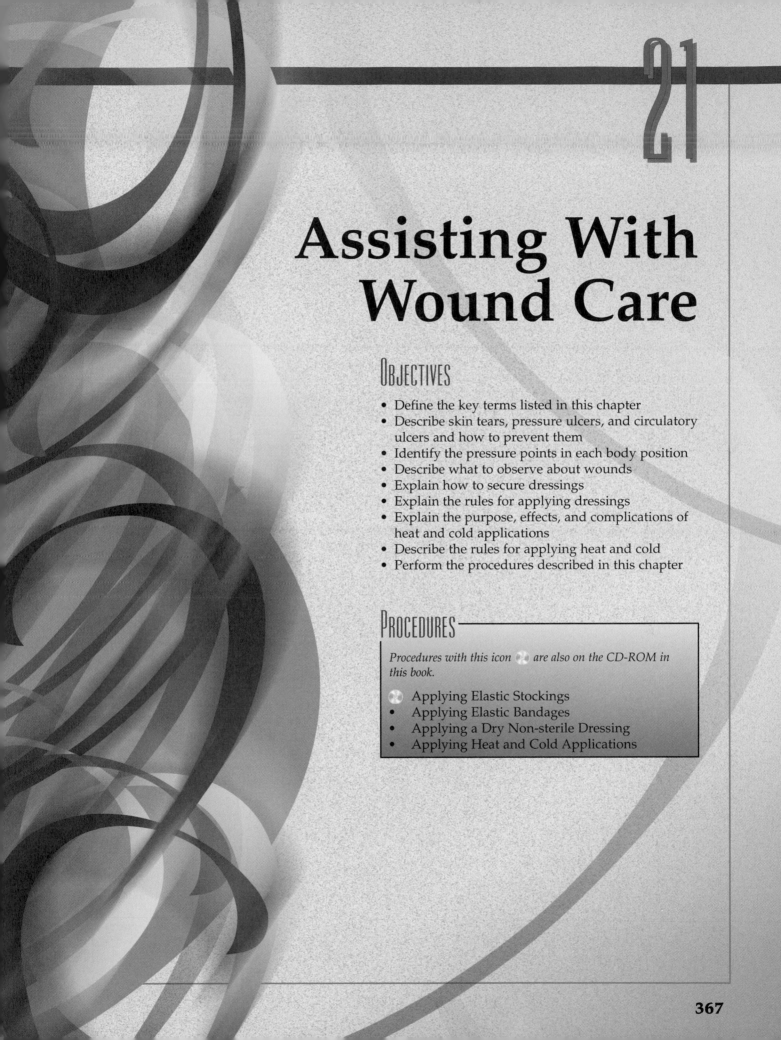

Assisting With Wound Care

OBJECTIVES

- Define the key terms listed in this chapter
- Describe skin tears, pressure ulcers, and circulatory ulcers and how to prevent them
- Identify the pressure points in each body position
- Describe what to observe about wounds
- Explain how to secure dressings
- Explain the rules for applying dressings
- Explain the purpose, effects, and complications of heat and cold applications
- Describe the rules for applying heat and cold
- Perform the procedures described in this chapter

PROCEDURES

Procedures with this icon are also on the CD-ROM in this book.

- Applying Elastic Stockings
- Applying Elastic Bandages
- Applying a Dry Non-sterile Dressing
- Applying Heat and Cold Applications

KEY TERMS

bedsore A pressure ulcer, pressure sore, or decubitus ulcer

circulatory ulcer An open wound on the lower legs and feet caused by decreased blood flow through arteries or veins; vascular ulcer

constrict To narrow

decubitus ulcer A pressure ulcer, pressure sore, or bedsore

dilate To expand or open wider

pressure sore A bedsore, decubitus ulcer, or pressure ulcer

pressure ulcer Any injury caused by unrelieved pressure; decubitus ulcer, bedsore, or pressure sore

skin tear A break or rip in the skin; the epidermis (top skin layer) separates from the underlying tissues

wound A break in the skin or mucous membrane

 A **wound** is a break in the skin or mucous membrane. Wounds result from many causes.

Surgical incisions leave wounds. So does *trauma*—an accident or violent act that injures the skin, mucous membranes, bones, and internal organs. Pressure ulcers occur from poor skin care and immobility. Circulatory ulcers are caused by a decrease in blood flow through the arteries or veins (p. 373).

The wound is a portal of entry for microbes. Infection is a major threat. Wound care involves preventing infection and further injury to the wound and nearby tissues.

SKIN TEARS

A **skin tear** is a break or rip in the skin. The epidermis (top skin layer) separates from the underlying tissues. Skin tears are caused by friction and shearing (Chapter 11), pulling, or pressure on the skin.

Bumping a hand, arm, or leg on any hard or sharp surface can cause a skin tear. Beds, bed rails, chairs, wheelchair footplates, and tables are dangers. So is holding an arm or leg too tight.

Skin tears are painful. They are portals of entry for microbes. Tell the nurse at once if you cause or find a skin tear. To prevent skin tears:

- Keep the person's and your fingernails short and smoothly filed.
- Do not wear rings or bracelets.
- Follow the care plan and safety rules to move, position, transfer, bathe, and dress the person.
- Prevent shearing and friction.
- Use an assist device to move and turn the person in bed.

PRESSURE ULCERS

A **pressure ulcer (decubitus ulcer, bedsore,** or **pressure sore)** is any injury caused by unrelieved pressure. It usually occurs over a bony area—back of the head, the shoulder blades, elbows, hips, sacrum, knees, ankles, heels, and toes (Fig. 21-1).

Causes

Pressure, friction, and shearing are common causes of skin breakdown and pressure ulcers. Other factors include breaks in the skin, poor circulation to an area, moisture, dry skin, and irritation by urine and feces. Older and disabled persons are at great risk for pressure ulcers. Their skin is easily injured. Causes include age-related skin changes, chronic disease, and general debility.

Pressure occurs when the skin over a bony area is squeezed between hard surfaces. The bone is one hard surface. The other is usually the mattress or chair seat. Squeezing or pressure prevents blood flow to the skin and underlying tissues. Lack of blood flow means oxygen and nutrients cannot get to the cells. Therefore involved skin and tissues die (Fig. 21-2, p. 370).

Friction scrapes the skin, causing an open area. The open area needs to heal. A good blood supply is needed. A poor blood supply or an infection can lead to a pressure ulcer.

Shearing is when the skin sticks to a surface (usually the bed or chair) while deeper tissues move downward (Chapter 11). This occurs when the person slides down in the bed or chair. Blood vessels and tissues are damaged. Blood flow to the area is reduced.

Persons at Risk

Persons at risk for pressure ulcers are those who:
- Are confined to a bed or chair
- Need some or total help in moving
- Have loss of bowel or bladder control
- Have poor nutrition or fluid balance
- Have altered mental awareness
- Have problems sensing pain or pressure
- Have circulatory problems
- Are older, obese, or very thin

Signs of Pressure Ulcers

The first sign of a pressure ulcer is pale skin or a reddened area. Color changes may be hard to notice in persons with dark skin. The person may complain of pain, burning, or tingling in the area. Some do not feel anything unusual. Box 21-1 on p. 370 describes pressure ulcer stages.

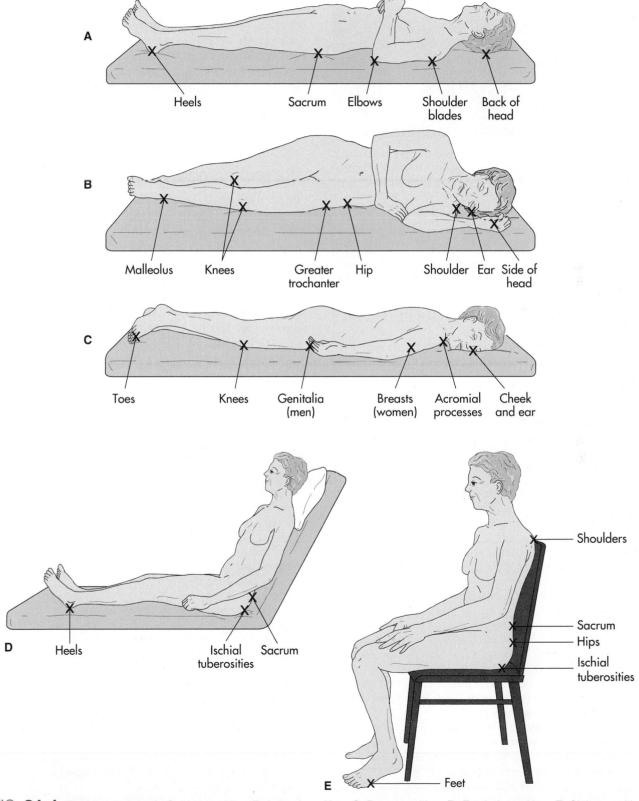

FIG. 21-1 Pressure points. **A,** Supine position. **B,** Lateral position. **C,** Prone position. **D,** Fowler's position. **E,** Sitting position.

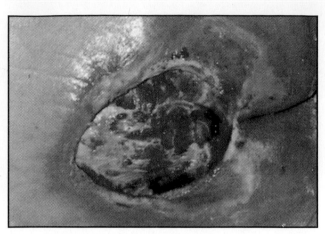

FIG. **21-2** A pressure ulcer. (Used with permission from "Proceedings from the November National V.A.C.®", *Ostomy Wound Management*, Feb 2005, Vol. 51, Issue 2A [Suppl] p. 7S, HMP Communications.)

BOX 21-1	Stages of Pressure Ulcers

Stage 1 The skin is red. The color does not return to normal when the skin is relieved of pressure (Fig. 21-3, *A*). The skin is intact.

Stage 2 The skin cracks, blisters, or peels (Fig. 21-3, *B*). There may be a shallow crater.

Stage 3 The skin is gone. Underlying tissues are exposed (Fig. 21-3, *C*). The exposed tissue is damaged. There may be drainage from the area.

Stage 4 Muscle and bone are exposed and damaged (Fig. 21-3, *D*). Drainage is likely.

Sites

Pressure ulcers usually occur over bony areas. The bony areas are called *pressure points*. This is because they bear the weight of the body in a certain position (see Fig. 21-1). Pressure from body weight can reduce the blood supply to the area.

In obese people, pressure ulcers can occur in areas where skin has contact with skin. Common sites are between abdominal folds, the legs, the buttocks, and under the breasts. Friction occurs in these areas.

The ears also are sites for pressure ulcers. This is from pressure of the ear on the mattress when in the side-lying position.

Prevention and Treatment

Preventing pressure ulcers is much easier than trying to heal them. Good nursing care, cleanliness, and skin care are essential. The measures in Box 21-2 help prevent skin breakdown and pressure ulcers. Follow the person's care plan.

The person at risk for pressure ulcers is placed on a surface that reduces or relieves pressure. Such surfaces include foam, air, alternating air, gel, or water mattresses. The health team decides on the best surface for the person.

BOX 21-2	Measures to Prevent Pressure Ulcers

- Follow the repositioning schedule in the person's care plan. The person is repositioned at least every 2 hours. Some persons are repositioned every 15 minutes.
- Position the person according to the care plan. Use pillows for support as instructed by the nurse. The 30-degree lateral position is recommended (Fig. 21-4, p. 372).
- Prevent shearing and friction during handling and moving procedures.
- Prevent shearing. Do not raise the head of the bed more than 30 degrees. Follow the care plan.
- Prevent friction by applying a thin layer of cornstarch to the bottom sheets.
- Provide good skin care. The skin is clean and dry after bathing. The skin is free of moisture from urine, stools, perspiration, and wound drainage.
- Minimize skin exposure to moisture. Check incontinent persons often. Also check persons who perspire heavily and those with wound drainage. Change linens and clothing as needed, and provide good skin care.
- Check with the nurse before using soap. Soap can dry and irritate the skin.
- Apply a moisturizer to dry areas—hands, elbows, legs, ankles, and heels. The nurse tells you what to use and what areas need attention.
- Give a back massage when repositioning the person. *Do not massage bony areas.*
- Keep linens clean, dry, and wrinkle-free.
- Apply powder where skin touches skin.
- Do not irritate the skin. Avoid scrubbing or vigorous rubbing when bathing or drying the person.
- Do not massage over pressure points. *Never rub or massage reddened areas.*
- Use pillows and blankets to prevent skin from being in contact with skin. They also reduce moisture and friction.
- Keep the heels off the bed. Use pillows or other devices as the nurse directs. Place the pillows or devices under the lower legs from mid-calf to the ankles.
- Use protective devices as the nurse and care plan direct (p. 372).
- Remind persons sitting in chairs to shift their positions every 15 minutes. This decreases pressure on bony points.
- Report any signs of skin breakdown or pressure ulcers at once.

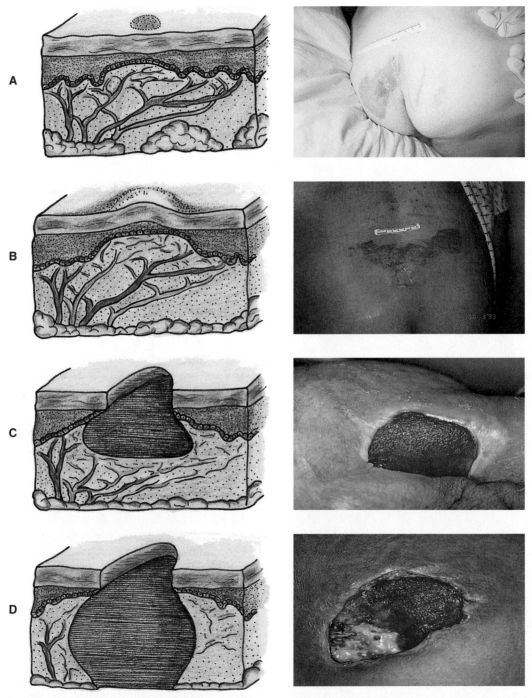

FIG. **21-3** Stages of pressure ulcers. **A,** Stage 1. **B,** Stage 2. **C,** Stage 3. **D,** Stage 4. (Courtesy Laurel Wiersema-Bryant, RN, MSN, Clinical Nurse Specialist, Barnes-Jewish Hospital, St Louis.)

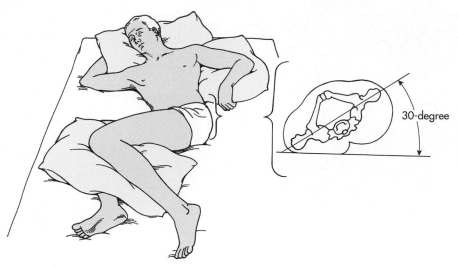

FIG. **21-4** The 30-degree lateral position. Pillows are placed under the head, shoulder, and leg. This position inclines (lifts up) the hip to avoid pressure on the hip. The person does not lie on the hip as in the side-lying position. (From Bryant and others: Pressure ulcers: in Bryant RA, editor: *Acute and chronic wounds: nursing management,* St Louis, 1992, Mosby.)

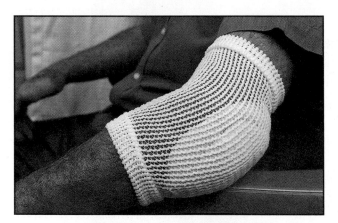

FIG. **21-5** Elbow protector.

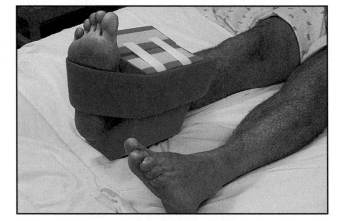

FIG. **21-6** Heel elevator.

The doctor orders wound care products, drugs, treatments, and special equipment to promote healing. The nurse and care plan tell you what to do. These protective devices are often used to prevent and treat pressure ulcers and skin breakdown.

- *Bed cradle*—A bed cradle is placed on the bed and over the person. Top linens are brought over the cradle to prevent pressure on the legs and feet (Chapter 20).
- *Elbow protectors*—These devices are made of foam or sheepskin. They fit the shape of the elbow (Fig. 21-5).
- *Heel elevators*—Pillows or special cushions are used to raise the heels off the bed (Fig. 21-6). Special braces and splints also are used to keep pressure off the heels.
- *Flotation pads*—Flotation pads or cushions (Fig. 21-7) are made of a gel-like substance. They are used for chairs and wheelchairs. The outer case is heavy plastic. The pad is placed in a cover or pillowcase to protect the skin.

- *Eggcrate-like mattress*—This is a foam pad that looks like an egg carton (Fig. 21-8). Peaks in the mattress distribute the person's weight more evenly. It is placed on top of the regular mattress. The eggcrate-like mattress is put in a special cover. The cover protects against moisture and soiling. Only a bottom sheet is used to cover the eggcrate-like mattress and cover. No other bottoms linens are used.
- *Special beds*—Some beds have air flowing through the mattresses (Fig. 21-9). The *person floats* on the mattress. Body weight is distributed evenly. There is little pressure on bony parts. Other beds allow repositioning without moving the person. The person is turned to the prone or supine position or tilted various degrees. Alignment does not change. Pressure points change as the position changes. There is little friction. Some beds constantly rotate from side to side. They are useful for persons with spinal cord injuries.
- *Other equipment*—Trochanter rolls and foot boards are also used (Chapter 20).

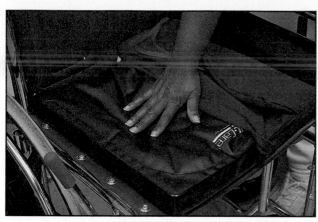

FIG. **21-7** Flotation pad.

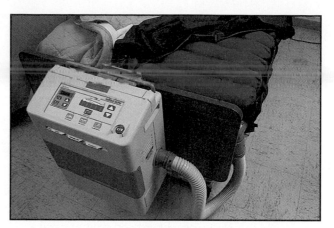

FIG. **21-9** Air flotation bed.

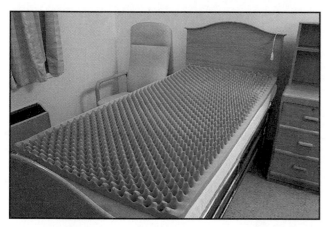

FIG. **21-8** Eggcrate-like mattress on the bed.

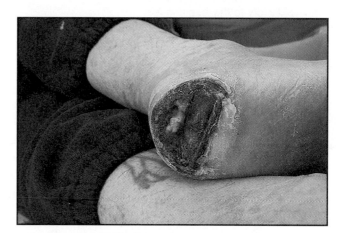

FIG. **21-10** Stasis ulcer.

CIRCULATORY ULCERS

Some people have diseases that affect blood flow to and from the legs and feet. Such poor circulation can lead to pain, open wounds, and swelling of tissues *(edema)*. Infection and gangrene can result from the open wound and poor circulation. *Gangrene* is a condition in which there is death of tissue.

Circulatory ulcers *(vascular ulcers)* are open wounds on the lower legs and feet caused by decreased blood flow through arteries or veins. Persons with diseases affecting the blood vessels are at risk. These wounds are painful and hard to heal.

■ *Stasis ulcers (venous ulcers)* are open wounds on the lower legs and feet caused by poor blood return through the veins (Fig. 21-10). The heels and inner aspect of the ankles are common sites. They can occur from skin injury. Scratching is a common cause. Or the ulcers occur spontaneously.

■ *Arterial ulcers* are open wounds on the lower legs and feet caused by poor arterial blood flow. They are found between the toes, on top of the toes, and on the outer side of the ankle. The heels are common sites for persons on bedrest. These ulcers can occur from shoes that fit poorly.

Prevention and Treatment

Circulatory ulcers are hard to heal. Preventing skin breakdown is important. Follow the person's care plan (Box 21-3). The doctor may order elastic stockings or elastic bandages to promote circulation.

BOX 21-3	Measures to Prevent Circulatory Ulcers

- Remind the person not to sit with the legs crossed.
- Position the person according to the care plan.
- Do not use elastic or rubber band type of garters to hold socks or hose in place.
- Do not dress the person in tight clothes.
- Keep the feet clean and dry. Clean and dry between the toes.
- Do not scrub or rub the skin during bathing and drying.
- Keep linens clean, dry, and wrinkle-free.
- Avoid injury to the legs and feet.
- Make sure shoes fit well.
- Keep pressure off the heels and other bony areas. Use pillows or other devices as the nurse and care plan direct.
- Check the person's legs and feet. Report skin breaks or changes in skin color.
- Do not massage over pressure points. *Never rub or massage reddened areas.*
- Follow the care plan for walking and exercise.

 Elastic Stockings

Elastic stockings exert pressure on the veins. The pressure promotes venous blood flow to the heart. By doing so, the stockings help prevent blood clots *(thrombi).* A blood clot is called a *thrombus.*

If blood flow is sluggish, blood clots may form. They can form in the deep leg veins (Fig. 21-11, *A*). A blood clot can break loose and travel through the bloodstream. It then becomes an embolus. An *embolus* is a blood clot that travels through the vascular system until it lodges in a distant vessel (Fig. 21-11, *B*). An embolus from a vein lodges in the lungs *(pulmonary embolus).* A pulmonary embolus can cause severe respiratory problems and death.

Elastic stockings also are called anti-embolism or anti-embolic (AE stockings). Persons at risk for thrombi include those who:

- Have heart and circulatory disorders
- Are on bedrest
- Have had surgery
- Are pregnant

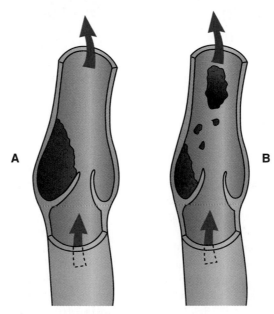

FIG. **21-11** **A,** A blood clot is attached to the wall of a vein. The arrows show the direction of blood flow. **B,** Part of the thrombus breaks off and becomes an embolus. The embolus will travel in the bloodstream until it lodges in a distant vessel.

DELEGATION GUIDELINES
Elastic Stockings

Before applying elastic stockings, you need this information from the nurse and care plan:
- What size to use—small, medium, or large
- What length to use—thigh-high or knee-high
- When to remove and re-apply them—usually every 8 hours for 30 minutes
- What observations to report and record:
  - When you applied the stockings
  - Skin color and temperature
  - Leg and foot swelling
  - Skin tears, wounds, or signs of skin breakdown
  - Complaints of pain, tingling, or numbness
  - When you removed the stockings and for how long
  - When you re-applied the stockings
  - When you washed the stockings

PROMOTING SAFETY AND COMFORT
Elastic Stockings

Safety

Stockings should not have twists, creases, or wrinkles after you apply them. Twists can affect circulation. Creases and wrinkles can cause skin breakdown.

Comfort

Stockings are applied before the person gets out of bed. Otherwise the legs can swell from sitting or standing. Stockings are hard to put on when the legs are swollen. The person lies in bed while they are off. This prevents the legs from swelling.

Gently handle and move the person's foot and leg. Do not force the joints (toes, foot, ankle, knee, and hip) beyond their range of motion or to the point of pain.

Applying Elastic Stockings

Quality of Life

Remember to:

- Knock before entering the person's room
- Address the person by name
- Introduce yourself by name and title

- Explain the procedure to the person before beginning and during the procedure
- Protect the person's rights during the procedure
- Handle the person gently during the procedure

Pre-Procedure

1. Follow *Delegation Guidelines: Elastic Stockings*. See *Promoting Safety and Comfort: Elastic Stockings*.
2. Practice hand hygiene.
3. Obtain elastic stockings in the correct size and length.
4. Identify the person. Check the ID bracelet against the assignment sheet. Call the person by name.
5. Provide for privacy.
6. Raise the bed for body mechanics. Bed rails are up if used.

Procedure

7. Lower the bed rail near you if up.
8. Position the person supine.
9. Expose the legs. Fan-fold top linens toward the thighs.
10. Turn the stocking inside out down to the heel.
11. Slip the foot of the stocking over the toes, foot, and heel (Fig. 21-12, *A*, p. 376).
12. Grasp the stocking top. Pull the stocking up the leg. It turns right side out as it is pulled up. The stocking is even and snug (Fig. 21-12, *B*, p. 376).
13. Remove twists, creases, or wrinkles.
14. Repeat steps 10 through 13 for the other leg.

Post-Procedure

15. Cover the person.
16. Provide for comfort. (See the inside of the front book cover.)
17. Place the signal light within reach.
18. Lower the bed to its lowest position.
19. Raise or lower bed rails. Follow the care plan.
20. Unscreen the person.
21. Complete a safety check of the room. (See the inside of the front book cover.)
22. Decontaminate your hands.
23. Report and record your observations.

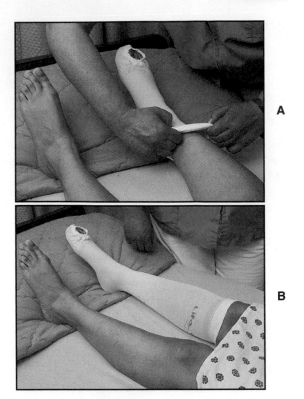

FIG. **21-12** Applying elastic stockings. **A,** The stocking is slipped over the toes, foot, and heel. **B,** The stocking turns right side out as it is pulled up over the leg.

Before applying an elastic bandage, you need this information from the nurse and the care plan:
- Where to apply the bandage
- What width and length to use
- When to remove the bandage and for how long
- What to do if the bandage is wet or soiled
- What observations to report and record:
  - When you applied the bandage
  - Skin color and temperature
  - Swelling of the part
  - Skin tears, wounds, or signs of skin breakdown
  - Complaints of pain, itching, tingling, or numbness
  - When you removed the bandage and for how long
  - When you re-applied the bandage

Elastic Bandages

Elastic bandages have the same purposes as elastic stockings. They also provide support and reduce swelling from injuries. Sometimes they are used to hold dressings in place. They are applied to arms and legs. When applying bandages:
- Use the correct size. Use the proper length and width to bandage the extremity.
- Position the part in good alignment.
- Face the person during the procedure.
- Start at the lower *(distal)* part of the extremity. Work upward to the top *(proximal)* part.
- Expose fingers or toes if possible. This allows circulation checks.
- Apply the bandage with firm, even pressure.
- Check the color and temperature of the extremity every hour.
- Re-apply a loose or wrinkled bandage.
- Replace a moist or soiled bandage.

Safety

Elastic bandages must be firm and snug. However, they must not be tight. A tight bandage can affect circulation.

Some agencies do not let nursing assistants apply elastic bandages. Know your agency's policy.

Comfort

A tight bandage can cause pain and discomfort. Apply it with firm, even pressure. If the person complains of pain, itching, tingling, or numbness, remove the bandage and tell the nurse at once.

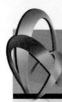

Applying Elastic Bandages

Quality of Life

Remember to:

- Knock before entering the person's room
- Address the person by name
- Introduce yourself by name and title

- Explain the procedure to the person before beginning and during the procedure
- Protect the person's rights during the procedure
- Handle the person gently during the procedure

Pre-Procedure

1 Follow *Delegation Guidelines: Elastic Bandages*. See *Promoting Safety and Comfort: Elastic Bandages*.
2 Practice hand hygiene.
3 Collect the following:
   - Elastic bandage as directed by the nurse
   - Tape or metal clips (unless the bandage has Velcro)

4 Identify the person. Check the ID bracelet against the assignment sheet. Call the person by name.
5 Provide for privacy.
6 Raise the bed for body mechanics. Bed rails are up if used.

Procedure

7 Lower the bed rail near you if up.
8 Help the person to a comfortable position. Expose the part you will bandage.
9 Make sure the area is clean and dry.
10 Hold the bandage so the roll is up. The loose end is on the bottom (Fig. 21-13, *A*).
11 Apply the bandage to the smallest part of the wrist, foot, ankle, or knee.
12 Make two circular turns around the part (Fig. 21-13, *B*).
13 Make overlapping spiral turns in an upward direction. Each turn overlaps about 2/3 of the previous turn (Fig. 21-13, *C*).

14 Apply the bandage smoothly, with firm, even pressure. It is not tight.
15 End the bandage with two circular turns.
16 Secure the bandage in place with Velcro, tape, or clips. The clips are not under the body part.
17 Check the fingers or toes for coldness or cyanosis (bluish color). Ask about pain, itching, numbness, or tingling. Remove the bandage if any are noted. Report your observations to the nurse.

Post-Procedure

18 Provide for comfort. (See the inside of the front book cover.)
19 Place the signal light within reach.
20 Lower the bed to its lowest position.
21 Raise or lower bed rails. Follow the care plan.

22 Unscreen the person.
23 Complete a safety check of the room. (See the inside of the front book cover.)
24 Decontaminate your hands.
25 Report and record your observations.

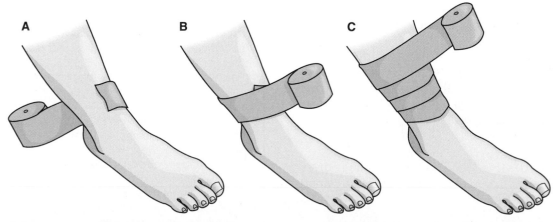

FIG. **21-13** Applying an elastic bandage. **A,** The roll of the bandage is up. The loose end is at the bottom. **B,** The bandage is applied to the smallest part with two circular turns. **C,** The bandage is applied with spiral turns in an upward direction.

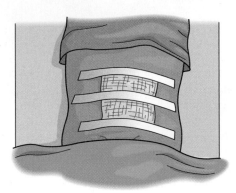

FIG. **21-14** Tape is applied at the top, middle, and bottom of the dressing. The tape extends several inches beyond both sides of the dressing.

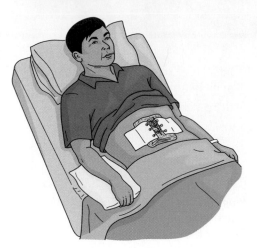

FIG. **21-15** Montgomery ties.

DRESSINGS

Wound dressings protect wounds from injury and microbes. They absorb drainage, remove dead tissue, and promote comfort. They also provide a moist environment for wound healing.

Securing Dressings

Dressings must be secured over wounds. Microbes can enter the wound, and drainage can escape if the dressing is dislodged. Tape and Montgomery ties are used to secure dressings. Binders also hold dressings in place.

Tape
Adhesive, paper, plastic, and elastic tapes are common. Adhesive tape sticks well to the skin. However, adhesive remaining on the skin is hard to remove. It can irritate the skin. Allergies to adhesive tape are common. Paper and plastic tapes usually do not cause allergic reactions. Elastic tape allows movement of the body part.

Tape is applied to secure the top, middle, and bottom of the dressing (Fig. 21-14). The tape extends several inches on each side of the dressing. *The tape must not circle the entire body part. If swelling occurs, circulation to the part is impaired.*

Montgomery Ties
Montgomery ties (Fig. 21-15) are used for large dressings and frequent dressing changes. A Montgomery tie has an adhesive strip and a cloth tie. When the

dressing is in place, the adhesive strips are placed on both sides of the dressing. Then the ties are secured over the dressing. They are untied for the dressing change. The adhesive strips are not removed unless soiled.

Applying Dressings

Some agencies let you apply simple, dry, non-sterile dressings to simple wounds. Box 21-4 lists the rules for applying dressings.

BOX 21-4	**Rules For Applying Dry Non-Sterile Dressings**

- Meet fluid and elimination needs before you begin.
- Collect needed equipment and supplies before you begin.
- Control your nonverbal communication. Wound odors, appearance, and drainage may be unpleasant. Do not communicate your thoughts and reactions to the person.
- Remove soiled dressings so the person cannot see the soiled side. The drainage and its odor may upset the person.
- Do not force the person to look at the wound. A wound can affect body image and self-esteem. The nurse helps the person deal with the wound.
- Remove tape by pulling it toward the wound.
- Remove dressings gently. They may stick to the wound, drain, or surrounding skin.
- Report and record your observations. *See Delegation Guidelines: Applying Dressings.*

DELEGATION GUIDELINES
Applying Dressings

Before applying a dressing, you need this information from the nurse and care plan:
- When to change the dressing
- When the person received a drug for pain relief; when it will take effect
- How to secure the dressing—tape or Montgomery ties
- What kind of tape to use—adhesive, paper, plastic, or elastic
- What observations to report and record:
  - A red or swollen wound
  - An area around the wound that is warm to touch
  - If wound edges are closed or separated
  - A wound that has broken open
  - Drainage appearance—clear, bloody, or watery and blood-tinged; thick and green, yellow, or brown
  - The amount of drainage
  - Wound or drainage odor
  - Intactness and color of surrounding tissues
  - Swelling of surrounding tissues

PROMOTING SAFETY AND COMFORT
Applying Dressings

Safety

Contact with blood, body fluids, secretions, or excretions is likely. Follow Standard Precautions and the Bloodborne Pathogen Standard. Wear personal protective equipment as needed.

Comfort

Some dressing changes can cause discomfort or pain. If so, the nurse gives a pain-relief drug before the dressing change. Allow 30 minutes for the drug to take effect. Then change the dressing.

Applying a Dry Non-Sterile Dressing

Quality of Life

Remember to:
- Knock before entering the person's room
- Address the person by name
- Introduce yourself by name and title

- Explain the procedure to the person before beginning and during the procedure
- Protect the person's rights during the procedure
- Handle the person gently during the procedure

Pre-Procedure

1 Follow *Delegation Guidelines: Applying Dressings.* See *Promoting Safety and Comfort: Applying Dressings.*
2 Practice hand hygiene.
3 Collect needed supplies and equipment:
   - Gloves
   - Personal protective equipment as needed
   - Tape or Montgomery ties
   - Dressings as directed by the nurse
   - Adhesive remover
   - Scissors

   - Plastic bag
   - Bath blanket
4 Identify the person. Check the ID bracelet against the assignment sheet. Call the person by name.
5 Provide for privacy.
6 Arrange your work area. You should not have to reach over or turn your back on the work area.
7 Raise the bed for body mechanics. Bed rails are up if used.

Continued

Applying a Dry Non-Sterile Dressing—cont'd

Procedure

8 Lower the bed rail near you if up.

9 Help the person to a comfortable position.

10 Cover the person with a bath blanket. Fan-fold top linens to the foot of the bed.

11 Expose the affected body part.

12 Make a cuff on the plastic bag. Place it within reach.

13 Decontaminate your hands.

14 Put on a gown and mask if needed.

15 Put on the gloves.

16 Undo Montgomery ties or remove tape:
   a Montgomery ties: fold ties away from the wound.
   b Tape: hold the skin down. Gently pull the tape toward the wound.

17 Remove adhesive from the skin if necessary. Wet a 4 × 4 gauze dressing with the adhesive remover. Clean away from the wound.

18 Remove gauze dressings. Start with the top dressing. The soiled side is away from the person's sight. Put dressings in the bag. They must not touch the outside of the bag.

19 Remove the dressing directly over the wound very gently. It may stick to the wound or drain.

20 Observe the wound, drain site, and wound drainage.

21 Remove the gloves, and put them into the bag. Decontaminate your hands.

22 Put on clean gloves.

23 Open the dressings.

24 Cut the length of tape needed.

25 Apply dressings as directed by the nurse.

26 Secure the dressings in place. Use tape or Montgomery ties.

27 Remove your gloves, and put them in the bag. Decontaminate your hands.

Post-Procedure

28 Provide for comfort. (See the inside of the front book cover.)

29 Place the signal light within reach.

30 Lower the bed to its lowest position.

31 Raise or lower bed rails. Follow the care plan.

32 Discard supplies into the bag. Tie the bag closed. Discard the bag according to agency policy. (Wear gloves for this step.)

33 Clean your work surface. Follow the Blood-borne Pathogen Standard.

34 Unscreen the person.

35 Complete a safety check of the room. (See the inside of the front book cover.)

36 Remove the gloves. Decontaminate your hands.

37 Report and record your observations.

BINDERS

Binders are applied to the abdomen, chest, or perineal areas. Binders promote healing because they support wounds and hold dressings in place. They also reduce or prevent swelling, promote comfort, and prevent injury. Binders are secured in place with Velcro, zippers, hooks, pins, or other closures.

Straight abdominal binders provide abdominal support and hold dressings in place (Fig. 21-16). The binder is applied with the person supine. The top part is at the person's waist. The lower part is over the hips.

Breast binders support the breasts after breast surgery (Fig. 21-17). The woman is supine when it is applied. It is pulled snugly across the chest and secured in place.

T-binders secure dressings in place after rectal and perineal surgeries. The single T-binder is for women (Fig. 21-18, *A*). The double T-binder is for men (Fig. 21-18, *B*). The waistbands are brought around the waist and pinned at the front. The tails are brought between the legs and up to the waistband. They are pinned in place at the waistband.

Apply a binder so there is firm, even pressure over the area. It should be snug but not interfere with breathing or circulation. Secure pins so they point away from the wound. Re-apply the binder if it becomes loose, wrinkled, or out of position or causes discomfort. Change binders that are moist, wet, or soiled.

PROMOTING SAFETY AND COMFORT
Binders

Safety

Binders must be applied properly. Otherwise, severe discomfort, skin irritation, and circulatory and respiratory complications can occur. The binder's effectiveness and the person's safety depend on correct application.

Comfort

A binder should promote comfort. Re-apply the binder if it causes pain or discomfort.

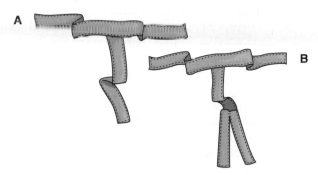

FIG. **21-18** **A,** Single T-binder. **B,** Double T-binder.

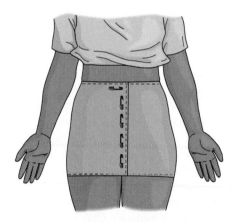

FIG. **21-16** Straight abdominal binder secured with pins.

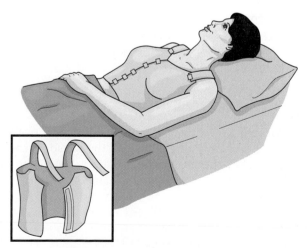

FIG. **21-17** Breast binder.

HEAT AND COLD APPLICATIONS

Heat and cold applications promote healing and comfort. They also reduce tissue swelling. Heat and cold have opposite effects on body function. Severe injuries and changes in body function can occur.

Heat Applications

Heat applications are often used for musculoskeletal injuries or problems (sprains, arthritis). They relieve pain, relax muscles, and decrease joint stiffness. They also promote healing and reduce tissue swelling.

When heat is applied to the skin, blood vessels in the area dilate. **Dilate** means to expand or open wider (Fig. 21-19). Blood flow increases. Tissues have more oxygen and nutrients for healing. Excess fluid is removed from the area faster.

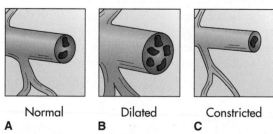

Normal   Dilated   Constricted
A   **B**   **C**

FIG. **21-19** **A,** Blood vessel under normal conditions. **B,** Dilated blood vessel. **C,** Constricted blood vessel.

Complications

High temperatures can cause burns. Report pain, excessive redness, and blisters at once.

Also observe for pale skin. When heat is applied too long, blood vessels **constrict** (narrow) (see Fig. 21-19). Blood flow decreases when vessels constrict. Tissues receive less blood. Tissue damage occurs, and the skin is pale.

Older and fair-skinned people have fragile skin that is easily burned. Persons with problems sensing heat or pain are also at risk. *(See Persons With Dementia: Complications From Heat Applications.)* Nervous system damage, loss of consciousness, and circulatory disorders and some drugs interfere with sensation.

Metal implants pose risks. Metal conducts heat. Deep tissues can be burned. Pacemakers and joint replacements are made of metal. Do not apply heat in the implant area.

Moist and Dry Heat Applications

With a *moist heat application,* water is in contact with the skin. Water conducts heat. Moist heat has greater and faster effects than dry heat. Heat penetrates deeper with a moist application. To prevent injury, moist heat applications have lower (cooler) temperatures than dry heat applications. Moist heat applications include:

- Hot compresses (Fig. 21-20, *A*)—a *compress* is a soft pad applied over a body area. It is usually made of cloth.
- Hot soaks (Fig. 21-20, *B*)—a body part is put into water.
- Sitz baths (Fig. 21-20, *C* and *D*)—the perineal and rectal areas are immersed in warm or hot water. (*Sitz* means *seat* in German.)
- Hot packs (Fig. 21-20, *E*)—a *pack* involves wrapping a body part.

With *dry heat applications,* water is not in contact with the skin. A dry heat application stays at the desired temperature longer. Dry heat does not penetrate as deeply as moist heat. Because water is not used, dry heat needs higher (hotter) temperatures to achieve the desired effect. Therefore burns are still a risk.

Hot packs and the aquathermia pad (Aqua-K, K-Pad) are dry heat applications (Fig. 21-21, p. 384). The aquathermia pad is an electric device used for dry heat. Tubes inside the pad are filled with distilled water. Heated water flows to the pad through a hose. Another hose returns water to the heating unit. The water is reheated and returned back into the pad.

Persons With Dementia

Complications From Heat Applications

Confused persons and those with dementia may not recognize pain. Look for changes in the person's behavior. Behavior changes can signal pain.

Cold Applications

Cold applications reduce pain, prevent swelling, and decrease circulation and bleeding. Cold has the opposite effect of heat. When cold is applied to the skin, blood vessels constrict (see Fig. 21-19). Blood flow decreases. Less oxygen and nutrients are carried to the tissues. Cold applications are useful right after an injury. Decreased blood flow reduces the amount of bleeding. Less fluid collects in the tissues. Cold has a numbing effect on the skin. This helps reduce or relieve pain in the part.

Complications

Complications include pain, burns, and blisters. Burns and blisters occur from intense cold. They also occur when dry cold is in direct contact with the skin.

When cold is applied for a long time, blood vessels dilate. Blood flow increases. The prolonged application of cold has the same effect as heat applications.

Older and fair-skinned persons have fragile skin. They are at great risk for complications. So are persons with mental or sensory impairments.

Moist and Dry Cold Applications

Moist cold applications penetrate deeper than dry ones. Therefore moist applications are not as cold as dry applications.

The cold compress is a moist cold application (see Fig. 21-20, *A*). Dry cold applications include ice bags, ice collars, and ice gloves (Fig. 21-22, p. 384). Cold packs can be moist or dry applications (see Fig. 21-20, *E*).

FOCUS ON THE PERSON

The wound can affect the person's basic needs. However, it is only one aspect of the person's care. Remember, the *person* has the wound. See *Focus on the Person: Assisting With Wound Care* on p. 386.

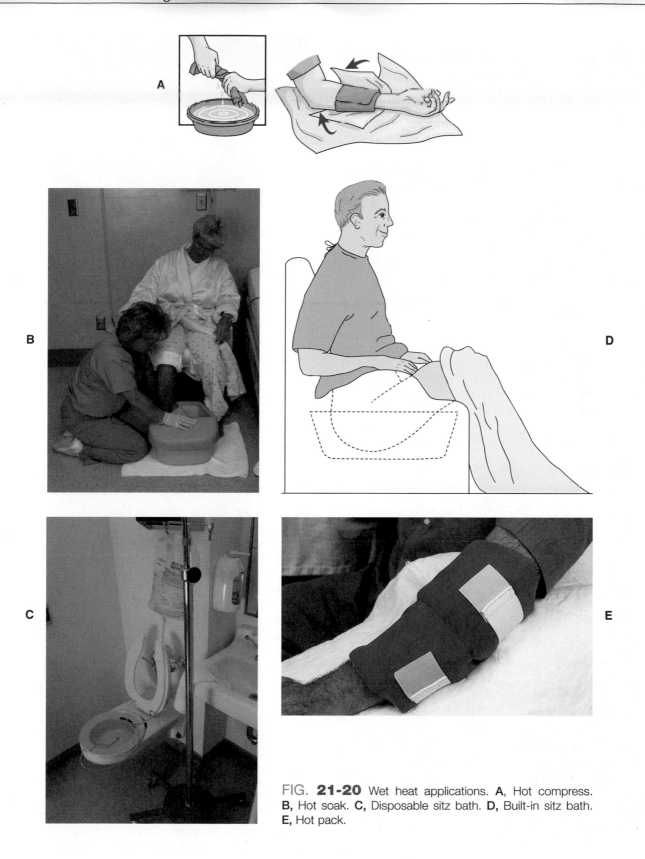

FIG. **21-20** Wet heat applications. **A,** Hot compress. **B,** Hot soak. **C,** Disposable sitz bath. **D,** Built-in sitz bath. **E,** Hot pack.

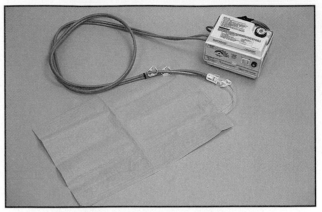

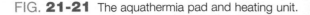

FIG. **21-21** The aquathermia pad and heating unit.

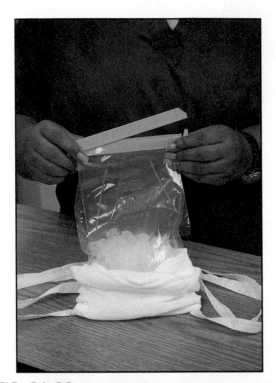

FIG. **21-22** The ice bag is filled ½ to ⅔ full with ice.

DELEGATION GUIDELINES
Applying Heat and Cold

Before applying heat and cold, you need this information from the nurse and care plan:
- The type of application—hot compress or pack, commercial compress, hot soak, sitz bath, aquathermia pad; ice bag, ice collar, ice glove, cold pack, or cold compress
- How to cover the application
- The application site
- What temperature to use (Table 21-1)
- How long to leave the application in place
- What observations to report and record:
  - Complaints of pain, numbness, or burning
  - Excessive redness
  - Blisters
  - Pale, white, or gray skin
  - Cyanosis (bluish skin color)
  - Shivering
  - Time, site, and length of the application
- What observations to report at once

PROMOTING SAFETY AND COMFORT
Applying Heat and Cold

Safety

Protect the person from injury during heat and cold applications. Practice the rules in Box 21-5 to prevent burns and other complications. Also follow these safety measures:
- *Sitz bath.* Blood flow increases to the perineum and rectum. Therefore less blood flows to other body parts. The person may become weak or feel faint. Drowsiness can occur from the bath's relaxing effect. Observe for signs of weakness, faintness, or fatigue. Also protect the person from injury. Check the person often. Keep the signal light within reach, and prevent chills and burns.
- *Commercial hot and cold packs.* Read warning labels and follow the manufacturer's instructions to safely use a commercial hot pack.
- *Aquathermia pad:*
  - Follow electrical safety precautions (Chapter 8).
  - Check the device for damage or other flaws.
  - Follow the manufacturer's instructions.
  - Place the heating unit on an even, uncluttered surface. This prevents it from being knocked over or knocked off of the surface.
  - Use a flannel cover to insulate the pad. It absorbs perspiration at the application site. (Some agencies use a towel or pillowcase.)
  - Secure the pad in place with ties, tape, or rolled gauze. Do not use pins. They can puncture the pad and cause leaks.
  - Do not place the pad under the person or under a body part. This prevents the escape of heat. Burns can result if heat cannot escape.

Comfort

Cold applications may cause chilling and shivering. Provide for warmth.

TABLE 21-1	Heat and Cold Temperature Ranges	
Temperature	**Fahrenheit Range**	**Centigrade Range**
Very hot	106° to 115° F	41.1° to 46.1° C
Hot	98° to 106° F	36.6° to 41.1° C
Warm	93° to 98° F	33.8° to 36.6° C
Tepid	80° to 93° F	26.6° to 33.8° C
Cool	65° to 80° F	18.3° to 26.6° C
Cold	50° to 65° F	10.0° to 18.3° C

Modified from Perry AG, Potter PA: *Clinical nursing skills and techniques*, ed 5, St Louis, 2002, Mosby.

BOX 21-5 Rules For Applying Heat and Cold

- Know how to use the equipment.
- Measure the temperature of moist applications. Use a bath thermometer. Or follow agency policy for measuring temperature.
- Follow agency policies for safe temperature ranges. See Table 21-1 for guidelines.
- Do not apply *very hot* (above 106° to 115° F [41.1° to 46.1° C]) applications. Tissue damage can occur. A nurse applies *very hot* applications.
- Ask the nurse what the temperature of the application should be.
  - Heat—cooler temperatures are needed for persons at risk.
  - Cold—warmer temperatures are needed for persons at risk.
- Know the precise site of the application. Ask the nurse to show you the site.
- Cover dry heat or cold applications before applying them. Use a flannel cover, towel, or pillowcase. Follow agency policy.
- Observe the skin every 5 minutes for signs of complications. See *Delegation Guidelines: Applying Heat and Cold*.
- Do not let the person change the temperature of the application.
- Ask the nurse how long to leave the application in place. Carefully watch the time. Heat and cold are applied for no longer than 15 to 20 minutes.
- Follow the rules of electrical safety when using electrical appliances to apply heat.
- Provide for privacy. Properly drape and screen the person. Expose only the body part where you will apply heat or cold.
- Place the signal light within the person's reach.

Applying Heat and Cold Applications

Quality of Life

Remember to:

- Knock before entering the person's room
- Address the person by name
- Introduce yourself by name and title

- Explain the procedure to the person before beginning and during the procedure
- Protect the person's rights during the procedure
- Handle the person gently during the procedure

Pre-Procedure

1 Follow *Delegation Guidelines: Applying Heat and Cold*. See *Promoting Safety and Comfort: Applying Heat and Cold*.
2 Practice hand hygiene.
3 Collect needed equipment.
4 Identify the person. Check the ID bracelet against the assignment sheet. Call the person by name.
5 Provide for privacy.

Continued

Applying Heat and Cold Applications—cont'd

Procedure

6 Prepare the application. Follow agency procedures and the manufacturer's instructions.
7 Place a dry application in a cover.
8 Place the application on the affected part. Note the time.
9 Secure the application in place with ties, tape, or rolled gauze. Do not use pins.
10 Place the signal light within reach. Unscreen the person.
11 Raise or lower bed rails. Follow the care plan.
12 Check the person every 5 minutes. Check for signs and symptoms of complications (see *Delegation Guidelines: Applying Heat and Cold*). Remove the application if any occur. Tell the nurse at once.
13 Remove the application at the specified time. (If bed rails are up, lower the near one for this step.)

Post-Procedure

14 Provide for comfort. (See the inside of the front book cover.)
15 Place the signal light within reach.
16 Raise or lower bed rails. Follow the care plan.
17 Unscreen the person.
18 Complete a safety check of the room. (See the inside of the front book cover.)
19 Clean the sitz bath with disinfectant solution. Wear utility gloves.
20 Clean and return reusable items to their proper place. Follow agency policy for soiled linen. Wear gloves for this step.
21 Discard the gloves. Decontaminate your hands.
22 Report and record your observations.

Focus on the PERSON

Assisting With Wound Care

Providing comfort—A wound can cause pain and discomfort. The wound and the pain may affect breathing and moving. Turning, repositioning, and walking may be painful. Handle the person gently. Allow pain drugs time to take effect before giving care.

Ethical behavior—Wound drainage may have odors. Some wounds are large and disfiguring. Love, belonging, and self-esteem needs are affected. You must be sensitive to the person's feelings. The person may be sad and tearful or angry and hostile. Adjustment may be hard and rehabilitation necessary. Be gentle and kind, give thoughtful care, and practice good communication. Do not judge the person by the size, site, odor, or cause of the wound.

Remaining independent—Amputation of a finger, hand, arm, toe, foot, or leg can affect function, everyday activities, and the person's job. Eye injuries can affect vision. Abdominal trauma and surgery can affect eating and elimination. Rehabilitation may be necessary.

Speaking up—The person may not tell you about pain or discomfort. Therefore, you need to ask these questions:

For elastic bandages:
- "Does the bandage feel too tight?"
- "Do you feel pain, itching, tingling, or numbness?"

For dressings:
- "Is the dressing comfortable?"
- "Does the tape cause pain or itching?"

For binders:
- "Is the binder too tight or too loose?"
- "Does the binder cause pain?"
- "Do you feel pressure from the binder?" If yes: "Where? Please show me."

For heat and cold applications:
- "Does the application feel too hot or too cold?"
- "Do you feel any pain, numbness, or burning?"
- "Are you warm enough?"

OBRA and other laws—Before applying an elastic bandage, changing a dressing, or applying heat and cold, make sure that:
- Your state allows you to perform the procedure
- The procedure is in your job description
- You have the necessary training
- You are familiar with the equipment
- You review the procedure with the nurse
- A nurse is available to answer questions and to supervise you

Nursing teamwork—The entire nursing team must prevent pressure ulcers. As you walk down hallways, look into rooms to see if a person has slid down in bed or in a chair. Do the same when people are in dining and lounge areas. Help reposition the person. Ask a co-worker to help you as needed. Report the repositioning to the nurse.

REVIEW QUESTIONS

Circle the **BEST** answer.

1 Which can cause skin tears?
   a Keeping your nails trim and smooth
   b Dressing the person in soft clothing
   c Wearing rings
   d Handling the person gently

2 Which can cause pressure ulcers?
   a Repositioning the person every 2 hours
   b Scrubbing and rubbing the skin
   c Applying lotion to dry areas
   d Keeping linens clean, dry, and wrinkle-free.

3 Which are *not* used to treat pressure ulcers?
   a Special beds
   b Waterbeds and flotation pads
   c Plastic drawsheets and waterproof pads
   d Heel elevators and elbow protectors

4 A person has a circulatory ulcer. Which measure should you question?
   a Use elastic garters to hold socks in place.
   b Do not cut or trim toenails.
   c Prevent injury to the person's legs.
   d Apply elastic stockings.

5 Elastic stockings
   a Prevent blood clots
   b Hold dressings in place
   c Reduce swelling after injury
   d Prevent pressure ulcers

6 When applying an elastic bandage
   a The part is in good alignment
   b Cover the fingers or toes if possible
   c Apply it from the largest to smallest part of the extremity
   d Apply it from the upper to the lower part of the extremity

7 A dressing does the following *except*
   a Protect the wound from injury
   b Absorb drainage
   c Provide moisture for wound healing
   d Support the wound and reduce swelling

8 To secure a dressing, apply tape
   a Around the entire part
   b To the top and bottom of the dressing
   c To the top, middle, and bottom of the dressing
   d As the person prefers

9 An abdominal binder is used to
   a Prevent blood clots
   b Prevent wound infection
   c Provide support and hold dressings in place
   d Decrease circulation and swelling

10 The greatest threat from heat applications is
   a Infection
   b Burns
   c Chilling
   d Pressure ulcers

11 Mrs. Parks is using an aquathermia pad. Which is *false*?
   a It is a dry heat application.
   b A flannel cover is used to insulate the pad.
   c Electric safety precautions are practiced.
   d Pins secure the pad in place.

12 Which is *not* a complication of cold applications?
   a Pain
   b Burns and blisters
   c Cyanosis
   d Infection

13 Before applying an ice bag
   a Place the bag in a freezer
   b Measure the temperature of the bag
   c Place the bag in a cover
   d Provide perineal care

14 Moist, cold compresses are left in place no longer than
   a 20 minutes
   b 30 minutes
   c 45 minutes
   d 60 minutes

Answers to these questions are on p. 469.

Assisting With Oxygen Needs

22

OBJECTIVES

- Define the key terms listed in this chapter
- Describe hypoxia and abnormal respirations
- Explain the measures that promote oxygenation
- Describe the devices used in oxygen therapy
- Explain how to safely assist with oxygen therapy
- Perform the procedure described in this chapter

PROCEDURES

Procedures with this icon 🔆 *are also on the CD-ROM in this book.*

- Assisting With Coughing and Deep Breathing Exercises

KEY TERMS

apnea The lack or absence (*a*) of breathing (*pnea*)

bradypnea Slow (*brady*) breathing (*pnea*); respirations are less than 12 per minute

Cheyne-Stokes respirations Respirations gradually increase in rate and depth and then become shallow and slow; breathing may stop (*apnea*) for 10 to 20 seconds

dyspnea Difficult, labored, or painful (*dys*) breathing (*pnea*)

hyperventilation Respirations are rapid (*hyper*) and deeper than normal

hypoventilation Respirations are slow (*hypo*), shallow, and sometimes irregular

hypoxia Cells do not have enough (*hypo*) oxygen (*oxia*)

orthopnea Breathing (*pnea*) deeply and comfortably only when sitting (*ortho*)

orthopneic position Sitting up (*ortho*) and leaning over a table to breathe

tachypnea Rapid (*tachy*) breathing (*pnea*); respirations are 24 or more per minute

---

BOX 22-1	Signs and Symptoms of Hypoxia

- Restlessness
- Dizziness
- Disorientation and confusion
- Behavior and personality changes
- Problems concentrating and following directions
- Anxiety and apprehension
- Fatigue
- Agitation
- Increased pulse rate and respirations
- Sitting position, often leaning forward
- Cyanosis (bluish color to the skin, lips, mucous membranes, and nail beds)
- Dyspnea

Oxygen (O_2) is a gas. It has no taste, odor, or color. It is a basic need required for life. Death occurs within minutes if breathing stops. Serious illnesses occur without enough oxygen. Illness, surgery, and injuries affect the amount of oxygen in the blood and cells.

ALTERED RESPIRATORY FUNCTION

Hypoxia means that cells do not have enough (*hypo*) oxygen (*oxia*). Cells do not receive enough oxygen. They cannot function properly. Hypoxia is life-threatening. Anything that affects respiratory function can cause hypoxia. The brain is very sensitive to inadequate O_2. Restlessness is an early sign. So are dizziness and disorientation. Report the signs and symptoms in Box 22-1 to the nurse at once.

Adults normally have 12 to 20 respirations per minute. Normal respirations are quiet, effortless, and regular. Both sides of the chest rise and fall equally. The following breathing patterns are abnormal:

- **Tachypnea**—Rapid (*tachy*) breathing (*pnea*). Respirations are 24 or more per minute.
- **Bradypnea**—Slow (*brady*) breathing (*pnea*). Respirations are fewer than 12 per minute.
- **Apnea**—Lack or absence (*a*) of breathing (*pnea*).

- **Hyperventilation**—Respirations are rapid (*hyper*) and deeper than normal.
- **Hypoventilation**—Respirations are slow (*hypo*), shallow, and sometimes irregular.
- **Dyspnea**—Difficult, labored, or painful (*dys*) breathing (*pnea*).
- **Cheyne-Stokes respirations**—Respirations gradually increase in rate and depth. Then they become shallow and slow. Breathing may stop (apnea) for 10 to 20 seconds.
- **Orthopnea**—Breathing (*pnea*) deeply and comfortably only when sitting (*ortho*).

PROMOTING OXYGENATION

Disease and injury can prevent oxygen from reaching the alveoli. Pain, immobility, and some drugs interfere with deep breathing and coughing up secretions. Oxygen needs must be met. The following measures are common in care plans.

Positioning

Breathing is usually easier in semi-Fowler's and Fowler's position. Persons with difficulty breathing often prefer sitting up and leaning over a table to breathe. This is called the **orthopneic position.** (*Ortho* means sitting or standing. *Pnea* means breathing.) Place a pillow on the table to increase the person's comfort (Fig. 22-1, p. 390).

Position changes are needed at least every 2 hours. Follow the care plan.

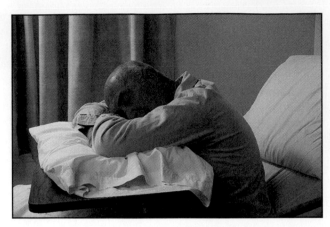

FIG. **22-1** The person is in the orthopneic position. A pillow is on the overbed table for the person's comfort.

Coughing and Deep Breathing

Coughing removes mucus. Deep breathing moves air into most parts of the lungs. Coughing and deep-breathing exercises help persons with respiratory problems. They are done after surgery and during bedrest. The exercises are painful after surgery or injury. Breaking an incision open while coughing is a fear.

Some doctors order coughing and deep breathing every 2 hours while the person is awake. Others want them done every hour while the person is awake.

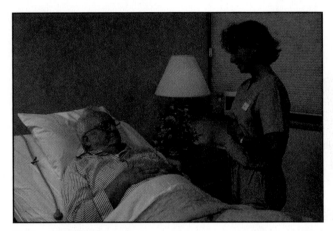

FIG. **22-2** The hands are over the rib cage for deep breathing.

DELEGATION GUIDELINES
Coughing and Deep Breathing

When delegated coughing and deep-breathing exercises, you need this information from the nurse and the care plan:
- When to do them
- How many deep breaths and coughs the person needs to do
- What observations to report and record:
  - The number of times the person coughed and took deep breaths
  - How the person tolerated the procedure

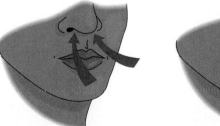

FIG. **22-3** The person inhales through the nose and exhales through pursed lips during the deep-breathing exercise.

Assisting With Coughing and Deep-Breathing Exercises

Pre-Procedure

1 Follow *Delegation Guidelines: Coughing and Deep Breathing.*

2 Practice hand hygiene.

3 Identify the person. Check the ID bracelet against the assignment sheet. Call the person by name.

4 Provide for privacy.

Procedure

5 Help the person to a comfortable sitting position: dangling, semi-Fowler's, or Fowler's.

6 Have the person deep breathe:
   a Have the person place the hands over the rib cage (Fig. 22-2).
   b Ask the person to exhale. Explain that the ribs should move as far down as possible.
   c Have the person take a deep breath. It should be as deep as possible. Remind the person to inhale through the nose (Fig. 22-3).
   d Ask the person to hold the breath for 3 seconds.
   e Ask the person to exhale slowly through pursed lips (see Fig. 22-3). The person should

   exhale until the ribs move as far down as possible.
   f Repeat this step 4 more times.

7 Ask the person to cough:
   a Have the person interlace the fingers over the incision (Fig. 22-4, *A*). The person can also hold a pillow or folded towel over the incision (Fig. 22-4, *B*).
   b Have the person take in a deep breath as in step 6.
   c Ask the person to cough strongly twice with the mouth open.

Post-Procedure

8 Provide for comfort. (See the inside of the front book cover.)

9 Place the signal light within reach.

10 Raise or lower bed rails. Follow the care plan.

11 Unscreen the person.

12 Complete a safety check of the room. (See the inside of the front book cover.)

13 Decontaminate your hands.

14 Report and record your observations.

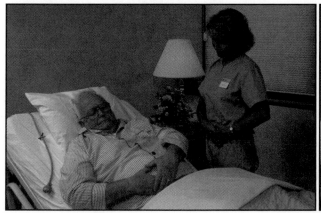
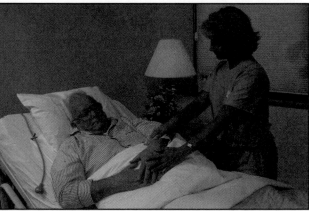

A   B

FIG. **22-4** The person supports an incision for the coughing exercise. **A,** Fingers are interlaced over the incision. **B,** A pillow is held over the incision.

OXYGEN THERAPY

Disease, injury, and surgery often interfere with breathing. The amount of oxygen in the blood may be less than normal. If so, the doctor orders oxygen therapy.

Oxygen is treated as a drug. The doctor orders the amount of oxygen to give, the device to use, and when to give it. Some people need oxygen constantly. Others need it for symptom relief—chest pain or shortness of breath. Oxygen helps relieve chest pain. Persons with respiratory diseases may have enough oxygen at rest. With mild exercise or activity, they become short of breath. Oxygen helps to relieve the shortness of breath.

Oxygen Sources

Oxygen is supplied as follows:
- *Wall outlet.* Oxygen is piped into each person's unit (Fig. 22-5).
- *Oxygen tank.* The oxygen tank is placed at the bedside. Small tanks are used by persons who walk or use wheelchairs (Fig. 22-6). A gauge tells how much oxygen is left (Fig. 22-7). Tell the nurse if the tank is low.
- *Oxygen concentrator.* The machine removes oxygen from the air (Fig. 22-8). A power source is needed. A portable oxygen tank is needed for power failures and mobility.
- *Liquid oxygen system.* A portable unit is filled from a stationary unit (Fig. 22-9). A dial shows the amount of oxgyen in the unit. Tell the nurse if the unit is low.

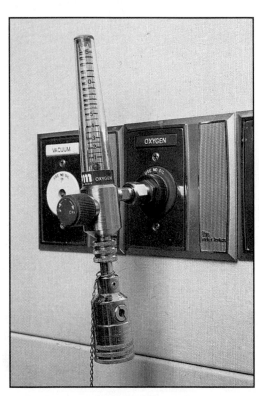

FIG. **22-5** Wall oxygen outlet with flow-meter. The flow-meter is used to set the flow rate.

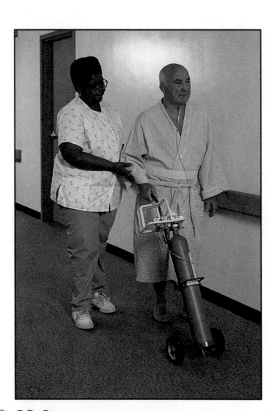

FIG. **22-6** A portable oxygen tank is used when walking.

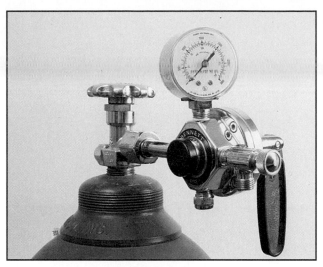

FIG. **22-7** The gauge shows the amount of oxygen In the tank.

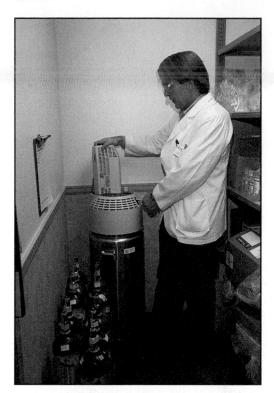

FIG. **22-9** Liquid oxygen system.

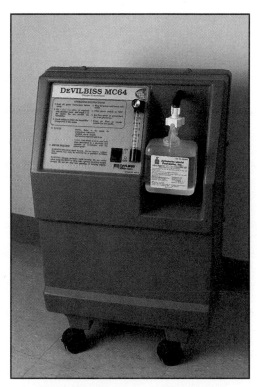

FIG. **22-8** Oxygen concentrator.

PROMOTING SAFETY AND COMFORT
Oxygen Sources

Safety

Liquid oxygen is very cold. If touched, it can freeze the skin. Never tamper with the equipment. Doing so is unsafe and could damage the equipment. Follow agency procedures and the manufacturer's instructions when working with liquid oxygen.

Oxygen Devices

The doctor orders the device used to give oxygen. These devices are common.

■ *Nasal cannula* (Fig. 22-10, p. 394). The prongs are inserted into the nostrils. A band goes over the ears and under the chin to keep the device in place. Tight prongs can irritate the nose. Pressure ulcers on the ears and cheekbones are possible.

■ *Simple face mask* (Fig. 22-11, p. 394). Covers the nose and mouth. The mask has small holes in the sides. Carbon dioxide escapes when exhaling. Room air enters when inhaling. Talking and eating are hard to do with a mask. Listen carefully. Moisture can build up under masks. Keep the face clean and dry. This helps prevent irritation from the mask. Masks are removed for eating. Usually oxygen is given by cannula during meals.

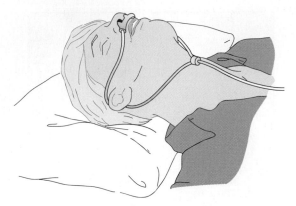

FIG. **22-10** Nasal cannula.

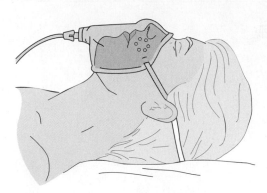

FIG. **22-11** Simple face mask.

Oxygen Flow Rates

The *flow rate* is the amount of oxygen given. It is measured in liters per minute (L/min). The doctor orders 2 to 15 liters of O_2 per minute. The nurse or respiratory therapist sets the flow rate (see Fig. 22-5).

The nurse and care plan tell you the person's flow rate. When giving care and checking the person, always check the flow rate. Tell the nurse at once if it is too high or too low. A nurse or respiratory therapist will adjust the flow rate. Some states and agencies let nursing assistants adjust oxygen flow rates. Know your agency's policy.

Oxygen Safety

You assist the nurse with oxygen therapy. You do not give oxygen. You do not adjust the flow rate unless allowed by your state and agency. However, you must give safe care. Follow the rules in Box 22-2.

FOCUS ON THE PERSON

You assist in the care of persons with oxygen needs. You must give safe and effective care. *See Focus on the Person: Assisting With Oxygen Needs.*

BOX 22-2   **Safety Rules For Oxygen Therapy**

- Never remove the oxygen device.
- Make sure the oxygen device is secure but not tight.
- Check for signs of irritation from the device. Check behind the ears, under the nose (cannula), and around the face (mask). Also check the cheekbones.
- Keep the face clean and dry when a face mask is used.
- Never shut off oxygen flow.
- Do not adjust the flow rate unless allowed by your state and agency.
- Tell the nurse at once if the flow rate is too high or too low.
- Tell the nurse at once if the humidifier is not bubbling.
- Secure connecting tubing in place. Tape or pin it to the person's garment following agency policy.
- Make sure there are no kinks in the tubing.
- Make sure the person does not lie on any part of the tubing.
- Report signs and symptoms of hypoxia and abnormal breathing patterns to the nurse at once.
- Give oral hygiene as directed. Follow the care plan.
- Make sure the device is clean and free of mucus.
- Follow the safety measures to prevent equipment accidents (Chapter 8).
- Follow the safety measures for fire and the use of oxygen (Chapter 8).

Focus on the PERSON

Assisting With Oxygen Needs

Providing comfort—Elastic bands on oxygen cannulas and face masks must be snug but not tight. Tight bands on a cannula cause discomfort and pressure on the face and nostrils.

Ethical behavior—A person may complain about not being able to breathe or about not "getting enough air." Yet you see the person breathing. Do not dismiss the person's complaint. Tell the nurse at once. You cannot feel what the person does. You must rely on what the person tells you. This is the right thing to do.

Remaining independent—Portable oxygen sources increase the person's independence. Small oxygen tanks are examples. The person can wheel the tank (see Fig. 22-6) or attach it to a wheelchair. A portable liquid oxygen unit can be worn over the shoulder.

Speaking up—The questions you ask the person can help promote comfort and safety. They also aid the nurse in the assessment step of the nursing process. For example:
- "Do you need more pillows?"
- "Do you want the head of your bed raised more?"
- "How often are you coughing?"
- "Are you coughing anything up?"
- "Please remember to cover your nose and mouth when coughing. I'll put these tissues where you can reach them."
- "Please use a tissue when you cough up mucus, then put on your signal light. The nurse needs to observe the mucus."

OBRA and other laws—Oxygen is treated as a drug. State nurse practice acts allow nurses to give drugs. Therefore, you do not start and maintain oxygen therapy. You assist the nurse in providing safe care.

Nursing teamwork—Oxygen tanks and liquid oxygen systems only contain a certain amount of oxygen. When the oxygen level is low, another tank is needed or the liquid oxygen system is refilled. Always check the oxygen level when you are with or near persons using these oxygen sources. Report at once a low oxygen level to the co-worker assigned to the person.

REVIEW QUESTIONS

Circle the **BEST** answer.

1 Hypoxia is
a Not enough oxygen in the blood
b The amount of hemoglobin that contains oxygen
c Not enough oxygen in the cells
d The lack of carbon dioxide

2 An early sign of hypoxia is
a Cyanosis
b Increased pulse and respiratory rates
c Restlessness
d Dyspnea

3 A person can breathe deeply and comfortably only while sitting. This is called
a Dyspnea   c Bradypnea
b Orthopnea   d Cheyne-Stokes respirations

4 A person's respirations are 28 per minute. This is called
a Tachypnea   c Hyperventilation
b Apnea   d Hypoventilation

5 To promote oxygenation, position changes are needed at least every
a 30 minutes   c 90 minutes
b Hour   d 2 hours

6 You are assisting with coughing and deep breathing. Which is *false?*
a The person inhales through pursed lips.
b The person sits in a comfortable sitting position.
c The person inhales deeply through the nose.
d The person holds a pillow over an incision.

7 When assisting with oxygen therapy, you can
a Turn the oxygen on and off
b Start the oxygen
c Decide what device to use
d Keep connecting tubing secure and free of kinks

8 These statements are about oxygen flow rates. Which is *true?*
a You can check the flow rate.
b The flow rate is measured in milliliters (ml).
c The flow rate is the amount of oxygen given in 1 minute.
d The flow rate is the same for all persons.

Answers to these questions are on p. 469.

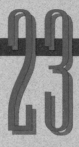

Assisting With Rehabilitation and Restorative Care

OBJECTIVES

- Define the key terms listed in this chapter
- Describe how rehabilitation involves the whole person
- Identify the complications to prevent
- Explain your role in rehabilitation and restorative care
- Explain how to promote quality of life

Key Terms

activities of daily living (ADL) The activities usually done during a normal day in a person's life

disability Any lost, absent, or impaired physical or mental function

prosthesis An artificial replacement for a missing body part

rehabilitation The process of restoring the person to his or her highest possible level of physical, psychological, social, and economic function

restorative aide A nursing assistant with special training in restorative nursing and rehabilitation skills

restorative nursing care Care that helps persons regain their health, strength, and independence

Disease, injury, birth defects, and surgery can affect body function. Often more than one function is lost. A **disability** is any lost, absent, or impaired physical or mental function. Disabilities are short-term or long-term. Some are permanent. Daily activities are hard or seem impossible. The person may depend totally or in part on others for basic needs. The degree of disability affects how much function is possible.

Rehabilitation is the process of restoring the person to his or her highest possible level of physical, psychological, social, and economic function. The focus is on improving abilities to the greatest extent possible. For some persons, the goal is to return to work. For others, self-care is the goal. Sometimes improved function is not possible. Then the goal is to prevent further loss of function. This helps the person maintain the best possible quality of life.

Some people have suffered strokes, fractures, amputations, or other injuries. They need to regain function or adjust to a long-term disability. Some need home care or nursing center care.

RESTORATIVE NURSING

Some persons are weak. Many cannot perform everyday activities. **Restorative nursing care** is care that helps persons regain their health, strength, and independence. Some people have more progressive illnesses. They become more and more disabled. Restorative nursing programs prevent unnecessary decline in function. They may involve measures that promote:

- Self-care
- Elimination
- Positioning
- Mobility
- Communication
- Cognitive function

Many persons need restorative nursing and rehabilitation. Often it is hard to separate them. In many agencies, they mean the same thing. Both focus on the whole person.

Restorative Aides

Some agencies have restorative aides. A **restorative aide** is a nursing assistant with special training in restorative nursing and rehabilitation skills. These aides assist the nursing and health teams as needed.

Usually nursing assistants are promoted to restorative aide positions. Those chosen have excellent work ethics, job performance, and skills. Required training varies among states. If there are no state requirements, the center provides needed training.

REHABILITATION AND THE WHOLE PERSON

An illness or injury has physical, psychological, and social effects. So does a disability. The person with a disability needs to adjust physically, psychologically, socially, and economically. Abilities—what the person can do—are stressed. Complications are prevented. They can lead to further disability.

Rehabilitation often takes longer in older persons than in other age groups. Long or fast-paced rehabilitation programs are hard for them. They often have many chronic health problems that can slow and complicate recovery. They also are at risk for injuries.

Physical Aspects

Rehabilitation starts when the person seeks health care. Complications are prevented. They can occur from bedrest, a long illness, or recovery from surgery or injury. Bowel and bladder problems are prevented. So are contractures and pressure ulcers.

Self-care is a major goal. **Activities of daily living (ADL)** are the activities usually done during a normal day in a person's life. ADL include bathing, oral hygiene, dressing, eating, elimination, and moving about. The health team evaluates the person's ability to perform ADL. They also consider the need for self-help devices.

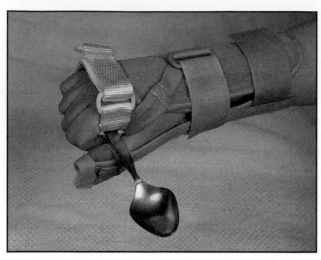

FIG. **23-1** Eating device attached to a splint.

Sometimes the hands, wrists, and arms are affected. Self-help devices are often needed. Equipment is changed, made, or bought to meet the person's needs.

■ Eating devices include glass holders, plate guards, and silverware with curved handles or cuffs (Chapter 17). Some devices attach to splints (Fig. 23-1).

■ Electric toothbrushes are helpful. Some persons cannot perform back-and-forth brushing motions for oral hygiene.

■ Longer handles attach to combs, brushes, and sponges (Fig. 23-2).

■ Some self-help devices for cooking, dressing, writing, phone calls, and other tasks are shown in Figure 23-3.

The person may need crutches or a walker, cane, or brace. Physical therapy is common after musculoskeletal and nervous system diseases, injuries, and surgeries. Some people need wheelchairs. If possible, they learn wheelchair transfers. Such transfers include to and from the bed, toilet, bathtub, sofa, chair, and in and out of cars (Fig. 23-4, p. 400).

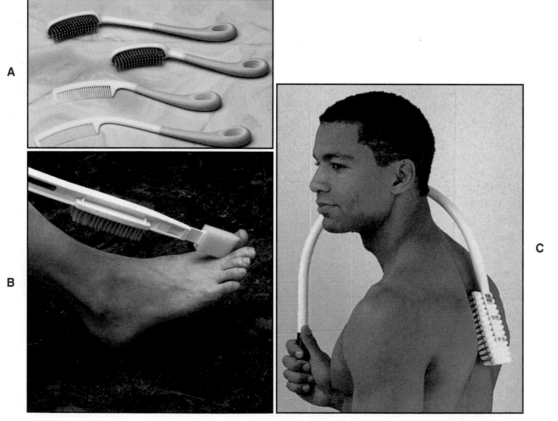

FIG. **23-2** A, Long-handled combs and brushes for hair care. B, Long-handled brush for bathing. C, Brush with a curved handle. (A and B courtesy Northcoast Medical, Inc., Morgan Hill, Calif.; C courtesy Sammons Preston Roylan, An AbilityOne Company, Bolingbrook, Ill.)

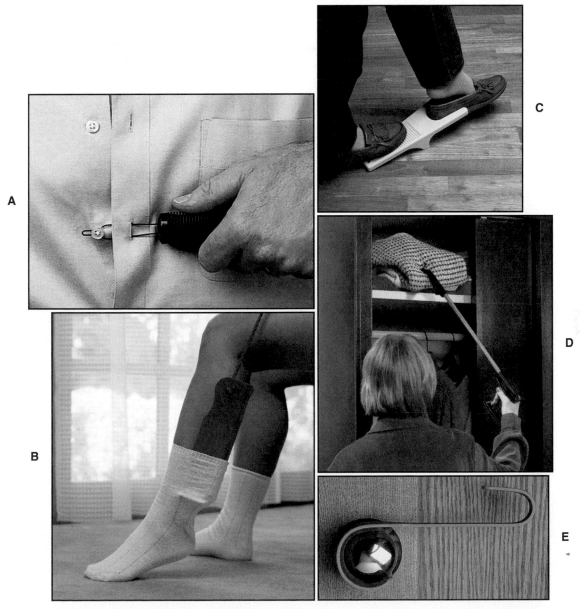

FIG. **23-3** **A,** A button hook is used to button and zip clothing. **B,** A sock assist is used to pull on socks and stockings. **C,** A shoe remover is used to take off shoes. **D,** Reachers are helpful to remove items from high shelves. **E,** A doorknob turner increases leverage to help turn the knob. (**A, B, C,** and **E** courtesy Northcoast Medical, Inc., Morgan Hill, Calif.; **D,** courtesy Sammons Preston Roylan, An AbilityOne Company, Bolingbrook, Ill.)

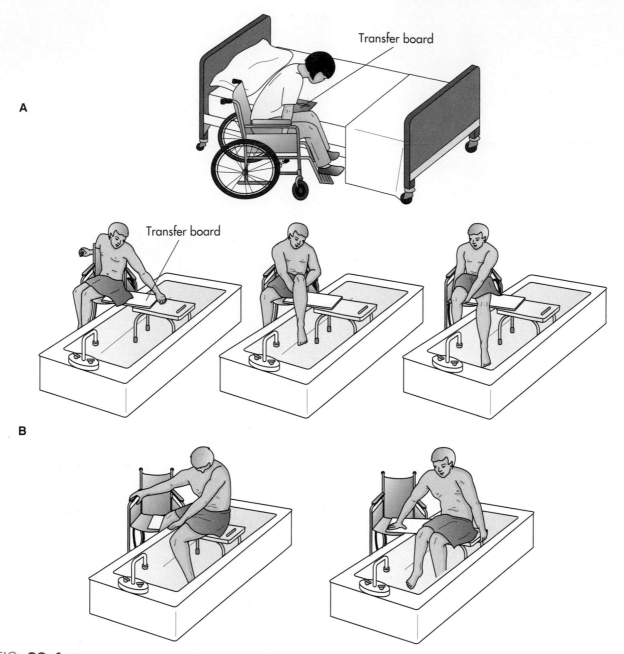

FIG. **23-4** The person uses a transfer board. **A,** The person transfers from the wheelchair to bed. **B,** The person transfers from the wheelchair to the bathtub.

A **prosthesis** is an artificial replacement for a missing body part. The person learns how to use an artificial arm or leg (Chapter 24). The goal is for the prosthesis to be like the missing body part in function and appearance.

Difficulty swallowing (*dysphagia*) and the inability to speak (*aphasia*) may occur after a stroke. The person may need a dysphagia diet (Chapter 17). When possible, exercises are taught to improve swallowing. Speech therapy and communication devices (Chapter 5) are helpful.

BOX 23-1	Assisting With Rehabilitation and Restorative Care

- Follow the nurse's instructions carefully.
- Follow the person's care plan.
- Follow the person's daily routine.
- Provide for safety (Chapter 8).
- Protect the person's rights. Privacy and personal choice are very important.
- Report early signs and symptoms of complications. They include pressure ulcers, contractures, and bowel and bladder problems.
- Keep the person in good alignment at all times (Chapter 11).
- Use safe transfer methods (Chapter 11).
- Practice measures to prevent pressure ulcers (Chapter 21).
- Turn and reposition the person as directed.
- Perform range-of-motion exercises as instructed.
- Apply assistive devices as ordered.
- Do not pity the person or give sympathy.
- Encourage the person to perform ADL to the extent possible.

- Allow time for the person to complete tasks. Do not rush the person.
- Give praise when even a little progress is made.
- Provide emotional support and reassurance.
- Try to understand and appreciate the person's situation, feelings, and concerns.
- Provide for spiritual needs.
- Practice the methods developed by the rehabilitation team when assisting the person.
- Practice the task that the person must do. This helps you guide and direct the person.
- Know how to apply the person's self-help devices.
- Know how to use and operate special equipment used by the person.
- Stress what the person can do. Focus on abilities and strengths, not disabilities and weaknesses.
- Remember that muscles will atrophy if not used.
- Have a hopeful outlook.

Psychological and Social Aspects

A disability can affect function and appearance. Self-esteem and relationships may suffer. The person may feel unwhole, useless, unattractive, unclean, or undesirable. The person may deny the disability. The person may expect therapy to correct the problem. He or she may be depressed, angry, and hostile.

Successful rehabilitation depends on the person's attitude. The person must accept his or her limits and be motivated. The focus is on abilities and strengths. Despair and frustration are common. Progress may be slow. Learning a new task is a reminder of the disability.

Remind persons of their *progress*. They need help accepting disabilities and limits. Give support, reassurance, and encouragement. Meeting psychological and social needs is part of the care plan. Spiritual support helps some persons.

THE REHABILITATION TEAM

Rehabilitation is a team effort. The person, family, doctor, nursing team, and other health team members are involved in setting goals and planning care. All help the person regain function and independence.

The team meets often to discuss the person's progress. Changes in the rehabilitation plan are made as needed. The person and family attend the meetings when possible. Families members are key members of the team. They provide support and encouragement. Often they help with care when the person returns home.

Your Role

Every part of your job focuses on promoting the person's independence. Preventing decline in function also is a goal. The many procedures, care measures, and rules in this book apply. Safety, communication, legal, and ethical aspects apply. So do the measures in Box 23-1.

QUALITY OF LIFE

Successful rehabilitation and restorative care improve the person's quality of life. A hopeful and winning outlook is helpful. Promoting quality of life helps the person's attitude. The more the person can do alone, the better his or her quality of life. To promote quality of life:

- *Protect the right to privacy.* The person relearns old or practices new skills in private. Others do not need to see mistakes, falls, spills, or clumsiness. Nor do they need to see anger or tears. Privacy protects dignity and promotes self-respect.
- *Encourage personal choice.* This gives the person control. Not being able to control body movements or functions is very frustrating. Persons are allowed and encouraged to control their lives to the extent possible. Persons who are sad and depressed may not want to make choices. Encourage them to do so. It can help them feel in control of those things that affect them.
- *Protect the right to be free from abuse and mistreatment.* Sometimes improvement is not seen for weeks. What seems simple is often very hard for the person. Repeated explanations and demonstrations may have no or little results. You may become upset and short-tempered. Or other staff or the family may have such behaviors. Protect the person from physical and mental abuse and mistreatment. Report signs of abuse or mistreatment to the nurse.

- *Learn to deal with your anger and frustration.* The person does not choose loss of function. If the process upsets you, think how the person must feel. Discuss your feelings with the nurse.
- *Encourage activities.* Often persons worry about how others view the disability. Provide support and reassurance. Remind the person that others have disabilities. They can give support and understanding.
- *Provide a safe setting.* It must meet the person's needs. Needed changes are made. The overbed table, bedside stand, and signal light are moved to the person's strong side. The person may need a special chair. If unable to use the signal light, another way is needed to communicate with the staff. The rehabilitation team suggests these and other changes.
- *Show patience, understanding, and sensitivity.* Progress may be slow and hard to see. The person may be upset and discouraged. Give support, encouragement, and praise when needed. Stress the person's abilities and strengths. Do not give pity or sympathy.

FOCUS ON THE PERSON

Loss of function affects the person's life. Some people cannot work. Some cannot take care of children or family. Others cannot meet their own needs. You must help promote quality of life. *See Focus on the Person: Assisting With Rehabilitation and Restorative Care.*

Focus on the PERSON

Assisting With Rehabilitation and Restorative Care

Providing comfort—Some diseases and injuries result in chronic pain. The pain is constant or occurs on and off. Always follow the person's care plan (Chapter 12).

Mental comfort also is important. The person may be angry, sad, frustrated, or depressed because of a loss of function or loss of a body part. Practice good communication skills. Often you do not need to say anything. Just be there and listen.

Ethical behavior—The person may not want to practice rehabilitation procedures or methods. He or she may want you to provide care instead. Personal choice is important. However, the person needs to follow the rehabilitation plan. Otherwise, he or she will not make progress. Do not let the person control you. Letting the person control you is the wrong thing to do. Report any problems to the nurse.

Remaining independent—The more the person can do for himself or herself, the better his or her quality of life. Independence to the greatest extent possible is the goal of rehabilitation and restorative care.

Some people have very limited function. Remember to focus on what the person can do. Do not focus on what the person cannot do.

Speaking up—You may need to guide and direct the person as he or she performs care measures. First listen to how the nurse or therapist guides and directs. Use their words. Hearing the same thing helps the person learn and remember what to do.

OBRA and other laws—OBRA requires that nursing centers provide services required by the person's comprehensive care plan. If a person requires physical therapy, it must be provided. If occupational therapy is required, it must be provided. The same holds for speech and other therapies. All services require a doctor's order.

Nursing teamwork—The rehabilitation process can frustrate the person, you, and other nursing team members. Nursing teamwork is not just about helping with care. It is also about providing emotional support to each other. Sometimes it helps to talk about your feelings. The nursing team can help you control or express your feelings. Sometimes it is helpful to assist with other patients and residents for a while.

REVIEW QUESTIONS

Circle the **BEST** answer.

1. Rehabilitation and restorative care focus on
   a. What the person cannot do
   b. What the person can do
   c. The whole person
   d. The person's rights

2. Mr. Olson's rehabilitation begins with preventing
   a. Angry feelings
   b. Contractures and pressure ulcers
   c. Illness and injury
   d. Loss of self-esteem

3. Mr. Olson has weakness on his right side. ADL are
   a. Done by him to the extent possible
   b. Done by you
   c. Postponed until he can use his right side
   d. Supervised by a therapist

4. Persons with disabilities are likely to feel the following *except*
   a. Undesirable
   b. Angry and hostile
   c. Depressed
   d. Relief

5. Which statement is *false*?
   a. Sympathy and pity help the person adjust to the disability.
   b. You should know how to apply self-help devices.
   c. You should know how to use equipment used in the person's care.
   d. You need to convey hopefulness to the person.

6. Mr. Olson is learning to use a walker. He asks to have music played. You should
   a. Tell him music is not allowed
   b. Choose some music
   c. Ask him to choose some music
   d. Ask a therapist to choose some music

7. Mr. Olson's right side is weak. The signal light is on his right side. You move it to the left side. You have promoted his quality of life by
   a. Protecting him from abuse and mistreatment
   b. Allowing personal choice
   c. Providing for his safety
   d. Taking part in his activities

Circle **T** if the statement is true and **F** if the statement is false.

8. **T F** A person's speech therapy should be done in private.

9. **T F** You tell Mr. Olson that he cannot have dessert until he does his exercises. This is abuse and mistreatment.

10. **T F** Rehabilitation programs for older persons are usually slower paced than those for younger persons.

11. **T F** Only the doctor and physical therapist make up the rehabilitation team.

12. **T F** Nursing assistants and restorative aides are involved in the person's rehabilitation program.

Answers to these questions are on p. 469.

Caring For Persons With Common Health Problems

Objectives

- Define the key terms listed in this chapter
- Describe how cancer is treated
- Describe musculoskeletal disorders and the care required
- Describe nervous system disorders and the care required
- Describe hearing loss and the care required
- Describe eye disorders and the care required
- Describe respiratory disorders and the care required
- Describe cardiovascular disorders and the care required
- Describe urinary system disorders and the care required
- Describe digestive disorders and the care required
- Describe diabetes and the care required
- Describe communicable diseases and the care required
- Describe mental health disorders and the care required

KEY TERMS

anxiety A vague, uneasy feeling in response to stress
aphasia The inability (*a*) to speak (*phasia*)
arthroplasty The surgical replacement (*plasty*) of a joint (*arthro*)
benign tumor A tumor that grows slowly and within a local area
fracture A broken bone
hemiplegia Paralysis on one side of the body
malignant tumor A tumor that grows fast and invades other tissues; cancer
metastasis The spread of cancer to other body parts
paraplegia Paralysis from the waist down
quadriplegia Paralysis from the neck down
tumor A new growth of abnormal cells; tumors are benign or malignant

Understanding common health problems gives meaning to the required care. The nurse gives you more information as needed. Refer to Chapter 6 while you study this chapter.

CANCER

A **tumor** is a new growth of abnormal cells. Tumors are benign or malignant (Fig. 24-1).

A **benign tumor** grows slowly and within a local area. It does not spread to other body parts. A **malignant tumor** (cancer) grows fast. It invades other tissues. **Metastasis** is the spread of cancer to other body parts (Fig. 24-2, p. 406).

Common cancer sites are the skin, lungs, colon, rectum, breast, prostate, uterus, and urinary tract. Cancer is the second leading cause of death in the United States. It occurs in all ages.

Exact causes are unknown. The National Cancer Institute cites these risk factors:

- Tobacco—smoking tobacco, chewing tobacco and snuff, and second-hand smoke.
- Exposure to radiation—sun, sunlamps, tanning booths, x-ray procedures.
- Alcohol.
- Diet—high-fat diet, being seriously overweight.
- Chemicals and other substances—metals, pesticides, asbestos, and others.
- Hormone replacement therapy (HRT).
- Diethylstilbestrol—a synthetic form of estrogen used between the early 1940s and 1971. It was given during pregnancy to prevent certain problems.
- Close relatives with certain types of cancer—melanoma and cancers of the breast, ovary, prostate, and colon.

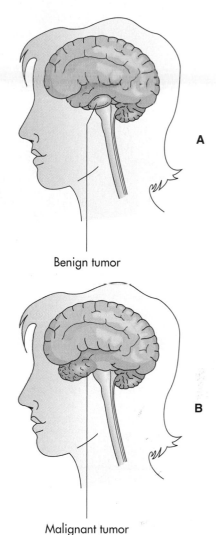

Benign tumor

Malignant tumor

FIG. **24-1** **A,** Benign tumors grow within a local area. **B,** Malignant tumors invade other tissues.

If detected early, cancer can be treated and controlled (Box 24-1, p. 406). Surgery, radiation therapy, and chemotherapy are the most common cancer treatments.

- *Surgery.* Tumors are removed to cure or control cancer. Surgery also is done to relieve pain from advanced cancer.
- *Radiation therapy.* X-ray beams are aimed at the tumor. Cancer cells and normal cells receive radiation. Both are destroyed. Burns, skin breakdown, and hair loss can occur at the treatment site. Discomfort, nausea and vomiting, diarrhea, and loss of appetite (*anorexia*) are other side effects.
- *Chemotherapy.* Drugs are given that kill cancer cells and normal cells. Side effects can be severe. The gastrointestinal tract is irritated. Nausea, vomiting, and diarrhea result. *Stomatitis,* an inflammation (*itis*) of the mouth (*stomat*), may occur. Hair loss (*alopecia*) may occur. Bleeding and infection are risks from decreased blood cell production.

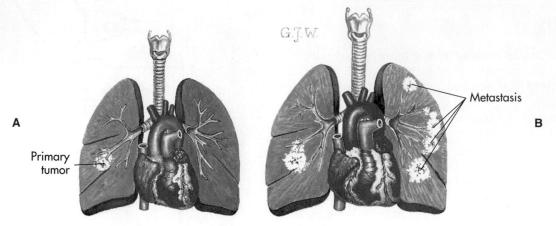

FIG. **24-2** **A,** Tumor in the lung. **B,** Tumor has metastasized to the other lung. (Modified from Belcher AE: *Cancer nursing,* St Louis, 1992, Mosby.)

BOX 24-1	Some Signs and Symptoms of Cancer

- Thickening or lump in the breast or any other part of the body
- A new mole or a change in an existing mole
- A sore that does not heal
- Hoarseness or a cough that does not go away
- Changes in bowel or bladder habits
- Discomfort after eating
- Difficulty swallowing
- Weight gain or loss with no reason
- Unusual bleeding or discharge
- Feeling weak or tired

Modified from National Cancer Institute: *What you need to know about cancer: an overview,* NIH Publication No. 00-1566, June 17, 2005 posted.

Persons with cancer have many needs. They include:

- Pain relief or control
- Rest and exercise
- Fluids and nutrition
- Preventing skin breakdown
- Preventing bowel problems (Pain relief drugs cause constipation. Radiation therapy and chemotherapy cause diarrhea.)
- Dealing with treatment side effects

Psychological, social, and spiritual needs are great. Anger, fear, and depression are common. Some surgeries are disfiguring. The person may feel unwhole, unattractive, or unclean.

Provide needed support. Do not avoid the person. Listen and use touch to show that you care. Often the person needs to talk and have someone listen. You may not have to say anything. Just listen. A spiritual leader may provide comfort.

MUSCULOSKELETAL DISORDERS

Musculoskeletal disorders affect movement. Injury and age-related changes are common causes.

Arthritis

Arthritis means joint *(arth)* inflammation *(itis).* Pain and decreased mobility occur in the affected joints.

Osteoarthritis (Degenerative Joint Disease)

This occurs with aging, joint injury, and obesity. The hips, knees, spine, fingers, and thumbs are commonly affected. Joint stiffness occurs with rest and lack of motion. Pain occurs with weight-bearing and joint motion. Severe pain affects rest, sleep, and mobility. Cold weather and dampness seem to increase symptoms.

Treatment involves relieving pain and stiffness. Doctors often order drugs and heat or cold applications. Exercise decreases pain, increases flexibility, and improves blood flow. Regular rest protects the joints from overuse. Canes and walkers provide support. Weight loss is stressed for persons who are obese. Falls are prevented. Help is given with activities of daily living (ADL) as needed. Toilet seat risers are helpful when hips and knees are affected. Some people need joint replacement surgery.

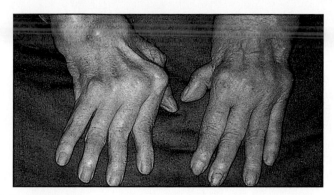

FIG. **24-3** Deformities caused by rheumatoid arthritis. (From Stevens A, Lowe J: *Pathology: Illustrated review in color,* ed. 2, London, 2000, Mosby.)

Rheumatoid Arthritis

Rheumatoid arthritis (RA) is a chronic inflammatory disease. It causes joint pain, swelling, and stiffness. Most common in women, it can occur at any age.

RA occurs on both sides of the body. For example, if the right wrist is involved, so is the left wrist. The wrist and finger joints closest to the hand are often affected (Fig. 24-3). Neck, shoulders, elbows, hips, knees, ankles, and feet joints can be affected. So can other body parts.

Treatment goals are to relieve pain, reduce inflammation, and slow down or stop joint damage. The care plan may include:

- Rest balanced with exercise.
- Good alignment. The person is positioned to prevent contractures and promote comfort. The person is turned and repositioned at least every 2 hours.
- 8 to 10 hours of sleep each night. Morning and afternoon rest periods are needed.
- An exercise program. It includes range-of-motion exercises.
- Walking aids, self-help devices, and splints as needed.
- Safety measures to prevent falls.

Drugs are ordered for pain relief and to reduce inflammation. Heat or cold applications may be ordered. Some persons need joint replacement surgery.

Emotional support is needed. A good outlook and being active are important. The more that persons can do for themselves, the better off they are. Give encouragement and praise. Listen when the person needs to talk.

Total Joint Replacement

Arthroplasty is the surgical replacement *(plasty)* of a joint *(arthro)*. Ankle, knee, hip, shoulder, wrist, finger, and toe joints can be replaced. The diseased joint is removed and replaced with a prosthesis. Pain is relieved and joint motion restored.

Osteoporosis

With osteoporosis, the bone *(osteo)* becomes porous and brittle *(porosis)*. Bones are fragile and break easily. Spine, hip, and wrist fractures are common.

Older persons are at risk. So are women after menopause. The lack of estrogen after menopause causes bone changes. So do low levels of dietary calcium. Tobacco use, alcoholism, lack of exercise, bedrest, and immobility are risk factors. Exercise and activity are needed for bone strength. For bone to form properly, it must bear weight. If not, calcium is absorbed. The bone becomes porous and brittle.

Back pain, gradual loss of height, and stooped posture occur. Fractures are a major threat. With brittle bones, even slight activity can cause a fracture. Turning in bed, getting up from a chair, or coughing can cause fractures. They are great risks from falls and accidents.

Prevention is important. Doctors often order calcium and vitamin supplements. Estrogen is ordered for some women. Weight-bearing exercise (walking, jogging, stair climbing, and so on) and strength training (lifting weights) are needed. Smoking and alcohol are avoided. Some people wear back braces or corsets for good posture. Others need walking aids. Protect the person from falls and accidents (Chapter 8). Turn and reposition the person gently.

Fractures

A **fracture** is a broken bone (Fig. 24-4). A *closed fracture (simple fracture)* means the bone is broken but the skin is intact. In an *open fracture (compound fracture)*, the broken bone has come through the skin.

Falls, accidents, cancer, and osteoporosis are causes. Signs and symptoms include pain, swelling, limited movement, loss of function, bruising, and bleeding.

For healing, bone ends are brought into normal position. This is called *reduction*. *Closed reduction* involves moving the bone back into place. The skin is not opened. *Open reduction* involves surgery. The bone is exposed and brought back into alignment. Nails, rods, pins, screws, plates, or wires keep the bone in place. After reduction, movement of the bone ends is prevented with a cast or traction.

Plastic and fiberglass casts dry quickly. A plaster of paris cast dries in 24 to 48 hours. It is odorless, white, and shiny when dry. When wet, it is gray, cool, and has a musty smell. You can assist the nurse with care (Box 24-2).

With traction, a steady pull from two directions keeps the bone in place. Weights, ropes, and pulleys are used (Fig. 24-7). Traction is applied to the neck, arms, legs, or pelvis. The nurse may ask you to assist with the person's care (Box 24-3, p. 410).

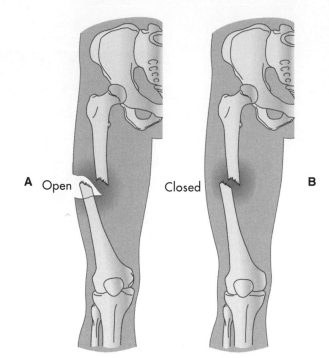

FIG. **24-4** **A,** Open Fracture. **B,** Closed fracture. (From Thibodeau GA, Patton KT: *The human body in health & disease*, ed 3, St Louis, 2002, Mosby.)

BOX 24-2 Rules For Cast Care

- Do not cover the cast with blankets, plastic, or other material. A cast gives off heat as it dries. Covers prevent the escape of heat. Burns can occur if the heat cannot escape.
- Turn the person every 2 hours. All cast surfaces are exposed to the air at one time or another. Turning promotes even drying.
- Do not place a wet cast on a hard surface. It flattens the cast. The cast must keep its shape. Use pillows to support the entire length of the cast (Fig. 24-5).
- Support a wet cast with your palms when turning and positioning the person (Fig. 24-6). Fingertips can dent the cast. The dents can cause pressure areas that can lead to skin breakdown.
- Report rough cast edges. The nurse will need to cover the cast edges with tape.
- Keep the cast dry. A wet cast loses its shape. Some casts are near the perineal area. The nurse may apply a waterproof material around the perineal area after the cast dries.
- Do not let the person insert anything into the cast. Itching under the cast causes an intense desire to scratch. Items used for scratching (pencils, coat hangers, knitting needles, back scratchers) can open the skin. An infection can develop. Scratching items can wrinkle the

stockinette or be lost into the cast. Both can cause pressure and lead to skin breakdown.
- Elevate a casted arm or leg on pillows. This reduces swelling.
- Have enough help when turning and repositioning the person. Plaster casts are heavy and awkard. Balance is lost easily.
- Position the person as directed.
- Report these signs and symptoms at once:
  - Pain: pressure ulcer, poor circulation, or nerve damage
  - Swelling and a tight cast: reduced blood flow to the part
  - Pale skin: reduced blood flow to the part
  - Cyanosis: reduced blood flow to the part
  - Odor: infection
  - Inability to move the fingers or toes: pressure on a nerve
  - Numbness: pressure on a nerve or reduced blood flow to the part
  - Temperature changes: cool skin means poor circulation; hot skin means inflammation
  - Drainage on or under the cast: infection
  - Chills, fever, nausea, and vomiting: infection
- Complete a safety check before leaving the room. (See the inside of the front book cover.)

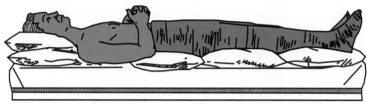

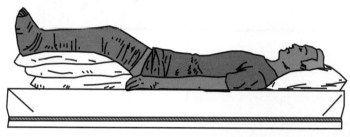

FIG. **24-5** Pillows support the entire length of the wet cast. (From Harkness GH, Dincher JR: *Medical-surgical nursing: Total patient care,* ed 10, St Louis, 1999, Mosby.)

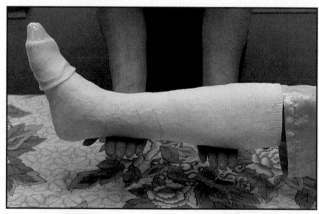

FIG. **24-6** The cast is supported with the palms during lifting.

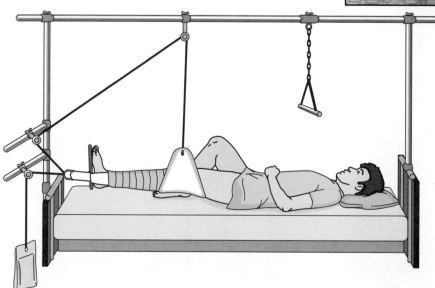

FIG. **24-7** Traction set-up. Note the weights, pulleys, and ropes. (From Phipps WJ and others: *Medical-surgical nursing: heath and illness perspectives,* ed 7, St Louis, 2003, Mosby.)

BOX 24-3   Caring For Persons in Traction

- Keep the person in good body alignment.
- Do not remove the traction.
- Keep weights off the floor. Weights must hang freely from the traction set-up (see Fig. 24-7).
- Do not add or remove weights from the traction set-up.
- Perform range-of-motion exercises for the uninvolved body parts as directed.
- Position the person as directed. Usually only the back-lying position is allowed. Sometimes slight turning is allowed.
- Provide the fracture pan for elimination.
- Give skin care as directed.
- Put bottom linens on the bed from the top down. The person uses the trapeze to raise the body off the bed.
- Check pin, nail, wire, or tong sites for redness, drainage, or odors. Report any observations to the nurse at once.
- Observe for the signs and symptoms listed under cast care (see Box 24-2). Report these observations to the nurse at once.
- Complete a safety check before leaving the room. (See the inside of the front book cover.)

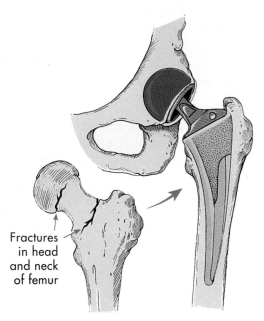

Fractures in head and neck of femur

FIG. **24-8** Hip fracture repaired with a prosthesis. (Modified from Christensen BL, Kockrow EO: *Adult health nursing,* ed 4, St Louis, 2003, Mosby.)

Hip Fractures

Fractured hips are common in older persons (Fig. 24-8). Surgery is done to fix the fracture in position with a pin, nail, plate, screw, or prosthesis. Rehabilitation is needed after surgery. Slow healing and other health problems affect the person's condition and care. Post-operative problems present life-threatening risks. They include pneumonia, urinary tract infections, and thrombi in the leg veins. Pressure ulcers, constipation, and confusion are other risks. Box 24-4 describes the care required.

BOX 24-4   Care of the Person With a Hip Fracture

- Give good skin care. Skin breakdown can occur rapidly.
- Encourage coughing and deep-breathing exercises as directed.
- Turn and reposition the person as directed. Usually the person is not positioned on the operative side.
- Keep the operated leg abducted at all times. The leg is abducted when the person is supine, being turned, or in a side-lying position. Use pillows (Fig. 24-9) or abductor splints as directed.
- Prevent external rotation of the hip (turning outward). Use trochanter rolls, pillows, sandbags, or abductor splints as directed.
- Perform range-of-motion exercises as directed. Do not exercise the affected leg.
- Provide a straight-backed chair with armrests. The person needs a high, firm seat. A low, soft chair is not used.
- Place the chair on the unaffected side.
- Assist the nurse in transferring the person.
- Do not let the person stand on the operated leg unless allowed by the doctor.
- Support and elevate the leg as directed when the person is in the chair.
- Apply elastic stockings as directed.
- Remind the person not to cross his or her legs.
- Complete a safety check before leaving the room. (See the inside of the front book cover.)

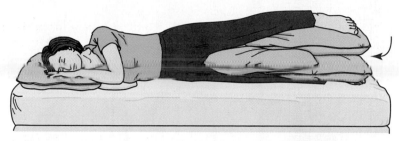

FIG. **24-9** Pillows are used to keep the hip in abduction. (From Phipps WJ and others: *Medical-surgical nursing: health and illness perspectives*, ed 7, St Louis, 2003, Mosby.)

NERVOUS SYSTEM DISORDERS

Nervous system disorders can affect mental and physical functions. They can affect the ability to speak, understand, feel, see, hear, touch, think, control bowels and bladder, or move.

Stroke

Stroke is a disease affecting the blood vessels that supply blood to the brain. It also is called a *cerebrovascular accident (CVA)*. The main causes are:

- *A ruptured blood vessel.* Bleeding occurs in the brain.
- *Blood clots.* A blood clot blocks blood flow to the brain.

Brain cells in the area affected do not get oxygen and nutrients. Brain damage occurs. Functions controlled by that part of the brain are lost or impaired.

Stroke is the third leading cause of death in the United States. It is the leading cause of disability in adults. See Box 24-5 for warning signs. The person needs emergency care.

Reproduced with permission of the American Heart Association, http://www.strokeassociation.org/presenter.jhtml?identifier=1020, Learn to Recognize a Stroke© 2005, American Heart Association.

Stroke can occur suddenly. The person may have warning signs (see Box 24-5). The person also may have nausea, vomiting, and memory loss. Unconsciousness, noisy breathing, high blood pressure, slow pulse, redness of the face, and seizures may occur. So can paralysis on one side of the body **(hemiplegia)**. The person may lose bowel and bladder control and the ability to speak. **Aphasia** is the inability *(a)* to speak *(phasia)*.

If the person survives, some brain damage is likely. Functions lost depend on the area of brain damage (Fig. 24-10, p. 412). The effects of a stroke include:

- Loss of face, hand, arm, leg, or body control
- Hemiplegia
- Changing emotions (crying easily or mood swings, sometimes for no reason)
- Difficulty swallowing *(dysphagia)*
- Aphasia or slow or slurred speech
- Changes in sight, touch, movement, and thought
- Impaired memory
- Urinary frequency, urgency, or incontinence
- Depression and frustration

Rehabilitation starts at once. The person may depend in part or totally on others for care. The health team helps the person regain the highest possible level of function (Box 24-6, p. 412).

BOX 24-5 **Warning Signs of Stroke**

- Sudden numbness or weakness of the face, arm, or leg especially on one side of the body
- Sudden confusion, trouble speaking, or understanding
- Sudden trouble seeing in one or both eyes
- Sudden trouble walking, dizziness, or loss of balance or coordination
- Sudden, severe headaches with no known cause

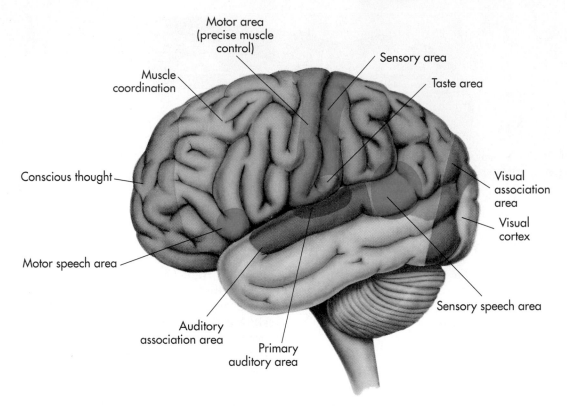

FIG. 24-10 Functions lost from a stroke depend on the area of brain damage. (From Thibodeau GA, Patton KT: *The human body in health & disease,* ed 3, St Louis, 2002, Mosby.)

BOX 24-6 Care of the Person With a Stroke

- The lateral position prevents aspiration.
- Coughing and deep breathing are encouraged.
- The bed is kept in semi-Fowler's position.
- Turning and repositioning are done at least every 2 hours.
- Food and fluid needs are met.
- Elastic stockings prevent thrombi (blood clots) in the legs.
- Range-of-motion exercises prevent contractures.
- A catheter is inserted, or a bladder training program is started.
- A bowel training program may be needed.
- Safety precautions are practiced. Use bed rails according to the care plan.
- Keep the signal light within reach. It is on the person's unaffected side. If unable to use the signal light, check the person often.

- The person does as much self-care as possible. Assist as needed.
- Communication methods are established. Magic slates, pencil and paper, a picture board, or other methods are used. Limit questions to those that have "yes" or "no" answers. Speak slowly. Allow the person time to respond (Chapter 5).
- Good skin care prevents pressure ulcers.
- Speech, physical, and occupational therapies are ordered.
- Assistive and self-help devices are used as needed (Chapter 23).
- Support, encouragement, and praise are given.
- Complete a safety check before leaving the room. (See the inside of the front book cover.)

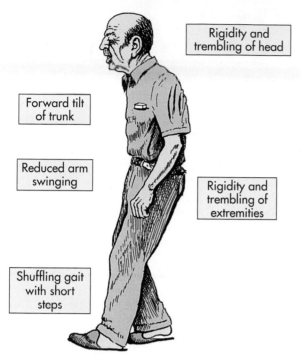

Rigidity and trembling of head

Forward tilt of trunk

Reduced arm swinging

Rigidity and trembling of extremities

Shuffling gait with short steps

FIG. **24-11** Signs of Parkinson's disease. (From Thibodeau GA, Patton KT: *The human body in health & disease*, ed 3, St Louis, 2002, Mosby.)

Aphasia

Expressive aphasia is difficulty expressing or sending out thoughts. Thinking is clear. There are problems speaking, spelling, counting, gesturing, or writing. The person thinks one thing but says another. For example, the person thinks about food but asks for a book. The person may call others the wrong names. Sometimes only sounds, not words, are uttered. The person may cry or swear for no reason.

Receptive aphasia relates to difficulty receiving information. The person has trouble understanding what is said or read. People and common objects are not recognized. The person may not know how to use a fork, toilet, cup, TV, phone, or other items.

Some people have expressive and receptive aphasia. This is called *expressive-receptive aphasia.*

Parkinson's Disease

Parkinson's disease is a slow, progressive disorder with no cure. Degeneration of a part of the brain occurs. Persons over 50 years old are at risk. Some signs and symptoms are shown in Figure 24-11. Pill-rolling movements (rubbing of the thumb and index finger) are common. So is a mask-like expression—the person cannot blink and smile. A fixed stare is common.

Other signs and symptoms develop over time. They include swallowing and chewing problems, constipation, and bladder problems. Sleep problems and depression can occur. So can memory loss, slow thinking, and emotional changes. Speech changes occur. They include slurred, monotone, and soft speech.

The doctor orders drugs for Parkinson's disease. Exercise and physical therapy are ordered to improve strength, posture, balance, and mobility. Therapy is needed for speech and swallowing problems. The person may need help with eating and self-care. Normal elimination is a goal. Safety measures prevent injury.

Multiple Sclerosis

Multiple sclerosis (MS) is a chronic disease. *Multiple* means many. *Sclerosis* means hardening or scarring. The myelin (which covers nerve fibers) in the brain and spinal cord are destroyed. Nerve impulses are not sent to and from the brain in a normal manner. There is no cure.

Symptoms usually start between the ages of 20 and 40. Some people have little or no symptom progress after the first attack. For others, symptoms lessen or disappear (remission). At some point, there are flare-ups (relapses). With each flare-up, more symptoms can occur. Some people have no remissions. Their conditions gradually decline. New attacks leave new symptoms and more damage.

Symptoms depend on the damaged area. Vision problems may occur. Muscle weakness and balance problems affect standing and walking. Paralysis can occur. Tremors, numbness and tingling, loss of feeling, speech problems, dizziness, and poor coordination are common. Problems with concentration, attention, memory, judgment, and behavior may occur. Fatigue increases such problems. Bowel, bladder, and sexual function problems occur. Respiratory muscle weakness is common. So are anger and depression.

Persons with MS are kept active as long as possible. The care plan reflects the person's changing needs. Skin care, hygiene, and range-of-motion exercises are important. So are turning, positioning, coughing, and deep breathing. Bowel and bladder elimination is promoted. Injuries are prevented. So are complications from bedrest.

Spinal Cord Injuries

Spinal cord injuries can permanently damage the nervous system. Common causes are stab or bullet wounds, accidents, falls, and sports injuries. Cervical traction is often needed to keep the spine straight.

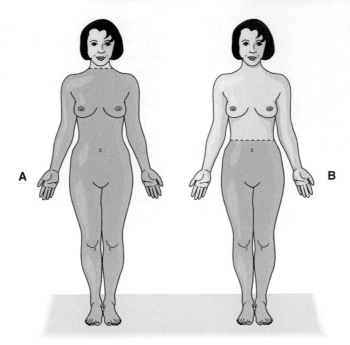

FIG. **24-12** The shaded areas show the areas of paralysis. **A,** Quadriplegia. **B,** Paraplegia.

The higher the level of injury, the more functions lost (Fig. 24-12). With lumbar injuries, leg function is lost. Injuries at the thoracic level cause loss of muscle function below the chest. Injuries at the lumbar or thoracic levels cause paraplegia. **Paraplegia** is paralysis from the waist down. Cervical injuries cause loss of function to the arms, chest, and below the chest. **Quadriplegia** is paralysis from the neck down.

If the person survives, rehabilitation is necessary. Care measures are listed in Box 24-7.

HEARING LOSS

Hearing losses range from mild to severe. *Deafness* is hearing loss in which it is impossible for the person to understand speech through hearing alone. Clear speech, responding to others, safety, and awareness of surroundings require hearing.

A person may not notice gradual hearing loss. Others may see changes in the person's behavior or attitude. Symptoms of hearing loss include:

- Speaking too loudly
- Leaning forward to hear
- Turning and cupping the better ear toward the speaker
- Answering questions or responding inappropriately
- Asking for words to be repeated

BOX 24-7   **Care of Persons With Paralysis**

- Prevent falls. Follow the care plan for safety measures and bed rail use.
- Keep the bed in the low position.
- Keep the signal light within reach. If unable to use the signal light, check the person often.
- Prevent burns. Check bath water, heat applications, and food for proper temperature.
- Turn and reposition at least every 2 hours.
- Prevent pressure ulcers. Follow the care plan.
- Maintain good alignment at all times. Use supportive devices according to the care plan.
- Follow bowel and bladder training programs.
- Maintain muscle function and prevent contractures. Assist with range-of-motion and other exercises as directed.
- Assist with food and fluids as needed. Provide self-help devices as ordered.
- Give emotional and psychological support.
- Follow the person's rehabilitation plan.
- Complete a safety check before leaving the room. (See the inside of the front book cover.)

Hearing-impaired persons may wear hearing aids or read lips. They watch facial expressions, gestures, and body language. Follow the measures in Box 24-8 to help the person hear or lip-read (speech-read). Some people learn sign language (Fig. 24-13, p. 416).

Some people have *hearing assistance* dogs (hearing guide dogs). The dog alerts the person to sounds. Examples include phones, doorbells, smoke detectors, alarm clocks, sirens, or on-coming cars.

Hearing Aids

A *hearing aid* makes sounds louder (Fig. 24-14, p. 416). It does not correct or cure the hearing problem. The person hears better because the device makes sounds louder. Background noise and speech are louder. The measures in Box 24-8 apply.

Sometimes hearing aids do not seem to work properly. Try these simple measures:

- Check if the hearing aid is *on*. It has an *on* and *off* switch.
- Check the battery position.
- Insert a new battery if needed.
- Clean the earmold if necessary.

Hearing aids are costly. Handle and care for them properly. Report lost or damaged hearing aids to the nurse at once. *Check with the nurse before washing a hearing aid. Also follow the manufacturer's instructions.* Remove the battery at night. When not in use, turn the hearing aid off.

BOX 24-8   Communicating With the Hearing Impaired Person

- Gain attention. Alert the person to your presence. Raise an arm or hand or lightly touch the person's arm. Do not startle or approach the person from behind.
- Position yourself at the person's level. If the person is sitting, you sit. If the person is standing, you stand.
- Face the person when speaking. Do not turn or walk away while you are talking. Do not talk to the person from the doorway or another room.
- Make sure the person is wearing his or her hearing aid. Make sure it is turned on and working.
- Stand or sit in good light. Shadows and glares affect the person's ability to see your face clearly.
- Make sure the person is wearing needed eyeglasses or contact lenses. This helps the person see your face for speech-reading.
- Speak clearly, distinctly, and slowly.
- Speak in a normal tone of voice. Do not shout.
- Adjust the pitch of your voice as needed. Ask the person if he or she can hear you better.
  - If the person does not wear a hearing aid, lower the pitch if you are a female. Women's voices are higher pitched and are harder to hear than lower pitched male voices.
  - If the person wears a hearing aid, raise the pitch slightly.

- Do not cover your mouth, smoke, eat, or chew gum while talking. Mouth movements are affected.
- Keep your hands away from your face. The person must be able to clearly see your face.
- Stand or sit on the side of the better ear.
- State the topic of conversation first.
- Tell the person when you are changing the subject. State the new subject of conversation.
- Use short sentences and simple words.
- Use gestures and facial expressions to give useful clues.
- Write out important names and words.
- Say things in another way if the person does not seem to understand.
- Keep conversations and discussions short. This avoids tiring the person.
- Repeat and rephrase statements as needed.
- Be alert to the messages sent by your facial expressions, gestures, and body language.
- Reduce or eliminate background noises. For example, turn off radios, stereos, TVs, air conditioners, and fans.

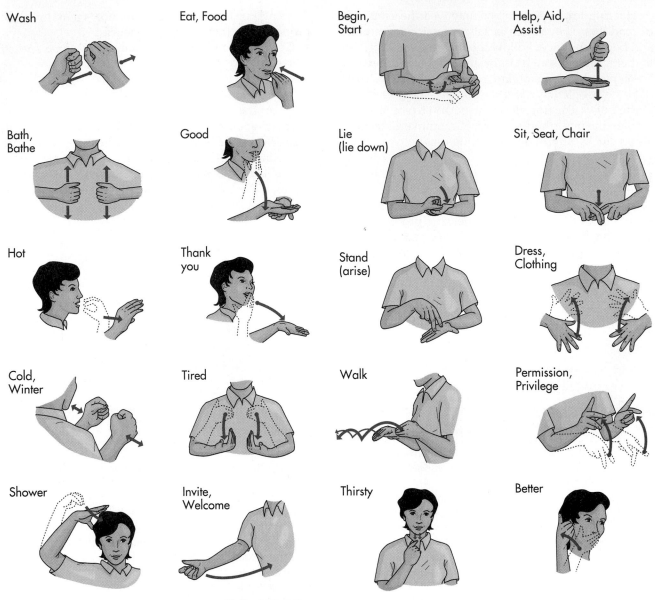

Wash

Eat, Food

Begin, Start

Help, Aid, Assist

Bath, Bathe

Good

Lie (lie down)

Sit, Seat, Chair

Hot

Thank you

Stand (arise)

Dress, Clothing

Cold, Winter

Tired

Walk

Permission, Privilege

Shower

Invite, Welcome

Thirsty

Better

FIG. **24-13** Sign language examples.

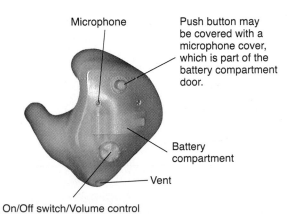

Microphone

Push button may be covered with a microphone cover, which is part of the battery compartment door.

Battery compartment

Vent

On/Off switch/Volume control

FIG. **24-14** A hearing aid. (Courtesy Siemens Hearing Instruments, Piscataway, NJ)

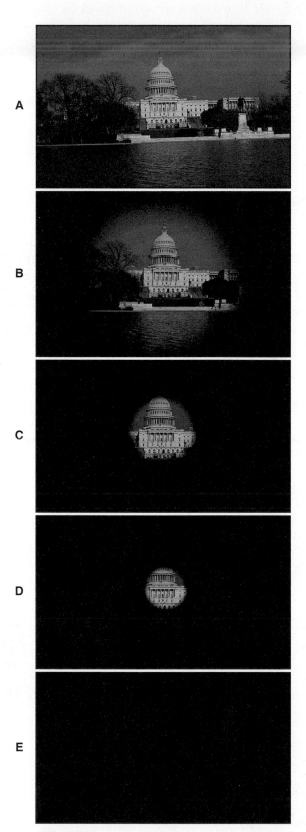

FIG. **24-15** **A,** Normal vision. **B,** Loss of peripheral vision begins. **C, D, E,** Vision loss continues, with eventual blindness.

EYE DISORDERS

Vision loss occurs at all ages. Vision loss is sudden or gradual in onset. One or both eyes are affected.

Glaucoma

Fluid pressure within the eye increases. This damages the optic nerve. Vision loss with eventual blindness occurs. Onset is gradual or sudden. Peripheral vision is lost. The person sees through a tunnel (Fig. 24-15), has blurred vision, and see halos around lights. With sudden onset, the person has severe eye pain, nausea, and vomiting. Persons over 40 are at risk. African-Americans and Asian-Americans are at greater risk than white Americans.

Treatment involves drug therapy and possibly surgery. The goal is to prevent further damage to the optic nerve. Prior damage cannot be reversed.

Cataract

The lens of the eye becomes cloudy. Light cannot enter the eye (Fig. 24-16). Vision blurs and dims. The person is sensitive to light and glares. A cataract can occur in one or both eyes. Aging is the most common cause.

Surgery is the only treatment. The lens is removed. A plastic lens is put in the eye. After surgery, protect the eye from injury:

■ Keep the eye shield in place as directed. Some doctors allow the shield off during the day if eyeglasses are worn. The shield is worn for sleep, including naps.

■ Follow measures for the blind person when an eye shield is worn (p. 418). The person may have vision loss in the other eye.

■ Remind the person not to rub or press the affected eye.

■ Do not bump the eye.

■ Do not shower or shampoo the person without a doctor's order.

■ Report eye drainage or complaints of pain at once.

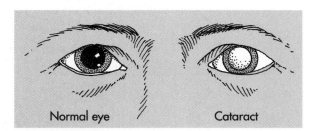

FIG. **24-16** One eye is normal. The other has a cataract. (From Phipps WJ and others: *Medical-surgical nursing: concepts and clinical practice,* ed 5, St Louis, 1995, Mosby.)

Corrective Lenses

Eyeglasses and contact lenses can correct many vision problems. Some people wear glasses for reading or seeing at a distance. Others wear them for all activities. Contact lenses are usually worn while awake.

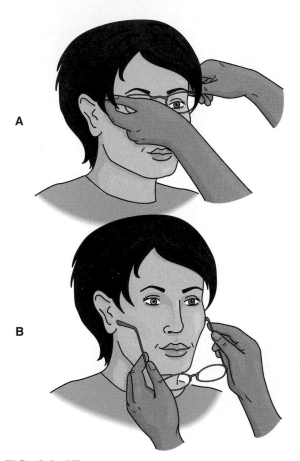

A

B

FIG. **24-17** **A,** To remove eyeglasses, hold the frames in front of the ear on both sides. **B,** Lift the frames from the ears. Bring the glasses down away from the face.

Protect glasses from breakage or other damage (Fig. 24-17). When not worn, put them in the eyeglass case. Put the case in the drawer of the bedside stand or overbed table. To prevent loss, nursing centers label eyeglasses with the person's name.

Clean glasses daily and as needed. Use warm water for glass lenses. Dry them with soft tissue. Plastic lenses scratch easily. Use special cleaning solutions, tissues, and cloths.

Contact lenses fit on the eye. They are easily lost. To remove and clean them, follow the manufacturer's instructions and agency procedures.

Blindness

Birth defects, accidents, and eye diseases are among the many causes of blindness. It is also a complication of some diseases. Some people are totally blind. Others sense some light, but have no usable vision. Still others have some usable vision, but cannot read newsprint.

Loss of sight is serious. Adjustments are hard and long. Moving about, daily activities, reading braille, and using a guide dog (seeing-eye dog) all require training.

Braille is a writing system that uses raised dots. Dots are arranged for each letter of the alphabet. The first 10 letters also represent 0 through 9 (Fig. 24-18). Braille is read with the fingers.

Blind persons learn to move about using a white cane with a red tip or a guide dog. Both are used worldwide by persons who are blind. The guide dog sees for the person. The dog is aware of danger and guides the person through traffic.

Treat the blind person with respect and dignity—not with pity. Most blind people adjust well and lead independent lives. Follow the practices in Box 24-9.

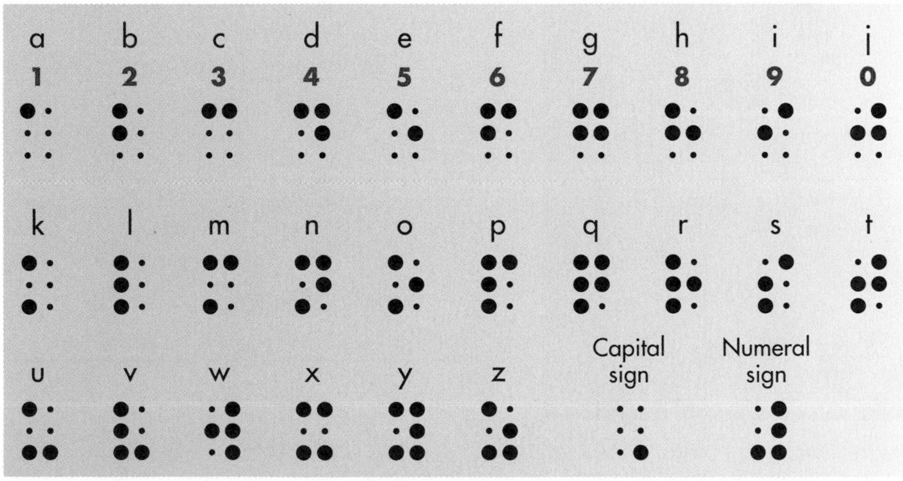

FIG. **24-18** Braille.

BOX 24-9	Caring For the Blind Person

- Ask the person how much he or she can see. Do not assume the person is totally blind or that the person has some vision.
- Provide lighting as the person prefers. Tell the person when the lights are on or off.
- Adjust drapes, blinds, and shades to prevent glares.
- Face the person when speaking. Speak slowly and clearly.
- Do not shout or speak loudly. Blindness does not mean the person has hearing loss.
- Identify yourself. Give your name, title, and reason for being there. Do not touch the person until you have indicated your presence.
- Identify others. Explain where each person is located and what the person is doing.
- Address the person by name. This tells the person that you are directing a comment or question to him or her.
- Do not avoid using the words "see," "look," or "read."
- Orient the person to the room. Describe the layout. Also describe the location and purpose of furniture and equipment.
- Let the person move about. Let him or her touch and find furniture and equipment.
- Do not leave the person in the middle of a room. Make sure the person can reach a wall or furniture.
- Do not rearrange furniture and equipment.
- Keep doors open or shut. Never leave them partly open.
- Give step-by-step explanations of procedures as you perform them. Tell the person when the procedure is over.

- Offer assistance. Simply say, "May I help you?" Respect the person's answer.
- Tell the person when you are leaving the room.
- Assist the person in walking. Walk slightly ahead of him or her (Fig. 24-19). Tell the person which arm is offered. Never push, pull, or guide the person in front of you. Walk at a normal pace.
- Tell the person when you are coming to a curb or steps. State if the steps are up or down.
- Inform the person of doors, turns, furniture, and other obstructions when assisting with walking.
- Give specific directions. Say "right behind you," "on your left," or "in front of you." Avoid phrases like "over here" or "over there."
- Keep hallways and walkways free of carts, equipment, toys, and other items.
- Assist in food selection. Read menus to the person.
- Explain the location of food and beverages. Use the face of a clock (Chapter 17). Or guide the person's hand to each item on the tray.
- Cut meat, open containers, butter bread, and perform other similar activities if needed.
- Keep the signal light within the person's reach.
- Provide a radio, compact disks or audiotapes, audio books, TV, and braille books.
- Let the person perform self-care if able.
- Complete a safety check before leaving the room. (See the inside of the front book cover.)

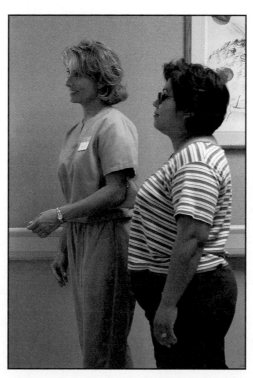

FIG. **24-19** The blind person walks slightly behind the nursing assistant. She touches the assistant's arm lightly.

RESPIRATORY DISORDERS

The respiratory system brings oxygen (O_2) into the lungs and removes carbon dioxide (CO_2) from the body. Respiratory disorders interfere with this function and threaten life.

Chronic Obstructive Pulmonary Disease

Three disorders are grouped under chronic obstructive pulmonary disease (COPD). They are chronic bronchitis, emphysema, and asthma. They interfere with the exchange of O_2 and CO_2 in the lungs. They obstruct airflow.

Chronic Bronchitis

Chronic bronchitis occurs after repeated episodes of bronchitis. Bronchitis means inflammation *(itis)* of the bronchi *(bronch)*. Smoking is the major cause.

Smoker's cough in the morning is often the first symptom. At first the cough is dry. Over time the person coughs up mucus. Mucus may contain pus. The cough becomes more frequent. The person has difficulty breathing and tires easily. Mucus and inflamed breathing passages *obstruct* airflow into the lungs. The body cannot get normal amounts of oxygen.

The person must stop smoking. Oxygen therapy and breathing exercises are often ordered. Respiratory tract infections are prevented. If one occurs, prompt treatment is needed.

Emphysema

In emphysema, the alveoli enlarge. They become less elastic. They do not expand and shrink normally with breathing in and out. Some air is trapped in the alveoli when exhaling. Trapped air is not exhaled. Over time, more alveoli are involved. As more air is trapped in the lungs, the person develops a *barrel chest* (Fig. 24-20). Breathing is easier when the person sits upright and slightly forward (Chapter 22).

Smoking is the most common cause. The person has shortness of breath and a cough. At first, shortness of breath occurs with exertion. Over time, it occurs at rest. Sputum may contain pus. The person must stop smoking. Respiratory therapy, breathing exercises, oxygen, and drug therapy are ordered.

Asthma

The airway narrows with asthma. Dyspnea results. Allergies and emotional stress are common causes. Symptoms are mild to severe. Wheezing and coughing are common. Sudden attacks *(asthma attacks)* can occur. There is shortness of breath, wheezing, coughing, rapid pulse, sweating, and cyanosis. Asthma is treated with drugs.

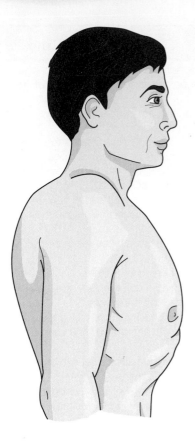

FIG. **24-20** Barrel chest from emphysema.

Pneumonia

Pneumonia is an inflammation and infection of lung tissue. Bacteria, viruses, aspiration, and immobility are causes. The person is very ill. Fever, chills, painful cough, chest pain on breathing, and a rapid pulse occur. Cyanosis may be present. Sputum is thick and green, yellowish, or rust colored.

Drugs are ordered for infection and pain. Fluid intake is increased because of fever and to thin secretions. Thin secretions are easier to cough up. IV fluids and oxygen may be needed. Semi-Fowler's position eases breathing. Standard Precautions are followed. Isolation Precautions are used depending on the cause.

Tuberculosis

Tuberculosis (TB) is a bacterial infection in the lungs. TB is spread by airborne droplets with coughing, sneezing, speaking, and singing (Chapter 10). Nearby persons can inhale the bacteria. Those who have close, frequent contact with an infected person are at risk. TB is more likely to occur in close, crowded areas. Age, poor nutrition, and HIV infection are other risk factors.

Risk Factors For Hypertension

Factors You Cannot Change

- Age—45 or older for men; 55 or older for women
- Gender—younger men are at greater risk than younger women; the risk increases for women after menopause
- Race—African-Americans are at greater risk than whites
- Family history—tends to run in families

Factors You Can Change

- Being overweight—related to diet, lack of exercise, and atherosclerosis
- Stress—increased sympathetic nervous system activity
- Tobacco use—nicotine narrows blood vessels
- High-salt diet—sodium causes fluid retention; increased fluid raises the blood volume
- Excessive alcohol—increases chemical substances in the body that increase blood pressure
- Lack of exercise—increases risk of being overweight
- Atherosclerosis—arteries narrow because of fatty build-up in the vessels

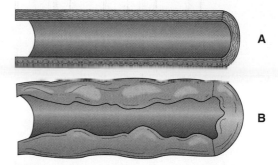

FIG. **24-21** **A,** Normal artery. **B,** Fatty deposits collect on the artery walls in atherosclerosis.

heart pumps with more force to move blood through narrowed vessels. Kidney disorders, head injuries, some pregnancy problems, and adrenal gland tumors are other causes.

Signs and symptoms develop over time. Headache, blurred vision, dizziness, and nose bleeds occur. Hypertension can lead to stroke, heart attack, heart failure, kidney failure, and blindness.

Certain drugs can lower blood pressure. A diet low in fat and salt, a healthy weight, and regular exercise are needed. No smoking is allowed. Alcohol and caffeine are limited. Managing stress and sleeping well also lower blood pressure.

Coronary Artery Disease

The coronary arteries supply the heart with blood. In coronary artery disease (CAD), one or all of the coronary arteries narrow. Therefore the heart muscle gets less blood. The most common cause is atherosclerosis (Fig. 24-21). The narrowed arteries block blood flow. Blockage may be total or partial.

CAD is the leading cause of death in the United States. It is more common in men, older persons, and persons with a family history of CAD. Such risk factors cannot be controlled. Other risk factors can be controlled—smoking, obesity, lack of exercise, hypertension, high cholesterol, and diabetes.

Treatment involves reducing risk factors. Major complications of CAD are angina pectoris and myocardial infarction (heart attack).

Angina Pectoris

Angina (*pain*) pectoris (*chest*) means chest pain. The chest pain is from reduced blood flow to a part of the heart muscle (myocardium). It is commonly called *angina*. It occurs when the heart needs more oxygen. Normally blood flow to the heart increases when the need for oxygen increases. Exertion, a heavy meal, stress, and excitement increase the heart's need for oxygen. In CAD, narrowed vessels prevent increased blood flow.

An active infection may not occur for many years. Chest x-ray and TB testing can detect the disease. Signs and symptoms are tiredness, loss of appetite, weight loss, fever, and night sweats. Cough and sputum production increase over time. Chest pain occurs.

Drugs for TB are given. The mouth and nose are covered with tissues when coughing or sneezing. Tissues are flushed down the toilet. Or they are placed in a paper bag and burned. In health care agencies, tissues are placed in a biohazard bag. Hand washing after contact with sputum is essential. Standard Precautions and Isolation Precautions are practiced.

CARDIOVASCULAR DISORDERS

Cardiovascular disorders are the leading causes of death in the United States. Problems occur in the heart or blood vessels.

Hypertension

With hypertension (*high blood pressure*), the resting blood pressure is too high. The systolic pressure is 140 mm Hg or higher. Or the diastolic pressure is 90 mm Hg or higher. Such measurements must occur two or more times. *Prehypertension* is when the systolic pressure is between 120 and 139 mm Hg or the diastolic pressure is between 80 and 89 mm Hg. See Box 24-10 for risk factors.

Narrowed blood vessels are a common cause. The

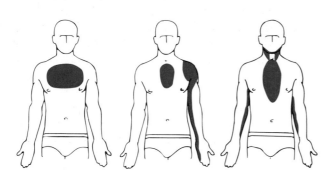

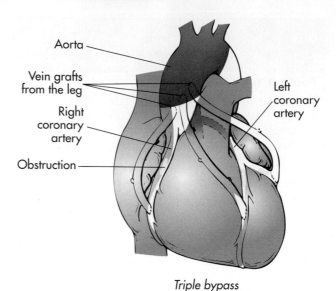

Triple bypass

FIG. **24-22** Shaded areas show where the pain of angina is located. (From Phipps WJ and others: *Medical-surgical nursing: concepts and clinical practice,* ed 5, St Louis, 1995, Mosby.)

FIG. **24-23** Coronary artery bypass surgery. (From Thibodeau GA, Patton KT: *The human body in health & disease,* ed 3, St Louis, 2002, Mosby.)

Chest pain is described as a tightness or pressure. Some complain of discomfort in the chest (Fig. 24-22). Pain in the jaw, neck, and down one or both arms is common. The person may be pale, feel faint, and perspire. Dyspnea is common. Rest often relieves symptoms in 3 to 15 minutes.

Besides rest, a *nitroglycerin* tablet is taken when an angina attack occurs. It is placed under the tongue. There it dissolves and is rapidly absorbed into the bloodstream. Tablets are kept with the person at all times. The person takes a tablet and then tells the nurse.

Things that cause angina are avoided. The person needs to stay indoors during cold weather or during hot, humid weather. Doctor-supervised exercise programs are helpful.

Surgery can open or bypass the diseased part of the artery (Fig. 24-23). Increased blood flow to the heart is the goal. Angina pectoris often leads to heart attack. Chest pain not relieved by rest and nitroglycerin may signal a heart attack. The person needs emergency care.

Myocardial Infarction

Myocardial refers to the heart muscle. *Infarction* means tissue death. With myocardial infarction (MI), part of the heart muscle dies. Blood flow to the heart muscle is suddenly blocked. Sudden cardiac death *(cardiac arrest)* can occur (Chapter 26).

BOX 24-11   **Signs and Symptoms of Myocardial Infarction**

- Sudden, severe chest pain (usually on the left side)
- Pain is described as crushing, stabbing, or squeezing; some describe pain in terms of someone sitting on the chest
- Pain may radiate to the neck and jaw, and down the arm or to other sites
- Pain is more severe and lasts longer than angina pectoris
- Pain is not relieved by rest and nitroglycerin
- Indigestion and nausea
- Dyspnea
- Dizziness
- Perspiration and cold, clammy skin
- Pallor or cyanosis
- Low blood pressure and a weak, irregular pulse
- Fear, apprehension, and a feeling of doom

Signs and symptoms are listed in Box 24-11. MI is an emergency. Life-threatening complications are prevented. Cardiac rehabilitation is planned. The goal is to prevent another heart attack. The program includes exercise, dietary changes, and lifestyle changes. The person may need surgery to open or bypass the diseased artery.

Heart Failure

Heart failure or congestive heart failure (CHF) occurs when the heart cannot pump blood normally. Blood backs up. Tissue congestion occurs.

- *Left-sided failure.* The left side of the heart cannot pump blood normally. Blood backs up into the lungs. The person has dyspnea, increased sputum, and cough. Also, the rest of the body does not get enough blood. Signs and symptoms occur from effects on the organs. Poor blood flow to the brain causes confusion, dizziness, and fainting. The kidneys produce less urine. The skin is pale. Blood pressure falls.
- *Right-sided failure.* The right side of the heart cannot pump blood normally. Blood backs up into the venous system. Feet and ankles swell. Neck veins bulge. Liver congestion affects liver function. The abdomen becomes congested with fluid. The right side of the heart pumps less blood to the lungs. Normal blood flow does not occur from the lungs to the left side of the heart. The left side has less blood to pump to the body. As with left-sided heart failure, organs receive less blood. The signs and symptoms described for left-sided failure occur.

Drugs strengthen the heart. They also reduce the amount of fluid in the body. A sodium-controlled diet is ordered. Fluids are restricted. Oxygen is given. Semi-Fowler's or Fowler's position is preferred for breathing. Bedrest, intake and output, daily weight, elastic stockings, and range-of-motion exercises are part of the care plan.

URINARY SYSTEM DISORDERS

The kidneys, ureters, bladder, and urethra are the major urinary system structures. Disorders can occur in these structures.

- *Urinary tract infection (UTI).* Urinary tract infections are common. Microbes can enter the system through the urethra. Catheters, poor perineal hygiene, immobility, and poor fluid intake are common causes.
  - *Cystitis* is a bladder (*cyst*) infection (*itis*). Urinary frequency, urgency, pain or burning on urination, blood or pus in the urine, foul-smelling urine, and fever may occur. Antibiotics are ordered. Fluids are encouraged. If untreated, cystitis can lead to pyelonephritis.
  - *Pyelonephritis* is inflammation (*itis*) of the kidney (*nephr*) pelvis (*pyelo*). Cloudy urine may contain pus, mucus, and blood. Chills, fever, back pain, and nausea and vomiting occur. So do the signs and symptoms of cystitis. Treatment involves antibiotics and fluids.

- *Renal calculi.* These are kidney (*renal*) stones (*calculi*). Bedrest, immobility, and poor fluid intake are risk factors. The person has severe, cramping pain in the back and side just below the ribs and pain in the abdomen, thigh, and urethra. Nausea, vomiting, fever, chills, and blood in the urine are common. Voiding is painful, frequent, and urgent. Drugs are given for pain relief. The person needs 2000 to 3000 ml of fluid a day. Increased fluids help stones pass through the urine. All urine is strained. Surgical removal of the stone may be necessary. Some dietary changes can prevent stones.
- *Renal failure.* The kidneys do not function or are severely impaired. Waste products are not removed from the blood. The body retains fluid. Heart failure and hypertension easily result. Renal failure may be acute or chronic. The person is very ill.

THE ENDOCRINE SYSTEM

The endocrine system is made up of glands. The endocrine glands secrete hormones that affect other organs and glands. Diabetes is the most common endocrine disorder.

Diabetes

In this disorder the body cannot produce or use insulin properly. Insulin is needed for sugar use. The pancreas secretes insulin. Sugar builds up in the blood. Cells do not have enough sugar for energy and cannot function. There are three types of diabetes:

- *Type 1*—occurs most often in children and young adults. The pancreas produces little or no insulin. Onset is rapid. There is increased thirst and urination, constant hunger, weight loss, blurred vision, and extreme fatigue.
- *Type 2*—occurs in adults. Persons over 40 years of age are at risk. Obesity and hypertension are risk factors. The pancreas secretes insulin. However, the body cannot use it well. Onset is slow. The person has fatigue, nausea, frequent urination, increased thirst, weight loss, and blurred vision. Infections are frequent. Wounds heal slowly.
- *Gestational diabetes*—develops during pregnancy. (Gestation comes from *gestare*. It means *to bear*.) It usually goes away after the baby is born. However, the woman is at risk for type 2 diabetes later in life.

BOX 24-12	Hypoglycemia and Hyperglycemia

Hypoglycemia (Low blood sugar)
   Causes: Too much insulin or diabetic drugs, omitting a meal, delayed meal, eating too little food, increased exercise, vomiting
   Signs and Symptoms: Hunger, weakness, trembling and shakiness, sweating, headache, dizziness, faintness, rapid pulse, low blood pressure, rapid and shallow respirations, clumsy or jerky movements, tingling around the mouth, confusion, changes in vision, cold and clammy skin, convulsions, unconsciousness

Hyperglycemia (High blood sugar)
   Causes: Undiagnosed diabetes, not enough insulin or diabetic drugs, eating too much food, too little exercise, physical or emotional stress
   Signs and symptoms: Weakness; drowsiness; thirst; very dry mouth; hunger; frequent urination; leg cramps; flushed face; sweet breath odor; slow, deep, and labored respirations; rapid, weak pulse; low blood pressure; dry skin; blurred vision; headache; nausea and vomiting; convulsions; coma

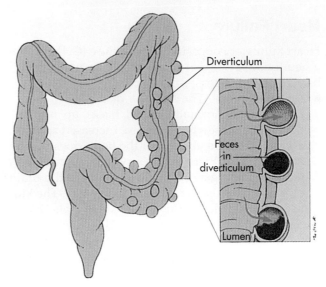

FIG. **24-24** Diverticulosis. (From Christensen BL, Kockrow EO: *Adult health nursing,* ed 4, St Louis, 2003, Mosby.)

Diabetes must be controlled to prevent complications. They include blindness, renal failure, nerve damage, hypertension, and circulatory disorders. Circulatory disorders can lead to stroke, heart attack, and slow healing. Foot and leg wounds are very serious. Infection and gangrene can occur. Sometimes amputation is needed.

Risk factors include a family history of the disease. For type 1, whites are at greater risk than nonwhites. Type 2 is more common in older and overweight persons.

Type 1 is treated with daily insulin therapy, healthy eating (Chapter 17), and exercise. Type 2 is treated with healthy eating and exercise. Many persons with type 2 take oral drugs. Some need insulin. Overweight persons need to lose weight.

Both types require blood glucose monitoring. Good foot care is needed. Corns, blisters, and calluses can lead to an infection and amputation.

The person's blood sugar level can fall too low or go too high:

- *Hypoglycemia* means low *(hypo)* sugar *(glyc)* in the blood *(emia).*
- *Hyperglycemia* means high *(hyper)* sugar *(glyc)* in the blood *(emia).*

See Box 24-12 for their causes, signs, and symptoms. Both can lead to death if not corrected. You must call for the nurse at once.

DIGESTIVE DISORDERS

The digestive system breaks down food so the body can absorb it. Solid wastes are eliminated. Diarrhea, constipation, flatulence, and fecal incontinence are discussed in Chapter 16. So is care of persons with colostomies and ileostomies.

Diverticular Disease

Many people have small pouches in their colons (Fig. 24-24). Each pouch is called a *diverticulum. (Diverticulare* means *to turn inside out.)* The condition of having these pouches is called *diverticulosis. (Osis* means *condition of.)* The pouches can become infected or inflamed. This is called *diverticulitis. (Itis* means *inflammation.)* It is common in older persons. A low-fiber diet and constipation also are risk factors.

When feces enter the pouches, they can become inflamed and infected. The person has abdominal pain and tenderness in the lower left abdomen. Fever, nausea and vomiting, chills, cramping, and constipation are likely. Bloating, rectal bleeding, frequent urination, and pain while voiding can occur.

The doctor orders needed dietary changes. Sometimes antibiotics are ordered. Surgery is needed for severe disease, obstruction, and ruptured pouches. The diseased part of the bowel is removed. Sometimes a colostomy is necessary (Chapter 16).

Vomiting

Vomiting means expelling stomach contents through the mouth. It signals illness or injury. Aspirated vomitus can obstruct the airway. Vomiting large amounts of blood can lead to shock. These measures are needed:

■ Follow Standard Precautions and the Bloodborne Pathogen Standard.
■ Turn the person's head well to one side. This prevents aspiration.
■ Place a kidney basin under the person's chin.
■ Move vomitus away from the person.
■ Provide oral hygiene. This helps remove the bitter taste of vomitus.
■ Observe vomitus for color, odor, and undigested food. If it looks like coffee grounds, it contains digested blood. This signals bleeding. Report your observations.
■ Measure, report, and record the amount of vomitus. Note the amount on the I&O record.
■ Save a specimen for laboratory study.
■ Dispose of vomitus after the nurse observes it.
■ Provide for comfort. (See the inside of the front book cover.)

COMMUNICABLE DISEASES

Communicable diseases are contagious or infectious diseases. They can be transmitted from one person to another. Standard Precautions and Isolation Precautions are followed. Assist the person with hygiene and hand washing as needed.

Hepatitis

Hepatitis is an inflammation of the liver. It can be mild or cause death. Signs and symptoms are listed in Box 24-13. Treatment involves rest, a healthy diet, fluids, and no alcohol. Recovery takes about 8 weeks. There are five major types of hepatitis:

■ *Hepatitis A* is spread by the fecal-oral route. The virus is ingested when eating or drinking food or water contaminated with feces. It is also ingested when eating or drinking from a vessel contaminated with feces. Causes include poor sanitation, crowded living conditions, poor nutrition, and poor hygiene. Anal sex and IV drug abuse also are causes. Handle bedpans, feces, and rectal thermometers carefully. Good hand washing is needed by everyone, including the person.

BOX 24-13	Signs and Symptoms of Hepatitis

- Loss of appetite and weight loss
- Weakness, fatigue, exhaustion
- Nausea and vomiting
- Fever and chills
- Skin rash and itching
- Dark urine
- Jaundice (yellowish color to the skin and whites of the eyes)
- Light-colored stools
- Diarrhea or constipation
- Headache
- Abdominal pain or discomfort
- Muscle aches

■ *Hepatitis B* is caused by the hepatitis B virus (HBV). It is present in the blood and body fluids (saliva, semen, vaginal secretions) of infected persons. It is spread by contaminated blood products, IV drug use, and sexual contact, especially anal sex.
■ *Hepatitis C* is spread by blood contaminated with the virus. A person may have the virus but no symptoms. Serious liver disease and damage may show up years later. Even without symptoms, the person can transmit the disease. The virus is spread by:
  □ Contaminated blood products
  □ IV drug use; inhaling cocaine through contaminated straws
  □ Contaminated needles used for tattooing and body piercing
  □ High-risk sexual activity
■ *Hepatitis D* occurs in persons infected with the hepatitis B virus (HBV). It is spread the same way as HBV.
■ *Hepatitis E* occurs in countries with contaminated water supplies. It is spread by the fecal-oral route.

Acquired Immunodeficiency Syndrome

Acquired immunodeficiency syndrome (AIDS) is caused by a virus. The virus is called the *human immunodeficiency virus (HIV)*. It attacks the immune system. The ability to fight other diseases is affected. Many new drugs help reduce complications and prolong life. AIDS has no vaccine and no cure at present. It is a life-threatening disease.

BOX 24-14	Signs and Symptoms of AIDS

- Loss of appetite
- Weight loss
- Fever
- Headache
- Night sweats
- Diarrhea
- Painful or difficulty swallowing
- Tiredness, extreme or constant
- Skin rashes
- Swollen glands in the neck, underarms, and groin
- Cough
- Shortness of breath
- Sores or white patches in the mouth or on the tongue
- Purple blotches or bumps on the skin that look like bruises but do not disappear
- Blurred vision
- Confusion
- Forgetfulness
- Dementia (Chapter 25)

BOX 24-15	Caring For the Person With AIDS

- Practice Standard Precautions.
- Follow the Bloodborne Pathogen Standard.
- Provide daily hygiene. Avoid irritating soaps.
- Provide oral hygiene before meals and at bedtime. A toothbrush with soft bristles is best.
- Provide oral fluids as ordered.
- Measure and record intake and output.
- Measure weight daily.
- Encourage deep-breathing and coughing exercises as ordered.
- Prevent pressure ulcers.
- Assist with range-of-motion exercises and ambulation as ordered.
- Encourage self-care as able. The person may need assistive devices (walker, commode, eating devices).
- Encourage the person to be as active as possible.
- Change linens and garments as often as needed when fever is present.
- Be a good listener. Provide emotional support.

The virus is spread through body fluids—blood, semen, vaginal secretions, and breast milk. HIV is not spread by saliva, tears, sweat, sneezing, coughing, insects, or casual contact. The virus is transmitted mainly by:

- Unprotected anal, vaginal, or oral sex with an infected person ("Unprotected" is without a new latex or polyurethane condom.)
- Needle and syringe sharing among IV drug users
- HIV-infected mothers before or during childbirth and through breast-feeding

Box 24-14 lists the signs and symptoms of AIDS. Some persons infected with HIV are symptom free for 8 to 10 years. However, they carry the virus. They can spread it to others.

Persons with AIDS are at risk for pneumonia, TB, and Kaposi's sarcoma (a cancer). Memory loss, loss of coordination, paralysis, mental health disorders, and dementia may occur.

You may care for persons with AIDS or those who are HIV carriers (Box 24-15). Protect yourself and others from the virus. Follow Standard Precautions and the Bloodborne Pathogen Standard. In some persons, HIV or AIDS is not yet diagnosed.

Persons age 50 years and older also get AIDS. They get and spread HIV through sexual contact and IV drug use. Aging and other diseases can mask the signs and symptoms of AIDS. Often the person dies without the disease being diagnosed.

Sexually Transmitted Diseases

Sexually transmitted diseases (STDs) are spread by oral, vaginal, or anal sex. Some people do not have signs and symptoms or are not aware of an infection. Others know but do not seek treatment because of embarrassment.

STDs often occur in the genital and rectal areas. They also occur in the ears, mouth, nipples, throat, tongue, eyes, and nose. Using condoms helps prevent the spread of STDs, especially HIV and AIDS. Some STDs are also spread through skin breaks, by contact with infected body fluids (blood, semen, saliva), or by contaminated blood or needles.

Standard Precautions and the Bloodborne Pathogen Standard are also followed.

MENTAL HEALTH DISORDERS

Mental relates to the mind. Therefore mental health involves the mind. Mental health and mental illness involve stress. *Stress* is the response or change in the body caused by any emotional, physical, social, or economic factor.

- *Mental health* means that the person copes with and adjusts to everyday stresses in ways accepted by society.
- *Mental illness* is a disturbance in the ability to cope with or adjust to stress. Behavior and function are impaired.

Mental health disorders have many causes. Sometimes a person cannot cope or adjust to stress. Chemical imbalances and genetics are other causes. So are drug or substance abuse. Social and cultural factors also can lead to mental illness.

Anxiety Disorders

Anxiety is a vague, uneasy feeling in response to stress. The person senses danger or harm—real or imagined. The person acts to relieve the unpleasant feeling. Often anxiety occurs when needs are not met.

Some anxiety is normal. Persons with mental health problems have higher levels of anxiety. Signs and symptoms depend on the degree of anxiety (Box 24-16).

Coping and defense mechanisms relieve anxiety. Some are healthy. Others are not. Coping mechanisms include eating, drinking, smoking, exercising, fighting, and talking about the problem. Some people play music, go for a walk, take a hot bath, or want to be alone.

Defense mechanisms are unconscious reactions that block unpleasant or threatening feelings (Box 24-17). Some use of defense mechanisms is normal. With mental health problems, they are used poorly.

Some common anxiety disorders are:

- *Panic disorder*—Panic is an intense and sudden feeling of fear, anxiety, terror, or dread. Onset is sudden with no obvious reason. The person cannot function. Signs and symptoms of anxiety are severe. *Panic attacks* can last for a few minutes or for hours.
- *Phobias*—Phobia means fear, panic, or dread. The person has an intense fear of an object, situation, or activity.
- *Obsessive-compulsive disorder*—An *obsession* is a recurrent, unwanted thought or idea. *Compulsion* is repeating an act over and over again (a ritual). The act may not make sense, but the person has much anxiety if the act is not done.

BOX 24-16	**Signs and Symptoms of Anxiety**

- A "lump" in the throat
- "Butterflies" in the stomach
- Rapid pulse and respirations; increased blood pressure
- Rapid speech and voice changes
- Dry mouth
- Sweating
- Nausea and diarrhea
- Urinary frequency and urgency
- Poor attention span; difficulty following directions
- Difficulty sleeping
- Loss of appetite

BOX 24-17	**Defense Mechanisms**

Compensation. *Compensate* means to make up for, replace, or substitute. The person makes up for or substitutes a strength for a weakness.

EXAMPLE: A boy is not good in sports. But he learns to play music.

Conversion. *Convert* means to change. An emotion is shown or changed into a physical symptom.

EXAMPLE: A girl does not want to read out loud in school. She complains of a headache.

Denial. *Deny* means refusing to accept or believe something that is true. The person refuses to face or accept unpleasant or threatening things.

EXAMPLE: A man had a heart attack. He continues to smoke after being told to quit.

Displacement. *Displace* means to move or take the place of. An individual moves behaviors or emotions from one person, place, or thing to a safe person, place, or thing.

EXAMPLE: You are angry with your boss. You yell at a friend.

Projection. *Project* means to blame another. An individual blames another person or object for unacceptable behaviors, emotions, ideas, or wishes.

EXAMPLE: A girl fails a test. She blames a friend for not helping her study.

Rationalization. *Rational* means sensible, reasonable, or logical. An acceptable reason or excuse is given for one's behavior or actions. The real reason is not given.

EXAMPLE: A man is often late for work. He did not get a raise. He says that the boss does not like him.

Regression. *Regress* means to move back or to retreat. The person retreats or moves back to an earlier time or condition.

EXAMPLE: A 3-year-old wants a baby bottle when a new baby comes into the family.

Repression. *Repress* means to hold down or keep back. The person keeps unpleasant or painful thoughts or experiences from the conscious mind. They cannot be recalled or remembered.

EXAMPLE: A child was sexually abused. Now 33 years old, she has no memory of the event.

Schizophrenia

Schizophrenia means split *(schizo)* mind *(phrenia)*. It is a severe, chronic, disabling brain disease. It involves:

- *Psychosis*—a state of severe mental impairment. The person does not view the real or unreal correctly.
- *Delusion*—a false belief. For example, a person believes he is God. Or a person believes she is a movie star.
- *Hallucination*—seeing, hearing, or feeling something that is not real. A person may see animals, insects, or people that are not real.
- *Paranoia*—a disorder *(para)* of the mind *(noia)*. The person has false beliefs (delusions). He or she is suspicious about a person or situation. For example, a woman believes her food is poisoned.
- *Delusion of grandeur*—an exaggerated belief about one's importance, wealth, power, or talents. For example, a man believes he is Superman. Or a woman believes she is the Queen of England.
- *Delusion of persecution*—the false belief that one is being mistreated, abused, or harassed. For example, a person believes that someone is "out to get" him or her.

Thinking and behavior are disturbed. The person has delusions and hallucinations. The person has problems relating to others. He or she may be paranoid. Responses are inappropriate. Communication is disturbed. The person may withdraw. The person may sit for hours alone without moving, speaking, or responding. Some persons regress (see Box 24-17). An adult may act like an infant or child.

Affective Disorders

Affect relates to feelings and emotions. Affective disorders involve feelings, emotions, and moods.

Bipolar Disorder

Bipolar means two *(bi)* poles or ends *(polar)*. The person has severe extremes in mood, energy, and ability to function. There are emotional lows *(depression)* and emotional highs *(mania)*. The disorder also is called manic-depressive illness.

The disorder tends to run in families. When depressed, the person is very sad and feels hopeless, helpless, and worthless. Self-esteem is low. Suicide is a risk. During mania, the person is excited, has much energy, and is very busy. Little sleep is needed. The person jumps from one idea to another. Delusions of grandeur are common.

Major Depression

Depression involves the body, mood, and thoughts. The person is very sad. He or she loses interest in daily activities. Body functions are depressed.

BOX 24-18	Signs and Symptoms of Depression in Older Persons

- Fatigue and lack of interest
- Inability to experience pleasure
- Feelings of uselessness, hopelessness, and helplessness
- Decreased sexual interest
- Increased dependency
- Anxiety
- Slow or unreliable memory
- Paranoia
- Agitation
- Focus on the past
- Thoughts of death and suicide
- Difficulty completing activities of daily living
- Changes in sleep patterns
- Poor grooming
- Withdrawal from people and interests
- Muscle aches, abdominal pain, and headaches
- Nausea and vomiting
- Dry mouth

From Lueckenotte AG: *Gerontologic nursing*, ed 2, St Louis, 2002, Mosby.

Depression is common in older persons. They have many losses—death of family and friends, loss of health, loss of body functions, loss of independence. Loneliness and the side effects of some drugs also are causes. See Box 24-18 for the signs and symptoms of depression in older persons. Often the person is thought to have a cognitive disorder (Chapter 25). Therefore the depression often is untreated.

Personality Disorders

Personality disorders involve rigid and maladaptive behaviors. To *adapt* means to change or adjust. *Mal* means bad, wrong, or ill. *Maladaptive* means to change or adjust in the wrong way. Because of their behaviors, those with personality disorders cannot function well in society. Personality disorders include:

- *Abusive personality.* The person copes with anxiety by abusing others. Behavior may be violent.
- *Paranoid personality.* The person is very suspicious. There is distrust of others.
- *Antisocial personality.* The person has poor judgment. He or she lacks responsibility and is hostile. Morals and ethics are lacking. Others are blamed for actions and behaviors. The person has no guilt. He or she does not learn from experiences or punishment. The person is often in trouble with the police.

Care and Treatment

Treatment of mental health problems involves having the person explore thoughts and feelings. This is done through psychotherapy and group, occupational, art, and family therapies. Often drugs are ordered.

The RN uses the nursing process to meet the person's needs. The needs of the total person must be met. This includes physical, safety and security, and emotional needs.

Communication is important. Be alert to the person's nonverbal communication and your own.

FOCUS ON THE PERSON

A person may have one or more health problems. The care you give affects the person's quality of life. See *Focus on the Person: Caring for Persons With Common Health Problems.*

Focus on the PERSON

Caring For Persons With Common Health Problems

Providing comfort—Comfort needs depend on the disorder. Some persons have little or no pain or discomfort. Others have severe pain. To provide comfort, follow the care plan and the measures listed on the inside of the front book cover.

Ethical behavior—Some disorders, accidents, and injuries result from life-style choices. Poor diet, lack of exercise, and alcohol and drug abuse are examples. Whatever the cause or contributing factors, do not judge the person or the person's actions. Always treat the person with dignity and respect.

Remaining independent—Many people require rehabilitation after illness, injury, or surgery. The goal is for the person to function at his or her highest possible level. Follow the rehabilitation plan (Chapter 23).

Speaking up—Only the common health problems were presented in this chapter. And only basic information was given. You may want to know more about a health problem. Or a person may have a disorder not discussed in this chapter. Ask the nurse to explain the problem and the care required. Also look up the problem in a medical dictionary.

OBRA and other laws—You must protect the person's privacy and confidentiality. This is required by OBRA and the Health Insurance Portability and Accountability Act of 1996 (HIPAA). HIPAA is described in Chapter 2.

A patient or resident may be your family member or friend. If you are not involved in that person's care, you have no right to information about that person. Or friends or family members may ask you about patients and residents whom they know. You cannot share information with them. Simply say: "I'm sorry. I cannot tell you. That would be unprofessional, illegal, and unethical conduct."

Nursing teamwork—A person's condition can change very quickly. A person with angina pectoris may have a myocardial infarction. A person with hypertension may have a stroke. A person may develop complications after surgery. Sudden changes in a person's condition require the nurse's attention. You need to help as the nurse directs. You may need to assist the nurse. Or you may need to help with other patients or residents. Always help willingly. The entire nursing team may need to make that "extra effort" to meet patient and resident needs.

REVIEW QUESTIONS

Circle the **BEST** answer.

1 Which is *not* a warning sign of cancer?
   a Painful, swollen joints
   b A sore that does not heal
   c Unusual bleeding or discharge
   d Discomfort after eating

2 A person has arthritis. Care includes the following *except*
   a Preventing contractures
   b Range-of-motion exercises
   c A cast or traction
   d Assisting with ADL

3 After a hip pinning, the operated leg is
   a Abducted at all times
   b Adducted at all times
   c Externally rotated at all times
   d Flexed at all times

4 A person with osteoporosis is at risk for
   a Fractures
   b An amputation
   c Phantom limb pain
   d Paralysis

5 A person had a stroke. Which measure should you question?
   a Semi-Fowler's position
   b Range-of-motion exercises every 2 hours
   c Turn, reposition, and give skin care every 2 hours
   d Bed in the highest horizontal position

6 Receptive aphasia means that the person has trouble
   a Talking
   b Writing
   c Understanding messages
   d Using gestures

7 A person has Parkinson's disease. Which is *false?*
   a Part of the brain is affected.
   b Mental function is affected first.
   c Stiff muscles, slow movements, and a shuffling gait occur.
   d The person is protected from injury.

8 A person has hearing loss. You should do the following *except*
   a Speak clearly, distinctly, and slowly
   b Sit or stand where there is good light
   c Shout
   d Stand or sit on the side of the better ear

9 A hearing aid
   a Corrects the hearing problem
   b Makes sounds louder
   c Makes speech clearer
   d Lowers background noise

10 A hearing aid does not seem to be working. First, you should
   a See if it is turned on
   b Wash it with soap and water
   c Have it repaired
   d Remove the batteries

11 When eyeglasses are not being worn, they should be
   a Soaked in a cleansing solution
   b Kept within the person's reach
   c Put in the case and in the bedside stand
   d Placed on the overbed table

12 A person is blind. You should do the following *except*
   a Identify yourself
   b Move equipment and furniture to provide variety
   c Explain procedures step-by-step
   d Have the person walk behind you

13 A person has emphysema. Which is *false?*
   a The person has dyspnea only with activity.
   b Smoking is the most common cause.
   c Breathing is usually easier sitting upright and slightly forward.
   d Sputum may contain pus.

14 A person has hypertension. Treatment will likely include the following *except*
   a No smoking and regular exercise
   b A high-sodium diet
   c A low-calorie diet if the person is obese
   d Drugs to lower the blood pressure

15 A person has angina pectoris. Which is *true?*
   a Damage to the heart muscle occurs.
   b The pain is described as crushing, stabbing, or squeezing.
   c The pain is relieved with rest and nitroglycerin.
   d The pain is always on the left side of the chest.

Review Questions

16 A person is having a myocardial infarction. Which is *false*?
  a The person is having a heart attack.
  b This is an emergency.
  c The person may have a cardiac arrest.
  d The person does not have enough blood to supply the body with needed oxygen.

17 A person has heart failure. Which measure should you question?
  a Encourage fluids
  b Measure intake and output
  c Measure weight daily
  d Perform range-of-motion exercises

18 A person has cystitis. This is
  a A kidney infection
  b Kidney stones
  c An ostomy
  d A bladder infection

19 Which is *not* a sign of diabetes?
  a Increased urine production
  b Weight gain
  c Hunger
  d Increased thirst

20 A person with diabetes needs the following *except*
  a Exercise
  b Good foot care
  c A sodium-controlled diet
  d Healthy eating

21 Vomiting is dangerous because of
  a Aspiration
  b Diverticular disease
  c Constipation
  d Stroke

22 AIDS and hepatitis require
  a Sterile gloves
  b Double bagging
  c Standard Precautions
  d Masks, gowns, and goggles

23 AIDS is spread by contact with infected
  a Blood
  b Urine
  c Tears
  d Saliva

24 These statements are about HIV and AIDS. Which is *false*?
  a The Blood Pathogen Standard is followed.
  b The person may have nervous system damage.
  c The person is at risk for infection.
  d The person always shows some signs and symptoms.

25 These statements are about STDs. Which statement is *false*?
  a They are usually spread by sexual contact.
  b They can affect the genital area and other parts of the body.
  c Signs and symptoms are always obvious.
  d Some result in death.

26 Stress is
  a The way a person copes with and adjusts to everyday living
  b A response or change in the body caused by some factor
  c A mental or emotional disorder
  d A thought or idea

27 Defense mechanisms are used to
  a Blame others
  b Make excuses for behavior
  c Return to an earlier time
  d Block unpleasant feelings

28 A phobia is
  a A serious mental health problem
  b A false belief
  c An intense fear of something
  d Feelings and emotions

29 A person cleans and cleans the bathroom. This behavior is:
  a A delusion
  b A hallucination
  c A compulsion
  d An obsession

30 Bipolar disorder means that the person
  a Is very suspicious
  b Has anxiety
  c Is very unhappy and feels unwanted
  d Has severe mood swings

Answers to these questions are on p. 469.

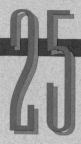

Caring For Persons With Confusion and Dementia

OBJECTIVES

- Define the key terms listed in this chapter
- Describe confusion and its causes
- List the measures that help confused persons
- Explain the difference between delirium, depression, and dementia
- Describe Alzheimer's disease (AD)
- Describe the signs, symptoms, and behaviors of AD
- Explain the care required by persons with AD and other dementias
- Describe the effects of AD on the family

KEY TERMS

delirium A state of temporary but acute mental confusion
delusion A false belief
dementia The loss of cognitive function and social function caused by changes in the brain
hallucination Seeing, hearing, or feeling something that is not real
pseudodementia False *(pseudo)* dementia
sundowning Signs, symptoms, and behaviors of AD increase during hours of darkness

Changes in the brain and nervous system occur with aging (Box 25-1). Certain diseases affect the brain. Changes in the brain can affect cognitive function. (*Cognitive* relates to knowledge.) Quality of life is affected. Cognitive function involves memory, thinking, reasoning, ability to understand, judgment, and behavior.

CONFUSION

Confusion has many causes. Diseases, infections, hearing and vision loss, and drug side effects are some causes. So is brain injury. With aging, there is reduced blood supply to the brain. Brain cells are lost. Personality and mental changes can result. Memory and the ability to make good judgments are lost. A person may not know people, the time, or the place. Some people gradually lose the ability to perform daily activities. Behavior changes are common. The person may be angry, restless, depressed, and irritable.

Acute confusion *(delirium)* occurs suddenly. It is usually temporary. Causes include infection, illness, injury, drugs, and surgery. Treatment is aimed at the cause.

BOX 25-1	**Changes in the Nervous System From Aging**

- Brain cells are lost.
- Nerve conduction slows.
- Response and reaction times are slower.
- Reflexes are slower.
- Vision and hearing decrease.
- Taste and smell decrease.
- Touch and sensitivity to pain decrease.
- Blood flow to the brain is reduced.
- Sleep patterns change.
- Memory is shorter.
- Forgetfulness occurs.
- Dizziness can occur.

Confusion caused by physical changes cannot be cured. Some measures help to improve function (Box 25-2, p. 434). You must meet the person's basic needs.

DEMENTIA

Dementia is the loss of cognitive function and social function. It is caused by changes in the brain. (*De* means from. *Mentia* means mind.) Dementia is not a normal part of aging. Most older people do not have dementia. Some early warning signs include:

- Recent memory loss that affects job skills
- Problems with common tasks (for example, dressing, cooking, driving)
- Problems with language; forgetting simple words
- Getting lost in familiar places
- Misplacing things and putting things in odd places (for example, putting a watch in the oven)
- Personality changes
- Poor or decreased judgment (for example, going outdoors in the snow without shoes)
- Loss of interest in life

Some dementias can be reversed. When the cause is removed, so are the signs and symptoms. Treatable causes include:

- Drugs and alcohol
- Delirium and depression
- Tumors
- Heart, lung, and blood vessel problems
- Head injuries
- Infection
- Vision and hearing problems

Permanent dementias result from changes in the brain. They have no cure. Function declines over time. Parkinson's disease causes changes in the brain. So does cardiovascular disease. Multi-infarct dementia (MID) is caused by many *(multi)* strokes. The stroke leaves an area of damage called an *infarct*. Alzheimer's disease is the most common type of permanent dementia.

Pseudodementia means false *(pseudo)* dementia. The person has the signs and symptoms of dementia. However, there are no changes in the brain. This can occur with delirium and depression.

Delirium and Depression

Delirium and depression can be mistaken for dementia. **Delirium** is a state of temporary but acute mental confusion. Onset is sudden. It is common in older persons with acute or chronic illnesses. Infections, heart and lung diseases, and poor nutrition are common causes. So are hormone disorders. Hypoglycemia is also a cause (Chapter 24). Alcohol and

---

BOX 25-2   **Caring For the Confused Person**

- Follow the person's care plan.
- Provide for safety.
- Face the person. Speak clearly and slowly.
- Call the person by name every time you are in contact with him or her.
- State your name. Show your name tag.
- Give the date and time each morning. Repeat as needed during the day or evening.
- Explain what you are going to do and why.
- Give clear, simple directions and answers to questions.
- Ask clear and simple questions. Give the person time to respond.
- Keep calendars and clocks with large numbers in the person's room and in nursing areas (Fig. 25-1). Remind the person of holidays, birthdays, and special events.
- Have the person wear eyeglasses and hearing aids as needed.
- Use touch to communicate (Chapter 5).
- Place familiar objects and pictures within the person's view.

- Provide newspapers, magazines, TV, and radio. Read to the person if appropriate.
- Discuss current events with the person.
- Maintain the day-night cycle. Open curtains, shades, blinds, and drapes during the day. Close them at night. Use a night-light at night. The person wears regular clothes during the day—not sleepwear.
- Provide a calm, relaxed, and peaceful setting. Prevent loud noises, rushing, and congested hallways and dining rooms.
- Follow the person's routine. Meals, bathing, exercise, TV, and other activities have a schedule. This promotes a sense of order and what to expect.
- Break tasks into small steps when helping the person.
- Do not rearrange furniture or the person's belongings.
- Encourage the person to take part in self-care.
- Be consistent.

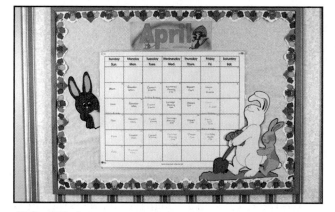

FIG. **25-1** A large calendar can help confused persons.

many drugs can cause delirium. Delirium has a short course. It can last for a few hours to as long as 1 month.

Delirium signals physical illness in older persons and in persons with dementia. It is an emergency. The cause must be found and treated. Signs and symptoms of delirium include:

- Anxiety
- Disorientation
- Tremors
- Hallucinations (p. 436)
- Delusions (p. 436)
- Attention problems
- Decline in level of consciousness
- Memory problems

Depression is the most common mental health problem in older persons. It is often overlooked. Depression, aging, and some drug side effects have similar signs and symptoms. See Chapter 24 for the signs and symptoms of depression in older persons.

ALZHEIMER'S DISEASE

Alzheimer's disease (AD) is a brain disease. Brain cells that control intellectual and social function are damaged. These functions are affected: memory, thinking, reasoning, judgment, language, behavior, mood, and personality.

The person has problems with work and everyday functions. Problems with family and social relationships occur. There is a steady decline in memory and mental function.

The disease is gradual in onset. It gets worse and worse over 3 to 20 years. AD occurs in both men and women. Some people in their 40s and 50s have AD. However, it usually occurs after the age of 65. It is often diagnosed around the age of 80. The cause is unknown. A family history of AD and Down syndrome are risk factors.

Signs of AD

The classic sign of AD is *gradual loss of short-term memory*. See Box 25-3 for the warning signs and other signs of AD.

BOX 25-3	Signs of AD

Warning Signs

- Asking the same question over and over again.
- Repeating the same story—word for word, again and again.
- Forgetting how to cook, or how to make repairs, or how to play cards. The person forgets activities that were once done regularly and with ease.
- Losing the ability to pay bills or balance a checkbook.
- Getting lost in familiar places. Or misplacing household objects.
- Neglecting to bathe. Or wearing the same clothes over and over again. Meanwhile, the person insists that a bath was taken or that clothes are clean.
- Relying on someone else to make decisions or answer questions that he or she would have handled.

Other Signs

- Forgets recent events, conversations, and appointments
- Forgets simple directions
- Forgets names (including family members)
- Forgets the names of everyday things (clock, radio, TV, and so on)
- Forgets words; loses train of thought
- Substitutes unusual words and names for what is forgotten
- Speaks in a native language

- Curses or swears
- Misplaces things; puts things in odd places
- Has problems writing checks
- Gives away large amounts of money
- Does not recognize or understand numbers
- Has problems following conversations
- Has problems reading and writing
- Becomes lost in familiar settings
- Forgets where he or she is
- Does not know how to get back home
- Wanders from home
- Cannot tell or understand time or dates
- Cannot solve everyday problems (iron is left on, stove burners left on, food burning on the stove, and so on)
- Cannot perform everyday tasks (dressing, bathing, brushing teeth, and so on)
- Distrusts others
- Is stubborn
- Withdraws socially
- Is restless
- Becomes suspicious
- Becomes fearful
- Does not want to do things
- Sleeps more than usual

Warning signs from The Alzheimer's Disease Education and Referral Center (ADEAR), a service of the National Institute on Aging, *The Seven Warning Signs of Alzheimer's Disease, http://www.alzheimers.org/pubs/sevensigns.htm.*

Problems with complex tasks appear first. The person has problems using the phone, driving, managing money, planning meals, and working. Over time, problems occur with simple tasks. These include bathing, dressing, eating, using the toilet, and walking.

Stages of AD

AD is often described in terms of 3 stages (Box 25-4, p. 436). Sometimes it is described as having seven stages:

- No cognitive decline
- Very mild cognitive decline
- Mild cognitive decline
- Moderate cognitive decline
- Moderately severe cognitive decline
- Severe cognitive decline
- Very severe cognitive decline

Signs and symptoms become more severe with each stage. The disease ends in death.

Behaviors

The following behaviors are common with AD.

Wandering

Persons with AD are not oriented to person, time, and place. They may wander away and not find their way back. Wandering may be by foot, car, bicycle, or other means. They may be with you one moment and gone the next.

Judgment is poor. They cannot tell what is safe or dangerous. Life-threatening accidents are great risks. They can walk into traffic or into a nearby river, lake, ocean, or forest. If not properly dressed, heat or cold exposure is a risk.

Wandering may have no cause. Or the person may be looking for something or someone—the bathroom, the bedroom, a child, or a partner. Pain, drug side effects, stress, restlessness, and anxiety are possible causes. Sometimes finding the cause prevents wandering.

For persons living at home, the Alzheimer's Association has a Safe Return Program. The program is nationwide. It serves to identify and safely return persons who wander or become lost. A small fee is charged. A family member completes a form and provides a picture. These are entered into a national database. The person receives an ID (wallet card,

---

BOX 25-4   Stages of Alzheimer's Disease

Stage 1: Mild

- Memory loss—forgetfulness; forgets recent events
- Problems finding words, finishing thoughts, following directions, and remembering names
- Poor judgment; bad decisions (including when driving)
- Disoriented to time and place
- Lack of spontaneity—less outgoing or interested in things
- Blames others for mistakes, forgetfulness, and other problems
- Moodiness
- Problems performing every day tasks

Stage 2: Moderate

- Restlessness—increases during the evening hours
- Sleep problems
- Memory loss increases—may not know family and friends
- Dulled senses—cannot tell the difference between hot and cold; cannot recognize dangers
- Fecal and urinary incontinence
- Needs help with activities of daily living (ADL)—bathing, feeding, and dressing self; afraid of bathing; will not change clothes
- Loses impulse control—foul language, poor table manners, sexual aggression, rudeness

- Movement and gait problems—walks slowly, has a shuffling gait
- Communication problems—cannot follow directions; problems with reading, writing, and math; speaks in short sentences or single words; statements may not make sense
- Repeats motions and statements—moves things back and forth constantly; says the same thing over and over again
- Agitation—behavior may be violent

Stage 3: Severe

- Seizures (Chapter 26)
- Cannot speak—may groan, grunt, or scream
- Does not recognize self or family members
- Depends totally on others for all activities of daily living
- Disoriented to person, time, and place
- Totally incontinent of urine and feces
- Cannot swallow—choking and aspiration are risks
- Sleep problems increase
- Becomes bed bound—cannot sit or walk
- Coma
- Death

---

bracelet or necklace, clothing labels). Anyone finding a person can call the Safe Return number on the ID. Safe Return then calls the family member or caregiver. Some persons are reported missing. Safe Return can provide the person's information and photo to the police.

Sundowning

With **sundowning,** signs, symptoms, and behaviors of AD increase during hours of darkness. It occurs in the late afternoon and evening hours. As daylight ends and darkness starts, confusion and restlessness increase. So do anxiety, agitation, and other symptoms. Behavior is worse after the sun goes down. It may continue throughout the night.

Sundowning may relate to being tired or hungry. Poor light and shadows may cause the person to see things that are not there. Persons with AD may be afraid of the dark.

Hallucinations

A **hallucination** is seeing, hearing, or feeling something that is not real. Senses are dulled. Affected persons see animals, insects, or people that are not present. Some hear voices. They may feel bugs crawling or feel that they are being touched.

Sometimes the problem is caused by impaired vision or hearing. The person needs to wear eyeglasses and hearing aids as prescribed.

Delusions

Delusions are false beliefs. People with AD may think they are some other person. Some believe they are in jail, are being killed, or are being attacked. A person may believe that the caregiver is someone else. Many other false beliefs can occur.

Catastrophic Reactions

These are extreme responses. The person reacts as if there is a disaster or tragedy. The person may scream, cry, or be agitated or combative. These reactions are common from too many stimuli. Eating, music or TV playing, and being asked questions all at once can overwhelm the person.

Agitation and Restlessness

The person may pace, hit, or yell. Common causes are pain or discomfort, anxiety, lack of sleep, and too many or too few stimuli. Hunger and the need to eliminate also are causes. A calm, quiet setting helps calm the person. So does meeting basic needs.

Caregivers can cause these behaviors. A caregiver may rush the person or be impatient. Or mixed verbal and nonverbal messages are sent. Caregivers always need to look at how their behaviors affect other persons.

Aggression and Combativeness

These behaviors include hitting, pinching, grabbing, biting, or swearing. They may result from agitation and restlessness. They frighten others.

Sometimes these behaviors are part of the individual's personality. Or pain, fatigue, too much stimulation, caregiver stress, and feeling lost or abandoned are causes. The behaviors can occur during care measures (bathing, dressing) that upset or frighten the person. See Chapter 5 for dealing with the angry person. See Chapter 8 for workplace violence. Also follow the person's care plan.

Screaming

Persons with AD have communication problems. At first, it is hard to find the right words. As AD progresses, the person speaks in short sentences or in words. Often speech is not understandable.

The person screams to communicate. It is common in persons who are very confused and have poor communication skills. The person may scream a word or a name. Or the person just makes screaming sounds.

Possible causes include hearing and vision problems, pain or discomfort, fear, and fatigue. Too much or not enough stimulation is another cause. The person may react to a caregiver or family member by screaming.

Sometimes these measures are helpful:

- Providing a calm, quiet setting
- Playing soft music
- Having the person wear hearing aids and eyeglasses
- Having a family member or favorite caregiver comfort and calm the person
- Using touch to calm the person

Abnormal Sexual Behaviors

Sexual behaviors are labeled abnormal because of how and when they occur. Persons with AD are not oriented to person, time, and place. Sexual behaviors may involve the wrong person, the wrong place, and the wrong time. They also cannot control behavior. Healthy persons do not undress or expose themselves in front of others. They do not masturbate or engage in sexual pleasures in public. They know their sexual partners. Persons with AD often mistake someone else for a sexual partner. The person kisses and hugs the other person.

Some behaviors are not sexual. Touching, scratching, and rubbing the genitals can signal infection, pain, or discomfort in the urinary or reproductive systems. Poor hygiene is another cause. So is being wet or soiled from urine or feces.

The nurse encourages the person's sexual partner to show affection. Their normal practices are encouraged. Examples include hand holding, hugging, kissing, and touching. When a person masturbates in public, lead the person to his or her room. Provide for privacy and safety. Good hygiene prevents itching. Clean the person quickly and thoroughly after elimination. Do not let the person stay wet or soiled.

The RN assesses the person for urinary or reproductive system problems. The doctor is contacted as necessary.

Repetitive Behaviors

Repetitive means to repeat over and over again. Persons with AD repeat the same motions over and over again. For example, the person folds the same napkin over and over. Or the person says the same words over and over. Or the same question is asked. Such behaviors do not harm the person. However, they can annoy caregivers and the family.

Harmless acts are allowed. Music, picture books, exercise, and movies are distracting. Taking the person for a walk can help. Such measures also help when words or questions are repeated.

CARE OF PERSONS WITH AD AND OTHER DEMENTIAS

Usually the person is cared for at home until symptoms are severe. Adult day care may help. Often nursing center care is required. Sometimes hospital care is needed for other illnesses. You may care for persons with AD or other dementias in any of these settings. The person and family need your support and understanding.

People with AD do not choose to be forgetful, incontinent, agitated, or rude. Nor do they choose to have other behaviors, signs, and symptoms of the disease. They cannot control what is happening to them. The disease causes the behaviors. *The disease is responsible, not the person.*

Currently AD has no cure. Symptoms worsen over many years. The rate varies from person to person. Over time, persons with AD depend on others for care. Safety, hygiene, nutrition and fluids, elimination, and activity needs must be met. So must comfort and sleep needs. The person's care plan will include many of the measures listed in Box 25-5 on p. 438.

Comfort and safety are important. Good skin care and alignment prevent skin breakdown and contractures. You must take special care to treat these persons with dignity and respect. They have the same rights as persons who are alert and active. Talk to them in a calm voice. Always explain what you are going to do. Massage, soothing touch, music, and aromatherapy are comforting and relaxing. The person may need hospice care as death nears (Chapter 27).

Text continued on p. 440

BOX 25-5	**Care of Persons With AD and Other Dementias**

Environment

- Follow established routines.
- Avoid changing rooms or roommates.
- Place picture signs on rooms, bathrooms, dining rooms, and other areas (Fig. 25-2).
- Keep personal items where the person can see them.
- Stay within the person's sight to the extent possible.
- Place memory aids (large clocks and calendars) where the person can see them.
- Keep noise levels low.
- Play music and show movies from the person's past.
- Select tasks and activities specific to the person's cognitive abilities and interests.

Communication

- Approach the person in a calm, quiet manner.
- Approach the person from the front. Do not approach the person from the side or the back. This can startle the person.
- Call the person by name.
- Identify other people by their names. Avoid pronouns (he, she, them, and so on).
- Follow the rules of communication (Chapters 4 and 5).
- Practice measures to promote communication (Chapter 5).
- Use gestures or cues. Point to objects.
- Speak in a calm, gentle voice.
- Speak slowly. Use simple words and sentences.
- Let the person speak. Do not interrupt or rush the person.
- Give the person time to respond.
- Do not criticize, correct, or argue with the person.
- Present one idea, question, or instruction at a time.
- Ask simple questions having simple answers. Do not ask complex questions.
- Do not present the person with many choices.
- Provide simple explanations of all procedures and activities.
- Give consistent responses.

Safety

- Remove harmful, sharp, and breakable objects from the area. This includes knives, scissors, glass, dishes, razors, and tools.
- Provide plastic eating and drinking utensils. This helps prevent breakage and cuts.
- Place safety plugs in electric outlets.
- Keep cords and electric equipment out of reach.
- Remove electric appliances from the bathroom. Examples include hair dryers, curling irons, make-up mirrors, and electric shavers.
- Store personal care items (shampoo, deodorant, lotion, and so on) in a safe place.
- Keep childproof caps on medicine containers and household cleaners.
- Store household cleaners and drugs in locked storage areas.
- Store dangerous equipment and tools in a safe place.
- Remove knobs from stoves or place childproof covers on the knobs.

- Remove dangerous appliances and power tools from the home.
- Remove firearms from the home.
- Store car keys in a safe place.
- Supervise the person who smokes.
- Store cigarettes, cigars, pipes, matches, and other smoking materials in a safe place.
- Practice safety measures to prevent falls (Chapter 8).
- Practice safety measures to prevent fires (Chapter 8).
- Practice safety measures to prevent burns (Chapter 8).
- Practice safety measures to prevent poisoning (Chapter 8).
- Keep all doors to kitchens, utility rooms, and housekeeping closets locked.

Wandering

- Follow agency policy for locking doors and windows. Locks are often placed at the top and bottom of doors (Fig. 25-3, p. 440). The person is not likely to look for a lock in such places.
- Keep door alarms and electronic doors turned on. The alarm goes off when the door is opened. Respond to door alarms at once.
- Follow agency policy for fire exits. Everyone must be able to leave the building if there is a fire.
- Make sure the person wears an ID bracelet or Safe Return ID at all times.
- Exercise the person as ordered. Adequate exercise often reduces wandering.
- Involve the person in activities—folding napkins, dusting a table, sorting socks, rolling yarn, sweeping, sanding blocks of wood, or watering plants.
- Do not use restraints. Restraints require a doctor's order. They also tend to increase confusion and disorientation.
- Do not argue with the person who wants to leave. The person does not understand what you are saying.
- Go with the person who insists on going outside. Make sure he or she is properly dressed. Guide the person inside after a few minutes (Fig. 25-4, p. 440).
- Let the person wander in enclosed areas. Many nursing centers have enclosed areas where residents can walk about (Fig. 25-5, p. 440). They provide a safe place for the person to wander.

Sundowning

- Complete treatments and activities early in the day.
- Provide a calm, quiet setting late in the day.
- Do not restrain the person.
- Encourage exercise and activity early in the day.
- Meet nutrition needs. Hunger can increase restlessness.
- Promote elimination. The need to eliminate can increase restlessness.
- Do not try to reason with the person. He or she cannot understand what you are saying.
- Do not ask the person to tell you what is bothering him or her. Communication is impaired. The person does not understand what you are asking. He or she cannot think or speak clearly.

BOX 25-5　Care of Persons With AD and Other Dementias—cont'd

Hallucinations and Delusions

- Make sure the person wears eyeglasses and hearing aids as needed. Follow the care plan.
- Do not argue with the person. He or she does not understand what you are saying.
- Reassure the person. Tell him or her that you will provide protection from harm.
- Distract the person with some item or activity. Taking the person for a walk may be helpful.
- Use touch to calm and reassure the person.
- Eliminate noises that the person could misinterpret. TV, radio, stereos, furnaces, air conditioners, and other things could affect the person.
- Check lighting. Make sure there are no glares, shadows, or reflections.
- Cover or remove mirrors. The person could misinterpret his or her reflection.

Sleep

- Follow bedtime rituals.
- Use night-lights so the person can see. They help prevent accidents and disorientation.
- Limit caffeine during the day.
- Discourage naps during the day.
- Encourage exercise during the day.
- Reduce noises.

Basic Needs

- Meet food and fluid needs (Chapter 17). Provide finger foods. Cut food and pour liquids as needed.
- Provide good skin care (Chapters 13 and 21). Keep the person's skin free of urine and feces.
- Promote urinary and bowel elimination (Chapters 15 and 16).
- Provide incontinence care as needed (Chapters 15 and 16).

- Promote exercise and activity during the day (Chapter 20). This helps reduce wandering and sundowning behaviors. The person may also sleep better.
- Reduce intake of coffee, tea, and cola drinks. These contain caffeine. Caffeine is a stimulant. It can increase restlessness, confusion, and agitation.
- Provide a quiet, restful setting. Soft music is better than loud TV programs.
- Play music during care activities, such as bathing and during meals.
- Promote personal hygiene (Chapter 13). Do not force the person into a shower or tub. People with AD are often afraid of bathing. Try bathing the person when he or she is calm. Use the person's preferred bathing method (tub bath, shower, bed bath). Provide privacy and keep the person warm. Do not rush the person.
- Provide oral hygiene (Chapter 13).
- Choose clothing that is comfortable and simple to put on. Front opening garments are easy to put on. Pullover tops are harder to put on. And the person may become frightened when his or her head is inside the pullover top.
- Select clothing that closes with Velcro. Such items are easy to put on and take off. Buttons, zippers, snaps, and other closures can frustrate the person.
- Offer simple clothing choices (Fig. 25-6, p. 440). Let the person choose between two shirts or two blouses, two pants or two slacks, and so on.
- Lay clothing out in the order it will be put on. Hand the person one clothing item at a time. Tell or show the person what to do. Do not rush him or her.
- Have equipment ready for any procedure. This reduces the amount of time the person is involved in care measures.
- Observe for signs and symptoms of health problems (Chapter 4).
- Prevent infection (Chapter 10).

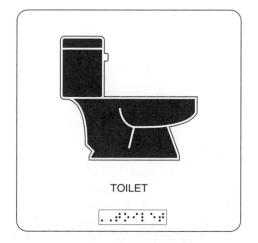

TOILET

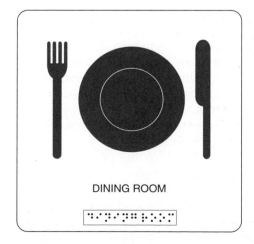

DINING ROOM

FIG. **25-2** Signs give cues to persons with dementia.

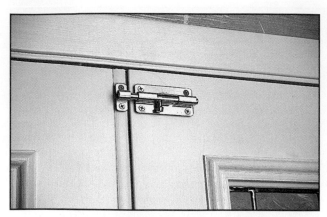

FIG. **25-3** A slide lock is at the top of the door.

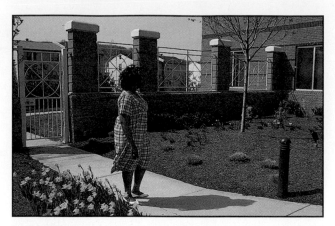

FIG. **25-5** An enclosed garden allows persons with AD to wander in a safe setting.

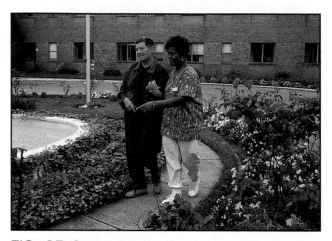

FIG. **25-4** Walk outside with the person who wanders. Then guide the person back inside after a few minutes.

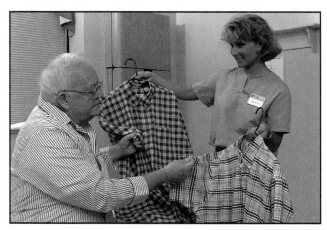

FIG. **25-6** The person with AD is offered simple clothing choices.

The person can have other health problems and injuries. However, the person may not know there is pain, fever, constipation, incontinence, or other signs and symptoms. Carefully observe the person. Report any change in the person's usual behavior to the nurse.

Infection is a major risk. The person cannot fully tend to self-care. Infection can occur from poor hygiene. This includes poor skin care, oral hygiene, and perineal care after bowel and bladder elimination. Inactivity and immobility can cause pneumonia and pressure ulcers.

The person needs to feel useful, worthwhile, and active. This promotes self-esteem. Therapists work with one person, a small group, or a large group. Therapies and activities focus on the person's strengths and past successes. For example:

- A woman used to cook. She helps clean fruit.
- A man was a good dancer. Activities are planned so he can dance.
- A man likes to clean. He helps with dusting.

Supervised activities meet the person's needs and cognitive abilities. The person's interests are considered. Activities are based on what the person enjoys and can do. Some people like crafts, exercise, gardening, and listening and moving to music. Others like sing-alongs, reminiscing, and board games. Some like to string beads, fold towels, or roll dough. Massage, range-of-motion exercises, and touch are also important therapies.

Special Care Units

Many nursing centers have special care units for persons with AD and other dementias. Some units are secured. This means that entrances and exits are locked. Persons in these units have a safe setting to move about in. They cannot wander away. Some persons have aggressive behaviors that disrupt or threaten others. They may need a secured unit.

At some point, the secured unit is no longer needed for safe care. For example, the person's condition progresses from stage 2 to stage 3. The person cannot sit or walk. Wandering is not a concern. The person is transferred to another unit.

The Family

The person may live at home or with a partner, children, or other family members. The family gives care Or someone stays with the person. Health care is sought when the family cannot deal with the situation or meet the person's needs. Home health care may help for a while. Adult day care is an option. Long-term care is needed when:

- Family members cannot meet the person's needs
- The person no longer knows the caregiver
- Family members have health problems
- Money problems occur
- The person's behaviors present dangers to self or others

Diagnostic tests, doctor's visits, drugs, and home care are costly. So is long-term care. The person's medical care can drain family finances.

The family has special needs. Caring for the person at home or in a nursing center is stressful. There are physical, emotional, social, and financial stresses. Adult children are in the *sandwich generation.* They are caught between their own children who need attention and an ill parent who needs care. Caring for two families is stressful. Often adult children have jobs too.

Caregivers can suffer from anger, anxiety, depression, and sleeplessness. Some cannot concentrate or are irritable. They can develop health problems. They need to take care of their own health. A healthy diet, exercise, and plenty of rest are needed. Asking for help is important. The caregiver needs to feel free to ask family and friends for help.

Caregivers need much support and encouragement. Many join AD support groups. The groups are sponsored by hospitals, nursing centers, and the Alzheimer's Association. The Alzheimer's Association has chapters in cities and towns across the country. Support groups offer encouragement and advice. People in similar situations share their feelings, anger, frustration, guilt, and other emotions. They also share coping and caregiving ideas.

The family often feels helpless. No matter what is done, the person only gets worse. Much time, money, energy, and emotion are needed to care for the person. Anger and resentment may result. Guilt feelings are common. The family also knows that the person did not choose the disease. They know that the person does not choose to have its signs, symptoms, and behaviors. Sometimes behaviors are embarrassing. The family may be upset and angry that the loved one cannot show love or affection.

The family is an important part of the health team. They help plan the person's care whenever possible. They need to learn how to bathe, feed, dress, and give oral hygiene to the person. They also need to learn how to provide a safe setting. The RN and support group will help the family learn to give necessary care.

Validation Therapy

Validation therapy may be part of the person's care plan. The therapy is based on the following principles:

- All behavior has meaning.
- Development occurs in a sequence, order, and pattern (Chapter 7). Certain tasks must be completed during a stage of development. A stage cannot be skipped. Each stage is the basis for the next stage.
- If a person does not successfully complete a stage of development, unresolved issues and emotions may surface later in life.
- A person may return to the past to resolve such issues and emotions.
- Caregivers need to listen and provide empathy.
- Attempts are not made to correct the person's thoughts or bring the person back to reality. For example:
  - While going from room to room, Mrs. Bell calls for her babies. In reality, her babies died shortly after birth. The caregiver does not tell Mrs. Bell that her babies died after they were born. Instead, the caregiver says: "Tell me about your babies."
  - Mrs. Brown sits all day on a bench by the window. She says that she is at the train station waiting to meet her husband. In reality, her husband was killed during World War II. Buried in England, he never returned home. The caregiver does not remind Mrs. Brown of what happened. Instead, the caregiver encourages Mrs. Brown to talk about her husband.
  - Mr. Garcia was 3 years old when his father died. He holds a ball constantly. He is very upset when anyone tries to remove it from his hand. He calls for his father and repeats "play ball, play ball." The caregiver does not remind Mr. Garcia that he is 80 years old and that his father died many years ago. Instead, the caregiver says, "Tell me about playing ball."

The health team decides if validation therapy might help a person. If so, it will be part of the person's care plan. Proper use of validation therapy requires special training. If the therapy is used in your agency, you will receive the training needed to use it correctly.

QUALITY OF LIFE

Quality of life is important for all persons with confusion and dementia. Nursing center residents have rights under OBRA. They may not know or be able to exercise their rights. However, the family knows the person's rights. They want those rights protected. They want respect and dignity for the loved one.

The person has the right to privacy and confidentiality. Protect the person from exposure. Only those involved in the person's care are present for care and procedures. The person is allowed to visit in private. Space is provided for a private visit. Protect confidentiality. Do not share information about the person's care and condition with others.

Personal choice is important. If able, simple choices are encouraged. For example, a person chooses to wear a dress or slacks. Watching or not watching TV may be a simple choice. The family makes choices if the person cannot. They choose bath times, menus, clothing, activities, and other care.

The person has the right to keep and use personal items. Some items provide comfort. A pillow, blanket, afghan, or sweater may have meaning to the person. The person may not know why or even recognize the item. Still, it is important. Personal items are kept safe. Protect the person's property from loss or damage.

These persons must be kept free from abuse, mistreatment, and neglect. Caring for persons with confusion and dementia is often very frustrating. Some behaviors are hard to deal with. Family and staff can become short-tempered and angry. Protect the person from abuse (Chapter 2). Report any signs of abuse to the nurse at once. Be patient and calm when caring for these persons. Talk with the nurse if you are becoming upset. Sometimes an assignment change is needed for a while.

All persons have the right to be free from restraints. Restraints require a doctor's order. They are used only if it is the best way to protect the person. They are not used for staff convenience. Restraints can make confusion and demented behaviors worse. The nurse tells you when to use restraints.

Activity and a safe setting promote quality of life (see Box 25-5). Safe, calm, and quiet activities are needed. The recreational therapist and other health team members will find activities that are best for each person. These are part of the person's care plan.

FOCUS ON THE PERSON

Confusion and dementia affect quality of life. The problem may be short-term or long-term. The person needs to be treated with dignity and respect. *See Focus on the Person: Caring for Persons with Confusion and Dementia.*

Focus on the PERSON

Caring For Persons With Confusion and Dementia

Providing comfort—The person with dementia may not be able to recognize pain or discomfort. The person may not be able to communicate symptoms. Report signs of pain (Chapters 4 and 18) to the nurse. Also report changes in the person's behavior.

To promote comfort, follow the person's care plan. Also practice the comfort measures listed on the inside of the front book cover.

Ethical behavior—As AD progresses, the family will need to make decisions for the person. You may not agree with their decisions. However, you must respect their decisions. The person still deserves quality care. The person and family still deserve kindness and respect.

Remaining independent—Persons with dementia have problems with activities of daily living. Eating, bathing, dressing, and elimination are examples. The care plan will include measures to help the person remain independent as long as possible. Maintaining the person's routines is an example. For example, Mrs. Lund follows this order after getting out of bed: uses the bathroom, washes hands, brushes teeth, showers, puts on make-up, brushes hair, dresses, and has breakfast. You may need to break down each task into simple steps. Allow extra time for the person to complete a task. Let the person do as much for himself or herself as possible.

Speaking up—Impaired communication is a common problem among persons with AD and other dementias. Communication abilities decline over time. Some persons can have brief conversations. To promote communication, practice the measures in Box 25-5. Avoid the following:
- Giving orders. For example: "Sit down and eat." Such a statement is bossy. It does not show respect for the person.
- Wanting the truth. For example, avoid saying: "Don't you remember?" "What's my name?" "What day is it?"
- Correcting the person's errors. For example, do not say: "No, that is your daughter Rose. That's not Mary." Or, "I just told you that it's time to get dressed. You already had breakfast."

OBRA and other laws—According to OBRA, secured nursing units are physical restraints. Centers must follow OBRA rules. The center must use the least-restrictive approach to care. The person's rights are always protected.

Nursing teamwork—The entire staff must protect the person from harm. Always look for dangers in the person's room, and in hallways, lounges, dining areas, and other areas on the nursing unit. Remove the danger if you can, and tell the nurse at once. If you cannot remove the danger, also tell the nurse at once.

Every staff member must be alert to persons who wander. Such persons are allowed to wander in safe areas. However, you may see a person wander into another person's room or unsafe area. Kitchens, shower rooms, and utility rooms are examples. Or a person may try to wander to another nursing unit or out of the agency. Gently guide the person back to a safe area. Report the problem to the nurse.

REVIEW QUESTIONS

Circle the **BEST** answer.

1 Cognitive function relates to the following *except*
   a Memory loss and personality
   b Thinking and reasoning
   c Ability to understand
   d Judgment and behavior

2 A person is confused after surgery. The confusion is likely to be
   a Permanent
   b Temporary
   c Caused by an infection
   d Caused by a brain injury

3 A person is confused. The care plan includes the following. Which should you question?
   a Restrain in bed at night.
   b Give clear, simple directions.
   c Use touch to communicate.
   d Open drapes during the day.

4 A person has delusions. A delusion is
   a A false belief
   b An illness caused by changes in the brain
   c Seeing, hearing, or feeling something that is not real
   d Alzheimer's disease

5 A person has AD. Which is *true?*
   a AD occurs only in older persons.
   b Diet and drugs can cure the disease.
   c AD and delirium are the same.
   d AD ends in death.

6 The following are common in persons with AD *except*
   a Memory loss, poor judgment, and sleep disturbances
   b Loss of impulse control and the ability to communicate
   c Wandering, delusions, and hallucinations
   d Paralysis, dyspnea, and pain

7 Sundowning means that
   a The person becomes sleepy when the sun sets
   b Behaviors become worse in the late afternoon and evening hours
   c Behavior improves at night
   d The person is in the third stage of the disease

8 A person with AD is screaming. You know that this is
   a An agitated reaction
   b A way to communicate
   c Caused by a delusion
   d A repetitive behavior

9 AD support groups do the following *except*
   a Provide care
   b Offer encouragement and care ideas
   c Provide support for the family
   d Promote the sharing of feelings and frustrations

10 A person with AD tends to wander. You should do the following *except*
    a Make sure doors alarms are turned on
    b Make sure the ID bracelet is worn
    c Assist with exercise as ordered
    d Tell the person where to wander safely

11 Safety is important for the person with AD. Which is *false?*
    a Safety plugs are placed in electric outlets.
    b Cleaners and drugs are kept locked up.
    c The person can keep smoking materials.
    d Sharp and breakable objects are removed from the environment.

12 You are caring for a person with AD. Which is *false?*
    a You can reason with the person.
    b Touch can calm and reassure the person.
    c A calm, quiet setting is important.
    d Help is needed with ADL.

Answers to these questions are on p. 470.

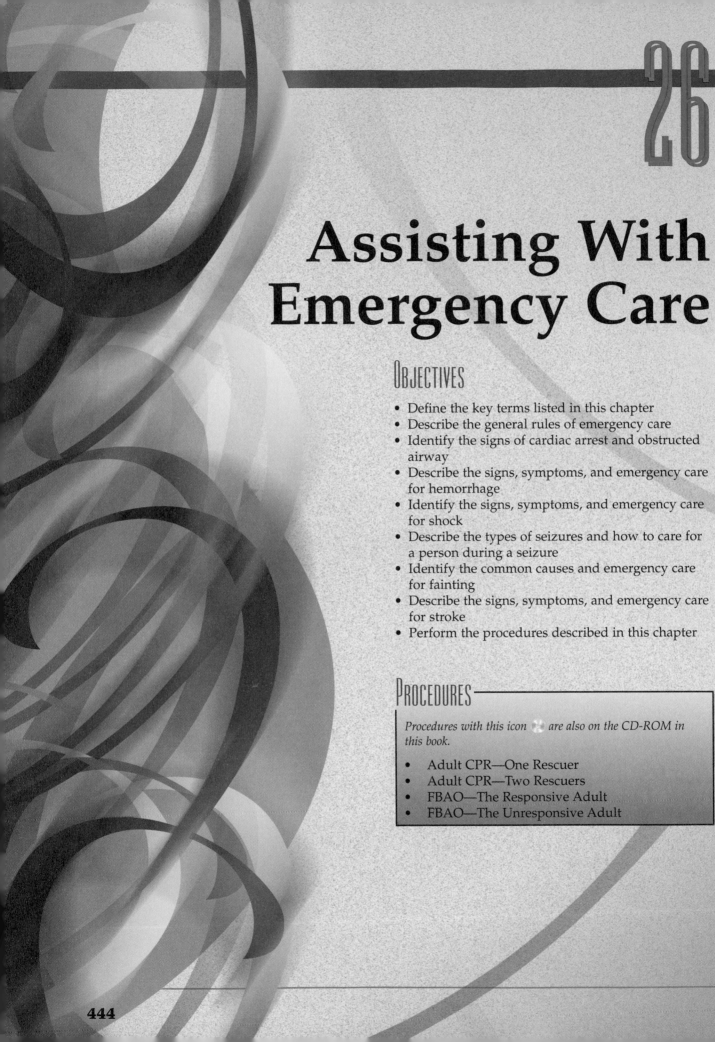

Assisting With Emergency Care

Objectives

- Define the key terms listed in this chapter
- Describe the general rules of emergency care
- Identify the signs of cardiac arrest and obstructed airway
- Describe the signs, symptoms, and emergency care for hemorrhage
- Identify the signs, symptoms, and emergency care for shock
- Describe the types of seizures and how to care for a person during a seizure
- Identify the common causes and emergency care for fainting
- Describe the signs, symptoms, and emergency care for stroke
- Perform the procedures described in this chapter

Procedures

Procedures with this icon ✼ are also on the CD-ROM in this book.

- Adult CPR—One Rescuer
- Adult CPR—Two Rescuers
- FBAO—The Responsive Adult
- FBAO—The Unresponsive Adult

Key Terms

cardiac arrest The heart and breathing stop suddenly and without warning

convulsion A seizure

fainting The sudden loss of consciousness from an inadequate blood supply to the brain

hemorrhage The excessive loss of blood in a short time

respiratory arrest Breathing stops but heart action continues for several minutes

seizure Violent and sudden contractions or tremors of muscle groups; convulsion

shock Results when organs and tissues do not get enough blood

Emergencies can occur anywhere. Sometimes you can save a life if you know what to do. You are encouraged to take a first aid course and a basic life support (BLS) course. These courses prepare you to give emergency care.

The basic life support procedures in this chapter are given as information. They do not replace certification training. You need a basic life support course for health care providers.

EMERGENCY CARE

In an emergency, the Emergency Medical Services (EMS) system is activated. Emergency personnel (paramedics, emergency medical technicians) rush to the scene. They treat, stabilize, and transport persons with life-threatening problems. To activate the EMS system, dial 911. Or call the local fire or police department or the telephone operator.

In nursing centers, a nurse decides when to activate the EMS system. The nurse tells you how to help. If a person has stopped breathing or is in

PROMOTING SAFETY AND COMFORT
Emergency Care

Safety

During emergencies, contact with blood, body fluids, secretions, and excretions is likely. Follow Standard Precautions and the Bloodborne Pathogen Standard to the extent possible.

Comfort

Psychological comfort is important in emergency situations. Help the person feel safe and secure. Provide reassurance and explanations about care. Use a calm approach.

cardiac arrest, the nurse may start cardiopulmonary resuscitation (CPR) (p. 446). Some centers allow nursing assistants to start CPR. Others do not. Know your center's policy about CPR.

Death is expected in persons suffering from terminal illnesses. Usually these persons are not resuscitated (Chapter 27). This information is in the care plan.

Each emergency is different. The rules in Box 26-1 apply to any emergency.

BASIC LIFE SUPPORT

When the heart and breathing stop, the person is clinically dead. Blood and oxygen are not circulated through the body. Brain and other organ damage occurs within minutes.

BOX 26-1 | General Rules of Emergency Care

- Know your limits. Do not do more than you are able. Do not perform an unfamiliar procedure. Do what you can under the circumstances.
- Stay calm. This helps the person feel more secure.
- Know where to find emergency supplies.
- Follow Standard Precautions and the Bloodborne Pathogen Standard to the extent possible.
- Check for life-threatening problems. Check for breathing, a pulse, and bleeding.
- Keep the person lying down or as you found him or her. Moving the person could make an injury worse.
- Perform necessary emergency measures.
- Call for help, or have someone activate the EMS system. *Do not hang up until the operator has hung up.* Give the operator the following information:
  - Your location: street address and city, cross streets or roads, and landmarks
  - Telephone number you are calling from
  - What happened (for example, heart attack, accident, fire)—police, fire equipment, and ambulances may be needed
  - How many people need help
  - Condition of victims, obvious injuries, and life-threatening situations
  - What aid is being given
- Do not remove clothes unless you have to. If you must remove clothing, tear or cut garments along the seams.
- Keep the person warm. Cover the person with a blanket, coats, or sweaters.
- Reassure the person. Explain what is happening and that help was called.
- Do not give the person food or fluids.
- Keep bystanders away. They invade privacy, and tend to stare, give advice, and comment about the person's condition. The person may think the situation is worse than it really is.

Cardiac arrest is when the heart and breathing stop suddenly and without warning. It can occur anywhere and at any time. Common causes include heart disease, drowning, electric shock, severe injury, foreign-body airway obstruction (FBAO), and drug overdose. The person has an abnormal heart rhythm called *ventricular fibrillation*. The heart cannot pump blood. A normal rhythm must be restored (p. 453). Otherwise the person will die.

Respiratory arrest is when breathing stops but heart action continues for several minutes. If breathing is not restored, cardiac arrest occurs. Causes of respiratory arrest include stroke, foreign-body airway obstruction (FBAO), drug overdose, injuries, suffocation, and heart attack.

Basic life support (BLS) procedures support breathing and circulation. They require speed and skill.

PROMOTING SAFETY AND COMFORT
Basic Life Support

Safety

The discussion and procedures that follow assume that the person does not have injuries from trauma. If injuries are present, special measures are needed to position the person and open the airway. Such measures are learned during a BLS certification course.

Chain of Survival

The American Heart Association's (AHA's) basic life support courses teach the adult Chain of Survival. Chain of Survival actions are:

- *Early access to the emergency response system.* This means activating the EMS system. Hospitals and nursing centers call special codes for life-threatening emergencies.
- *Early CPR.*
- *Early defibrillation.* See p. 453.
- *Early advanced care.* This is given by EMS staff, doctors, and nurses. They give drugs and perform life-saving measures.

Cardiopulmonary Resuscitation for Adults

Cardiopulmonary resuscitation (CPR) must be started at once when a person is in cardiac arrest. It provides oxygen to the brain and heart until advanced emergency care is given. There are three major signs of cardiac arrest: *no response, no breathing, and no pulse.* The person's skin is cool, pale, and gray. The person is not coughing or moving.

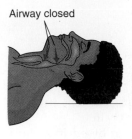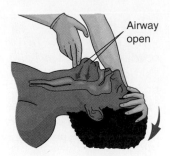

Airway closed   Airway open

FIG. 26-1 The head-tilt/chin-lift maneuver opens the airway. One hand is on the person's forehead. Pressure is applied to tilt the head back. The chin is lifted with the fingers of the other hand.

CPR has three basic parts (the ABCs of CPR)—**A**irway, **B**reathing, and **C**irculation.

Airway
The airway is often obstructed (blocked) during cardiac arrest. The person's tongue falls toward the back of the throat and blocks the airway. The *head-tilt/chin-lift maneuver* opens the airway (Fig. 26-1):

- Position the person supine on a hard, flat surface.
- Kneel or stand at the person's side.
- Place the palm of one hand on the forehead.
- Tilt the head back by pushing down on the forehead with your palm.
- Place the fingers of the other hand under the bony part of the chin.
- Lift the chin as you tilt the head backward with your other hand.

When the airway is open, check for vomitus, loose dentures, or other objects. These can obstruct the airway during rescue breathing. Remove dentures and wipe vomitus away with your index and middle fingers. Wear gloves or cover your fingers with a cloth.

Breathing
Before you start rescue breathing, check for adequate breathing (Fig. 26-2). It should take no more than 10 seconds to do the following:

- Maintain an open airway.
- Place your ear over the person's mouth and nose.
- Observe the person's chest.
- *Look* to see if the chest rises and falls.
- *Listen* for the escape of air.
- *Feel* for the flow of air on your cheek.

Mouth-to-mouth breathing (Fig. 26-3) involves placing your mouth over the person's mouth. To give mouth-to-mouth breathing:

- Keep the airway open.
- Pinch the person's nostrils shut. Use your thumb and index finger. Use the hand on the forehead. Shutting the nostrils prevents air from escaping through the nose.
- Take a deep breath.

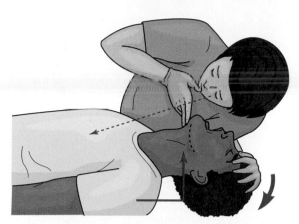

FIG. **26-2** Determining adequate breathing. *Look* to see if the chest rises and falls. *Listen* for the escape of air. *Feel* for the flow of air on your cheek.

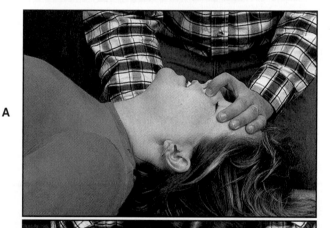

A

B

FIG. **26-3** Mouth-to-mouth breathing. **A,** The person's airway is opened. The nostrils are pinched shut. **B,** The person's mouth is sealed by the rescuer's mouth.

- Place your mouth tightly over the person's mouth.
- Blow air into the person's mouth slowly. You should see the chest rise as the lungs fill with air. You should also hear air escape when the person exhales.
- Remove your mouth from the person's mouth. Then take in a quick, deep breath.

Mouth-to-barrier device breathing is used in the

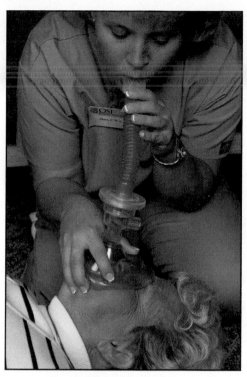

FIG. **26-4** Barrier device.

workplace. A barrier device is placed over the person's mouth and nose. It prevents contact with the person's mouth and blood, body fluids, secretions, or excretions (Fig. 26-4). The seal must be tight.

When you start CPR, give 2 breaths first. Allow exhalation after each breath. Then give breaths at a rate of 10 to 12 breaths per minute. During CPR, 2 breaths are given after every 15 chest compressions.

Circulation

Chest compressions force blood through the circulatory system. Before starting chest compressions, check for a pulse. Use the carotid artery on the side near you. To find the carotid pulse, place 2 fingers on the person's trachea (windpipe). Then slide your fingertips down off the trachea to the groove of the neck (Fig. 26-5, p. 448). While checking for a pulse, also look for signs of circulation. See if the person has started breathing or is coughing or moving.

The heart lies between the sternum (breastbone) and the spinal column. When pressure is applied to the sternum, the sternum is depressed. This compresses the heart between the sternum and spinal column (Fig. 26-6, p. 448). For effective chest compressions, the

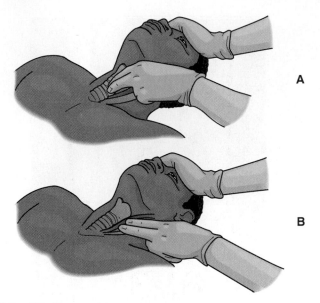

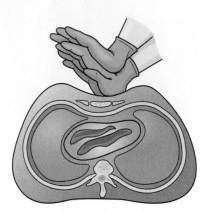

FIG. 26-5 Locating the carotid pulse. **A,** Two fingers are placed on the trachea. **B,** The fingers are moved down into the groove of the neck to the carotid pulse.

FIG. 26-6 The heart lies between the sternum and spinal column. The heart is compressed when pressure is applied to the sternum.

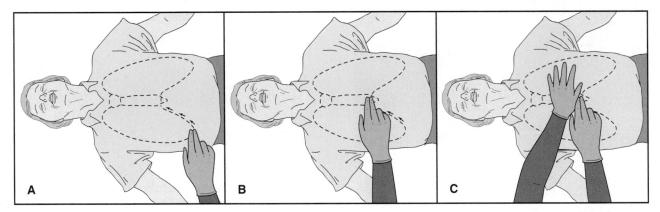

FIG. 26-7 Proper hand position for CPR. **A,** Find the rib cage. **B,** Move your fingers along the rib cage to the notch. **C,** Place the heel of your hand next to your index finger.

person must be supine and on a hard, flat surface, and proper hand position is needed (Fig. 26-7).

- Use 2 or 3 fingers to find the lower part of the person's rib cage on the side near you. Use the hand closest to the person's feet.
- Move your fingers up along the rib cage to the notch at the center of the chest.
- Place the heel of your other hand on the lower half of the sternum by your index finger.
- Remove your fingers from the notch.
- Place your other hand on the hand that is on the sternum.
- Extend or interlace your fingers. Keep them off the chest.

To give chest compressions, your arms are straight. Your shoulders are directly over your hands (Fig. 26-8). Exert firm downward pressure to depress the sternum about 1½ to 2 inches in an adult. Then release pressure without removing your hands from the chest. Give compressions in a regular rhythm at a rate of 100 per minute.

PROMOTING SAFETY AND COMFORT
Cardiopulmonary Resuscitation For Adults

Safety

Never practice CPR on another person. Serious damage can be done. Mannequins are used to learn and practice CPR.

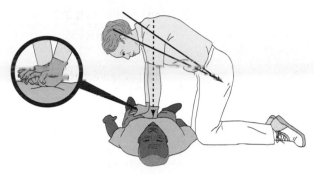

FIG. **26-8** To give chest compressions, the arms are straight and shoulders are over the hands.

Adult CPR—One Rescuer

Procedure

1 Check if the person is responding. Tap or gently shake the person, call the person by name, and shout "Are you OK?"

2 Call for help. Activate the EMS system or the agency's emergency response system.

3 Position the person supine. Logroll the person so there is no twisting of the spine. The person must be on a hard, flat surface. Place the person's arms alongside the body.

4 Open the airway. Use the head-tilt/chin-lift method.

5 Check for breathing. *Look* to see if the chest rises and falls. *Listen* for the escape of air. *Feel* for the flow of air on your cheek.

6 Give 2 slow breaths if the person is not breathing or is not breathing adequately. Each breath takes 2 seconds. Let the person's lungs deflate between breaths.

7 Check for a carotid pulse and for breathing, coughing, and moving. This should take 5 to 10 seconds. Use your other hand to keep the airway open with the head-tilt/chin-lift method. Start chest compressions if there are no signs of circulation.

8 Give chest compressions at a rate of 100 per minute. Give 15 compressions and then 2 slow breaths.

   a Establish a rhythm and count out loud. (Try: "1 and, 2 and, 3 and, 4 and, 5 and, 6 and, 7 and, 8 and, 9 and, 10 and, 11 and, 12 and, 13 and, 14 and, 15.")

   b Open the airway, and give 2 slow breaths.

   c Repeat this step until 4 cycles of 15 compressions and 2 breaths are given.

9 Check for a carotid pulse. Also check for breathing, coughing, and moving.

10 Continue CPR if the person has no signs of circulation. Begin with chest compressions. Continue the cycle of 15 compressions and 2 breaths. Check for circulation every few minutes.

11 Do the following if the person has signs of circulation:

   a Check for breathing.

   b Position the person in the recovery position (p. 453) if the person is breathing.

   c Monitor breathing and circulation.

12 Do the following if the person has signs of circulation but breathing is absent:

   a Give 1 rescue breath every 5 seconds. This is at a rate of 10 to 12 breaths per minute.

   b Monitor circulation.

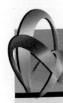

Adult CPR—Two Rescuers

Procedure

1 Check if the person is responding. Tap or gently shake the person, call the person by name, and shout "Are you OK?" One rescuer activates the EMS system or the agency's emergency response system.
2 Open the airway, and check for breathing. Use the head-tilt/chin-lift method.
3 Give 2 slow rescue breaths if the person is not breathing or if breathing is inadequate. Let the lungs deflate between breaths.
4 Check for a pulse using the carotid artery. Also check for breathing, coughing, and moving.
5 Perform 2-person CPR (Fig. 26-9) if there are no signs of circulation:
   a One rescuer gives chest compressions at a rate of 100 per minute. Count out loud in a rhythm. (Try: "1 and, 2 and, 3 and, 4 and, 5 and, 6 and, 7 and, 8 and, 9 and, 10 and, 11 and, 12 and, 13 and, 14 and, 15.")
   b The other rescuer gives 2 slow breaths after every 15 compressions. Pause for the breaths. Continue chest compressions after the breaths.
6 One rescuer does the following after 4 cycles of 15 compressions and 2 breaths:
   a Gives 2 slow breaths.
   b Checks for circulation—carotid pulse, breathing, coughing, and moving.
7 Continue with 15 compressions and 2 slow breaths if the person has no signs of circulation. Start with chest compressions.

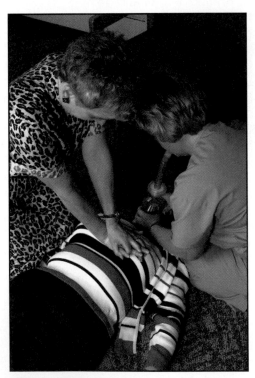

FIG. **26-9** Two people performing CPR.

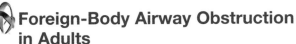

Foreign-Body Airway Obstruction in Adults

Foreign-body airway obstruction *(FBAO; choking)* can lead to cardiac arrest. Air cannot pass through the air passages to the lungs. The body does not get oxygen.

Foreign bodies can cause airway obstruction. This often occurs during eating. A large, poorly chewed piece of meat is the most common cause. Laughing and talking while eating also are common causes. So is excessive alcohol intake. Older persons are at risk from weakness, poorly fitting dentures, dysphagia, and chronic illnesses.

FBAO can occur in the unconscious person. Common causes are aspiration of vomitus and the tongue falling back into the airway.

Foreign bodies can cause partial or complete airway obstruction. With *partial obstruction*, some air moves in and out of the lungs. The person is conscious. Usually the person can speak. Often forceful coughing can remove the object.

With severe or *complete airway obstruction*, the conscious person clutches at the throat. The person cannot breathe, speak, or cough. The person appears pale and cyanotic (bluish color). Air does not move in and out of the lungs. The conscious person is very frightened. If the obstruction is not removed, the person will die. FBAO is an emergency.

The Heimlich maneuver is used to relieve FBAO. It involves abdominal thrusts. The maneuver is performed with the person standing, sitting, or lying down. The finger sweep is used with the Heimlich maneuver when an adult becomes unconscious.

The Heimlich maneuver is not effective in very obese persons or pregnant women. Chest thrusts are used (Box 26-2).

BOX 26-2 **Obstructed Airway: Chest Thrusts For Obese or Pregnant Persons**

The Victim Is Sitting or Standing

1 Stand behind the person.
2 Place your arms under the person's underarms. Wrap your arms around the person's chest.
3 Make a fist. Place the thumb side of the fist on the middle of the sternum (breastbone).
4 Grasp the fist with your other hand.
5 Give backward chest thrusts until the object is expelled or the person becomes unconscious.

The Victim Is Lying Down or Unconscious

1 Position the person supine.
2 Kneel next to the person.
3 Position your hands as for external chest compressions.
4 Give chest thrusts until the object is expelled or the person becomes unconscious.

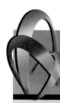

FBAO—The Responsive Adult

Procedure

1 Ask the person if he or she is choking.
2 Ask if the person can cough or speak.
3 Give abdominal thrusts (Fig. 26-10, p. 452):
  a Stand behind the person.
  b Wrap your arms around the person's waist.
  c Make a fist with one hand.
  d Place the thumb side of the fist against the abdomen. The fist is in the middle above the navel and below the end of the sternum (breastbone).
  e Grasp your fist with your other hand.
  f Press your fist and hand into the person's abdomen with a quick, upward thrust.
  g Repeat thrusts until the object is expelled or the person loses consciousness.
4 Lower the unresponsive person to the floor or ground. Position the person supine.
5 Activate the EMS system or the agency's emergency response system.
6 Do a finger sweep to check for a foreign object.
  a Open the person's mouth. Use the tongue-jaw lift method (Fig. 26-11, *A*, p. 452).
    (1) Grasp the tongue and lower jaw with your thumb and fingers.

    (2) Lift the lower jaw upward.
  b Insert your other index finger into the mouth along the side of the cheek and deep into the throat (Fig. 26-11, *B*, p. 452). Your finger should be at the base of the tongue.
  c Form a hook with your index finger.
  d Try to dislodge and remove the object. Do not push it deeper into the throat.
  e Grasp and remove the object if it is within reach.
7 Open the airway with the head-tilt/chin-lift method.
8 Give 1 or 2 rescue breaths.
9 Reposition the person's head if the chest did not rise. Give 1 or 2 rescue breaths.
10 Give up to 5 abdominal thrusts (See procedure: *FBAO—The Unresponsive Adult*, p. 452).
11 Repeat steps 6 through 10 (finger sweeps, rescue breathing, and abdominal thrusts) until rescue breathing is effective. Start CPR if necessary.

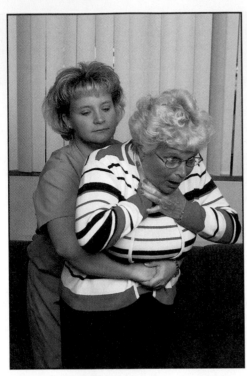

FIG. **26-10** Abdominal thrusts with the person standing.

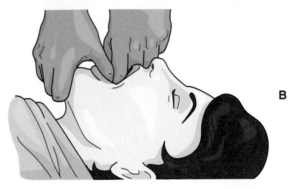

FIG. **26-11** Tongue-jaw lift maneuver. **A,** Grasp the person's tongue and lift the jaw upward with one hand. **B,** Use the index finger of the other hand to check for a foreign object.

 The Unresponsive Adult

You may find an adult who is unresponsive. You did not see the person lose consciousness, and you do not know the cause. Do not assume the cause is choking. Check for unresponsiveness and start rescue breathing. Abdominal thrusts are done if you cannot ventilate the person. Then use the finger sweep maneuver.

FBAO—The Unresponsive Adult

Procedure

1 Check to see if the person is responding.
2 Call for help. Activate the EMS system or the agency's emergency response system.
3 Logroll the person to the supine position with his or her face up. Arms are at the sides.
4 Open the airway. Use the head-tilt/chin-lift method.
5 Check for breathing.
6 Give 1 or 2 slow rescue breaths. Reposition the person's head and open the airway if the chest does not rise. Give 1 or 2 rescue breaths.
7 Give 5 abdominal thrusts (Fig. 26-12) if you cannot ventilate the person.
  a Straddle the person's thighs.

b Place the heel of one hand against the abdomen. It is in the middle above the navel and below the end of the sternum (breastbone).
c Place your second hand on top of your first hand.
d Press both hands into the abdomen with a quick, upward thrust. Give 5 thrusts.
8 Do a finger sweep to check for a foreign object. See step 6 in procedure: *FBAO—The Responsive Adult,* p. 451.
9 Repeat steps 6 through 8 until rescue breathing is effective. Start CPR if necessary.

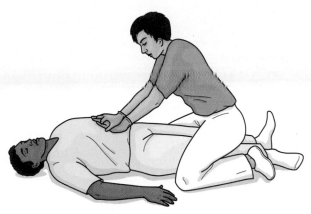

FIG. **26-12** Abdominal thrusts with the person lying down. The rescuer straddles the thighs.

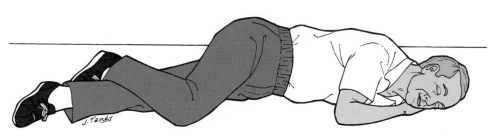

FIG. **26-13** Recovery position.

Recovery Position

The recovery position is used when the person is breathing and has a pulse but is not responding (Fig. 26-13). The position helps keep the airway open and prevents aspiration.

Logroll the person into the recovery position. Keep the head, neck, and spine straight. A hand supports the head. *Do not use this position if the person might have neck injuries or other trauma.*

Automated External Defibrillators

Ventricular fibrillation (VF, V-fib) is an abnormal heart rhythm. It causes cardiac arrest. Rather than beating in a regular rhythm, the heart shakes and quivers like a bowl of Jell-O. The heart does not pump blood. The heart, brain, and other organs do not receive blood and oxygen.

A *defibrillator* is used to deliver a shock to the heart. The shock stops the VF. This allows the return of a regular heart rhythm. Defibrillation as soon as possible after the onset of VF increases the person's chance of survival.

Automated external defibrillators (AEDs) are found in hospitals, nursing centers, dental offices, and other health care agencies. They are on airplanes and in airports, health clubs, malls, and many other public places. A basic life support course teaches health care providers how to use them. Remember, the goal is early defibrillation.

HEMORRHAGE

If a blood vessel is torn or cut, bleeding occurs. **Hemorrhage** is the excessive loss of blood in a short time. If the bleeding is not stopped, the person will die.

With internal hemorrhage, bleeding occurs inside the body into tissues and body cavities. Pain, shock (p. 455), vomiting blood, coughing up blood, and loss of consciousness signal internal hemorrhage. There is little you can do for internal bleeding. Activate the EMS system. Then keep the person warm, flat, and quiet until medical help arrives. Do not give fluids.

If not hidden by clothing, external bleeding is usually seen. Bleeding from an artery occurs in spurts.

FIG. **26-14** Direct pressure is applied to the wound to stop bleeding. The hand is placed over the wound.

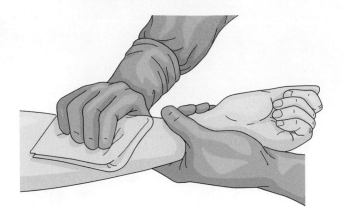

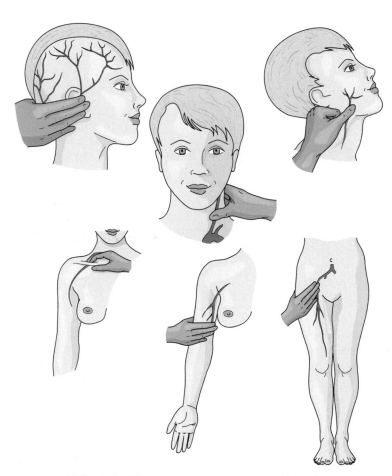

FIG. **26-15** Pressure points to control bleeding.

There is a steady flow of blood from a vein. To control external bleeding:

- Follow the rules in Box 26-1. This includes activating the EMS system.
- Do not remove any objects that have pierced or stabbed the person.
- Elevate the affected part—hand, arm, foot, or leg.
- Place a sterile dressing directly over the wound. Or use any clean material (handkerchief, towel, cloth, or sanitary napkin).

- Apply pressure with your hand directly over the bleeding site (Fig. 26-14). Do not release the pressure until the bleeding stops.
- If direct pressure does not control bleeding, apply pressure over the artery above the bleeding site (Fig. 26-15). Use your first three fingers. For example, if bleeding is from the lower arm, apply pressure over the brachial artery.
- Bind the wound when bleeding stops. Tape or tie the dressing in place. You can tie the dressing with such things as clothing, a scarf, a necktie, or a belt.

PROMOTING SAFETY AND COMFORT
Hemorrhage

Safety

Contact with blood is likely with hemorrhage. Follow Standard Precautions and the Bloodborne Pathogen Standard to the extent possible. Wear gloves if possible. Practice hand hygiene as soon as you can.

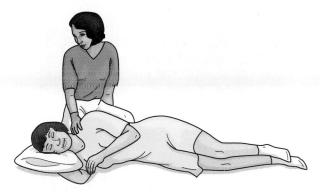

FIG. 26-16 A pillow protects the person's head during a seizure.

SHOCK

Shock results when organs and tissues do not get enough blood. Blood loss, heart attack (myocardial infarction), burns, and severe infection are causes. Signs and symptoms include low or falling blood pressure, rapid and weak pulse, and rapid respirations. The person is thirsty and has cold, moist, and pale skin. The person is restless. Confusion and loss of consciousness occur as shock worsens

Shock is possible in any person who is acutely ill or injured. Follow the rules in Box 26-1. Maintain an open airway and control bleeding.

SEIZURES

Seizures (convulsions) are violent and sudden contractions or tremors of muscle groups. They are caused by an abnormality in the brain. Causes include head injury, high fever, brain tumors, poisoning, seizure disorders, and nervous system infections. Lack of blood flow to the brain can also cause seizures.

The major types of seizures are *partial seizures* and *generalized seizures.* Only a part of the brain is involved with a partial seizure. A body part may jerk. Or the person has hearing or vision problems or stomach discomfort. The person does not lose consciousness.

With generalized seizures, the whole brain is involved. The *generalized tonic-clonic seizure (grand mal seizure)* has two phases. In the tonic phase, the person loses consciousness. If standing or sitting, the person falls to the floor. The body is rigid because all muscles contract at once. The clonic phase follows. Muscle groups contract and relax. This causes jerking and twitching movements. Urinary and fecal incontinence may occur. A deep sleep is common after the seizure. Confusion and headache may occur on awakening.

You cannot stop a seizure. However, you can protect the person from injury.

- Follow the rules in Box 26-1. This includes activating the EMS system.
- Do not leave the person alone.

- Lower the person to the floor. This protects the person from falling.
- Place a folded blanket, towel, cushion, pillow, or other soft item under the person's head (Fig. 26-16). Or cradle the person's head in your lap.
- Turn the person onto his or her side. Make sure the head is turned to the side.
- Loosen tight jewelry and clothing (ties, scarves, collars, necklaces) around the neck.
- Move furniture, equipment, and sharp objects away from the person.
- Do not give the person food or fluids.
- Do not try to restrain body movements during the seizure.
- Do not put any object or your fingers between the person's teeth.

FAINTING

Fainting is the sudden loss of consciousness from an inadequate blood supply to the brain. Hunger, fatigue, fear, and pain are common causes. Standing in one position for a long time and being in a warm, crowded room are other causes. Dizziness, perspiration, and blackness before the eyes are warning signals. The person looks pale. The pulse is weak. Respirations are shallow if consciousness is lost. For emergency care:

- Have the person sit or lie down before fainting occurs.
- If sitting, the person bends forward and places the head between the knees (Fig. 26-17, p. 456).
- If the person is lying down, raise the legs.
- Loosen tight clothing (belts, ties, scarves, collars, and so on).
- Keep the person lying down if fainting has occurred. Raise the legs.
- Do not let the person get up until symptoms have subsided for about 5 minutes.
- Help the person to a sitting position after recovery from fainting.

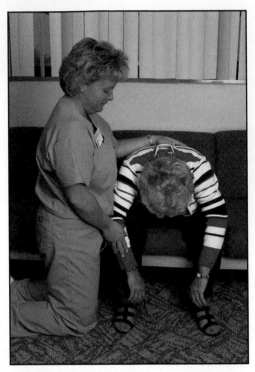

FIG. **26-17** The person bends forward and lowers her head between her knees to prevent fainting.

STROKE

Stroke (cerebrovascular accident) occurs when the brain is suddenly deprived of its blood supply (Chapter 24). Usually only part of the brain is affected. A stroke may be caused by a thrombus, an embolus, or hemorrhage if a blood vessel in the brain ruptures.

Signs of stroke vary. They depend on the size and location of brain injury. Loss of consciousness or semi-consciousness, rapid pulse, labored respirations, elevated blood pressure, and hemiplegia are signs of a stroke. The person may have slurred speech or aphasia (the inability to speak). Loss of vision in one eye, unsteadiness, and falling also are signs. Seizures may occur.

Emergency care includes the following:
- Follow the rules in Box 26-1. This includes activating the EMS system.
- Position the person in the recovery position on the affected side (see Fig. 26-13). The affected side is limp, and the cheek appears puffy.
- Elevate the head without flexing the neck.
- Loosen tight clothing (belts, ties, scarves, collars, and so on.)
- Keep the person quiet and warm.
- Reassure the person.
- Provide rescue breathing and CPR if necessary.
- Provide emergency care for seizures if necessary.

FOCUS ON THE PERSON

Protect quality of life during emergencies. Treat the person with dignity and respect. *See Focus on the Person: Assisting With Emergency Care.*

Focus on the **PERSON**

Assisting With Emergency Care

Providing comfort—The ill or injured person may have severe pain. Little can be done to relieve pain until medical help arrives. Reassure the person. Use a calm, soothing voice. Often holding the person's hand can bring great comfort.

Ethical behavior—People are curious. They want to know what happened, the extent of injuries or illness, and if the person will be okay. Do not discuss the situation. Do not offer ideas of what is wrong with the person. Only doctors diagnose. You can make observations about signs and symptoms. The doctor determines what is wrong with the person.

Remaining independent—Protect personal items from loss and damage. Dentures, eyeglasses, and hearing aids are often lost or broken in emergencies.

Speaking up—Some illnesses and injuries are life-threatening. To find out what happened and the person's condition, you can say:
- "Tell me what happened."
- "Where does it hurt?"
- "If you can, please point to where it hurts."
- "Is the pain constant or does it come and go?"
- "Tell me what's wrong."
- "Can you move your arms and legs?"

OBRA and other laws—Protect the right to privacy and confidentiality. Do not expose the person unnecessarily. You may be in a place where you cannot close doors, shades, and curtains. The person may be in a lounge, dining area, or public place. Do what you can to provide privacy.

Nursing teamwork—Onlookers can threaten privacy and confidentiality. During an emergency, your main concern is the person's illness or injuries. You cannot give care and manage onlookers at the same time. Ask someone else to deal with the onlookers. If someone else is giving care, keep onlookers away from the person.

REVIEW QUESTIONS

Circle the **BEST** answer.

1 When giving first aid, you should
   a Be aware of your own limits
   b Move the person
   c Give the person fluids
   d Perform needed emergency measures

2 Which is *not* a sign of cardiac arrest?
   a No pulse
   b No breathing
   c A sudden drop in blood pressure
   d Unconsciousness

3 Mouth-to-mouth rescue breathing involves the following *except*
   a Pinching the nostrils shut
   b Placing your mouth tightly over the person's mouth
   c Blowing air into the mouth as you exhale
   d Covering the nose with your mouth

4 Chest compressions are performed on an adult. The chest is compressed
   a ½ to 1 inch with the index and middle fingers
   b 1 to 1½ inches with the heel of one hand
   c 1½ to 2 inches with two hands
   d With one hand in the middle of the sternum

5 Which does *not* determine adequate breathing?
   a Looking to see if the chest rises and falls
   b Counting respirations for 30 seconds
   c Listening for the escape of air
   d Feeling for the flow of air

6 Which pulse is used during adult CPR?
   a The apical pulse
   b The brachial pulse
   c The carotid pulse
   d The femoral pulse

7 You are doing adult CPR alone. Which is *false?*
   a Give 2 breaths after every 15 compressions
   b Check for a pulse after 1 minute
   c Give 1 breath after every fifth compression
   d Count out loud

8 Adult CPR is being given by 2 people. Rescue breaths are given
   a After every 5 compressions
   b After every 15 compressions
   c After every compression
   d Only when the positions are changed

9 The most common cause of FBAO in adults is
   a A loose denture
   b Meat
   c Marbles
   d Candy

10 If airway obstruction occurs, the person usually
   a Clutches at the throat
   b Can speak, cough, and breathe
   c Is calm
   d Has a seizure

11 These statements are about the Heimlich maneuver. Which is *true?*
   a The person can be standing, sitting, or lying down.
   b Rescue breaths are given before the thrusts.
   c The finger sweep is used if the person is awake and alert.
   d The maneuver is used for pregnant women.

12 A person is hemorrhaging from the left forearm. The first action is to
   a Lower the body part
   b Apply pressure to the brachial artery
   c Apply direct pressure to the wound
   d Cover the person

13 A person in shock needs
   a Rescue breathing
   b To be kept lying down
   c Clothes removed
   d The recovery position

14 These statements relate to tonic-clonic seizures. Which is *false?*
   a There is contraction of all muscles at once.
   b Incontinence may occur.
   c The seizure usually lasts a few seconds.
   d There is loss of consciousness.

15 A person is about to faint. Which is *false?*
   a Take the person outside for fresh air.
   b Have the person sit or lie down.
   c Loosen tight clothing.
   d Raise the legs if the person is lying down.

16 A person is having a stroke. Emergency care includes the following *except*
   a Positioning the person on the affected side
   b Giving the person sips of water
   c Loosening tight clothing
   d Keeping the person quiet and warm

Answers to these questions are on p. 470.

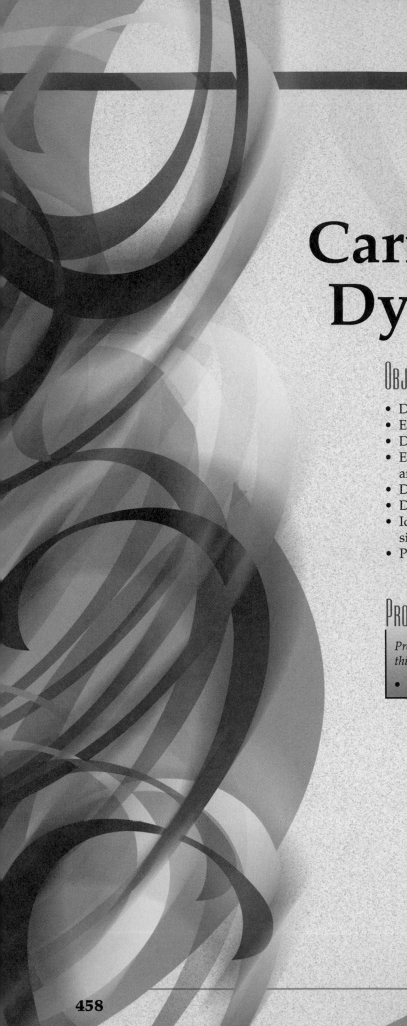

27

Caring For the Dying Person

OBJECTIVES

- Define the key terms listed in this chapter
- Explain the factors that affect attitudes about death
- Describe the five stages of dying
- Explain how to meet the needs of the dying person and family
- Describe hospice care
- Describe three advance directives and their purposes
- Identify the signs of approaching death and the signs of death
- Perform the procedure described in this chapter

PROCEDURES

Procedures with this icon ⊙ are also on the CD-ROM in this book.

- Assisting With Postmortem Care

KEY TERMS

advance directive A document stating a person's wishes about health care when that person cannot make his or her own decisions

postmortem After *(post)* death *(mortem)*

reincarnation The belief that the spirit or soul is reborn in another human body or in another form of life

rigor mortis The stiffness or rigidity *(rigor)* of skeletal muscles that occurs after death *(mortis)*

terminal illness An illness or injury for which there is no reasonable expectation of recovery

Some deaths are sudden; others are expected. Many illnesses and diseases have no cure. Some injuries are so serious that the body cannot function. The disease or injury ends in death. An illness or injury for which there is no reasonable expectation of recovery is a **terminal illness.**

Your feelings about death affect the care you give. You will help meet the dying person's physical, psychological, social, and spiritual needs. Therefore you must understand the dying process. Then you can approach the dying person with caring, kindness, and respect.

ATTITUDES ABOUT DEATH

Many people fear death. Some look forward to and accept death. Attitudes about death often change as a person grows older and with changing circumstances.

Culture and Religion

Practices and attitudes about death differ among cultures *(See Caring About Culture: Death Rites.)* In some cultures, dying people are cared for at home by the family. Some families prepare the body for burial.

Attitudes about death are closely related to religion. Some believe that life after death is free of suffering and hardship. They also believe in reunion with loved ones. Many believe sins and misdeeds are punished in the afterlife. Others believe there is no afterlife. To them, death is the end of life.

There also are religious beliefs about the body's form after death. Some believe the body keeps its physical form. Others believe that only the spirit or soul is present in the afterlife. **Reincarnation** is the belief that the spirit or soul is reborn in another human body or in another form of life.

Caring About Culture

Death Rites

In *Vietnam*, quality of life is more important than length of life because of beliefs in reincarnation. Less suffering in the next life is expected. Therefore dying persons are helped to recall past good deeds and to achieve a fitting mental state. Death at home is preferred over death in the hospital. Upon death, the body is washed and wrapped in clean, white sheets. In some areas a coin or jewels (a wealthy family) and rice (a poor family) are put in the dead person's mouth. This is from the belief that they will help the soul go through the encounters with gods and devils and the soul will be born rich in the next life. Relatives sew small pillows to place under the body's neck, feet, and wrists. The body is placed in a coffin for in-ground burial.

The *Chinese* have an aversion to death and to anything concerning death. Autopsy and disposal of the body are not prescribed by religion. Donating body parts is encouraged. The eldest son makes all arrangements. The body is buried in a coffin. After 7 years, the body is exhumed and cremated. The urn is reburied in the tomb. White or yellow and black clothing is worn for mourning.

In *India*, Hindu persons are often accepting of God's will. The person's desire to be clear-headed as death nears must be assessed in planning medical treatment. A time and place for prayer are essential for the family and the person. Prayer helps them deal with anxiety and conflict. The Hindu priest reads from Holy Sanskrit books. Some priests tie strings (meaning a blessing) around the neck or wrist. After death the son pours water into the mouth of the deceased. Blood transfusions, organ transplants, and autopsies are allowed. Cremation is preferred. Reincarnation is a Hindu belief.

From D'Avanzo CE, Geissler EM: *Pocket guide to cultural health assessment,* ed 3, St Louis, 2003, Mosby.

Age

Infants and toddlers have no concept of death. Between the ages of 3 and 5 years, children are curious and have ideas about death. They know when family members or pets die. They notice dead birds or bugs. They think death is temporary. Children often blame themselves when someone or something dies. To them, death is punishment for being bad. Answers to questions about death often cause fear and confusion.

Children between the ages of 5 and 7 years know death is final. To them, death happens to other people. It can be avoided. Children relate death to punishment and body mutilation. It also involves witches, ghosts, goblins, and monsters. These ideas come from fairy tales, cartoons, movies, video games, and TV.

Adults fear pain and suffering, dying alone, and the invasion of privacy. They also fear loneliness and separation from loved ones. They worry about the care and support of those left behind. Adults often resent death because it affects plans, hopes, dreams, and ambitions.

Older persons usually have fewer fears than younger adults. They know death will occur. Some welcome death as freedom from pain, suffering, and disability. Death also means reunion with those who have died. Like younger adults, they often fear dying alone.

THE STAGES OF DYING

Dr. Elisabeth Kübler-Ross described five stages of dying.

- *Denial* is the first stage. Persons refuse to believe they are dying. "No, not me" is a common response. The person believes a mistake was made.
- *Anger* is stage two. The person thinks "Why me?" There is anger and rage. Dying persons envy and resent those with life and health. Family, friends, and the health team are often targets of anger.
- *Bargaining* is the third stage. Anger has passed. The person now says "Yes, me, but. . . . " Often the person bargains with God for more time. Promises are made in exchange for more time. Bargaining is usually private and on a spiritual level.
- *Depression* is the fourth stage. The person thinks "Yes, me," and is very sad. The person mourns things that were lost and the future loss of life.
- *Acceptance* of death is the last stage. The person is calm and at peace. The person has said what needs to be said. Unfinished business is completed.

PSYCHOLOGICAL, SOCIAL, AND SPIRITUAL NEEDS

Dying people have psychological, social, and spiritual needs. They may want family and friends present. They may want to talk about their fears and worries. Some want to be alone. Often they need to talk during the night. Things are quiet. There are few distractions, and there is more time to think. You need to listen and use touch.

- *Listening*—The person needs to talk and share worries and concerns. Do not worry about saying the wrong thing or finding comforting words. You do not need to say anything. Being there for the person is what counts.
- *Touch*—Touch shows caring and concern when words cannot. Sometimes the person does not want to talk but needs you nearby.

Some people want to see a spiritual leader. Or they want to take part in religious practices. Provide privacy during prayer and spiritual moments. The person has the right to have religious objects nearby (medals, pictures, statues, or religious writings). Handle these valuables with care and respect.

PHYSICAL NEEDS

Every effort is made to promote physical and psychological comfort. The person is allowed to die in peace and with dignity.

Vision, Hearing, and Speech

Vision blurs and gradually fails. The person naturally turns toward light. A darkened room may frighten the person. The eyes may be half open. Secretions may collect in the corners of the eyes.

Because of failing vision, explain what you are doing to the person or in the room. The room should be well lit. However, avoid bright lights and glares. Good eye care is essential.

Hearing is one of the last functions lost. Many people hear until the moment of death. Even unconscious persons may hear. Always assume that the person can hear. Speak in a normal voice. Provide reassurance and explanations about care. Offer words of comfort. Avoid topics that could upset the person.

Speech becomes difficult. It may be hard to understand the person. Sometimes the person cannot speak. Anticipate the person's needs. Do not ask questions that need long answers. Ask "yes" or "no" questions. Despite the person's speech problems, you must talk to him or her.

Mouth, Nose, and Skin

Oral hygiene promotes comfort. Routine mouth care is given if the person can eat and drink. Frequent oral hygiene is given as death nears and when taking oral fluids is difficult. Oral hygiene is needed if mucus collects in the mouth and the person cannot swallow.

Crusting and irritation of the nostrils can occur. Nasal secretions, an oxygen cannula, or an NG tube are common causes. Carefully clean the nose. Apply lubricant as directed by the nurse and the care plan.

Circulation fails and body temperature rises as death nears. The skin feels cool, and looks pale and mottled (blotchy). Perspiration increases. Skin care, bathing, and preventing pressure ulcers are necessary. Linens and gowns are changed whenever needed. Although the skin feels cool, only light bed coverings are needed. Blankets may make the person feel warm and cause restlessness.

Elimination

Urinary and fecal incontinence may occur. Use incontinence products or bed protectors as directed. Give perineal care as needed. Constipation and urinary retention are common. Enemas and catheters may be needed (Chapters 15 and 16).

Comfort and Positioning

Skin care, personal hygiene, back massages, oral hygiene, and good alignment promote comfort. The nurse gives pain relief drugs ordered by the doctor. Frequent position changes and supportive devices also promote comfort. You may need help to turn the person slowly and gently. Semi-Fowler's position is usually best for breathing problems.

The Person's Room

The person's room should be comfortable and pleasant. It should be well lit and well ventilated. Unnecessary equipment is removed. Some equipment is upsetting to look at (suction machines, drainage containers). If possible, these items are kept out of the person's sight.

Mementos, pictures, cards, flowers, and religious items provide comfort. The person and family arrange the room as they wish. This helps meet love, belonging, and self-esteem needs. The room should reflect the person's choices.

THE FAMILY

This is a hard time for the family. It may be very hard to find comforting words. Show your feelings by being available, courteous, and considerate. Use touch to show your concern.

The health team helps make the family as comfortable as possible. You must respect the right to privacy. The person and family need time together. However, you cannot neglect care because the family is present. Most agencies let family members help give care. Or you can suggest that they take a break for a beverage or meal.

The family may be very tired, sad, and tearful. Watching a loved one die is very painful. So is dealing with the eventual loss of that person. The family needs support and understanding. A spiritual leader may provide comfort.

HOSPICE CARE

Hospice care focuses on physical, emotional, social, and spiritual needs. It is not concerned with cure or life-saving measures. Pain relief and comfort are stressed. The goal is to improve the dying person's quality of life.

Follow-up care and support groups for survivors are hospice services. So is support for health team members trying to deal with a person's death.

LEGAL ISSUES

Much attention is given to the right to die. Some people make end-of-life wishes known. The Patient Self-Determination Act and OBRA give persons the right to accept or refuse medical treatment and to make advance directives. An **advance directive** is a document stating a person's wishes about health care when that person cannot make his or her own decisions. Advance directives usually forbid certain care if there is no hope of recovery. These laws protect quality of care. Quality of care cannot be less because of the person's advance directives.

- *Living will*—is a document about measures that support or maintain life when death is likely. Tube feedings, ventilators, and CPR are examples. A living will may instruct doctors:
  - □ Not to start measures that prolong dying
  - □ To remove measures that prolong dying
- *Durable power of attorney*—gives the power to make health care decisions to another person. Usually this is a family member, friend, or lawyer.
- *"Do Not Resuscitate" order*—means that the person will not be resuscitated. The person is allowed to die with peace and dignity. The doctor writes the orders after consulting with the person and family. The family and doctor make the decision if the person is not mentally able to.

SIGNS OF DEATH

There are signs that death is near. These signs may occur rapidly or slowly.

- Movement, muscle tone, and sensation are lost. This usually starts in the feet and legs. It eventually spreads to other body parts. When mouth muscles relax, the jaw drops. The mouth may stay open. The facial expression is often peaceful.
- Peristalsis and other gastrointestinal functions slow down. Abdominal distention, fecal incontinence, fecal impaction, nausea, and vomiting are common.
- Body temperature rises. The person feels cool or cold, looks pale, and perspires heavily.
- Circulation fails. The pulse is fast, weak, and irregular. Blood pressure starts to fall.
- The respiratory system fails. Slow or rapid and shallow respirations are observed. Mucus collects in the airway. This causes the *death rattle* that is heard.
- Pain decreases as the person loses consciousness. However, some people are conscious until the moment of death.

The signs of death include no pulse, respirations, or blood pressure. The pupils are fixed and dilated. A doctor determines that death has occurred and pronounces the person dead.

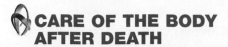 CARE OF THE BODY AFTER DEATH

Care of the body after *(post)* death *(mortem)* is called **postmortem** care. A nurse gives postmortem care. You may be asked to assist. The care begins when the doctor pronounces the person dead.

Postmortem care is done to maintain good appearance of the body. Discoloration and skin damage are prevented. Valuables and personal items are gathered for the family. The right to privacy and the right to be treated with dignity and respect apply after death.

Within 2 to 4 hours after death, rigor mortis develops. **Rigor mortis** is the stiffness or rigidity *(rigor)* of skeletal muscles that occurs after death *(mortis)*. The body is positioned in normal alignment before rigor mortis sets in. The family may want to see the body. The body should appear in a comfortable and natural position for this viewing.

In some agencies the body is prepared only for viewing. The funeral director completes postmortem care.

Postmortem care may involve repositioning the body. Moving the body can cause remaining air in the lungs, stomach, and intestines to be expelled. When air is expelled, sounds are produced. Do not let these sounds alarm or frighten you. They are normal and expected.

DELEGATION GUIDELINES
Postmortem Care

When assisting with postmortem care, you need this information from the nurse:

- If dentures will be inserted or placed in a denture cup
- If tubes will be removed or left in place
- If the family wants to view the body
- Special agency policies and procedures

PROMOTING SAFETY AND COMFORT
Postmortem Care

Safety

Standard Precautions and the Bloodborne Pathogen Standard are followed. You may have contact with blood, body fluids, secretions, or excretions.

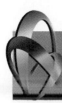

Assisting With Postmortem Care

Pre-Procedure

1 Follow *Delegation Guidelines: Postmortem Care.* See *Promoting Safety and Comfort: Postmortem Care.*
2 Practice hand hygiene.
3 Collect the following:
   • Postmortem kit (shroud or body bag, gown, ID tags, gauze squares, safety pins)
   • Bed protectors
   • Wash basin
   • Bath towels and washcloths
   • Denture cup
   • Tape
   • Dressings
   • Gloves
   • Cotton balls
   • Gown
   • Valuables envelope
4 Provide for privacy.
5 Raise the bed for body mechanics.
6 Make sure the bed is flat.

Procedure

7 Put on the gloves.
8 Position the body supine. Arms and legs are straight. A pillow is under the head and shoulders.
9 Close the eyes. Gently pull the eyelids over the eyes. Apply moist cotton balls gently over the eyelids if the eyes will not stay closed.
10 Insert dentures if it is agency policy. If not, put them in a labeled denture cup.
11 Close the mouth. If necessary, place a rolled towel under the chin to keep the mouth closed.
12 Follow agency policy about jewelry. Remove all jewelry, except for wedding rings if this is agency policy. List the jewelry that you removed. Place the jewelry and the list in a valuables envelope.
13 Place a cotton ball over the rings. Tape them in place.
14 Remove drainage containers. Leave tubes and catheters in place if there will be an autopsy. Ask the nurse about removing tubes.
15 Bathe soiled areas with plain water. Dry thoroughly.
16 Place a bed protector under the buttocks.
17 Remove soiled dressings. Replace them with clean ones.
18 Put a clean gown on the body. Position the body as in step 8.
19 Brush and comb the hair if necessary.
20 Cover the body to the shoulders with a sheet if the family will view the body.
21 Gather the person's belongings. Put them in a bag labeled with the person's name.
22 Remove supplies, equipment, and linens. Straighten the room. Provide soft lighting.
23 Remove the gloves. Decontaminate your hands.
24 Let the family view the body. Provide for privacy. Return to the room after they leave.
25 Decontaminate your hands. Put on gloves.
26 Fill out the ID tags. Tie one to the ankle or to the right big toe.
27 Place the body in the body bag or cover it with a sheet. Or apply the shroud (Fig. 27-1, p. 464).
   a Bring the top down over the head.
   b Fold the bottom up over the feet.
   c Fold the sides over the body.
   d Pin or tape the shroud in place.
28 Attach the second ID tag to the shroud, sheet, or body bag.
29 Leave the denture cup with the body.
30 Pull the privacy curtain around the bed. Or close the door.

Post-Procedure

31 Remove the gloves. Decontaminate your hands.
32 Strip the unit after the body has been removed. Wear gloves for this step.
33 Remove the gloves. Decontaminate your hands.
34 Report the following to the nurse:
   • The time the body was taken by the funeral director
   • What was done with jewelry and personal items
   • What was done with dentures

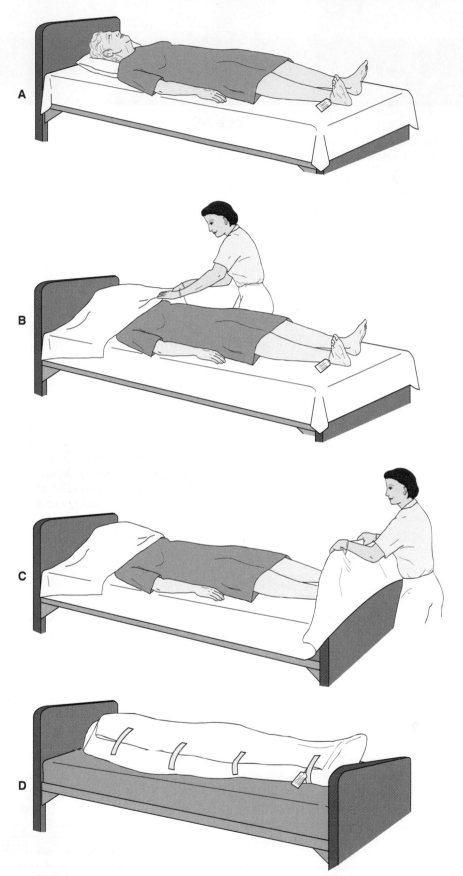

FIG. **27-1** Applying a shroud. **A,** Place the body on the shroud. **B,** Bring the top of the shroud down over the head. **C,** Fold the bottom up over the feet. **D,** Fold the sides over the body. Tape or pin the sides together. Attach the ID tag.

FOCUS ON THE PERSON

A person has the right to die in peace and with dignity. You assist the nurse with the dying person's care. *See Focus on the Person: Caring for the Dying Person.*

Focus on the PERSON

Caring For the Dying Person

Providing comfort—Many dying persons have severe pain. Pain from cancer, surgery, or injuries can be severe. Report complaints of pain or signs of pain to the nurse at once. Follow the comfort measures on the care plan. Gently turn and move the person. Also provide support and reassurance. The person's mental comfort also is important.

Ethical behavior—You may not agree with advance directives and resuscitation decisions. However, you must follow the person's or family's wishes and the doctor's orders. These may be against your personal, religious, and cultural values. If so, discuss the matter with the nurse. An assignment change may be needed.

Remaining independent—The person is encouraged to take part in his or her care to the extent possible. Some days the person can do more than on other days. Follow the nurse's directions and the care plan. Do not force the person to do more than he or she can physically or mentally do.

Speaking up—You may not know what to say to the dying person. That is hard for many experienced health team members. Unless you have been near death yourself, do not say "I understand what you are going through." Such a statement is a communication barrier. Instead you can say:
- "Would you like to talk? I have time to listen."
- "You seem sad. How can I help?"
- "Is it okay if I quietly sit with you for a while?"

OBRA and other laws—The dying person has rights under OBRA:
- *The right to privacy before and after death.* The person has the right not to have his or her body seen by others. Proper draping and screening are important.
- *The right to confidentiality before and after death.* The final moments and cause of death are kept confidential. So are statements, conversations, and family reactions.
- *The right to be free from abuse, mistreatment, and neglect.* The person has the right to receive kind and respectful care before and after death. Always report signs of abuse, mistreatment, or neglect to the nurse at once.
- *Freedom from restraint.* Restraints are used only if ordered by the doctor. Dying persons are often too weak to be dangerous to themselves or others.
- *The right to have personal possessions.* The person may want photos and religious items nearby. Protect the person's property from loss or damage before and after death. They may be family treasures or mementos.
- *The right to personal choice.* The person has the right to be involved in treatment and care. The dying person may refuse treatment. Advance directives are common. The health team must respect choices to refuse treatment or not prolong life.

Nursing teamwork—The nurse may need to spend a lot of time with the dying person. Often it is a busy time before and after someone dies. Offer to take equipment and supplies to and from the room. Also offer to help with other patients and residents.

REVIEW QUESTIONS

Circle the **BEST** answer.

1 Which is *true?*
   a Death from terminal illness is sudden and unexpected.
   b Doctors know when death will occur.
   c An illness is terminal when there is no reasonable hope of recovery.
   d All severe injuries result in death.

2 Reincarnation is the belief that
   a There is no afterlife
   b The spirit or soul is reborn into another human body or another form of life
   c The body keeps its physical form in the afterlife
   d Only the spirit or soul is present in the afterlife

3 Adults and older persons usually fear
   a Dying alone   c The five stages of dying
   b Reincarnation   d Advance directives

4 Persons in the stage of denial
   a Are angry
   b Make "deals" with God
   c Are sad and quiet
   d Refuse to believe they are dying

5 A dying person tries to gain more time during the stage of
   a Anger   c Depression
   b Bargaining   d Acceptance

6 When caring for a dying person, you should
   a Use touch and listen
   b Do most of the talking
   c Keep the room darkened
   d Speak in a loud voice

7 As death nears, the last sense lost is
   a Sight   c Smell
   b Taste   d Hearing

8 The dying person's care includes the following *except*
   a Eye care
   b Mouth care
   c Active range-of-motion exercises
   d Position changes

9 The dying person is positioned in
   a The supine position
   b The Fowler's position
   c Good body alignment
   d The dorsal recumbent position

10 A "Do Not Resuscitate" order was written. This means that
   a CPR will not be done
   b The person has a living will
   c No life-prolonging measures will be carried out
   d The person is kept alive as long as possible

11 The signs of death are
   a Convulsions and incontinence
   b No pulse, respirations, or blood pressure
   c Loss of consciousness and convulsions
   d The eyes stay open, no muscle movements, and the body is rigid

12 Postmortem care is done
   a After rigor mortis sets in
   b After the doctor pronounces the person dead
   c When the funeral director arrives for the body
   d After the family has viewed the body

Answers to these questions are on p. 470.

REVIEW QUESTION ANSWERS

Chapter 1: INTRODUCTION TO HEALTH CARE AGENCIES

1 b
2 b
3 c
4 b
5 a
6 a
7 a
8 c
9 d
10 T
11 T
12 F
13 F
14 F
15 T
16 F
17 F
18 T
19 T
20 T
21 F
22 T
23 F
24 T
25 T

Chapter 2: THE NURSING ASSISTANT

1 a
2 a
3 b
4 a
5 c
6 b
7 c
8 d
9 a
10 a
11 b
12 a
13 a
14 c

Chapter 3: WORK ETHICS

1 c
2 d
3 d
4 d
5 c
6 c
7 d
8 c
9 a
10 c
11 d
12 a
13 d
14 c

Chapter 4: COMMUNICATING WITH THE HEALTH TEAM

1 a
2 d
3 d
4 d
5 c
6 c
7 c
8 c
9 d
10 d
11 b
12 c
13 d
14 b

Chapter 5: UNDERSTANDING THE PERSON

1 c
2 d
3 b
4 d
5 d
6 b

7 d
8 c
9 a
10 d
11 c
12 b

Chapter 6: UNDERSTANDING BODY STRUCTURE AND FUNCTION

1 a
2 b
3 c
4 c
5 a
6 b
7 c
8 d
9 d
10 b
11 a
12 b
13 b
14 b
15 c
16 d
17 a
18 b

Chapter 7: CARING FOR THE OLDER PERSON

1 a
2 d
3 b
4 c
5 a
6 b
7 b
8 a
9 a
10 c
11 a
12 a

13 c
14 b
15 a

Chapter 8: PROMOTING SAFETY

1   T
2   F
3   T
4   T
5   F
6   T
7   F
8   T
9   T
10 T
11 F
12 c
13 c
14 d
15 c
16 d
17 d
18 c
19 b
20 c
21 b
22 d
23 b
24 d
25 b
26 c
27 a
28 d

Chapter 9: RESTRAINT ALTERNATIVES AND SAFE RESTRAINT USE

1   F
2   F
3   F
4   T
5   T
6   T
7   T
8   T
9   F
10 F
11 F
12 T
13 F
14 T
15 F
16 d
17 a

18 c
19 b
20 c
21 a
22 d
23 a
24 c
25 c
26 d

Chapter 10: PREVENTING INFECTION

1   T
2   F
3   F
4   F
5   F
6   b
7   d
8   d
9   d
10 c
11 a
12 d
13 c
14 a
15 d
16 d

Chapter 11: USING BODY MECHANICS

1   d
2   b
3   a
4   b
5   a
6   a
7   b
8   a
9   b
10 a
11 a
12 a
13 a
14 b
15 b
16 a
17 d
18 b
19 c
20 c
21 b
22 a

Chapter 12: ASSISTING WITH COMFORT

1   d
2   a
3   d
4   b
5   c
6   b
7   c
8   b
9   b
10 a
11 a
12 d
13 c
14 a
15 b
16 T
17 F
18 F
19 T
20 F

Chapter 13: ASSISTING WITH HYGIENE

1   T
2   T
3   F
4   F
5   F
6   F
7   F
8   F
9   F
10 T
11 T
12 T
13 d
14 b
15 c
16 c
17 d

Chapter 14: ASSISTING WITH GROOMING

1   d
2   b
3   c
4   a
5   d
6   d
7   b
8   d

9 b
10 F
11 F
12 T
13 T
14 F

Chapter 15: ASSISTING WITH URINARY ELIMINATION

1 b
2 d
3 a
4 b
5 b
6 a
7 a
8 d
9 c
10 d

Chapter 16: ASSISTING WITH BOWEL ELIMINATION

1 a
2 b
3 d
4 a
5 c
6 d
7 b
8 c
9 d
10 c

Chapter 17: ASSISTING WITH NUTRITION AND FLUIDS

1 a
2 a
3 d
4 d
5 c
6 a
7 c
8 d
9 d
10 a
11 c
12 c
13 b
14 a
15 c
16 a

Chapter 18: ASSISTING WITH ASSESSMENT

1 b
2 a
3 a
4 b
5 d
6 b
7 c
8 a
9 b
10 b
11 c
12 c
13 c
14 d

Chapter 19: ASSISTING WITH SPECIMENS

1 d
2 b
3 c
4 d
5 c
6 a
7 b

Chapter 20: ASSISTING WITH EXERCISE AND ACTIVITY

1 a
2 b
3 c
4 b
5 b
6 c
7 a
8 b
9 c
10 b
11 F
12 F
13 T
14 F
15 T

Chapter 21: ASSISTING WITH WOUND CARE

1 c
2 b
3 c
4 a
5 a

6 a
7 d
8 c
9 c
10 b
11 d
12 d
13 c
14 a

Chapter 22: ASSISTING WITH OXYGEN NEEDS

1 c
2 c
3 b
4 a
5 d
6 a
7 d
8 a

Chapter 23: ASSISTING WITH REHABILITATION AND RESTORATIVE CARE

1 c
2 b
3 a
4 d
5 a
6 c
7 c
8 T
9 T
10 T
11 F
12 T

Chapter 24: CARING FOR PERSONS WITH COMMON HEALTH PROBLEMS

1 a
2 c
3 a
4 a
5 d
6 c
7 b
8 c
9 b
10 a
11 c
12 b

13 a
14 b
15 c
16 d
17 a
18 d
19 b
20 c
21 a
22 c
23 a
24 d
25 c
26 b
27 d
28 c
29 c
30 d

Chapter 25: CARING FOR PERSONS WITH CONFUSION AND DEMENTIA

1 a
2 b
3 a

4 a
5 d
6 d
7 b
8 b
9 a
10 d
11 c
12 a

Chapter 26: ASSISTING WITH EMERGENCY CARE

1 a
2 c
3 d
4 c
5 b
6 c
7 c
8 b
9 b
10 a
11 a
12 c
13 b

14 c
15 a
16 b

Chapter 27: CARING FOR THE DYING PERSON

1 c
2 b
3 a
4 d
5 b
6 a
7 d
8 c
9 c
10 a
11 b
12 b

Appendix A

NATIONAL NURSE AIDE ASSESSMENT PROGRAM (NNAAP™) WRITTEN EXAMINATION CONTENT OUTLINE

The NNAAP Written Examination is comprised of seventy (70) multiple choice questions. Ten (10) of these questions are pre-test (non-scored) questions on which statistical information will be collected.

I. Physical Care Skills

A. Activities of Daily Living ..... 14% of exam
   1. Hygiene
   2. Dressing and Grooming
   3. Nutrition and Hydration
   4. Elimination
   5. Rest/Sleep/Comfort
B. Basic Nursing Skills .... 35% of exam
   1. Infection Control
   2. Safety/Emergency
   3. Therapeutic/Technical Procedures
   4. Data Collection and Reporting
C. Restorative Skills .... 8% of exam
   1. Prevention
   2. Self Care/Independence

II. Psychosocial Care Skills

A. Emotional and Mental Health
   Needs .... 10% of exam
B. Spiritual and Cultural
   Needs .... 4% of exam

III. Role of the Nurse Aide

A. Communication .... 7% of exam
B. Client Rights .... 7% of exam
C. Legal and Ethical Behavior .... 5% of exam
D. Member of the Health Care
   Team .... 10% of exam

NATIONAL NURSE AIDE ASSESSMENT PROGRAM (NNAAP™) SKILLS EVALUATION

List of Skills

1. Washes hands
2. Measures and records weight of ambulatory client
3. Provides mouth care
4. Dresses client with affected (weak) right arm
5. Transfers client from bed to wheelchair
6. Assists client to ambulate
7. Cleans and stores dentures
8. Performs passive range-of-motion (ROM) on one shoulder
9. Performs passive range-of-motion (ROM) on one knee and one ankle
10. Measures and records urinary output
11. Assists clients with use of bedpan
12. Provides perineal care (peri-care) for incontinent client
13. Provides catheter care
14. Measures and records oral temperature with a glass thermometer
15. Counts and records radial pulse
16. Counts and records respirations
17. Measures and records blood pressure
18. Puts one knee-high elastic stocking on client
19. Makes an occupied bed
20. Provides foot care on one foot
21. Provides fingernail care on one hand
22. Feeds client who cannot feed self
23. Positions client on side
24. Gives modified bed bath (face, and one arm, hand, and underarm)
25. Shampoos client's hair in bed

Appendix B

MINIMUM DATA SET (MDS) — *VERSION 2.0*
FOR NURSING HOME RESIDENT ASSESSMENT AND CARE SCREENING

BASIC ASSESSMENT TRACKING FORM

SECTION AA. IDENTIFICATION INFORMATION

1.	RESIDENT NAME⊙				
		a. (First)	b. (Middle Initial)	c. (Last)	d. (Jr/Sr)
2.	GENDER⊙	1. Male	2. Female		
3.	BIRTHDATE⊙	Month	Day	Year	
4.	RACE/ ETHNICITY⊙	1. American Indian/Alaskan Native 2. Asian/Pacific Islander 3. Black, not of Hispanic origin	4. Hispanic 5. White, not of Hispanic origin		
5.	SOCIAL SECURITY AND MEDICARE NUMBERS⊙ [C in 1st box if non med. no.]	a. Social Security Number b. Medicare number (or comparable railroad insurance number)			
6.	FACILITY PROVIDER NO.⊙	a. State No. b. Federal No.			
7.	MEDICAID NO. ["+" if pending, "N" if not a Medicaid recipient] ⊙				
8.	REASONS FOR ASSESS- MENT	[Note—Other codes do not apply to this form] **a.** Primary reason for assessment 1. Admission assessment (required by day 14) 2. Annual assessment 3. Significant change in status assessment 4. Significant correction of prior full assessment 5. Quarterly review assessment 10. Significant correction of prior quarterly assessment 0. *NONE OF ABOVE* **b.** *Codes for assessments required for Medicare PPS or the State* *1. Medicare 5 day assessment* *2. Medicare 30 day assessment* *3. Medicare 60 day assessment* *4. Medicare 90 day assessment* *5. Medicare readmission/return assessment* *6. Other state required assessment* *7. Medicare 14 day assessment* *8. Other Medicare required assessment*			

9. Signatures of Persons who Completed a Portion of the Accompanying Assessment or Tracking Form

I certify that the accompanying information accurately reflects resident assessment or tracking information for this resident and that I collected or coordinated collection of this information on the dates specified. To the best of my knowledge, this information was collected in accordance with applicable Medicare and Medicaid requirements. I understand that this information is used as a basis for ensuring that residents receive appropriate and quality care, and as a basis for payment from federal funds. I further understand that payment of such federal funds and continued participation in the government-funded health care programs is conditioned on the accuracy and truthfulness of this information, and that I may be personally subject to or may subject my organization to substantial criminal, civil, and/or administrative penalties for submitting false information. I also certify that I am authorized to submit this information by this facility on its behalf.

Signature and Title	Sections	Date
a.		
b.		
c.		
d.		
e.		
f.		
g.		
h.		
i.		
j.		
k.		
l.		

GENERAL INSTRUCTIONS

Complete this information for submission with all full and quarterly assessments (Admission, Annual, Significant Change, State or Medicare required assessments, or Quarterly Reviews, etc.)

⊙ = Key items for computerized resident tracking

☐ = When box blank, must enter number or letter   a. ☐ = When letter in box, check if condition applies

MDS 2.0 September, 2000

From Centers for Medicare and Medicaid Services, http://cms.ohhs.gov/medicaid/mds20.

Resident_____   Numeric Identifier_____

MINIMUM DATA SET (MDS) — *VERSION 2.0*
FOR NURSING HOME RESIDENT ASSESSMENT AND CARE SCREENING
BACKGROUND (FACE SHEET) INFORMATION AT ADMISSION

SECTION AB. DEMOGRAPHIC INFORMATION

1.	DATE OF ENTRY	*Date the stay began. Note — Does not include readmission if record was closed at time of temporary discharge to hospital, etc. In such cases, use prior admission date* ☐☐ — ☐☐ — ☐☐☐☐ Month — Day — Year
2.	ADMITTED FROM (AT ENTRY)	1. Private home/apt. with no home health services 2. Private home/apt. with home health services 3. Board and care/assisted living/group home 4. Nursing home 5. Acute care hospital 6. Psychiatric hospital, MR/DD facility 7. Rehabilitation hospital 8. Other
3.	LIVED ALONE (PRIOR TO ENTRY)	0. No 1. Yes 2. In other facility
4.	ZIP CODE OF PRIOR PRIMARY RESIDENCE	☐☐☐☐☐
5.	RESIDEN-TIAL HISTORY 5 YEARS PRIOR TO ENTRY	(*Check all settings resident **lived in** during 5 years prior to date of entry given in item AB1 above*) Prior stay at this nursing home — a. Stay in other nursing home — b. Other residential facility—board and care home, assisted living, group home — c. MH/psychiatric setting — d. MR/DD setting — e. *NONE OF ABOVE* — f.
6.	LIFETIME OCCUPA-TION(S) [Put "/" between two occupations]	☐☐☐☐☐☐☐☐☐☐☐☐☐☐☐
7.	EDUCATION (*Highest Level Completed*)	1. No schooling 5. Technical or trade school 2. 8th grade/less 6. Some college 3. 9-11 grades 7. Bachelor's degree 4. High school 8. Graduate degree
8.	LANGUAGE	(*Code for correct response*) **a.** Primary Language 0. English 1. Spanish 2. French 3. Other **b. If other, specify** ☐☐☐☐☐☐☐☐
9.	MENTAL HEALTH HISTORY	Does resident's RECORD indicate any history of mental retardation, mental illness, or developmental disability problem? 0. No 1. Yes

10.	CONDITIONS RELATED TO MR/DD STATUS	(*Check all conditions that are related to MR/DD status that were manifested before age 22, and are likely to continue indefinitely*)
		Not applicable—no MR/DD (Skip to AB11) — a.
		MR/DD with organic condition
		    Down's syndrome — b.
		    Autism — c.
		    Epilepsy — d.
		    Other organic condition related to MR/DD — e.
		MR/DD with no organic condition — f.

11.	DATE BACK-GROUND INFORMA-TION COMPLETED	☐☐ — ☐☐ — ☐☐☐☐ Month — Day — Year

SECTION AC. CUSTOMARY ROUTINE

1.	CUSTOMARY ROUTINE (*In year prior to DATE OF ENTRY to this nursing home, or year last in community if now being admitted from another nursing home*)	(*Check all that apply. If all information UNKNOWN, check last box only.*)

CYCLE OF DAILY EVENTS

Stays up late at night (e.g., after 9 pm)	a.
Naps regularly during day (at least 1 hour)	b.
Goes out 1+ days a week	c.
Stays busy with hobbies, reading, or fixed daily routine	d.
Spends most of time alone or watching TV	e.
Moves independently indoors (with appliances, if used)	f.
Use of tobacco products at least daily	g.
NONE OF ABOVE	h.

EATING PATTERNS

Distinct food preferences	i.
Eats between meals all or most days	j.
Use of alcoholic beverage(s) at least weekly	k.
NONE OF ABOVE	l.

ADL PATTERNS

In bedclothes much of day	m.
Wakens to toilet all or most nights	n.
Has irregular bowel movement pattern	o.
Showers for bathing	p.
Bathing in PM	q.
NONE OF ABOVE	r.

INVOLVEMENT PATTERNS

Daily contact with relatives/close friends	s.
Usually attends church, temple, synagogue (etc.)	t.
Finds strength in faith	u.
Daily animal companion/presence	v.
Involved in group activities	w.
NONE OF ABOVE	x.
UNKNOWN—Resident/family unable to provide information	y.

SECTION AD. FACE SHEET SIGNATURES

SIGNATURES OF PERSONS COMPLETING FACE SHEET:

a. Signature of RN Assessment Coordinator   Date

I certify that the accompanying information accurately reflects resident assessment or tracking information for this resident and that I collected or coordinated collection of this information on the dates specified. To the best of my knowledge, this information was collected in accordance with applicable Medicare and Medicaid requirements. I understand that this information is used as a basis for ensuring that residents receive appropriate and quality care, and as a basis for payment from federal funds. I further understand that payment of such federal funds and continued partici-pation in the government-funded health care programs is conditioned on the accuracy and truthful-ness of this information, and that I may be personally subject to or may subject my organization to substantial criminal, civil, and/or administrative penalties for submitting false information. I also certify that I am authorized to submit this information by this facility on its behalf.

	Signature and Title	Sections	Date
b.			
c.			
d.			
e.			
f.			
g.			

☐ = When box blank, must enter number or letter   ☐a. = When letter in box, check if condition applies   MDS 2.0 September, 2000

Resident_____ Numeric Identifier_____

MINIMUM DATA SET (MDS) — *VERSION 2.0*
FOR NURSING HOME RESIDENT ASSESSMENT AND CARE SCREENING
FULL ASSESSMENT FORM
(Status in last 7 days, unless other time frame indicated)

SECTION A. IDENTIFICATION AND BACKGROUND INFORMATION

1. RESIDENT NAME
a. (First) b. (Middle Initial) c. (Last) d. (Jr/Sr)

2. ROOM NUMBER

3. ASSESSMENT REFERENCE DATE
a. Last day of MDS observation period
Month — Day — Year
b. Original (0) or corrected copy of form (enter number of correction)

4a. DATE OF REENTRY
Date of reentry from most recent temporary discharge to a hospital in last 90 days (or since last assessment or admission if less than 90 days)
Month — Day — Year

5. MARITAL STATUS
1. Never married 3. Widowed 5. Divorced
2. Married 4. Separated

6. MEDICAL RECORD NO.

7. CURRENT PAYMENT SOURCES FOR N.H. STAY
(Billing Office to indicate; *check all that apply in last 30 days*)
- Medicaid per diem — a.
- Medicare per diem — b.
- Medicare ancillary part A — c.
- Medicare ancillary part B — d.
- CHAMPUS per diem — e.
- VA per diem — f.
- Self or family pays for full per diem — g.
- Medicaid resident liability or Medicare co-payment — h.
- Private insurance per diem (including co-payment) — i.
- Other per diem — j.

8. REASONS FOR ASSESSMENT
a. Primary reason for assessment
1. Admission assessment (required by day 14)
2. Annual assessment
3. Significant change in status assessment
4. Significant correction of prior full assessment
5. Quarterly review assessment
6. Discharged—return not anticipated
7. Discharged—return anticipated
8. Discharged prior to completing initial assessment
9. Reentry
10. Significant correction of prior quarterly assessment
0. NONE OF ABOVE

[Note—If this is a discharge or reentry assessment, only a limited subset of MDS items need be completed]

b. *Codes for assessments required for Medicare PPS or the State*
1. Medicare 5 day assessment
2. Medicare 30 day assessment
3. Medicare 60 day assessment
4. Medicare 90 day assessment
5. Medicare readmission/return assessment
6. Other state required assessment
7. Medicare 14 day assessment
8. Other Medicare required assessment

9. RESPONSIBILITY/ LEGAL GUARDIAN
(*Check all that apply*)
- Legal guardian — a.
- Other legal oversight — b.
- Durable power of attorney/health care — c.
- Durable power attorney/financial — d.
- Family member responsible — e.
- Patient responsible for self — f.
- NONE OF ABOVE — g.

10. ADVANCED DIRECTIVES
(For those items with supporting *documentation* in the medical record, *check all that apply*)
- Living will — a.
- Do not resuscitate — b.
- Do not hospitalize — c.
- Organ donation — d.
- Autopsy request — e.
- Feeding restrictions — f.
- Medication restrictions — g.
- Other treatment restrictions — h.
- NONE OF ABOVE — i.

SECTION B. COGNITIVE PATTERNS

1. COMATOSE
(*Persistent vegetative state/no discernible consciousness*)
0. No 1. Yes (**If yes, skip to Section G**)

2. MEMORY
(*Recall of what was learned or known*)
a. Short-term memory OK—seems/appears to recall after 5 minutes
0. Memory OK 1. Memory problem
b. Long-term memory OK—seems/appears to recall long past
0. Memory OK 1. Memory problem

3. MEMORY/ RECALL ABILITY
(*Check all that resident was **normally able to recall** during last 7 days*)
- Current season — a.
- Location of own room — b.
- Staff names/faces — c.
- That he/she is in a nursing home — d.
- NONE OF ABOVE are recalled — e.

4. COGNITIVE SKILLS FOR DAILY DECISION-MAKING
(*Made decisions regarding tasks of daily life*)
0. INDEPENDENT—decisions consistent/reasonable
1. MODIFIED INDEPENDENCE—some difficulty in new situations only
2. MODERATELY IMPAIRED—decisions poor; cues/supervision required
3. SEVERELY IMPAIRED—never/rarely made decisions

5. INDICATORS OF DELIRIUM— PERIODIC DISORDERED THINKING/ AWARENESS
(*Code for behavior in the last 7 days.*) [**Note:** Accurate assessment requires conversations with staff and family who have direct knowledge of resident's behavior over this time].
0. Behavior not present
1. Behavior present, not of recent onset
2. Behavior present, over last 7 days appears different from resident's usual functioning (e.g., new onset or worsening)

a. EASILY DISTRACTED—(e.g., difficulty paying attention; gets sidetracked)
b. PERIODS OF ALTERED PERCEPTION OR AWARENESS OF SURROUNDINGS—(e.g., moves lips or talks to someone not present; believes he/she is somewhere else; confuses night and day)
c. EPISODES OF DISORGANIZED SPEECH—(e.g., speech is incoherent, nonsensical, irrelevant, or rambling from subject to subject; loses train of thought)
d. PERIODS OF RESTLESSNESS—(e.g., fidgeting or picking at skin, clothing, napkins, etc; frequent position changes; repetitive physical movements or calling out)
e. PERIODS OF LETHARGY—(e.g., sluggishness; staring into space; difficult to arouse; little body movement)
f. MENTAL FUNCTION VARIES OVER THE COURSE OF THE DAY—(e.g., sometimes better, sometimes worse; behaviors sometimes present, sometimes not)

6. CHANGE IN COGNITIVE STATUS
Resident's cognitive status, skills, or abilities have changed as compared to status of **90 days ago** (or since last assessment if less than 90 days)
0. No change 1. Improved 2. Deteriorated

SECTION C. COMMUNICATION/HEARING PATTERNS

1. HEARING
(*With hearing appliance, if used*)
0. HEARS ADEQUATELY—normal talk, TV, phone
1. MINIMAL DIFFICULTY when not in quiet setting
2. HEARS IN SPECIAL SITUATIONS ONLY—speaker has to adjust tonal quality and speak distinctly
3. HIGHLY IMPAIRED/absence of useful hearing

2. COMMUNICATION DEVICES/ TECHNIQUES
(*Check all that apply* during last 7 days)
- Hearing aid, present and used — a.
- Hearing aid, present and not used regularly — b.
- Other receptive comm. techniques used (e.g., lip reading) — c.
- NONE OF ABOVE — d.

3. MODES OF EXPRESSION
(*Check all used* by resident to make needs known)
- Speech — a.
- Writing messages to express or clarify needs — b.
- American sign language or Braille — c.
- Signs/gestures/sounds — d.
- Communication board — e.
- Other — f.
- NONE OF ABOVE — g.

4. MAKING SELF UNDERSTOOD
(*Expressing information content—however able*)
0. UNDERSTOOD
1. USUALLY UNDERSTOOD—difficulty finding words or finishing thoughts
2. SOMETIMES UNDERSTOOD—ability is limited to making concrete requests
3. RARELY/NEVER UNDERSTOOD

5. SPEECH CLARITY
(*Code for speech in the last 7 days*)
0. CLEAR SPEECH—distinct, intelligible words
1. UNCLEAR SPEECH—slurred, mumbled words
2. NO SPEECH—absence of spoken words

6. ABILITY TO UNDERSTAND OTHERS
(*Understanding verbal information content—however able*)
0. UNDERSTANDS
1. USUALLY UNDERSTANDS—may miss some part/intent of message
2. SOMETIMES UNDERSTANDS—responds adequately to simple, direct communication
3. RARELY/NEVER UNDERSTANDS

7. CHANGE IN COMMUNICATION/ HEARING
Resident's ability to express, understand, or hear information has changed as compared to status of **90 days ago** (or since last assessment if less than 90 days)
0. No change 1. Improved 2. Deteriorated

☐ = When box blank, must enter number or letter ⬚a. = When letter in box, check if condition applies

MDS 2.0 September, 2000

Resident _____   Numeric Identifier _____

SECTION D. VISION PATTERNS

1.	VISION	(Ability to see in adequate light and with glasses if used) 0. ADEQUATE—sees fine detail, including regular print in newspapers/books 1. IMPAIRED—sees large print, but not regular print in newspapers/books 2. MODERATELY IMPAIRED—limited vision, not able to see newspaper headlines, but can identify objects 3. HIGHLY IMPAIRED—object identification in question, but eyes appear to follow objects 4. SEVERELY IMPAIRED—no vision or sees only light, colors, or shapes; eyes do not appear to follow objects	
2.	VISUAL LIMITATIONS/ DIFFICULTIES	Side vision problems—decreased peripheral vision (e.g., leaves food on one side of tray, difficulty traveling, bumps into people and objects, misjudges placement of chair when seating self)	a.
		Experiences any of following: sees halos or rings around lights; sees flashes of light; sees "curtains" over eyes	b.
		NONE OF ABOVE	c.
3.	VISUAL APPLIANCES	Glasses; contact lenses; magnifying glass 0. No 1. Yes	

SECTION E. MOOD AND BEHAVIOR PATTERNS

1.	INDICATORS OF DEPRES- SION, ANXIETY, SAD MOOD	(Code for indicators observed in last 30 days, irrespective of the assumed cause) 0. Indicator not exhibited in last 30 days 1. Indicator of this type exhibited up to five days a week 2. Indicator of this type exhibited daily or almost daily (6, 7 days a week)

VERBAL EXPRESSIONS OF DISTRESS

a. Resident made negative statements—e.g., "Nothing matters; Would rather be dead; What's the use; Regrets having lived so long; Let me die"

b. Repetitive questions—e.g., "Where do I go; What do I do?"

c. Repetitive verbalizations— e.g., calling out for help, ("God help me")

d. Persistent anger with self or others—e.g., easily annoyed, anger at placement in nursing home; anger at care received

e. Self deprecation—e.g., "I am nothing; I am of no use to anyone"

f. Expressions of what appear to be unrealistic fears—e.g., fear of being abandoned, left alone, being with others

g. Recurrent statements that something terrible is about to happen—e.g., believes he or she is about to die, have a heart attack

h. Repetitive health complaints—e.g., persistently seeks medical attention, obsessive concern with body functions

i. Repetitive anxious complaints/concerns (non-health related) e.g., persistently seeks attention/ reassurance regarding schedules, meals, laundry, clothing, relationship issues

SLEEP-CYCLE ISSUES

j. Unpleasant mood in morning

k. Insomnia/change in usual sleep pattern

SAD, APATHETIC, ANXIOUS APPEARANCE

l. Sad, pained, worried facial expressions—e.g., furrowed brows

m. Crying, tearfulness

n. Repetitive physical movements—e.g., pacing, hand wringing, restlessness, fidgeting, picking

LOSS OF INTEREST

o. Withdrawal from activities of interest—e.g., no interest in long standing activities or being with family/friends

p. Reduced social interaction

2.	MOOD PERSIS- TENCE	One or more indicators of depressed, sad or anxious mood were not easily altered by attempts to "cheer up", console, or reassure the resident over last 7 days 0. No mood 1. Indicators present, 2. Indicators present, indicators easily altered not easily altered
3.	CHANGE IN MOOD	Resident's mood status has changed as compared to status of 90 days ago (or since last assessment if less than 90 days) 0. No change 1. Improved 2. Deteriorated
4.	BEHAVIORAL SYMPTOMS	(A) Behavioral symptom frequency in last 7 days 0. Behavior not exhibited in last 7 days 1. Behavior of this type occurred 1 to 3 days in last 7 days 2. Behavior of this type occurred 4 to 6 days, but less than daily 3. Behavior of this type occurred daily (B) Behavioral symptom alterability in last 7 days 0. Behavior not present OR behavior was easily altered 1. Behavior was not easily altered

		(A)	(B)
a. WANDERING (moved with no rational purpose, seemingly oblivious to needs or safety)			
b. VERBALLY ABUSIVE BEHAVIORAL SYMPTOMS (others were threatened, screamed at, cursed at)			
c. PHYSICALLY ABUSIVE BEHAVIORAL SYMPTOMS (others were hit, shoved, scratched, sexually abused)			
d. SOCIALLY INAPPROPRIATE/DISRUPTIVE BEHAVIORAL SYMPTOMS (made disruptive sounds, noisiness, screaming, self-abusive acts, sexual behavior or disrobing in public, smeared/threw food/feces, hoarding, rummaged through others' belongings)			
e. RESISTS CARE (resisted taking medications/ injections, ADL assistance, or eating)			

5.	CHANGE IN BEHAVIORAL SYMPTOMS	Resident's behavior status has changed as compared to status of 90 days ago (or since last assessment if less than 90 days) 0. No change 1. Improved 2. Deteriorated	

SECTION F. PSYCHOSOCIAL WELL-BEING

1.	SENSE OF INITIATIVE/ INVOLVE- MENT	At ease interacting with others	a.
		At ease doing planned or structured activities	b.
		At ease doing self-initiated activities	c.
		Establishes own goals	d.
		Pursues involvement in life of facility (e.g., makes/keeps friends; involved in group activities; responds positively to new activities; assists at religious services)	e.
		Accepts invitations into most group activities	f.
		NONE OF ABOVE	g.
2.	UNSETTLED RELATION- SHIPS	Covert/open conflict with or repeated criticism of staff	a.
		Unhappy with roommate	b.
		Unhappy with residents other than roommate	c.
		Openly expresses conflict/anger with family/friends	d.
		Absence of personal contact with family/friends	e.
		Recent loss of close family member/friend	f.
		Does not adjust easily to change in routines	g.
		NONE OF ABOVE	h.
3.	PAST ROLES	Strong identification with past roles and life status	a.
		Expresses sadness/anger/empty feeling over lost roles/status	b.
		Resident perceives that daily routine (customary routine, activities) is very different from prior pattern in the community	c.
		NONE OF ABOVE	d.

SECTION G. PHYSICAL FUNCTIONING AND STRUCTURAL PROBLEMS

1. (A) ADL SELF-PERFORMANCE—(Code for resident's PERFORMANCE OVER ALL SHIFTS during last 7 days—Not including setup)

0. INDEPENDENT—No help or oversight —OR— Help/oversight provided only 1 or 2 times during last 7 days

1. SUPERVISION—Oversight, encouragement or cueing provided 3 or more times during last 7 days —OR— Supervision (3 or more times) plus physical assistance provided only 1 or 2 times during last 7 days

2. LIMITED ASSISTANCE—Resident highly involved in activity; received physical help in guided maneuvering of limbs or other nonweight bearing assistance 3 or more times — OR—More help provided only 1 or 2 times during last 7 days

3. EXTENSIVE ASSISTANCE—While resident performed part of activity, over last 7-day period, help of following type(s) provided 3 or more times:
—Weight-bearing support
— Full staff performance during part (but not all) of last 7 days

4. TOTAL DEPENDENCE—Full staff performance of activity during entire 7 days

8. ACTIVITY DID NOT OCCUR during entire 7 days

(B) ADL SUPPORT PROVIDED—(Code for MOST SUPPORT PROVIDED OVER ALL SHIFTS during last 7 days; code regardless of resident's self-performance classification)

0. No setup or physical help from staff
1. Setup help only
2. One person physical assist   8. ADL activity itself did not
3. Two+ persons physical assist   occur during entire 7 days

			(A) SELF-PERF	(B) SUPPORT
a.	BED MOBILITY	How resident moves to and from lying position, turns side to side, and positions body while in bed		
b.	TRANSFER	How resident moves between surfaces—to/from: bed, chair, wheelchair, standing position (EXCLUDE to/from bath/toilet)		
c.	WALK IN ROOM	How resident walks between locations in his/her room		
d.	WALK IN CORRIDOR	How resident walks in corridor on unit		
e.	LOCOMO- TION ON UNIT	How resident moves between locations in his/her room and adjacent corridor on same floor. If in wheelchair, self-sufficiency once in chair		
f.	LOCOMO- TION OFF UNIT	How resident moves to and returns from off unit locations (e.g., areas set aside for dining, activities, or treatments). If facility has only one floor, how resident moves to and from distant areas on the floor. If in wheelchair, self-sufficiency once in chair		
g.	DRESSING	How resident puts on, fastens, and takes off all items of street clothing, including donning/removing prosthesis		
h.	EATING	How resident eats and drinks (regardless of skill). Includes intake of nourishment by other means (e.g., tube feeding, total parenteral nutrition)		
i.	TOILET USE	How resident uses the toilet room (or commode, bedpan, urinal); transfer on/off toilet, cleanses, changes pad, manages ostomy or catheter, adjusts clothes		
j.	PERSONAL HYGIENE	How resident maintains personal hygiene, including combing hair, brushing teeth, shaving, applying makeup, washing/drying face, hands, and perineum (EXCLUDE baths and showers)		

Resident _____   Numeric Identifier _____

2.	BATHING	How resident takes full-body bath/shower, sponge bath, and transfers in/out of tub/shower (EXCLUDE washing of back and hair.) *Code for most dependent in self-performance and support.* **(A)** BATHING SELF-PERFORMANCE codes appear below	(A)	(B)
		0. Independent—No help provided		
		1. Supervision—Oversight help only		
		2. Physical help limited to transfer only		
		3. Physical help in part of bathing activity		
		4. Total dependence		
		8. Activity itself did not occur during entire 7 days *(Bathing support codes are as defined in **Item 1, code B above**)*		

3.	TEST FOR BALANCE (see training manual)	*(Code for ability during test in the **last 7 days**)* 0. Maintained position as required in test 1. Unsteady, but able to rebalance self without physical support 2. Partial physical support during test; or stands (sits) but does not follow directions for test 3. Not able to attempt test without physical help	
		a. Balance while standing	
		b. Balance while sitting—position, trunk control	

4.	FUNCTIONAL LIMITATION IN RANGE OF MOTION (see training manual)	*(Code for limitations during **last 7 days** that interfered with daily functions or placed resident at risk of injury)* **(A)** *RANGE OF MOTION* 0. No limitation 1. Limitation on one side 2. Limitation on both sides **(B)** *VOLUNTARY MOVEMENT* 0. No loss 1. Partial loss 2. Full loss	(A)	(B)
		a. Neck		
		b. Arm—Including shoulder or elbow		
		c. Hand—Including wrist or fingers		
		d. Leg—Including hip or knee		
		e. Foot—Including ankle or toes		
		f. Other limitation or loss		

5.	MODES OF LOCOMOTION	*(**Check all that apply** during last 7 days)*	
		Cane/walker/crutch — a.	Wheelchair primary mode of locomotion — d.
		Wheeled self — b.	
		Other person wheeled — c.	NONE OF ABOVE — e.

6.	MODES OF TRANSFER	*(**Check all that apply** during last 7 days)*	
		Bedfast all or most of time — a.	Lifted mechanically — d.
		Bed rails used for bed mobility or transfer — b.	Transfer aid (e.g., slide board, trapeze, cane, walker, brace) — e.
		Lifted manually — c.	NONE OF ABOVE — f.

7.	TASK SEGMENTA-TION	Some or all of ADL activities were broken into subtasks during **last 7 days** so that resident could perform them 0. No 1. Yes	

8.	ADL FUNCTIONAL REHABILITA-TION POTENTIAL	Resident believes he/she is capable of increased independence in at least some ADLs	a.
		Direct care staff believe resident is capable of increased independence in at least some ADLs	b.
		Resident able to perform tasks/activity but is very slow	c.
		Difference in ADL Self-Performance or ADL Support, comparing mornings to evenings	d.
		NONE OF ABOVE	e.

9.	CHANGE IN ADL FUNCTION	Resident's ADL self-performance status has changed as compared to status of **90 days ago** (or since last assessment if less than 90 days) 0. No change 1. Improved 2. Deteriorated	

SECTION H. CONTINENCE IN LAST 14 DAYS

1.	CONTINENCE SELF-CONTROL CATEGORIES *(**Code for resident's PERFORMANCE OVER ALL SHIFTS**)*
	0. *CONTINENT*—Complete control *[includes use of indwelling urinary catheter or ostomy device that does not leak urine or stool]*
	1. *USUALLY CONTINENT*—BLADDER, incontinent episodes once a week or less; BOWEL, less than weekly
	2. *OCCASIONALLY INCONTINENT*—BLADDER, 2 or more times a week but not daily; BOWEL, once a week
	3. *FREQUENTLY INCONTINENT*—BLADDER, tended to be incontinent daily, but some control present (e.g., on day shift); BOWEL, 2-3 times a week
	4. *INCONTINENT*—Had inadequate control BLADDER, multiple daily episodes; BOWEL, all (or almost all) of the time

a.	BOWEL CONTI-NENCE	Control of bowel movement, with appliance or bowel continence programs, if employed	
b.	BLADDER CONTI-NENCE	Control of urinary bladder function (if dribbles, volume insufficient to soak through underpants), with appliances (e.g., foley) or continence programs, if employed	

2.	BOWEL ELIMINATION PATTERN	Bowel elimination pattern regular—at least one movement every three days — a.	Diarrhea — c.
		Constipation — b.	Fecal impaction — d.
			NONE OF ABOVE — e.

3.	APPLIANCES AND PROGRAMS	Any scheduled toileting plan — a.	Did not use toilet room/commode/urinal — f.
		Bladder retraining program — b.	Pads/briefs used — g.
		External (condom) catheter — c.	Enemas/irrigation — h.
		Indwelling catheter — d.	Ostomy present — i.
		Intermittent catheter — e.	NONE OF ABOVE — j.

4.	CHANGE IN URINARY CONTI-NENCE	Resident's urinary continence has changed as compared to status of **90 days ago** (or since last assessment if less than 90 days) 0. No change 1. Improved 2. Deteriorated	

SECTION I. DISEASE DIAGNOSES

Check only those diseases that have a relationship to current ADL status, cognitive status, mood and behavior status, medical treatments, nursing monitoring, or risk of death. (Do not list inactive diagnoses)

1.	DISEASES	*(If none apply, **CHECK the NONE OF ABOVE box**)*

ENDOCRINE/METABOLIC/NUTRITIONAL			Hemiplegia/Hemiparesis	v.	
Diabetes mellitus	a.		Multiple sclerosis	w.	
Hyperthyroidism	b.		Paraplegia	x.	
Hypothyroidism	c.		Parkinson's disease	y.	
HEART/CIRCULATION			Quadriplegia	z.	
Arteriosclerotic heart disease (ASHD)	d.		Seizure disorder	aa.	
Cardiac dysrhythmias	e.		Transient ischemic attack (TIA)	bb.	
Congestive heart failure	f.		Traumatic brain injury	cc.	
Deep vein thrombosis	g.		**PSYCHIATRIC/MOOD**		
Hypertension	h.		Anxiety disorder	dd.	
Hypotension	i.		Depression	ee.	
Peripheral vascular disease	j.		Manic depression (bipolar disease)	ff.	
Other cardiovascular disease	k.		Schizophrenia	gg.	
MUSCULOSKELETAL			**PULMONARY**		
Arthritis	l.		Asthma	hh.	
Hip fracture	m.		Emphysema/COPD	ii.	
Missing limb (e.g., amputation)	n.		**SENSORY**		
Osteoporosis	o.		Cataracts	jj.	
Pathological bone fracture	p.		Diabetic retinopathy	kk.	
NEUROLOGICAL			Glaucoma	ll.	
Alzheimer's disease	q.		Macular degeneration	mm.	
Aphasia	r.		**OTHER**		
Cerebral palsy	s.		Allergies	nn.	
Cerebrovascular accident (stroke)	t.		Anemia	oo.	
Dementia other than Alzheimer's disease	u.		Cancer	pp.	
			Renal failure	qq.	
			NONE OF ABOVE	rr.	

2.	INFECTIONS	*(If none apply, **CHECK the NONE OF ABOVE box**)*

Antibiotic resistant infection (e.g., Methicillin resistant staph)	a.		Septicemia	g.	
Clostridium difficile (c. diff.)	b.		Sexually transmitted diseases	h.	
Conjunctivitis	c.		Tuberculosis	i.	
HIV infection	d.		Urinary tract infection **in last 30 days**	j.	
Pneumonia	e.		Viral hepatitis	k.	
Respiratory infection	f.		Wound infection	l.	
			NONE OF ABOVE	m.	

3.	OTHER CURRENT OR MORE DETAILED DIAGNOSES AND ICD-9 CODES	a. _____		•	
		b. _____		•	
		c. _____		•	
		d. _____		•	
		e. _____		•	

SECTION J. HEALTH CONDITIONS

1.	PROBLEM CONDITIONS	*(**Check all problems present** in last 7 days unless other time frame is indicated)*

INDICATORS OF FLUID STATUS			Dizziness/Vertigo	f.	
Weight gain or loss of 3 or more pounds within a 7 day period	a.		Edema	g.	
			Fever	h.	
			Hallucinations	i.	
Inability to lie flat due to shortness of breath	b.		Internal bleeding	j.	
Dehydrated; output exceeds input	c.		Recurrent lung aspirations in **last 90 days**	k.	
			Shortness of breath	l.	
Insufficient fluid; did **NOT** consume all/almost all liquids provided during **last 3 days**	d.		Syncope (fainting)	m.	
			Unsteady gait	n.	
OTHER			Vomiting	o.	
Delusions	e.		NONE OF ABOVE	p.	

Resident _____   Numeric Identifier _____

2.	PAIN SYMPTOMS	(*Code the **highest level of pain** present in the last 7 days*)	
		a. FREQUENCY with which resident complains or shows evidence of pain	**b. INTENSITY** of pain
		0. No pain (***skip to J4***)	1. Mild pain
		1. Pain less than daily	2. Moderate pain
		2. Pain daily	3. Times when pain is horrible or excruciating

3.	PAIN SITE	(*If pain present, **check all sites** that apply in last 7 days*)			
		Back pain	a.	Incisional pain	f.
		Bone pain	b.	Joint pain (other than hip)	g.
		Chest pain while doing usual activities	c.	Soft tissue pain (e.g., lesion, muscle)	h.
		Headache	d.	Stomach pain	i.
		Hip pain	e.	Other	j.

4.	ACCIDENTS	(***Check all that apply***)			
		Fell in **past 30 days**	a.	Hip fracture in **last 180 days**	c.
		Fell in **past 31-180 days**	b.	Other fracture in **last 180 days**	d.
				NONE OF ABOVE	e.

5.	STABILITY OF CONDITIONS	Conditions/diseases make resident's cognitive, ADL, mood or behavior patterns unstable—(fluctuating, precarious, or deteriorating)	a.
		Resident experiencing an acute episode or a flare-up of a recurrent or chronic problem	b.
		End-stage disease, 6 or fewer months to live	c.
		NONE OF ABOVE	d.

SECTION K. ORAL/NUTRITIONAL STATUS

1.	ORAL PROBLEMS	Chewing problem	a.
		Swallowing problem	b.
		Mouth pain	c.
		NONE OF ABOVE	d.

2.	HEIGHT AND WEIGHT	Record (*a.*) height in inches and (*b.*) weight in pounds. *Base weight on most recent measure in **last 30 days**; measure weight consistently in accord with standard facility practice—e.g., in a.m. after voiding, before meal, with shoes off, and in nightclothes*		
		a. HT (in.)	**b.** WT (lb.)	

3.	WEIGHT CHANGE	**a. Weight loss**—5 % or more in **last 30 days**; or 10 % or more in **last 180 days**	
		0. No 1. Yes	
		b. Weight gain—5 % or more in **last 30 days**; or 10 % or more in **last 180 days**	
		0. No 1. Yes	

4.	NUTRITIONAL PROBLEMS	Complains about the taste of many foods	a.	Leaves 25% or more of food uneaten at most meals	c.
		Regular or repetitive complaints of hunger	b.	*NONE OF ABOVE*	d.

5.	NUTRITIONAL APPROACHES	(***Check all that apply in last 7 days***)			
		Parenteral/IV	a.	Dietary supplement between meals	f.
		Feeding tube	b.		
		Mechanically altered diet	c.	Plate guard, stabilized built-up utensil, etc.	g.
		Syringe (oral feeding)	d.	On a planned weight change program	h.
		Therapeutic diet	e.		
				NONE OF ABOVE	i.

6.	PARENTERAL OR ENTERAL INTAKE	(*Skip to Section L if neither 5a nor 5b is checked*)	
		a. Code the proportion of **total calories** the resident received through parenteral or tube feedings in the **last 7 days**	
		0. None 3. 51% to 75%	
		1. 1% to 25% 4. 76% to 100%	
		2. 26% to 50%	
		b. Code the average **fluid intake** per day by IV or tube in **last 7 days**	
		0. None 3. 1001 to 1500 cc/day	
		1. 1 to 500 cc/day 4. 1501 to 2000 cc/day	
		2. 501 to 1000 cc/day 5. 2001 or more cc/day	

SECTION L. ORAL/DENTAL STATUS

1.	ORAL STATUS AND DISEASE PREVENTION	Debris (soft, easily movable substances) present in mouth prior to going to bed at night	a.
		Has dentures or removable bridge	b.
		Some/all natural teeth lost—does not have or does not use dentures (or partial plates)	c.
		Broken, loose, or carious teeth	d.
		Inflamed gums (gingiva); swollen or bleeding gums; oral abcesses; ulcers or rashes	e.
		Daily cleaning of teeth/dentures or daily mouth care—by resident or staff	f.
		NONE OF ABOVE	g.

SECTION M. SKIN CONDITION

1.	ULCERS (Due to any cause)	(*Record the number of ulcers at each ulcer stage—regardless of cause. If none present at a stage, record "0" (zero). Code all that apply during **last 7 days**. Code 9 = 9 or more.*) **[Requires full body exam.]**	Number at Stage
		a. Stage 1. A persistent area of skin redness (without a break in the skin) that does not disappear when pressure is relieved.	
		b. Stage 2. A partial thickness loss of skin layers that presents clinically as an abrasion, blister, or shallow crater.	
		c. Stage 3. A full thickness of skin is lost, exposing the subcutaneous tissues - presents as a deep crater with or without undermining adjacent tissue.	
		d. Stage 4. A full thickness of skin and subcutaneous tissue is lost, exposing muscle or bone.	

2.	TYPE OF ULCER	(*For each type of ulcer, **code for the highest stage in the last 7 days** using scale in item M1—i.e., 0=none; stages 1, 2, 3, 4*)	
		a. Pressure ulcer—any lesion caused by pressure resulting in damage of underlying tissue	
		b. Stasis ulcer—open lesion caused by poor circulation in the lower extremities	

3.	HISTORY OF RESOLVED ULCERS	Resident had an ulcer that was resolved or cured in LAST 90 DAYS	
		0. No 1. Yes	

4.	OTHER SKIN PROBLEMS OR LESIONS PRESENT	(***Check all that apply** during **last 7 days***)	
		Abrasions, bruises	a.
		Burns (second or third degree)	b.
		Open lesions other than ulcers, rashes, cuts (e.g., cancer lesions)	c.
		Rashes—e.g., intertrigo, eczema, drug rash, heat rash, herpes zoster	d.
		Skin desensitized to pain or pressure	e.
		Skin tears or cuts (other than surgery)	f.
		Surgical wounds	g.
		NONE OF ABOVE	h.

5.	SKIN TREATMENTS	(***Check all that apply** during **last 7 days***)	
		Pressure relieving device(s) for chair	a.
		Pressure relieving device(s) for bed	b.
		Turning/repositioning program	c.
		Nutrition or hydration intervention to manage skin problems	d.
		Ulcer care	e.
		Surgical wound care	f.
		Application of dressings (with or without topical medications) other than to feet	g.
		Application of ointments/medications (other than to feet)	h.
		Other preventative or protective skin care (other than to feet)	i.
		NONE OF ABOVE	j.

6.	FOOT PROBLEMS AND CARE	(***Check all that apply** during **last 7 days***)	
		Resident has one or more foot problems—e.g., corns, callouses, bunions, hammer toes, overlapping toes, pain, structural problems	a.
		Infection of the foot—e.g., cellulitis, purulent drainage	b.
		Open lesions on the foot	c.
		Nails/calluses trimmed during **last 90 days**	d.
		Received preventative or protective foot care (e.g., used special shoes, inserts, pads, toe separators)	e.
		Application of dressings (with or without topical medications)	f.
		NONE OF ABOVE	g.

SECTION N. ACTIVITY PURSUIT PATTERNS

1.	TIME AWAKE	(***Check appropriate time periods over last 7 days***) Resident awake all or most of time (i.e., naps no more than one hour per time period) in the:			
		Morning	a.	Evening	c.
		Afternoon	b.	*NONE OF ABOVE*	d.

(If resident is comatose, skip to Section O)

2.	AVERAGE TIME INVOLVED IN ACTIVITIES	(**When awake and not receiving treatments or ADL care**)	
		0. Most—more than 2/3 of time 2. Little—less than 1/3 of time	
		1. Some—from 1/3 to 2/3 of time 3. None	

3.	PREFERRED ACTIVITY SETTINGS	(***Check all settings** in which activities are **preferred***)			
		Own room	a.		
		Day/activity room	b.	Outside facility	d.
		Inside NH/off unit	c.	*NONE OF ABOVE*	e.

4.	GENERAL ACTIVITY PREFERENCES (adapted to resident's current abilities)	(***Check all PREFERENCES** whether or not activity is currently available to resident*)			
		Cards/other games	a.	Trips/shopping	g.
		Crafts/arts	b.	Walking/wheeling outdoors	h.
		Exercise/sports	c.	Watching TV	i.
		Music	d.	Gardening or plants	j.
		Reading/writing	e.	Talking or conversing	k.
		Spiritual/religious activities	f.	Helping others	l.
				NONE OF ABOVE	m.

Resident_____   Numeric Identifier_____

5.	PREFERS CHANGE IN DAILY ROUTINE	Code for resident preferences in daily routines 0. No change 1. Slight change 2. Major change **a.** Type of activities in which resident is currently involved **b.** Extent of resident involvement in activities	

SECTION O. MEDICATIONS

1.	NUMBER OF MEDICA-TIONS	(*Record the number of different medications used in the last 7 days;* enter "0" if none used)	
2.	NEW MEDICA-TIONS	(*Resident currently receiving medications that were initiated during the* **last 90 days**) 0. No 1. Yes	
3.	INJECTIONS	(*Record the number of DAYS injections of any type received during the* **last 7 days**; enter "0" if none used)	
4.	DAYS RECEIVED THE FOLLOWING MEDICATION	(*Record the number of DAYS during last 7 days; enter "0" if not used. Note—enter "1" for long-acting meds used less than weekly)* **a.** Antipsychotic **d.** Hypnotic **b.** Antianxiety **e.** Diuretic **c.** Antidepressant	

SECTION P. SPECIAL TREATMENTS AND PROCEDURES

1.	SPECIAL TREAT-MENTS, PROCE-DURES, AND PROGRAMS	**a. SPECIAL CARE**—*Check treatments or programs received during the* **last 14 days**

TREATMENTS

Chemotherapy	a.	Ventilator or respirator	l.
Dialysis	b.	**PROGRAMS**	
IV medication	c.	Alcohol/drug treatment program	m.
Intake/output	d.	Alzheimer's/dementia special care unit	n.
Monitoring acute medical condition	e.	Hospice care	o.
Ostomy care	f.	Pediatric unit	p.
Oxygen therapy	g.	Respite care	q.
Radiation	h.	Training in skills required to return to the community (e.g., taking medications, house work, shopping, transportation, ADLs)	r.
Suctioning	i.		
Tracheostomy care	j.		
Transfusions	k.	NONE OF ABOVE	s.

b. THERAPIES - *Record the number of days and total minutes each of the following therapies was administered (for at least 15 minutes a day) in the* **last 7 calendar days** *(Enter 0 if none or less than 15 min. daily)*
[Note—count only post admission therapies]
(A) = # of days administered for **15 minutes or more**
(B) = total # of minutes provided in **last 7 days**

	DAYS (A)	MIN (B)
a. Speech - language pathology and audiology services		
b. Occupational therapy		
c. Physical therapy		
d. Respiratory therapy		
e. Psychological therapy (by any licensed mental health professional)		

2.	INTERVEN-TION PROGRAMS FOR MOOD, BEHAVIOR, COGNITIVE LOSS	(*Check all interventions or strategies used in last 7 days*—no matter where received)	
		Special behavior symptom evaluation program	a.
		Evaluation by a licensed mental health specialist in **last 90 days**	b.
		Group therapy	c.
		Resident-specific deliberate changes in the environment to address mood/behavior patterns—e.g., providing bureau in which to rummage	d.
		Reorientation—e.g., cueing	e.
		NONE OF ABOVE	f.

3.	NURSING REHABILITA-TION/ RESTOR-ATIVE CARE	*Record the NUMBER OF DAYS each of the following rehabilitation or restorative techniques or practices was* **provided to the resident for more than or equal to 15 minutes per day in the last 7 days** *(Enter 0 if none or less than 15 min. daily.)*

a. Range of motion (passive)		**f.** Walking	
b. Range of motion (active)		**g.** Dressing or grooming	
c. Splint or brace assistance		**h.** Eating or swallowing	
TRAINING AND SKILL PRACTICE IN:		**i.** Amputation/prosthesis care	
d. Bed mobility		**j.** Communication	
e. Transfer		**k.** Other	

4.	DEVICES AND RESTRAINTS	(*Use the following codes for* **last 7 days**:) 0. Not used 1. Used less than daily 2. Used daily Bed rails **a.** — Full bed rails on all open sides of bed **b.** — Other types of side rails used (e.g., half rail, one side) **c.** Trunk restraint **d.** Limb restraint **e.** Chair prevents rising	
5.	HOSPITAL STAY(S)	Record number of times resident was admitted to hospital with an overnight stay **in last 90 days** (or since last assessment if less than 90 days). (*Enter 0 if no hospital admissions*)	
6.	EMERGENCY ROOM (ER) VISIT(S)	Record number of times resident visited ER without an overnight stay **in last 90 days** (or since last assessment if less than 90 days). (*Enter 0 if no ER visits*)	
7.	PHYSICIAN VISITS	In the **LAST 14 DAYS** (or since admission if less than 14 days in facility) how many days has the physician (or authorized assistant or practitioner) examined the resident? (*Enter 0 if none*)	
8.	PHYSICIAN ORDERS	In the **LAST 14 DAYS** (or since admission if less than 14 days in facility) how many days has the physician (or authorized assistant or practitioner) changed the resident's orders? *Do not include order renewals without change.* (*Enter 0 if none*)	
9.	ABNORMAL LAB VALUES	Has the resident had any abnormal lab values during the **last 90 days** (or since admission)? 0. No 1. Yes	

SECTION Q. DISCHARGE POTENTIAL AND OVERALL STATUS

1.	DISCHARGE POTENTIAL	**a.** Resident expresses/indicates preference to return to the community 0. No 1. Yes	
		b. Resident has a support person who is positive towards discharge	
		c. Stay projected to be of a short duration— discharge projected **within 90 days** (do not include expected discharge due to death) 0. No 2. Within 31-90 days 1. Within 30 days 3. Discharge status uncertain	
2.	OVERALL CHANGE IN CARE NEEDS	Resident's overall self sufficiency has changed significantly as compared to status of **90 days ago** (or since last assessment if less than 90 days) 0. No change 1. Improved—receives fewer supports, needs less restrictive level of care 2. Deteriorated—receives more support	

SECTION R. ASSESSMENT INFORMATION

1.	PARTICIPA-TION IN ASSESS-MENT	**a.** Resident: 0. No 1. Yes **b.** Family: 0. No 1. Yes 2. No family **c.** Significant other: 0. No 1. Yes 2. None	

2. SIGNATURE OF PERSON COORDINATING THE ASSESSMENT:

a. Signature of RN Assessment Coordinator (sign on above line)

b. Date RN Assessment Coordinator signed as complete

	Month	Day	Year

Resident _____ Numeric Identifier _____

SECTION T. THERAPY SUPPLEMENT FOR MEDICARE PPS

1.	SPECIAL TREAT-MENTS AND PROCE-DURES	**a. RECREATION THERAPY**—*Enter number of days and total minutes of recreation therapy administered (**for at least 15 minutes a day**) in the **last 7 days** (Enter 0 if none)*

		DAYS (A)	MIN (B)
(A) = # of days administered for 15 minutes or more (B) = total # of minutes provided in last 7 days			

Skip unless this is a Medicare 5 day or Medicare readmission/return assessment.

b. ORDERED THERAPIES—*Has physician ordered any of following therapies to begin in FIRST 14 days of stay—physical therapy, occupational therapy, or speech pathology service?*
0. No   1. Yes

If not ordered, skip to item 2

c. Through day 15, provide an estimate of the number of days when at least 1 therapy service can be expected to have been delivered.

d. Through day 15, provide an estimate of the number of therapy minutes (across the therapies) that can be expected to be delivered?

2.	WALKING WHEN MOST SELF SUFFICIENT	*Complete item 2 if ADL self-performance score for TRANSFER (G.1.b.A) is 0,1,2, or 3 AND at least one of the following are present:*

- Resident received physical therapy involving gait training (P.1.b.c)
- Physical therapy was ordered for the resident involving gait training (T.1.b)
- Resident received nursing rehabilitation for walking (P.3.f)
- Physical therapy involving walking has been discontinued within the past 180 days

Skip to item 3 if resident did not walk in last 7 days

(FOR FOLLOWING FIVE ITEMS, BASE CODING ON THE EPISODE WHEN THE RESIDENT WALKED THE FARTHEST WITHOUT SITTING DOWN. INCLUDE WALKING DURING REHABILITATION SESSIONS.)

a. Furthest distance walked without sitting down during this episode.

0. 150+ feet	3. 10-25 feet
1. 51-149 feet	4. Less than 10 feet
2. 26-50 feet	

b. Time walked without sitting down during this episode.

0. 1-2 minutes	3. 11-15 minutes
1. 3-4 minutes	4. 16-30 minutes
2. 5-10 minutes	5. 31+ minutes

c. Self-Performance in walking during this episode.

0. *INDEPENDENT*—No help or oversight

1. *SUPERVISION*—Oversight, encouragement or cueing provided

2. *LIMITED ASSISTANCE*—Resident highly involved in walking; received physical help in guided maneuvering of limbs or other nonweight bearing assistance

3. *EXTENSIVE ASSISTANCE*—Resident received weight bearing assistance while walking

d. Walking support provided associated with this episode (code regardless of resident's self-performance classification).

0. No setup or physical help from staff
1. Setup help only
2. One person physical assist
3. Two+ persons physical assist

e. Parallel bars used by resident in association with this episode.

0. No   1. Yes

3.	CASE MIX GROUP	Medicare						State					

MDS 2.0 September, 2000

SECTION V. RESIDENT ASSESSMENT PROTOCOL SUMMARY   Numeric Identifier _____

Resident's Name:	Medical Record No.:

1. Check if RAP is triggered.

2. For each triggered RAP, use the RAP guidelines to identify areas needing further assessment. Document relevant assessment information regarding the resident's status.

   - Describe:
     — Nature of the condition (may include presence or lack of objective data and subjective complaints).
     — Complications and risk factors that affect your decision to proceed to care planning.
     — Factors that must be considered in developing individualized care plan interventions.
     — Need for referrals/further evaluation by appropriate health professionals.

   - Documentation should support your decision-making regarding whether to proceed with a care plan for a triggered RAP and the type(s) of care plan interventions that are appropriate for a particular resident.

   - Documentation may appear anywhere in the clinical record (e.g., progress notes, consults, flowsheets, etc.).

3. Indicate under the Location of RAP Assessment Documentation column where information related to the RAP assessment can be found.

4. For each triggered RAP, indicate whether a new care plan, care plan revision, or continuation of current care plan is necessary to address the problem(s) identified in your assessment. The Care Planning Decision column must be completed within 7 days of completing the RAI (MDS and RAPs).

A. RAP PROBLEM AREA	(a) Check if triggered	Location and Date of RAP Assessment Documentation	(b) Care Planning Decision—check if addressed in care plan
1. DELIRIUM	☐		☐
2. COGNITIVE LOSS	☐		☐
3. VISUAL FUNCTION	☐		☐
4. COMMUNICATION	☐		☐
5. ADL FUNCTIONAL/ REHABILITATION POTENTIAL	☐		☐
6. URINARY INCONTINENCE AND INDWELLING CATHETER	☐		☐
7. PSYCHOSOCIAL WELL-BEING	☐		☐
8. MOOD STATE	☐		☐
9. BEHAVIORAL SYMPTOMS	☐		☐
10. ACTIVITIES	☐		☐
11. FALLS	☐		☐
12. NUTRITIONAL STATUS	☐		☐
13. FEEDING TUBES	☐		☐
14. DEHYDRATION/FLUID MAINTENANCE	☐		☐
15. DENTAL CARE	☐		☐
16. PRESSURE ULCERS	☐		☐
17. PSYCHOTROPIC DRUG USE	☐		☐
18. PHYSICAL RESTRAINTS	☐		☐

B.

1. Signature of RN Coordinator for RAP Assessment Process   2. ☐☐ — ☐☐ — ☐☐☐☐ Month Day Year

3. Signature of Person Completing Care Planning Decision   4. ☐☐ — ☐☐ — ☐☐☐☐ Month Day Year

MDS 2.0 September, 2000

RESIDENT ASSESSMENT PROTOCOL TRIGGER LEGEND FOR REVISED RAPS (FOR MDS VERSION 2.0)

Key:
- ● = One item required to trigger
- ❷ = Two items required to trigger
- ★ = One of these three items, plus at least one other item required to trigger
- @ = When both ADL triggers present, maintenance takes precedence

Proceed to RAP Review once triggered

MDS ITEM		CODE	Delirium	Cognitive Loss/Dementia	Visual Function	Communication	ADL-Rehabilitation Trigger A @	ADL-Maintenance Trigger B @	Urinary Incontinence and Indwelling Catheter	Psychosocial Well-Being	Mood State	Behavioral Symptoms	Activities Trigger A	Activities Trigger B	Falls	Nutritional Status	Feeding Tubes	Dehydration/Fluid Maintenance	Dental Care	Pressure Ulcers	Psychotropic Drug Use	Physical Restraints	
B2a	Short term memory	1		●																			B2a
B2b	Long term memory	1		●																			B2b
B4	Decision making	1,2,3		●																			B4
B4	Decision making	3				●																	B4
B5a to B5f	Indicators of delirium	2	●																		●		B5a to B5f
B6	Change in cognitive status	2	●																		●		B6
C1	Hearing	1,2,3				●																	C1
C4	Understood by others	1,2,3				●																	C4
C6	Understand others	1,2,3		●		●																	C6
C7	Change in communication	2																			●		C7
D1	Vision	1,2,3			●																		D1
D2a	Side vision problem	√			●																		D2a
E1a to E1p	Indicators of depression, anxiety, sad mood	1,2									●												E1a to E1p
E1n	Repetitive movement	1,2																			●		E1n
E1o	Withdrawal from activities	1,2								●													E1o
E2	Mood persistence	1,2									●												E2
E3	Change in mood	2	●																		●		E3
E4aA	Wandering	1,2,3											●										E4aA
E4aA - E4eA	Behavioral symptoms	1,2,3										●											E4aA - E4eA
E5	Change in behavioral symptoms	1										●											E5
E5	Change in behavioral symptoms	2	●																		●		E5
F1d	Establishes own goals	√								●													F1d
F2a to F2d	Unsettled relationships	√								●													F2a to F2d
F3a	Strong id, past roles	√								●													F3a
F3b	Lost roles	√								●													F3b
F3c	Daily routine different	√								●													F3c
G1aA - G1jA	ADL self-performance	1,2,3,4					●																G1aA - G1jA
G1aA	Bed mobility	2,3,4,8																		●			G1aA
G2A	Bathing	1,2,3,4					●																G2A
G3b	Balance while sitting	1,2,3																		●			G3b
G6a	Bedfast	√																		●			G6a
G8a,b	Resident, staff believe capable	√					●																G8a,b
H1a	Bowel incontinence	1,2,3,4																		●			H1a
H1b	Bladder incontinence	2,3,4							●														H1b
H2b	Constipation	√																			●		H2b
H2d	Fecal impaction	√																			●		H2d
H3c,d,e	Catheter use	√							●														H3c,d,e
H3g	Use of pads/briefs	√							●														H3g
I1i	Hypotension	√																			●		I1i
I1j	Peripheral vascular disease	√																		●			I1j
I1ee	Depression	√																			●		I1ee
I1jj	Cataracts	√			●																		I1jj
I1ll	Glaucoma	√			●																		I1ll
I2j	UTI	√																●					I2j
I3	Dehydration diagnosis	276.5																●					I3
J1a	Weight fluctuation	√																●					J1a
J1c	Dehydrated	√																●					J1c
J1d	Insufficient fluid	√																●					J1d
J1f	Dizziness	√													●						●		J1f
J1h	Fever	√																●					J1h
J1i	Hallucinations	√																			●		J1i
J1j	Internal bleeding	√																●					J1j
J1k	Lung aspirations	√																			●		J1k
J1m	Syncope	√																			●		J1m

RESIDENT ASSESSMENT PROTOCOL TRIGGER LEGEND FOR REVISED RAPS (FOR MDS VERSION 2.0)

Key:
- ● = One item required to trigger
- ❷ = Two items required to trigger
- ★ = One of these three items, plus at least one other item required to trigger
- @ = When both ADL triggers present, maintenance takes precedence

Proceed to RAP Review once triggered

MDS ITEM	CODE	Delirium	Cognitive Loss/Dementia	Visual Function	Communication	ADL-Rehabilitation Trigger A @	ADL-Maintenance Trigger B @	Urinary Incontinence and Indwelling Catheter	Psychosocial Well-Being	Mood State	Behavioral Symptoms	Activities Trigger A	Activities Trigger B	Falls	Nutritional Status	Feeding Tubes	Dehydration/Fluid Maintenance	Dental Care	Pressure Ulcers	Psychotropic Drug Use	Physical Restraints
J1n — Unsteady gait	√													●							●
J4a,b — Fell	√													●							●
J4c — Hip fracture	√																				●
K1b — Swallowing problem	√																				●
K1c — Mouth pain	√																	●			
K3a — Weight loss	1														●						
K4a — Taste alteration	√														●						
K4c — Leave 25% food	√														●						
K5a — Parenteral/IV feeding	√														●		●				
K5b — Feeding tube	√															●	●				
K5c — Mechanically altered	√														●						
K5d — Syringe feeding	√														●						
K5e — Therapeutic diet	√														●						
L1a,c,d,e — Dental	√																	●			
L1f — Daily cleaning teeth	Not √																	●			
M2a — Pressure ulcer	2,3,4														●						
M2a — Pressure ulcer	1,2,3,4																		●		
M3 — Previous pressure ulcer	1																		●		
M4e — Impaired tactile sense	√																		●		
N1a — Awake morning	√												❷								
N2 — Involved in activities	0												❷								
N2 — Involved in activities	2,3											●									
N5a,b — Prefers change in daily routine	1,2											●									
O4a — Antipsychotics	1-7																			★	
O4b — Antianxiety	1-7													●						★	
O4c — Antidepressants	1-7													●						★	
O4e — Diuretic	1-7																●				
P4c — Trunk restraint	1,2													●							●
P4c — Trunk restraint	2																		●		
P4d — Limb restraint	1,2																				●
P4e — Chair prevents rising	1,2																				●

MDS 2.0 September, 2000

APPENDIX C

USEFUL SPANISH VOCABULARY AND PHRASES*

CHAPTER 2: THE NURSING ASSISTANT

Miss	señorita (seh-nyoh-ree-tah)
Mrs.	señora (seh-nyoh-rah)
Mr.	señor (seh-nyohr)
Hello!	¡Hola! (Oh-lah)
I am going to cover you.	Lo voy acubrir. (Loh boy ah-koo-breer)

CHAPTER 3: WORK ETHICS

Excuse me.	Con permiso. (kohn pehr-mee-soh)
Good morning, sir.	Buenos días, señor. (Boo-eh-nohs dee-ahs, seh-nyohr)
Good afternoon!	¡Buenas tardes! (Boo-eh-nahs tahr-dehs)
How may I help you?	¿En qué puedo servirle? (Ehn keh poo-eh-doh sehr-beer-leh)
Thank you for talking to me!	¡Gracias por hablar conmigo! (Grah-see-ahs pohr ah-blahr kohn-mee-goh)
Good morning, Mrs. Ortiz!	!Buenos días, señora Ortiz! (Boo-eh-nohs dee-ahs, seh-nyo-rah ohr-tees)
Good morning, doctor!	!Buenos días, doctor! (Boo-eh-nohs dee-ahs, dohk-tohr)
You are welcome.	De nada. (Deh nah-dah)
Good afternoon!	!Buenas tardes! (Boo-eh-nahs tahr-dehs)
employ	emplear (ehm-pleh-ahr)
My name is...	Mi nobres es.../Me llamo... (Mee nohm-breh ehs/ Meh yah-moh)
Please!	¡Por favor! (Pohr fah-bohr)
Thank you!	¡Gracias! (Grah-see-ahs)
Thank you very much!	¡Muchas gracias! (Moo-chahs grah-see-ahs)
What can I help you with?	¿En qué puedo ayudarlo? (Ehn keh poo-eh-doh ah-yoo-dahr-loh)
Yes, sir.	Sí, señor. (See, seh-nyohr)

---

*This appendix is presented for your convenience. Please note: This listing does not include all chapters; only those for which vocabulary and phrases directly relate to the content in this textbook.

Translations taken from Joyce EV, Villanueva ME: *Say it in Spanish: A Guide for Health Care Professionals*, ed 2, Philadelphia, 2000, WB Saunders.

CHAPTER 4: COMMUNICATING
WITH THE HEALTH TEAM

Number	English	Spanish	Pronunciation
1	one	uno	(oo-noh)
2	two	dos	(dohs)
3	three	tres	(trehs)
4	four	cuatro	(koo-ah-troh)
5	five	cinco	(seen-koh)
6	six	seis	(seh-ees)
7	seven	siete	(see-eh-teh)
8	eight	ocho	(oh-choh)
9	nine	nueve	(noo-eh-beh)
10	ten	diez	(dee-ehs)
11	eleven	once	(ohn-seh)
12	twelve	doce	(doh-seh)
13	thirteen	trece	(treh-seh)
14	fourteen	catorce	(kah-tohr-seh)
15	fifteen	quince	(keen-seh)
16	sixteen	dieciséis	(dee-ehs-ee-seh-ees)
17	seventeen	diecisiete	(dee-ehs-ee-see-eh-teh)
18	eighteen	dieciocho	(dee-ehs-ee-oh-choh)
19	nineteen	diecinueve	(dee-ehs-ee-noo-eh-beh)
20	twenty	veinte	(beh-een-teh)
30	thirty	treinta	(treh-een-tah)
40	forty	cuarenta	(koo-ah-rehn-tah)
50	fifty	cincuenta	(seen-koo-ehn-tah)
60	sixty	sesenta	(seh-sehn-tah)
70	seventy	setenta	(seh-tehn-tah)
80	eighty	ochenta	(oh-chehn-tah)
90	ninety	noventa	(noh-behn-tah)
100	one hundred	cien	(see-ehn)

Time	Standard	Military (hours P.M.)
one o'clock	la una (la oo-nah)	las trece horas (lahs treh-seh oh-rahs)
two o'clock	las dos (lahs dohs)	las catorce horas (lahs kah-tohr-seh oh-rahs)
three o'clock	las tres (lahs trehs)	las quince horas (lahs keen-seh oh-rahs)
four o'clock	las cuatro (lahs koo-ah-troh)	las dieciséis horas (lahs dee-ehs-ee-seh-ees oh-rahs)
five o'clock	las cinco (lahs seen-koh)	las diecisiete horas (lahs dee-ehs-ee-see-eh-teh oh-rahs)
six o'clock	las seis (lahs seh-ees)	las dieciocho horas (lahs dee-ehs-ee-oh-choh oh-rahs)
seven o'clock	las siete (lahs see-eh-teh)	las diecinueve horas (lahs dee-ehs-ee-noo-eh-beh oh-rahs)
eight o'clock	las ocho (lahs oh-choh)	las veinte horas (lahs beh-een-teh oh-rahs)
nine o'clock	las nueve (lahs noo-eh-beh)	las veintiuna horas (lahs beh-een-tee-oo-nah oh-rahs)

Time	Standard	Military (hours P.M.)
ten o'clock	las diez (lahs dee-ehs)	las veintidós horas (lahs beh-een-tee-dohs oh-rahs)
eleven o'clock	las once (lahs ohn-seh)	las veintitrés horas (lahs beh-een-tee-trehs oh-rahs)
twelve o'clock/ midnight	las doce/la media noche (lahs doh-seh/lah meh-dee-ah non-cheh)	las cero horas (lahs seh-roh-oh-rahs) las veinticuatro horas (lahs beh-een-tee-koo-ah-troh oh-rahs)

abdomen	abdomen (ahb-doh-mehn)
communication	comunicación (koh-moo-nee-kah-see-ohn)
black	negro (neh-groh)
blue	azul (ah-sool)
clear	claro (klah-roh)
green	verde (behr-deh)
red	rojo (roh-hoh)
yellow	amarillo (ah-mah-ree-yoh)
white	blanco (blahn-koh)
Monday	lunes (loo-nehs)
Tuesday	martes (mahr-tehs)
Wednesday	miércoles (mee-ehr-koh-lehs)
Thursday	jueves (hoo-eh-behs)
Friday	viernes (bee-ehr-nehs)
Saturday	sábado (sah-bah-doh)
Sunday	domingo (doh-meen-goh)
what?	¿qué?/¿qué tal? (keh/keh tahl)
when?	¿cuándo? (koo-ahn-doh)
where?	¿dónde? (dohn-deh)
why?	¿por qué? (pohr keh)
for whom?	¿para quién? (pah-rah kee-ehn)

for what?	¿para qué? (pah-rah keh)
which?	¿cuál? (koo-ahl)
who?	¿quién? (kee-ehn)
how many?	¿cuántos? (koo-ahn-tohs)
how much?	¿cuánto? (koo-ahn-toh)
no, not	no (noh)
no one, nobody	nadie (nah-dee-eh)
nothing	nada (nah-dah)
never, not ever	nunca, jamás (noon-kah, hah-mahs)
neither	tampoco (tahm-poh-koh)
neither....nor	ni....ni (nee....nee)
not one, not any	ninguno (neen-goo-noh)
without	sin (seen)
Every two hours.	Cada dos horas. (Kah-dah dohs oh-rahs)
Hello, I'm John Goodguy.	Hola, soy John Goodguy. (Oh-lah, soh-ee John Goodguy)
Hello, Mrs. Mora.	Hola, señora Mora. (Oh-lah, seh-nyoh-rah Moh-rah)
How are you?	¿Cómo está? (Koh-moh ehs-tah)
How do you feel?	¿Cómo te sientes? (Koh-moh teh see-ehn-tehs)
How do you feel now?	¿Cómo se siente ahora? (Koh-moh seh see-ehn-teh ah-oh-rah)

CHAPTER 5: UNDERSTANDING THE PERSON

Let me know how you feel.	Dígame cómo se siente. (Dee-gah-meh koh-moh seh see-ehn-teh)	grandmother	abuela (ah-boo-eh-lah)
My name is...	Mi nombre es.../Me llamo... (Mee nohm-breh ehs/ Meh yah-moh)	grandfather	abuelo (ah-boo-eh-loh)
Good-bye!	¡Hasta luego! (Ahs-tah loo-eh-goh)	grandparents	abuelos (ah-boo-eh-lohs)
Hi!	¡Hola! (Oh-lah)	aunt	tía (tee-ah)
Good morning.	Buenos días. (Boo-eh-nohs dee-ahs)	uncle	tío (tee-oh)
Good afternoon.	Buenas tardes. (Boo-eh-nahs tahr-dehs)	stepfather	padrastro (pah-drahs-troh)
Good evening.	Buenas noches. (Boo-eh-nahs noh-chehs)	stepmother	madrastra (mah-drahs-trah)
Do you speak English?	¿Habla inglés? (Ah-blah een-glehs)	stepson	hijastro (ee-hahs-troh)
Thank you!	¡Gracias! (Grah-see-ahs)	stepdaughter	hijastra (ee-hahs-trah)
Thank you very much!	¡Muchas gracias! (Moo-chahs grah-see-ahs)	children	hijos (eeh-hohs)
You are welcome.	De nada. (Deh nah-dah)	great-grandparents	bisabuelos (bee-sah-boo-eh-lohs)
respect	respeto (rehs-peh-toh)	mother-in-law	suegra (soo-eh-grah)
the family	la familia (lah fah-mee-lee-ah)	father-in-law	suegro (soo-eh-grah)
father	padre (pah-dreh)	sister-in-law	cuñada (koo-nyah-dah)
dad	papá (pah-pah)	brother-in-law	cuñado (koo-nyah-doh)
mother	madre (mah-dreh)	cousins	primos (pree-mohs)
mom	mamá (mah-mah)	cousin (female)	prima (pree-mah)
husband	esposo (ehs-poh-soh)	cousin (male)	primo (pree-moh)
wife	esposa (ehs-poh-sah)	grandchildren	nietos (nee-eh-tohs)
sister	hermana (ehr-mah-nah)	godparents	padrinos (pah-dree-nohs)
brother	hermano (ehr-mah-noh)	godfather	padrino (pah-dree-noh)
son	hijo (ee-hoh)	godmother	madrina (mah-dree-nah)
daughter	hija (ee-hah)	Do you understand?	¿Comprende?/¿Entiende? (Kohm-prehn-deh/ Ehn-tee-ehn-deh)
niece	sobrina (soh-bree-nah)	Are you cold?	¿Tiene frío? (Tee-eh-neh free-oh)
nephew	sobrino (soh-bree-noh)	Are you hot?	¿Tiene calor? (tee-eh-neh kah-lohr)
		Are you hungry?	¿Tiene hambre? (Tee-eh-neh ahm-breh)
		Are you sleepy?	¿Tiene sueño? (Tee-eh-neh soo-eh-nyoh)

Are you thirsty?	¿Tiene sed? (Tee-eh-neh sehd)
Is that enough?	¿Es suficiente? (Ehs soo-fee-see-ehn-teh)
Is that a lot?	¿Es mucho? (Ehs moo-choh)
Is that too much?	¿Es demasiado? (Ehs deh-mah-see-ah-doh)
Are you comfortable?	¿Está cómoda? (Ehs tah koh-moh-dah)
A nurse will see you.	Una enfermera la atenderá. (Ooh-nah ehn-fehr-meh-rah lah ah-tehn-deh-rah)
Good!	¡Bueno! (Boo-eh-noh)
Good afternoon, Miss González.	Buenas tardes, señorita González. (Boo-eh-nahs tahr-dehs, seh-nyoh-ree-tah Gohn-sah-lehs)
Good luck!	¡Buena suerte! (Boo-eh-nah soo-ehr-teh)
Have a good day!	¡Pase un buen día! (Pah-seh oon boo-ehn dee-ah)
Hello.	Hola (Oh-lah)
I am through.	Ya terminé. (Yah tehr-mee-neh)
I will see you tomorrow.	Le veré mañana. (Lah beh-reh mah-nyah-nah)
I will return shortly.	Regresaré en seguida. (Reh-greh-sah-reh ehn seh-ghee-dah)
If you don't understand, please let me know.	Si no entiende, dígame por favor. (See noh ehn-tee-ehn-deh, dee-gah-meh pohr fah-bohr)
Visiting hours are from nine in the morning to nine at night.	Las horas de visita son de las nueve de la mañana a las nueve de la noche. (Lahs oh-rahs deh bee-see-tah shon deh lahs noo-eh-beh deh lah mah-nyah-nah ah lahs noo-eh-beh deh lah noh-cheh)
Visiting hours are from two to eight P.M.	Las horas de visita son de las dos a las ocho de la noche. (Lahs oh-rahs deh bee-see-tah sohn deh lahs dohs ah loahs oh-choh deh lah noh-cheh)

CHAPTER 6: UNDERSTANDING BODY STRUCTURE AND FUNCTION

ligament	ligamento (lee-gah-mehn-toh)
organ	órgano (ohr-gah-noh)
pancreas	páncreas (pahn-kreh-ahs)
saliva	saliva (sah-lee-bah)

CHAPTER 8: PROMOTING SAFETY

What can I help you with?	¿En qué puedo ayudarlo? (Ehn keh poo-eh-doh ah-yoo-dahr-loh)
This is the call bell.	Este es el timbre. (Ehs-teh ehs ehl teem-breh)
coma	coma (koh-mah)
comatose	comatoso (koh-mah-toh-soh)
Call if you need help.	Llame si necesita ayuda. (Yah-meh see neh-seh-see-tah ah-yoo-dah)
No smoking.	No se permite fumar. (Noh seh pehr-mee-teh foo-mahr)
Wear this bracelet all the time.	Use esta pulsera todo el tiempo. (Oo-seh ehs-tah pool-seh-rah toh-doh ehl tee-ehm-poh)
You cannot smoke here.	No puede fumar aquí. (Noh poo-eh-deh foo-mahr ah-kee)
You cannot smoke in your room.	No puede fumar en el cuatro. (Noh poo-eh-deh foo-mahr ehn ehl koo-ahr-toh)

CHAPTER 10: PREVENTING INFECTION

Wash well all fruits and vegetables.	Lave bien frutas y verduras. (Lah-beh bee-ehn froo-tahs ee behr-doo-rahs)
Wash hands before eating.	Lave las manos antes de comer. (Lah-beh lahs mah-nohs ahn-tehs deh koh-mehr)
bacteria	bacteria (bahk-teh-ree-ah)
inflammation	inflamación (een-flah-mah-see-ohn)

pathogen

patogénico
(pah-toh-heh-nee-koh)

What causes AIDS?

¿Qué causa el SIDA?
(Keh kah-oo-sah ehl see-dah)

A virus known as HIV . . .

El virus causal del SIDA se conoce como VIH . . .
(Ehl bee-roos kah-oo-sahl dehl see-dah seh koh-noh-seh koh-moh beh-ee-ah-cheh[VIH])

Who is at risk of getting AIDS?

¿Quién está en riesgo de contraer el SIDA?
(Kee-ehn ehs-tah ehn ree-ehs-goh deh kohn-trah-ehr ehl see-dah)

sexually active homosexual and bisexual males or females

homosexuales activos y hombres o mujeres bisexuales
(oh-moh-sehx-oo-ah-lehs ahk-tee-bohs ee ohm-brehs oh moo-heh-rehs bee-sehx-oo-ah-lehs)

intravenous drug abusers

los que abusan de las drogas intravenosas
(lohs keh ah-boo-sah deh lahs droh-gahs een-trah-beh-noh-sahs)

hemophiliacs and recipients of blood/blood components

hemofílicos, donadores de sangre o transfusión con sangre contaminada
(eh-moh-fee-lee-kohs, doh-nah-doh-rehs deh sahn-greh oh trahns-foo-see-ohn kohn sahn-greh kohn-tah-mee-nah-dah)

fetus of infected mothers

fetos de madres contamnadas
(feh-tohs deh mah-drehs kohn-tah-mee-nah-dahs)

Infected persons can transmit the virus.

Las personas infectadas pueden transmitir el virus
(Lahs pehr-soh-nahs een fehk-tah-dahs poo-ehdehn-trahns-mee-teer ehl bee-roos)

Can casual contact cause AIDS?

¿Los contactos eventaules puden causar SIDA?
(Lohs kohn-tahk-tohs eh-behn-too-ah-lehs poo-eh-dehn kah-oo-sahr see-dah)

HIV is not transmissible by casual contact, nor . . .

El VIH no es transmitido en forma casual, ni por . . .
(Ehl VIH noh ehs trahns-mee-tee-doh ehn fohr-mah kah-soo-ahl, nee pohr:)

living in the same house as infected persons

vivir en la misma casa con personas infectadas
(bee-beer ehn lah mees-mah kah-sah kohn pehr-soh-nahs een-fehk-tah-dahs)

eating food handled by persons with AIDS

comer comida preparada por personas infectadas con SIDA
(koh-mehr koh-mee-dah preh-pah-rah-dah pohr pehr-soh-nahs een-fehk-tah-dahs kohn see-dah)

coughing, sneezing, kissing, or swimming with infected persons

tos, estornudo, besar, o nadar con personas infectadas
(tohs, ehs-tohr-noo-doh, beh-sahr oh nah-dahr kohn pehr-soh-nahs een-fehk-tah-dahs)

How serious is AIDS?

¿Qué tan serio es el SIDA?
(Keh tahn seh-ree-oh ehs-ehl see-dah)

Is there a danger from donated blood?

¿Qué peligro hay por sangre donada?
(Keh peh-lee-groh ah-ee pohr sahn-greh doh-nah-dah)

The risk of contracting HIV is not high. Blood banks and other centers use sterile equipment and disposable needles.

El riesgo de contraer VIH no es alto. Los bancos de sangre y otros centros usan equipos estériles y agujas desechables.
(Ehl ree-ehs-goh deh kohn-trah-ehr VIH noh ehs ahl-toh. Lohns bahn-kohs deh sahn-greh ee oh-trohs sehn-trohs oo-sahn eh-kée-pohs ehs-teh-ree-lehs ee ah-goo-hahs deh-seh-chah-blehs)

The U.S. Public Health Service recommends:

El Departamento de Salud Pública de los Estados Unidos recomienda:
(Ehl Deh-pahr-tah-mehn-toh deh Sah-lood Poo-blee-kah deh lohs Ehs-tah-dohs Oo-nee-dohs reh-koh-mee-ehn-dah)

1. Know sexual background/ habits of partners.

1. Conozca los hábitos sexuales de su pareja.
(Koh-nohs-kah lohs ah-bee-tohs sex-oo-ah-lehs deh soo pah-reh-hah)

2. Use a condom or prophylactic.

2. Use un condón o profiláctico.
(Oo-seh oon kohn-dohn oh proh-fee-lahk-tee-koh)

3. If your partner is in a high risk group, cease sexual relations.

3. Si su compañera está en el grupo de alto riesgo, suspenda las relaciones sexuales.
(See soo kohm-pah-nyeh-rah ehs-tah ehn ehl groo-pah deh ahl-toh ree-ehs-goh, soos-pehn-dah lahs reh-lah-see-ohn-ehs sehx-oo-ahl-ehs)

4. Eliminate multiple sexual partners.

4. Elimine múltiples compañeros sexuales.
(Eh-lee-mee-neh mool-tee-plehs kohm-pha-nyeh-rohs sehx-oo-ah-lehs)

5. Don't use intravenous drugs with contaminated needles; don't share needles or syringes.

5. No use drogas intravenosas con agujas contaminadas; no comparta aguijas o jeringas.
(Noh oos-eh droh-gahs een-trah-veh-noh-sahs kohn ah-goo-hahs kohn-tah-mee-nah-dahs; noh kohm-pahr-tah ah-goo-hahs oh hehr-een-gahs)

hepatitis

hepatits
(eh-pah-tee-tees)

CHAPTER 11: USING BODY MECHANICS

I will put you on the stretcher.

Voy a ponerlo en la camilla.
(Boy ah poh-nher-loh ehn lah kah-mee-yah)

Sit in the chair.

Siéntese en la silla.
(See-ehn-teh-seh ehn lah see-yah)

spinal

espinal
(ehs-pee-nahl)

Do you need the headboard up?

¿Necesita levantar más la cabecera?
(Neh-seh-see-tah leh-bahn-tahr mahs lah kah-beh-seh-rah)

I am going to help you lie down.

Voy a ayudarlo a acostarse.
(Boy ah ah-yoo-dahr-loh ah ah-kohs-tahr-seh)

I am going to help you lie on the stretcher.

Voy a ayudarlo a acostarse en la camilla.
(Boy ah ah-yoo-dahr-loh ah ah-kohs-tahr-seh ehn lah kah-mee-yah)

I will help you sit.

Le ayudaré a sentarse.
(Leh ah-yoo-dah-reh ah sehn-tahr-seh)

Turn on your side.

Voltéese de lado.
(Bhol-teh-eh-seh deh lah-doh)

Turn to your side.

Voltéate de lado.
(Bhol-teh-ah-teh deh lah-doh)

CHAPTER 12: ASSISTING WITH COMFORT

At what time do you get up?

¿A qué hora se levanta?
(Ah keh oh-rah seh leh-bahn-tah)

At what time do you go to bed?

¿A qué hora se acuesta?
(Ah keh oh-rah seh ah-koo-ehs-tah)

How many hours do you sleep?

¿Cuántas horas duerme?
(Koo-ahn-tahs oh–rahs doo-ehr-meh)

Do you sleep during the day?

¿Duerme durante el día?
(Doo-ehr-meh doo-rahn-teh ehl dee-ah)

How long?

¿Cuánto tiempo?
(Koo-ahn-toh tee-ehm-poh)

Rest now.

Descanse ahora.
(Dehs-kahn-seh ah-oh-rah)

At what time do you go to sleep?

¿A qué hora se acuesta a dormir?
(Ah keh oh-rah seh ah-koo-ehs-tah ah dohr-meer)

Do you wake up at night?

¿Se despierta en la noche?
(Seh dehs-pee-ehr-tah ehn lah noh-chen)

Are you cold?

¿Tiene frío?
(Tee-eh-neh free-oh)

Are you comfortable?

¿Está cómoda?
(Ehs-tah koh-moh-dah)

Are you hurting?

¿Tiene dolor?
(Tee-eh-neh doh-lohr)

Are you sleepy?

¿Tiene sueño?
(Tee-eh-neh soo-eh-nyoh)

Do you have chest pain?

¿Tiene dolor en el pecho?
(Tee-eh-neh doh-lohr ehn ehl peh-choh)

Does it still hurt?

¿Todavía le duele?
(Toh-dah-bee-ah leh doo-eh-leh)

Does the pain move from one place to another?

¿El dolor se mueve de un lugar a otro?
(Ehl doh-lohr seh moo-eh-beh deh oon loo-gahr ah oh-troh)

Has the pain gotten worse or gotten better?

¿Se ha puesto el dolor peor o mejor?
(Seh ah poo-ehs-toh ehl doh-lohr peh-ohr oh meh-hohr)

How often do you have the pain?	¿Qué tan seguido tiene el dolor? (Keh tahn seh-gee-doh tee-eh-neh ehl doh-lohr)
I am going to let you rest.	Voy a dejarlo descansar. (Boy ah deh-hahr-loh dehs-kahn-sahr)
If it hurts, tell me.	Si duele, avísame. (See doo-eh-leh, ah-bee-sah-meh)
On a scale from 1 [insignificant] to 10 [unbearable]. . .	En una escala del 1 [insignificante] al 10 [intolerable]. . . (Ehn oo-nah ehs-kah-lah dehl oo-noh [een-seeg-nee-gee-kahn-teh] ahl dee-ehs [een-toh-leh-rah-bleh])
Pain?	¿Dolor? (Doh-lohr)
Point when it hurts.	Señale cuando duela. (Seh-nyah-leh koo-ahn-doh doo-eh-lah)
Rest.	Descanse (Des-kahn-seh)

CHAPTER 13: ASSISTING WITH HYGIENE

I am going to clean your teeth.	Voy a limpairle los dientes. (Boy ah leem-pee-ahr-leh lohs dee-ehn-tehs)
Rinse your mouth.	Enjuague su boca. (Ehn-hoo ah-geh soo boh-kah)
Here is a glass of water to rinse with.	Aquí está un vaso de agua para que se enjuague. (Ah-kee-ehs-tah oon bah-soh deh ah-goo-ah pah-rah keh seh ehn-hoo-ah-geh)
Open your mouth, please.	Abra la boca, por favor. (Ah-brah lah boh-kah, pohr fah-bohr)
There is a shower.	Hay una ducha/regadera. (Ah-ee oo-nah doo-chah/reh-gah-deh-rah)
There is also a bathtub/tub.	También hay una bañera/tina. (Tahm-bee-ehn ah-ee oo-nah bah-nyeh-rah/tee-nah)
Use dental floss.	Use hilo dental. (Oo-seh ee-loh dehn-tahl)

CHAPTER 14: ASSISTING WITH GROOMING

Mrs. . . ., I need to help you change clothes.	Señora . . ., necesito ayudarle a cambiar su ropa. (Señora . . ., neh-seh-see-toh ah-yoo-dahr-leh ah kahm-bee-ahr soo roh-pah)

CHAPTER 15: ASSISTING WITH URINARY ELIMINATION

When was the last time you used the toilet?	¿Cuándo fue la última vez gue hizo del baño/que obró? (Koo-ahn doh foo-eh lah ool-tee-mah behs keh ee-soh dehl bah-nyoh/keh oh-broh)
How often do you urinate?	¿Cuántas veces ornia? (Koo-ahn-tahs beh-sehs oh-ree-nah)
Do you want the bedpan?	¿Quiere el pato/el bacín? (Kee-eh-reh ehl pah-toh/ehl bah-seen)
Do you have problems with starting to urinate?	¿Tiene dificultad para empezar a orinar? (Tee-eh-neh dee-fee-kool-tahd pah-rah ehm-peh-sahr ah oh-ree-nahr)
Do you want to pass urine?	¿Quiere orinar? (Kee-eh-reh oh-ree-nahr)
Everytime you go to the bathroom to void, you must place the urine in the container.	Cada vez que vaya al baño a orinar, debe poner la orina en el recipiente. (Kah-dah behs keh bah-yah ahl bah-nyoh ah oh-ree-nahr, deh-beh poh-nehr lah oh-ree-nah ehn ehl reh-see-pee-ehn-teh)
I will ask you to void.	Le diré que orine. (Leh dee-reh keh oh-ree-neh)

CHAPTER 16: ASSISTING WITH BOWEL ELIMINATION

Are you constipated?	¿Está esterñido? (Ehs-tah ehs-treh-nyee-doh)
Do you have diarrhea?	¿Tiene diarrea? (Tee-eh-neh dee-ah-reh-ah)
Do you wish to have a bowel movement?	¿Quiere evacuar/hacer del baño? (Kee-eh-reh eh-bah-koo-ahr/ah-sehr dehl bah-nyoh)

A bowel movement. | Hacer del baño. (Ah-sehr dehl bah-nyoh)

Do you want to have a bowel movement? | ¿Quiere evacuar?¿Quiere obrar? (Kee-eh-reh eh-bah-koo-ahr/Kee-eh-reh oh-brahr)

I will collect a sample of feces. | Voy a recoger una muestra de excremento. (Boy ah reh-koh-hehr oo-nah moo-ehs-trah deh ehx-kreh-mehn-toh)

CHAPTER 17: ASSISTING WITH NUTRITION AND FLUIDS

Have you eaten? | ¿Ha comido? (Ah koh-mee-doh)

What did you eat? | ¿Qué comido? (Keh koh-mee-doh)

Do you take a special diet? | ¿Toma dieta especial? (Toh-mah dee-eh-tah ehs-peh-see-ah-lehs)

What foods do you like? | ¿Qué alimentos le gustan? (Keh ah-lee-mehn-tohs leh goos-tahn)

What foods do you dislike? | ¿Qué alimentos le disgustan? (Keh ah-lee-mehn-tohs leh dees-goos-tahn)

How many times do you eat per day? | ¿Cuántas veces come por día? (Koo-ahn-tahs beh-sehs koh-meh pohr dee-ah)

What did you eat for breakfast? | ¿Qué comió en el desayuno? (Keh koh-mee-oh ehn ehl dch-sah-yoo-noh)

I am going to give you a list. | Voy a darle una lista. (Boy ah dahr-leh oo-nah lees-tah)

For breakfast: | Para el desayuno: (Pah-rah ehl deh-sah-yoo-noh)

eggs | huevos (oo-eh-bohs)

toast | pan tostado (pahn tohs-tah-doh)

coffee | café (kah-feh)

milk | leche (leh-cheh)

juice | jugo (joo-goh)

fruit | fruta (froo-tah)

How do you like your coffee? | ¿Comó le gusta el café? (Koh-moh leh goos-tah ehl kah-feh)

black | negro (neh-groh)

with cream | con crema (kohn kreh-mah)

with sugar | con azúcar (kohn ah-soo-kahr)

What kind of coffee? | ¿Qué clase de café? (Keh klah-seh deh kah-feh)

regular | regular (reh-goo-lahr)

decaffeinated | descafeinado (dehs-kah-feh-ee-nah-doh)

instant | instantáneo (eens-tahn-tah-neh-oh)

What kind of juices? | ¿Qué clase de jugos? (Keh klah-seh deh joo-gohs)

orange | naranja (nah-rah-hah)

grape | uva (oo-bah)

apple | manzana (mahn-sah-nah)

grapefruit | toronja (toh-rohn-hah)

prune | ciruela (see-roo-eh-lah)

tomato | tomate (toh-mah-teh)

How do you like the eggs fixed? | ¿Cómo le gustan los huevos? (Koh-moh lch goos-tahn lohs oo-eh-bohs)

scrambled | revueltos (reh-boo-ehl-tohs)

over-easy | volteados (bohl-teh-ah-dohs)

fried | fritos (free-tohs)

hard-boiled | duros (doo-rohs)

with ham | con jamón (kohn hah-mahn)

We have cereals. | Tenemos cereales. (Teh-neh-mohs seh-reh-ah-lehs)

oatmeal | avena (ah-beh-nah)

cream of wheat | crema de trigo (kreh-mah deh tree-goh)

corn flakes | hojitas de maíz/corn flakes (oh-hee-tahs de mah-ees/hohrn fleh-ee-ks)

Do you like them hot/cold?	¿Le gustan calientes/fríos? (Leh goos-tahn kah-lee-ehn-tehs/free-ohs)	corn	maíz/elote (mah-ees/eh-loh-teh)
We have meats:	Tenemos carnes: (Teh-nehmohs kahr-nehs)	beans	frijoles/habas (free-hoh-lehs/ah-bahs)
beef	res (rehs)	pinto beans	frijol pinto (free-hohl peen-toh)
hamburger	hamburguesa (ahm-boor-geh-sah)	refried	refritos (reh-free-tohs)
steak	bistec (bees-tehk)	salad	ensalada (ehn-sah-lah-dah)
roast	rostizado (rohs-tee-sah-doh)	lettuce	lechuga (leh-choo-gah)
pork	puerco (poo-ehr-koh)	We also have desserts:	También tenemos postres: (Tahm-bee-ehn teh-neh-mohs pohs-trehs)
chops	chuletas (choo-leh-tahs)	ice cream	nieve/helado (nee-eh-beh/eh-lah-doh)
ribs	costillas (kohs-tee-yahs)	vanilla	vainilla (bah-ee-nee-yah)
chicken	pollo (poh-yoh)	chocolate	chocolate (choh-koh-lah-teh)
fried chicken	pollo frito (poh-yoh free-toh)	strawberry	fresa (freh-sah)
baked chicken	pollo asado (poh-yoh ah-sah-doh)	pies	pasteles (pahs-teh-lehs)
breast	pechuga (peh-choo-gah)	pecan	nuez (noo-ehs)
leg	pierna (pee-ehr-nah)	apple	manzana (mahn-sah-nah)
wings	alas (ah-lahs)	cookies	galletas (gah-yeh-tahs)
fish	pescado (pehs-kah-doh)	candy	dulces (dool-sehs)
breaded	empanizado (ehm-pah-nee-sah-doh)	The water is in the glass/pitcher.	El aqua están en el vaso/la jarra. (Ehl ah-goo-ah ehs-tah ehn ehl bah-soh/lah hah-rah)
broiled fish	pescado al horno (pehs-kah-doh ahl ohr-noh)	Do you want water?	¿Quere agua? (Kee-eh-reh ah-goo-ah)
Among the vegetables that we serve are:	Entre los vegetales que servimos hay: (Ehn-treh lohs beh-heh-tah-lehs keh sehr-bee-mohs ah-ee)	Do you need ice?	¿Necesita hielo? (Neh-seh-see-tah ee-eh-loh)
potatoes	papas (pah-pahs)	The fork, spoon, and knife are wrapped in the napkin.	El tenedor, cuchara y cuchillo están envueltos en la servilleta. (Ehl teh-neh-dohr, koo-chah-rah ee koo-chee-yoh ehs-tahn ehn-boo-ehl-tohs ehn lah sehr-bee-yeh-tah)
baked potatoes	papas asadas (pah-pahs ah-sah-dahs)		
french fries	papas fritas (pah-pahs free-tahs)		
mashed potatoes	puré de papas (poo-reh deh pah-pahs)	There is a straw.	Hay un popote. (Ah-ee oon poh-poh-teh)
green beans	ejotes/habichuelas (eh-hoh-tehs/ah-bee-choo-eh-lahs)	The salt and pepper are in these packets.	La sal y pimienta están en estos paquetes. (Lah sahl ee pee-mee-ehn-tah ehs-tahn ehn ehs-tohn pah-keh-tehs)
peas	chícharos (chee-chah-rohs)		

The cover is hot. La cubeirta está caliente. (Lah koo-bee-ehr-tah ehs-tah kah-lee-ehn-teh)

It keeps the food warm. Guarda la comida tibia. (Goo-ahr-dah lah koh-mee-dah tee-bee-ah)

Select your foods from the menu after breakfast. Seleccione las comidas del menú después del desayuno. (Seh-lehk-see-oh-neh lahs koh-mee-dahs dehl meh-noo dehs-poo-ehs dehl deh-sah-yoo-noh)

dehydration deshidratación (deh-see-drah-tah-see-ohn)

nutrition nutrición (noo-tree-see-ohn)

salt sal (sahl)

Do you want: ¿Quiere: (Kee-eh-reh)

a glass of water? un vaso de agua? (oon bah-soh deh ah-goo-ah)

a glass of juice? un vaso de jugo? (oon bah-soh deh hoo-goh)

Do you want: ¿Quiere: (Kee-eh-reh)

something to eat? algo de comer? (ahl-goh deh koh-mehr)

something to drink? algo de tomar/beber? (ahl-goh deh toh-mahr/beh-behr)

something to read? algo de leer? (ahl-goh deh leh-ehr)

After meals. Después de las comidas. Dehs-poo-ehs deh lahs koh-mee-dahs)

Are you hungry? ¿Tiene hambre? (Tee-eh-neh ahm-breh)

Difficulty in swallowing... Diffcultad al tragar... (Dee-fee-kool-tahd ahl-trah-gahr)

Do you want a cup of coffee? ¿Quiere una taza de café? (Kee-eh-reh oo-nah tah-sah deh-kah-feh)

Do you want a glass of juice? ¿Quiere un vaso con jugo? (Kee-eh-reh oon bah-soh kohn hoo-goh)

Do you want a glass of water? ¿Quiere un vaso con agua? (Kee-eh-reh oon bah-soh kohn ah-goo-ah)

Do you want something to drink? ¿Quiere algo de tomar/beber? (Kee-eh-reh ahl-goh deh toh-mahr/beh-behr)

How do you like your eggs fixed? ¿Comó le gustan los huevos? (Koh-moh leh goos-tahn lohs oo-eh-bohs)

How do you like your coffee? ¿Cómo le gusta el café? (Koh-moh leh goos-tah ehl kah-feh)

How many glasses of water do you drink? ¿Cuántos vasos de agua toma? (Koo-ahn-tohs bah-sohs de ah-goo-ah toh-mah)

The meals are served at.... Los alimentos se sirven a... (Lohs ah-lee-mehn-tohs seh seer-behn ah)

When was the last time you ate? ¿Cuándo fue la última vez que comió? (Koo-ahn-doh foo-eh lah ool-tee-mah behs keh koh-mee-oh)

You have to choose three meals a day. Tiene que escoger tres comidas diarias. (Tee-eh-neh keh ehs-koh-hehr trehs koh-mee-dahs dee-ah-ree-ahs)

CHAPTER 18: ASSISTING WITH ASSESSMENT

I will start by taking vital signs. Voy a empezar por tomar los signos vitales. (Boy ah ehm-peh-sahr pohr toh-mahr lohs seeg-nohs bee-tah-lehs)

Take the temperature rectally. Tome la temperatura por el recto. (Toh-meh lah tehm-peh-rah-too-rah pohr ehl rehk-toh)

bradycardia bradicardia (brah-dee-kahr-dee-ah)

fever fatal (fah-tahl)

pulse pulso (pool-soh)

rectal rectal (rehk-tahl)

stethoscope estetoscopio (ehs-teh-tohs-koh-pee-oh)

systole sístole (sees-toh-leh)

thermometer termómetro (tehr-moh-meh-troh)

I will take the radial pulse. Voy a tomar su pulso radial. (Boy ah toh-mahr soo pool-soh rah-dee-ahl)

I will take your blood pressure. Voy a tomar tu presión de sangre. (Boy ah toh-mahr too preh-see-ohn deh sahn-greh)

CHAPTER 19: ASSISTING WITH SPECIMENS

I am going to explain how to collect the urine.	Le voy a explicar cómo juntar la orina. (Leh boy ah ehx-plee-kahr koh-moh hoon-tahr lah oh-ree-nah)
Every time you urinate, put it in the container.	Cada vez que orine, póngala en el frasco. (Kah-dah behs keh oh-ree-neh, pohn-gah-lah ehn ehl frahs-koh)
The container will be kept in the bucket with ice.	El frasco se mantendrá en una tina con hielo. (Ehl frahs-koh seh mahn-tehn-drah ehn oo-nah tee-nah kohn ee-eh-loh)
Remember that you will do this for 24 hours.	Recuerde que hará esto por veinticuatro horas. (Reh-koo-ehr-deh keh ah-rah ehs-toh pohr beh-een-tee-koo-ah-troh oh-rahs)
If there is no ice in the bucket, call me.	Si no hay hielo en la tina, llámeme. (See noh ah-ee ee-eh-loh ehn lah tee-nah, yah-meh-meh)
I also need a urine sample.	También necesito una muestra de orina. (Tahm-bee-ehn neh-seh-see-toh oo-nah moo-ehs-trah deh oh-ree-nah)
I am going to explain the collection of the urine.	Le voy a explicar la colección de orina. (Leh boy ah ehx-plee-kahr lah koh-lehk-see-ohn de oh-ree-nah)

CHAPTER 20: ASSISTING WITH EXERCISE AND ACTIVITY

Please stay/remain in bed.	Por favor, quédeses en la cama. (Pohr fah-bohr, keh-deh-seh ehn lah kan-mah)
Lift your arm.	Levanta tu brazo. (leh-bahn-tah too brah-soh)
Extend it.	Extiéndelo. (Ehx-tee-ehn-deh-loh)
Flex it.	Dóblalo. (Doh-blah-loh)
Rotate it.	Gíralo./Dale vuelta. (Hee-rah-loh/Dah-leh boo-ehl-tah)
Bend your elbow.	Dobla el codo. (doh-blah ehl koh-doh)
Turn your forearm.	Voltea el antebrazo. (Bohl-teh-ah ehl ahn-teh brah-soh)
Open your hand.	Abre tu mano. (Ah-breh too mah-noh)
Close it.	Ciérrala. (See-eh-rah-lah)
Open the fingers wide.	Separa bien los dedos. (Seh-pah-rah bee-ehn lohs deh-dohs)
Bend the wrist.	Dobla la muñeca. (Doh-blah lah moo-nyeh-kah)
Extend your wrist.	Extiende tu muñeca. (Ehx-tee-ehn-deh too moo-nyeh-kay)
Lift your leg.	Levanta la pierna. (Leh-bahn-tah lah pee-ehr-nah)
Bend it.	Dóblala. (Doh-blah-lah)
Bend your hip.	Dobla tu Cadera. (Doh-blah too kah-deh-rah)
Straighten your knee.	Endereza la rodilla. (Ehn-deh-reh-sah lah roh-dee-yah)
Move your leg.	Mueve tu pierna. (Moo-eh-beh too pee-ehr-nah)
Forward.	Adelante. (Ah-deh-lahn-teh)
Backward.	Atrás. (Ah-trahs)
Turn it to the left.	Voltéalo hacia la izquierda. (Bohl-teh-ah-loh ah-see-ah lah ees-kee-ehr-dah)
Turn it to the right.	Voltéalo hacia la derecha. (Bohl-teh-ah-loh ah-see-ah lah deh-reh-chah)
Lift your foot.	Levanta tu pie. (Leh-bahn-tah too pee-eh)
Bend your toes.	Dobla tus dedos (del pie). (Doh-blah toos deh-dohs (dehl pee-eh)
Lower your foot.	Baja el pie. (Bah-hah ehl pee-eh)
Flex the foot upward.	Dobla el pie hacia arriba. (Doh-blah ehl pee-eh ah-see-ah ah-ree-bah)
Straighten your leg.	Endereza tu pierna. (Ehn-deh-reh-sah too pee-ehr-nah)
Please walk.	Camina, por favor. (Kah-mee-nah, pohr fah-bohr)
exercise	ejercicio (eh-hehr-see-see-oh)

syncope	síncope (seen-koh-peh)
Activities are part of the plan.	Las actividades son parte del plan. (Lahs ahk-tee-bee-dah-dehs sohn pahr-teh dehl plahn)
Are you dizzy?	¿Tiene mareos? (Tee-eh-neh mah-reh-ohs)
Do you feel dizzy?	¿Se siente mareado? (Seh see-ehn-teh mah-reh-ah-doh)
Extend your arm.	Extiende tu brazo. (Ehx-tee-ehn-deh too brah-soh)
Extend your leg and foot.	Extiende tu pierna y pie. (Ehx-tee-ehn-deh too pee-ehr-nah ee pee-eh)
Flex your foot upward.	Dobla el pie para arriba. (Doh-blah ehl pee-eh pah-rah ah-ree-bah)
Flex your arm.	Dobla tu brazo. (Doh-blah too brah-soh)
Now raise the left arm.	Ahora levante el brazo izquierdo. (Ah-oh-rah leh-bahn-teh ehl brah-soh ees-kee-ehr-doh)
Turn the forearm.	Voltea el antebrazo. (Bhol-teh-ah ehl ahn-teh-brah-soh)

CHAPTER 21: ASSISTING WITH WOUND CARE

hematoma	hematoma (eh-mah-toh-mah)
ulcer	úlcera (ool-seh-rah)

CHAPTER 22: ASSISTING WITH OXYGEN NEEDS

Breathe in.	Respire. (Rehs-pee-reh)
Breathe out.	Saque el aire. (Sah-keh ehl ah-ee-reh)
Now, take a deep breath.	Ahora, respira hondo. (Ah-oh-rah, rehs-pee-rah ohn-doh)
Cough!	¡Tose! (Toh-seh)
Cough harder!	¡Tose más fuerte! (Toh-seh mahs foo-ehr-teh)
Let it out.	Exhala. (Ehx-ah-lah)
oxygen	oxígen (ohx-ee-heh-noh)

Are you having problems breathing?	¿Tiene problemas al respirar? (Tee-eh-neh proh-bleh-mahs ahl rehs-pee-rahr)
Cough deeply.	Tosa más fuerte. (Toh-sah mahs foo-ehr-teh)
Does it hurt to breathe?	¿Te duele al respirar? (Teh doo-eh-leh ahl toh-sehr)
Does it hurt to cough?	¿Te duele al toser? (Teh doo-eh-leh ahl toh-sehr)

CHAPTER 23: ASSISTING WITH REHABILITATION AND RESTORATIVE CARE

independence	independencia (een-deh-pehn-dehn-see-ah)

CHAPTER 24: CARING FOR PERSONS WITH COMMON HEALTH PROBLEMS

What causes AIDS?	¿Qué causa el SIDA? (Keh kah-oo-sah ehl see-dah)
A virus known as HIV . . .	El virus causal del SIDA se conoce como VIH . . . (Ehl bee-roos kah-oo-sahl dehl see-dah seh koh-noh-seh koh-moh beh-ee-ah-cheh[VIH])
Who is at risk of getting AIDS?	¿Quién está en riesgo de contraer el SIDA? (Kee-ehn ehs-tah ehn ree-ehs-goh deh kohn-trah-ehr ehl see-dah)
sexually active homosexual and bisexual males or females	homosexuales activos y hombres o mujeres bisexuales (oh-moh-sehx-oo-ah-lehs ahk-tee-bohs ee ohm-brehs oh moo-heh-rehs bee-sehx-oo-ah-lehs)
intravenous drug abusers	los que abusan de las drogas intravenosas (lohs keh ah-boo-sah deh lahs droh-gahs een-trah-beh-noh-sahs)
hemophiliacs and recipients of blood/blood components	hemofílicos, donadores de sangre o transfusión con sangre contaminada (eh-moh-fee-lee-kohs, doh-nah-doh-rehs deh sahn-greh oh trahns-foo-see-ohn kohn sahn-greh kohn-tah-mee-nah-dah)
fetus of infected mothers	fetos de madres contamnadas (feh-tohs deh mah-drehs kohn-tah-mee-nah-dahs)

Infected persons can transmit the virus.
Las personas infectadas pueden transmitir el virus
(Lahs pehr-soh-nahs een fehk-tah-dahs poo-ehdehn-trahns-mee-teer ehl bee-roos)

Can casual contact cause AIDS?
¿Los contactos eventaules puden causar SIDA?
(Lohs kohn-tahk-tohs eh-behn-too-ah-lehs poo-eh-dehn kah-oo-sahr see-dah)

HIV is not transmissible by casual contact, nor . . .
El VIH no es transmitido en forma casual, ni por . . .
(Ehl VIH noh ehs trahns-mee-tee-doh ehn fohr-mah kah-soo-ahl, nee pohr:)

living in the same house as infected persons
vivir en la misma casa con personas infectadas
(bee-beer ehn lah mees-mah kah-sah kohn pehr-soh-nahs een-fehk-tah-dahs)

eating food handled by persons with AIDS
comer comida preparada por personas infectadas con SIDA
(koh-mehr koh-mee-dah preh-pah-rah-dah pohr pehr-soh-nahs een-fehk-tah-dahs kohn see-dah)

coughing, sneezing, kissing, or swimming with infected persons
tos, estornudo, besar, o nadar con personas infectadas
(tohs, ehs-tohr-noo-doh, beh-sahr oh nah-dahr kohn pehr-soh-nahs een-fehk-tah-dahs)

How serious is AIDS?
¿Qué tan serio es el SIDA?
(Keh tahn seh-ree-oh ehs-ehl see-dah)

AIDS has a high fatality rate approaching 100%.
EL SIDA tiene una tasa cercana al 100 por ciento de mortalidad.
(Ehl see-dah tee-eh-neh oo-nah tah-sah sehr-kah-nah ahl see-ehn pohr see-ehn-toh deh mohr-tah-lee-dahd)

Is there a danger from donated blood?
¿Qué peligro hay por sangre donada?
(Keh peh-lee-groh ah-ee pohr sahn-greh doh-nah-dah)

The risk of contracting HIV is not high. Blood banks and other centers use
El riesgo de contraer VIH no es alto. Los bancos de sangre y otros centros usan equipos estériles y agujas desechables.

sterile equipment and disposable needles.
(Ehl ree-ehs-goh deh kohn-trah-ehr VIH noh ehs ahl-toh. Lohns bahn-kohs deh sahn-greh ee oh-trohs sehn-trohs oo-sahn eh-kee-pohs ehs-teh-ree-lehs ee ah-goo-hahs deh-seh-chah-blehs)

The U.S. Public Health Service recommends:
El Departamento de Salud Pública de los Estados Unidos recomienda:
(Ehl Deh-pahr-tah-mehn-toh deh Sah-lood Poo-blee-kah deh lohs Ehs-tah-dohs Oo-nee-dohs reh-koh-mee-ehn-dah)

1. Know sexual background/ habits of partners.
1. Conozca los hábitos sexuales de su pareja.
(Koh-nohs-kah lohs ah-bee-tohs sex-oo-ah-lehs deh soo pah-reh-hah)

2. Use a condom or prophylactic.
2. Use un condón o profiláctico.
(Oo-seh oon kohn-dohn oh proh-fee-lahk-tee-koh)

3. If your partner is in a high risk group, cease sexual relations.
3. Si su compañera está en el grupo de alto riesgo, suspenda las relaciones sexuales.
(See soo kohm-pah-nyeh-rah ehs-tah ehn ehl groo-pah deh ahl-toh ree-ehs-goh, soos-pehn-dah lahs reh-lah-see-ohn-ehs sehx-oo-ahl-ehs)

4. Eliminate multiple sexual partners.
4. Elimine múltiples compañeros sexuales.
(Eh-lee-mee-neh mool-tee-plehs kohm-pha-nyeh-rohs sehx-oo-ah-lehs)

5. Don't use intra-venous drugs with contami-nated needles; don't share needles or syringes.
5. No use drogas intravenosas con agujas contaminadas; no comparta agujas o jeringas.
(Noh oos-eh droh-gahs een-trah-veh-noh-sahs kohn ah-goo-hahs kohn-tah-mee-nah-dahs; noh kohm-pahr-tah ah-goo-hahs oh hehr-een-gahs)

asthma
asma
(ahs-mah)

cancer   cáncer
                          (kahn-sehr)
cardiac   cardíaco
                          (kahr-dee-ah-koh)
chemotherapy   quimioterapia
                          (kee-mee-oh-teh-rah-pee-ah)
hepatitis   hepatits
                          (eh-pah-tee-tees)
insulin   insulina
                          (een-soo-lee-nah)
venereal   venéreo
                          (beh-neh-reh-oh)
vomit   vómito
                          (boh-mee-toh)
Does the pain get   ¿Se mejora el dolor si se
  better if you   detiene y descansa?
  stop and rest?   (Seh meh-hoh-rah ehl doh-
                            lohr see-seh deh-tee-eh-neh
                            ee dehs-kahn-sah)
glaucoma   glaucoma
                          (glah-oo-koh-mah)
vertigo   vértigo
                          (behr-tee-goh)
vision   visión
                          (bee-see-ohn)

CHAPTER 25: CARING FOR PERSONS WITH CONFUSION AND DEMENTIA

delirious   delirio
                          (deh-lee-ree-oh)

CHAPTER 26: ASSISTING WITH EMERGENCY CARE

We are going to   Vamos al hospital.
  the hospital.   (Bah-mohs ahl ohs-pee-tahl)
We are going in   Vamos en la ambulancia.
  the ambulance.   (Bah-mohs ehn lah ahm-boo-
                            lahn-see-ah)
cardiac   cardíaco
                         (kahr-dee-ah-koh)

CHAPTER 27: CARING FOR THE DYING PERSON

cancer   cáncer
                         (kahn-sehr)

Glossary

abduction Moving a body part away from the midline of the body

abuse The intentional mistreatment or harm of another person

acetone A substance that appears in urine from the rapid breakdown of fat for energy; ketone body or ketone

active physical restraint A restraint attached to the person's body and to a fixed (non-movable) object; it restricts movement or body access

activities of daily living (ADL) The activities usually done during a normal day in a person's life

adduction Moving a body part toward the midline of the body

advance directive A document stating a person's wishes about health care when that person cannot make his or her own decisions

alopecia Hair loss

ambulation The act of walking

anorexia The loss of appetite

anxiety A vague, uneasy feeling in response to stress

aphasia The inability *(a)* to speak *(phasia)*

apnea The lack or absence *(a)* of breathing *(pnea)*

arthroplasty The surgical replacement *(plasty)* of a joint *(arthro)*

asepsis Being free of disease-producing microbes

aspiration Breathing fluid or an object into the lungs

assault Intentionally attempting or threatening to touch a person's body without the person's consent

assisted living facility Provides housing, support services, and health care to persons needing help with daily activities

atrophy The decrease in size or a wasting away of tissue

base of support The area on which an object rests

battery Touching a person's body without his or her consent

bedsore A pressure ulcer, pressure sore, or decubitus ulcer

benign tumor A tumor that grows slowly and within a local area

biohazardous waste Items contaminated with blood, body fluids, secretions, or excretions; *bio* means life, and *hazardous* means dangerous or harmful

blood pressure The amount of force exerted against the walls of an artery by the blood

board and care home Provides a room, meals, laundry, and supervision; residential care facility

body alignment The way the head, trunk, arms, and legs are aligned with one another; posture

body language Messages sent through facial expressions, gestures, posture, hand and body movements, gait, eye contact, and appearance

body mechanics Using the body in an efficient and careful way

body temperature The amount of heat in the body that is a balance between the amount of heat produced and the amount lost by the body

bradypnea Slow *(brady)* breathing *(pnea)*; respirations are less than 12 per minute

calorie The amount of energy produced when the body burns food

cardiac arrest The heart and breathing stop suddenly and without warning

carrier A human or animal that is a reservoir for microbes but does not have signs and symptoms of infection

catheter A tube used to drain or inject fluid through a body opening

cell The basic unit of body structure

chart The medical record

Cheyne-Stokes respirations Respirations gradually increase in rate and depth and then become shallow and slow; breathing may stop *(apnea)* for 10 to 20 seconds

circulatory ulcer An open wound on the lower legs and feet caused by decreased blood flow through arteries or veins; vascular ulcer

civil law Laws dealing with relationships between people

clean technique Medical asepsis

colostomy A surgically created opening *(stomy)* between the colon *(colo)* and abdominal wall

coma A state of being unaware of one's surroundings and being unable to react or respond to people, places, or things

communicable disease A disease caused by pathogens that spread easily; a contagious disease

communication The exchange of information—a message sent is received and interpreted by the intended person

comprehensive care plan A written guide giving direction for the resident's care (required by OBRA)

confidentiality Trusting others with personal and private information

constipation The passage of a hard, dry stool

constrict To narrow

contagious disease Communicable disease

contamination The process of becoming unclean

contracture The lack of joint mobility caused by abnormal shortening of a muscle

convulsion A seizure

crime An act that violates a criminal law

criminal law Laws concerned with offenses against the public and against society

culture The characteristics of a group of people—language, values, beliefs, habits, likes, dislikes, customs—passed from one generation to the next

dandruff Excessive amount of dry, white flakes from the scalp

decubitus ulcer A pressure ulcer, pressure sore, or bedsore

defamation Injuring a person's name and reputation by making false statements to a third person

defecation The process of excreting feces from the rectum through the anus; bowel movement

dehydration A decrease in the amount of water in body tissues

delegate To authorize another person to perform a task

delirium A state of temporary but acute mental confusion

delusion A false belief

dementia The loss of cognitive function and social function caused by changes in the brain

development Changes in mental, emotional, and social function

developmental task A skill that must be completed during a stage of development

diarrhea The frequent passage of liquid stools

diastolic pressure The pressure in the arteries when the heart is at rest

digestion The process of physically and chemically breaking down food so that it can be absorbed for use by the cells

dilate To expand or open wider

disability Any lost, absent, or impaired physical or mental function

disaster A sudden catastrophic event in which people are injured and killed and property is destroyed

disinfection The process of destroying pathogens

dorsal recumbent position The back-lying or supine position

dorsiflexion Bending the toes and foot up at the ankle

dysphagia Difficulty *(dys)* swallowing *(phagia)*

dyspnea Difficult, labored, or painful *(dys)* breathing *(pnea)*

dysuria Painful or difficult *(dys)* urination *(uria)*

edema The swelling of body tissues with water

enema The introduction of fluid into the rectum and lower colon

enteral nutrition Giving nutrients through the gastrointestinal tract *(enteral)*

ethics Knowledge of what is right conduct and wrong conduct

extension Straightening a body part

external rotation Turning the joint outward

fainting The sudden loss of consciousness from an inadequate blood supply to the brain

false imprisonment Unlawful restraint or restriction of a person's freedom of movement

fecal impaction The prolonged retention and buildup of feces in the rectum

fecal incontinence The inability to control the passage of feces and gas through the anus

feces The semi-solid mass of waste products in the colon that are expelled through the anus

fever Elevated body temperature

flatulence The excessive formation of gas in the stomach and intestines

flatus Gas or air passed through the anus

flexion Bending a body part

flow rate The number of drops per minute *(gtt/min)*

footdrop The foot falls down at the ankle; permanent plantar flexion

Fowler's position A semi-sitting position; the head of the bed is raised between 45 and 60 degrees

fracture A broken bone

fraud Saying or doing something to trick, fool, or deceive a person

friction The rubbing of one surface against another

full visual privacy Having the means to be completely free from public view while in bed

functional incontinence The person has bladder control but cannot use the toilet in time

gavage Tube feeding

geriatrics The care of aging people

gerontology The study of the aging process

glucosuria Sugar *(glucos)* in the urine *(uria)*; glycosuria

glycosuria Sugar *(glycos)* in the urine *(uria)*; glucosuria

gossip To spread rumors or talk about the private matters of others

growth The physical changes that are measured and that occur in a steady and orderly manner

hallucination Seeing, hearing, or feeling something that is not real

harassment To trouble, torment, offend, or worry a person by one's behavior or comments

hazardous substance Any chemical in the workplace that can cause harm

health team Staff members who work together to provide health care; called the *interdisciplinary health care team* in nursing centers

hematuria Blood *(hemat)* in the urine *(uria)*

hemiplegia Paralysis on one side of the body

hemoptysis Bloody *(hemo)* sputum *(ptysis* means "to spit")

hemorrhage The excessive loss of blood in a short time

hirsutism Excessive body hair in women and children

hormone A chemical substance secreted by the glands into the bloodstream

hospice An agency or program for persons who are dying

hyperextension Excessive straightening of a body part

hypertension Blood pressure measurements that remain above *(hyper)* a systolic pressure of 140 mm Hg or a diastolic pressure of 90 mm Hg

hyperventilation Respirations are rapid *(hyper)* and deeper than normal

hypotension When the systolic blood pressure is below *(hypo)* 90 mm Hg and the diastolic pressure is below 60 mm Hg

hypoventilation Respirations are slow *(hypo)*, shallow, and sometimes irregular

hypoxia Cells do not have enough *(hypo)* oxygen *(oxia)*

ileostomy A surgically created opening *(stomy)* between the ileum (small intestine *[ileo]*) and the abdominal wall

immunity Protection against a disease or condition; the person will not get or be affected by the disease

infection A disease resulting from the invasion and growth of microbes in the body

insomnia A chronic condition in which the person cannot sleep or stay asleep all night

internal rotation Turning the joint inward

intravenous (IV) therapy Giving fluids through a needle or catheter inserted into a vein; IV and IV infusion

invasion of privacy When a person's name, picture, or private affairs are exposed or made public without consent

job description A list of responsibilities and functions the agency expects you to perform

ketone Acetone; ketone body

ketone body Acetone; ketone

lateral position The side-lying position

law A rule of conduct made by a government body

libel Making false statements in print, writing, or through pictures or drawings

licensed practical nurse (LPN) A nurse who has completed a 1-year nursing program and has passed a licensing test; called *licensed vocational nurse* (*LVN*) in some states

licensed vocational nurse (LVN) Licensed practical nurse

logrolling Turning the person as a unit, in alignment, with one motion

malignant tumor A tumor that grows fast and invades other tissues; cancer

malpractice Negligence by a professional person

medical asepsis Practices used to remove or destroy pathogens and to prevent their spread from one person or place to another person or place; clean technique

medical record A written account of a person's condition and response to treatment and care; chart

menopause The time when menstruation stops and menstrual cycles end

metabolism The burning of food for heat and energy by the cells

metastasis The spread of cancer to other body parts

microbe A microorganism

microorganism A small (*micro*) living plant or animal (*organism*) seen only with a microscope; a microbe

need Something necessary or desired for maintaining life and mental well-being

neglect Failure to provide the person with goods or services needed to avoid physical harm, mental anguish, or mental illness

negligence An unintentional wrong in which a person did not act in a reasonable and careful manner and causes harm to a person or property

nocturia Frequent urination (*uria*) at night (*noct*)

non-pathogen A microbe that does not usually cause an infection

nonverbal communication Communication that does not use words

nursing assistant A person who gives basic nursing care under the supervision of a licensed nurse

nursing care plan A written guide about the person's care

nursing center Provides health care services to persons who need regular or continuous care; nursing home or nursing facility

nursing facility (NF) Nursing center or nursing home

nursing home Nursing center or nursing facility

nursing process The method RNs use to plan and deliver nursing care; its five steps are assessment, nursing diagnosis, planning, implementation, and evaluation

nursing team RNs, LPNs/LVNs, and nursing assistants

nutrient A substance that is ingested, digested, absorbed, and used by the body

nutrition The processes involved in the ingestion, digestion, absorption, and use of foods and fluids by the body

objective data Information that is seen, heard, felt, or smelled; signs

observation Using the senses of sight, hearing, touch, and smell to collect information

old Between 75 and 84 years of age

old-old 85 years of age and older

oliguria Scant amount (*olig*) of urine (*uria*); less than 500 ml in 24 hours

ombudsman Someone who supports or promotes the needs and interests of another person

Omnibus Budge Reconciliation Act of 1987 (OBRA) A law that requires nursing centers to provide care in a manner and a setting that maintains or improves a person's quality of life, health, and safety

optimal level of function A person's highest potential for mental and physical performance

oral hygiene Mouth care

organ Groups of tissues with the same function

orthopnea Breathing (*pnea*) deeply and comfortably only when sitting (*ortho*)

orthopneic position Sitting up (*ortho*) and leaning over a table to breathe

orthostatic hypotension Abnormally low (*hypo*) blood pressure when the person suddenly stands up (*ortho* and *static*); postural hypotension

ostomy A surgically created opening

overflow incontinence Urine leaks when the bladder is too full

paraplegia Paralysis from the waist down

passive physical restraint A restraint near but not directly attached to the person's body; it does not totally restrict freedom of movement and allows access to certain body parts

pathogen A microbe that is harmful and can cause an infection

pediculosis (lice) Infestation with lice

perineal care Cleaning the genital and anal areas; pericare

peristalsis Involuntary muscle contractions in the digestive system that move food through the alimentary canal

plantar flexion The foot (*plantar*) is bent (*flexion*); bending the foot down at the ankle

polyuria Abnormally large amounts (*poly*) of urine (*uria*)

postmortem After (*post*) death (*mortem*)

postural hypotension Orthostatic hypotension

posture Body alignment

pressure sore A bedsore, decubitus ulcer, or pressure ulcer

pressure ulcer Any injury caused by unrelieved pressure; decubitus ulcer, bedsore, or pressure sore

priority The most important thing at the time

pronation Turning the joint downward

prone position Lying on the abdomen with the head turned to one side

prosthesis An artificial replacement for a missing body part

pseudodementia False (*pseudo*) dementia

pulse The beat of the heart felt at an artery as a wave of blood passes through the artery

pulse rate The number of heartbeats or pulses felt in 1 minute

quadriplegia Paralysis from the neck down

range of motion (ROM) The movement of a joint to the extent possible without causing pain

recording The written account of care and observations; charting

reflex incontinence The loss of urine at predictable intervals when the bladder is full

registered nurse (RN) A nurse who has completed a 2-, 3-, or 4-year nursing program and has passed a licensing test

regurgitation The backward flow of food from the stomach into the mouth

rehabilitation The process of restoring the person to his or her highest possible level of physical, psychological, social, and economic function

reincarnation The belief that the spirit or soul is reborn in another human body or in another form of life

religion Spiritual beliefs, needs, and practices

reporting The oral account of care and observations

residential care facility A board and care home

respiration The process of supplying the cells with oxygen and removing carbon dioxide from them; breathing air into (inhalation) and out of (exhalation) the lungs

respiratory arrest Breathing stops but heart action continues for several minutes

restorative aide A nursing assistant with special training in restorative nursing and rehabilitation skills

restorative nursing care Care that helps persons regain their health, strength, and independence

restraint Any item, object, device, garment, material, or drug that limits or restricts a person's freedom of movement or access to one's body

reverse Trendelenburg's position The head of the bed is raised, and the foot of the bed is lowered

rigor mortis The stiffness or rigidity (*rigor*) of skeletal muscles that occurs after death (*mortis*)

rotation Turning the joint

seizure Violent and sudden contractions or tremors of muscle groups; convulsion

semi-Fowler's position The head of the bed is raised 30 degrees; or the head of the bed is raised 30 degrees and the knee portion is raised 15 degrees

semi-prone side position Sims' position

sexuality The physical, psychological, social, cultural, and spiritual factors that affect a person's feelings and attitudes about his or her sex

shearing When skin sticks to a surface while muscles slide in the direction the body is moving

shock Results when organs and tissues do not get enough blood

side-lying position The lateral position

signs Objective data

Sims' position A left side-lying position in which the upper leg is sharply flexed so it is not on the lower leg and the lower arm is behind the person; semi-prone side position

skilled nursing facility (SNF) A nursing center that provides complex care for persons with severe health problems

skin tear A break or rip in the skin; the epidermis (top skin layer) separates from the underlying tissues

slander Making false statements orally

sleep deprivation The amount and quality of sleep are decreased

sleepwalking The sleeping person leaves the bed and walks about

sputum Mucus from the respiratory system that is expectorated (expelled) through the mouth

sterile The absence of *all* microbes

sterilization The process of destroying *all* microbes

stoma An opening; see colostomy and ileostomy

stool Excreted feces

stress incontinence When urine leaks during exercise and certain movements

subacute care Complex medical care or rehabilitation for persons who no longer need hospital care

subjective data Things a person tells you about that you cannot observe through your senses; symptoms

suffocation When breathing stops from the lack of oxgyen

sundowning Signs, symptoms, and behaviors of Alzheimer's Disease increase during hours of darkness

supination Turning the joint upward

supine position The back-lying or dorsal recumbent position

suppository A cone-shaped, solid drug that is inserted into a body opening; it melts at body temperature

symptoms Subjective data

system Organs that work together to perform special functions

systolic pressure The amount of force needed to pump blood out of the heart into the arterial circulation

tachypnea Rapid *(tachy)* breathing *(pnea)*; respirations are 24 or more per minute

task A function, procedure, activity, or work that does not require an RN's professional knowledge or judgment

teamwork Staff members work together as a group; each person does his or her part to provide safe and effective care; staff members help each other as needed

terminal illness An illness or injury for which there is no reasonable expectation of recovery

tissue A group of cells with similar functions

transfer belt A belt used to support persons who are unsteady or disabled; a gait belt

Trendelenburg's position The head of the bed is lowered, and the foot of the bed is raised

tumor A new growth of abnormal cells; tumors are benign or malignant

urge incontinence Urine is lost in response to a sudden, urgent need to void; the person cannot get to a toilet in time

urinary frequency Voiding at frequent intervals

urinary incontinence The loss of bladder control

urinary urgency The need to void at once

urination The process of emptying urine from the bladder; voiding

verbal communication Communication that uses written or spoken words

vital signs Temperature, pulse, respirations, and blood pressure

voiding Urination

work ethics Behavior in the workplace

workplace violence Violent acts directed toward persons at work or while on duty

wound A break in the skin or mucous membrane

young-old Between 65 and 74 years of age

Index

A

Abbreviations, 47
Abdominal binders, straight, 380, *381*
Abdominal thrusts, 450, *452, 453*
Abduction, 350, *353*
Abuse, 8
  definition of, 12
  forms of, 19–20
  OBRA requirements and, 20
  in rehabilitation and restorative care, 402
  reporting on, 19–20
  signs of, *20*
Abusive personality, 428
Acetone, 337, 341
Acquired immunodeficiency syndrome
    (AIDS), 425–426
Activities, 8. *see also* Exercise and activity
  encouragement of, 402
  exercise and, 349–365 (*see also* Exercise
    and activity)
Activities of daily living
  flow sheet for, *37*
  rehabilitation and restorative care for,
    397, 398, *398–400,* 402
Acute illness, 2
Adduction, 350, *353*
Admission sheet, 34
Adrenal glands, 77, *78*
Advance directive, 459, *461*
Affective disorders, 428
Age, 91. *see also* Older persons
Aggressive behavior, 53, 437
Agitation, in Alzheimer's disease, 436
AIDS, 425–426
Airway, in CPR, 446, *446*
Airway obstruction, foreign-body,
    450–453
  chest thrusts in obese and pregnant for,
    451
  Heimlich maneuver (abdominal
    thrusts) for, 450, *452*
  recovery position for, 453, *453*
  in responsive adult, 451, *452*
  in unresponsive adult, 452, *453*
Alert oriented residents, 2
Alimentary canal, 72, *73*
Alopecia, 235
Alveoli, 72, *72*
Alzheimer's disease (AD), 434–437
  aggression and combativeness in, 437
  agitation and restlessness in, 436
  catastrophic reactions in, 436
  delusions in, 436, 439
  hallucinations in, 436, 439
  repetitive behaviors in, 437

Alzheimer's disease (AD) (*Continued*)
  screaming in, 437
  sexual behavior in, abnormal, 437
  signs of, 434–435
  stages of, 435, 436
  sundowning in, 433, 436, 438
  wandering in, 435–436, 438
Alzheimer's disease (AD) care, 437–442,
    439, 440
  family in, 441
  quality of life in, 441–442
  special care units for, 440
  validation therapy in, 441
Alzheimer's units, 4
Ambulation, 350, 359–364
  assisting procedure for, 360, *361*
  delegation guidelines in, 359
  falling person and, 361, *362*
  overview of, 359
  safety and comfort in, 359
  walking aids for, 362, *362–365, 364*
Anger, 53, 402
Angina pectoris, 421–422, *422*
Ankle exercises, 356, *358*
Anorexia, 291
Anterior, 46, *46*
Antibodies, 78
Antigen, 78
Antisocial personality, 428
Anus, 73, *74*
Anxiety, 405
Anxiety disorders, 427
Aorta, 71, *71*
Aphasia, 405, 411
  expressive, 413
  expressive-receptive, 413
  receptive, 413
Apnea, 389
Appearance, 23, *24, 26*
Appetite, 295
Aquathermia pad, 384
Arterial ulcers, 373. *see also* Circulatory
    ulcers
Arteries, 71, *71*
Arteriole, 71
Arthritis, 406–407
Arthroplasty, 405, 407
Asepsis, 123
Asepsis, medical
  definition of, 123
  hand hygiene in, 125, *126, 127*
  supplies and equipment in, 128, *128, 129*
Aspiration, 204, 291, 307, *307, 308*
Assault, 12, 18
Assessment, 39, *39–40,* 311–335
  focus on person in, 334
  height and weight measurement in,
    331–332, *332*
  intake and output in, *328,* 328–330, *329*

Assessment (*Continued*)
  pain in, 333, *333, 334*
  vital signs in, 312–327 (*see also* Vital
    signs)
Assignment sheets, 42, *42*
Assisted living facility, 2, *3*
Asthma, 420
Atherosclerosis, 421, *421*
Atria, 70, *70*
Atrophy, from bedrest, 350, *351*
Attendance, 28
Attitude, 28
Automated external defibrillators (AEDs),
    453

B

Back massage, 227
  circulatory ulcers and, *374*
  pressure ulcers and, *370*
Barrel chest, 420, *420*
Barrier device, in mouth-to-mouth
    breathing, 447, *447*
Base of support, 144, *145*
Basic life support (BLS), 445–453
  automated external defibrillators in, 453
  for cardiac arrest, 446
  cardiopulmonary resuscitation in,
    446–450 (*see also* Cardiopulmonary
    resuscitation [CPR])
  chain of survival in, 446
  focus on person in, 456
  for foreign-body airway obstruction,
    450–453 (*see also* Foreign-body
    airway obstruction)
  for respiratory arrest, 446
  safety and comfort in, 446
Bathing, 213–225
  complete bed bath in, 214–216, *217–219*
  delegation guidelines for, 214
  for dementia patients, 213
  partial bath in, *220,* 220–221
  in rehabilitation and restorative care,
    398, *398*
  rules for, *213*
  tub baths and showers in, *222,* 222–225,
    223
Bathroom, in personal unit, 185
Battery, 12, 18
B cells, 78
Beans, *293,* 294–295
Bed alarms, *93,* 94
Bed cradles, 351, *353,* 372
Bedmaking, 186–199
  closed, 189–190, *191–194*
  linens in, *187,* 187–188
  occupied beds in, 195–196, *197, 198*
  overview of, 186, *186*
  rules and guidelines for, 188, *188*
  surgical beds in, 199, *199*

Bedpans, *258*, 258–260, *260*, *261*
Bed rails, restraints and, *113*
Bedrest, 350–351
  complications of, 350, *350*, *351*
  positioning for, 351, *351*, *352*
Beds
  lifting and moving persons in, 146–153
    (see also under Body mechanics)
  positions for, 181–182, *182*, *183*
  for pressure ulcers, 372, *373*
  special, 372, *373*
Bedside stand, 183, *183*
Bedsore; see Pressure ulcers
Behavior issues, 52–53, *53*. *see also specific behaviors*
Belonging needs, 52, *52*
Belt restraints, *112*, *116*
Benign tumor, 405, *405*
Between-meal nourishment, 306
Bile, 73
Biohazardous waste, 123, 138, *139*
Bipolar disorder, 428
Bladder, 74, *74*
Bleeding, 445, 453–455, *454*
  pressure and pressure points for, 454, *454*
Blindness, *418*, 418–419, *419*
Blood, 69
Bloodborne pathogen standard, 139–140
Blood clot, 411
Blood pressure assessment, *325*, 325–327, *326*
Blood sugar, 424
Blood vessels, 71, *71*
  dilation of, 381, *381*
  ruptured, 411
Board and care home, 2, 3
Body, structure and function of, 60–80
  cells in, 61, *61*, 62
  circulatory system in, 69–71, *70*, *71*
  digestive system in, 72–74, *73*
  endocrine system in, 77, *77*–78
  immune system in, 78–79, *79*
  integumentary system in, 62–63, *63*
  musculoskeletal system in, 63–65, *64*, *65*
  nervous system in, 66–68, *66*–69
  organs in, 61, *62*
  reproductive system in, 74–77, *75*–77
  respiratory system in, 71–72, *72*
  tissues in, 61, *62*
  urinary system in, 74, *74*
Body alignment, 144
Body language, 55, *55*
Body mechanics, 143–178
  base of support in, 144, *145*, 146
  body alignment in, 144, *145*
  ergonomics in, 146
  focus on person in, 176, *177*
  positioning in, 172–176, *173*–176
  rules for, *144*
Body mechanics, for lifting and moving persons in bed, 146–153
  lift sheet in, 150, *150*, 151
  logrolling in, 156, *156*, 157
  moving up in bed in, 148, *148*, 149
  safety and comfort in, 147
  side moving in, 152, *152*, 153
  side of bed sitting in, 158, 159, *159*

Body mechanics, for lifting and moving persons in bed *(Continued)*
  skin protection in, 146, *147*
  turning persons in, 154, *154*, 155
Body mechanics, for transferring persons, 160–171
  bed to chair or wheelchair transfers in, *162*, 162–165, *164*, *165*
  delegation guidelines in, 160
  mechanical lifts in, 167, 168, *169*
  toilet transfers in, 170, *170*, 171
  transfer belts in, 160, 161, *161*
Body temperature, 312–319. *see also* Temperature, body
Bones, 63, *64*, 84. *see also* specific disorders
Bowel elimination, 276–289, *277*
  bowel training in, 279, *279*
  comfort and safety in, *278*
  enemas in, 280–286 (see also Enemas)
  factors in, 277–278, *278*
  focus on person in, 288
  normal bowel movements in, 277
  ostomy and, 286–287, *287*
  problems of, 278–279
Bowman's capsule, 74, *75*
Braces, 364, *365*
Bradypnea, 389
Braille, 418, *418*
Brain, *67*
Breaks, 29
Breast binders, 380, *381*
Breasts, 76, *77*
Breathing
  in CPR, 446–447, *447*
  deep, 390, *390*, 391
  mouth-to-mouth, 446–447, *447*
  rescue, 446, *447*
Bronchioles, 71, *72*
Bronchitis, chronic, 420
Bronchus, 71, *72*

C
Calculi, renal, 423
Call system, 183–185, *184*, *185*
Calorie, 291
Calorie counts, 306
Cancer, 405–406
Canes, 362, *363*
Capillaries, 71
Carbohydrates, 295
Cardiac arrest, 422, 445, 446
Cardiac muscle, 64
Cardiopulmonary resuscitation (CPR), 446–450
  airway in, 446, *446*
  breathing in, 446–447, *447*
  circulation in, 447–448, *448*, *449*
  with one rescuer, 449
  with two rescuers, 450, *450*
Cardiovascular disorders, 421–423
  angina pectoris, 421–422, *422*
  coronary artery disease, 421, *421*
  heart failure, 423
  hypertension, 421
  myocardial infarction, 422
Cardiovascular system, 69–71, *70*, *71*, 85
Caregivers, children as, 82

Caring, for whole person, 51, *51*
Carotid pulse, 447, *448*
Carrier, 123–124
Case management, 5
Case mix groups, 5
Cast care, 408, *409*
Cataract, 417, *417*
Catastrophic reactions, in Alzheimer's disease, 436
Catheters
  condom, for urinary incontinence, 271–273, *272*
  for intravenous therapy, 308
  for urinary incontinence, 257, *266*, 266–268, *267*, *269*
Cells, 61, *61*, 62
Central nervous system, 66, *66*–67, *67*
Cerebrovascular accident (CVA), 411, 445, 453, 456
Cervix, 76, *76*
Chain of survival, 446
Chairs
  bed to chair transfers for, *162*, 162–165, *164*, *165*
  chair to bed transfers for, 165, *166*, *167*
  in personal unit, 183
  positioning persons in, 174, *174*–176, 176
Chest compressions, 447–448, *448*, *449*
Chest thrusts, 450, *451*
Cheyne-Stokes respirations, 389
Childcare, 28
Children, as caregivers, 82
Choice, personal, 7, *7*, 9
  of foods, 295
  in rehabilitation and restorative care, 402
Chromosomes, 61, *62*
Chronic bronchitis, 420
Chronic illness, 2
Chronic obstructive pulmonary disease (COPD), 420
Chyme, 73
Circulation, in CPR, 447–448, *448*
Circulatory system, 69–71, *70*, *71*, 85
Circulatory ulcers, 368, 373–377. *see also* Pressure ulcers
  prevention and treatment of, *374*, 374–377, *376*–378
  types of, 373, *373*
Civil law, 12, 18
Clarifying, in communication, 56
Clean technique, 123
Clitoris, 76, *76*, 77
Clock, 24-hour, 44, *44*
Closed fracture, 408
Closed reduction, 408
Closet and drawer space, 185
Clot, blood, 411
Cold applications; see Heat and cold applications
Collecting tubule, 74, *75*
Colon, 73, *74*
Colostomy, 28, 277, 286, *287*
Coma, 91
Combativeness, in Alzheimer's disease, 437
Comfort, 179–202. *see also specific disorders*
  in ambulation, 359
  in basic life support, 446

Comfort (Continued)
  in bedmaking, 186–199 (see also
      Bedmaking)
  with binder application, 381
  in dressings application, 379
  with elastic bandages, 376
  with elastic stockings, 375
  in emergency care, 445
  in feeding, 304
  focus on person in, 201
  for heat and cold applications, 384
  in height and weight measurement, 331
  in intake and output assessment, 329
  in meal preparation, 300
  with meal trays, 302
  person's unit in, 180–185, 180–185
  for range-of-motion exercises, 354
  of sleep, 200, 200–201
  in sputum specimen collection, 345
  in stool specimen collection, 343
  in temperature taking, 314
  in urine specimen collection, 337
  in urine specimen testing, 341
Commodes, 263, 263, 264
Communicable disease, 123, 425–426
Communication
  barriers to, 57
  with comatose persons, 57
  definition of, 33
  methods of, 55–56, 56
  nonverbal, 55, 55
  with other cultures, 56, 57
  verbal, 54, 54
Communication with health team, 33–49
  abbreviations in, 47
  computers in, 47, 47
  conflict in, 48
  guidelines for, 33
  Kardex in, 33, 38
  medical record in, 33, 35–37
  medical terminology in, 44, 44–45, 46
  nursing process in, 39–42, 39–43
  phone in, 47, 47
  reporting and recording in, 43, 43–44, 44
  resident care conferences in, 43
Compensation, 427
Competency evaluation, 12
Complete care residents, 3
Compound fracture, 408
Comprehensive care plan, 441
Computers, 47, 47
Condom catheters, 271–273, 272
Confidentiality, 7, 23, 28–29
Conflicts, 48
Confusion, 3, 433, 434, 434. see also
      Alzheimer's disease (AD);
      Alzheimer's disease (AD) care
Connective tissue, 61
Consent, informed, 18, 110
Constipation, 277, 278
Constriction, 368, 381, 382
Contact lenses, 418, 418
Contagious disease, 123
Contamination, 123
Contracture, 350, 350
Conversion, 427
Convoluted tubule, 74, 75

Convulsion, 445, 455, 455
Coronary artery bypass surgery, 422, 422
Coronary artery disease, 421, 421
Corrective lenses, 418, 418
Cough, smoker's, 420
Coughing, assisting with, 390, 391, 391
Courtesies, 29
CPR; see Cardiopulmonary resuscitation
      (CPR)
Crime, 12
Criminal law, 12, 18
Crutches, 362
Culture, 52, 53
  in eating and nutrition, 295
Cystitis, 423
Cytoplasm, 61, 61

D

Daily care, 204–205
Dandruff, 235
Deafness, 414
Death; see also Dying
  attitudes about, 459–460
  care of body after, 462–463, 464
  of partner, 82
  signs of, 462
Decubitus ulcers, 368. see also Pressure
      ulcers
Deep breathing, 390, 390, 391
Defamation, 12, 18
Defecation, 277. see also Elimination; Stool
Defibrillators, 453
Degenerative joint disease, 406
Dehydration, 291, 299
Delegation, 12
Delirium, 433–434
Delusion, 428, 433
  in Alzheimer's disease, 436, 439
  of grandeur, 428
  of persecution, 428
Demanding behavior, 53
Dementia, 433
  in Alzheimer's disease, 434–437 (see also
      Alzheimer's disease [AD])
  focus on person in, 442
  lighting and noise with, 181
  quality of life with, 441–442
Dementia care, 437–442, 439, 440
  in Alzheimer's disease, 437–442, 439,
      440 (see also Alzheimer's disease
      [AD] care)
  family in, 441
  special care units for, 440
  validation therapy in, 441
Dementia care unit, 4
Dementia patients
  bathing of, 213
  definition of, 91
  falling of, 361
  feeding of, 304
  hygiene care for, 204
  lighting and, 181
  noise and, 181
  restraints and, 115
  sleep and, 201
  urinary incontinence in, 265
Denial, 427
Depression, 428, 434

Dermis, 62, 63
Development, 82, 83
Developmental disability, 3
Developmental skill, 82, 83
Diabetes, 78, 423–424
Diagnosis, nursing, 40, 41
Diagnosis-related groups, 5
Diaphragm, 72, 72
Diarrhea, 277, 278
Diastole, 70
Diastolic pressure, 312, 325
Diets, special, 297, 297t–298t
Digestive disorders, 424, 424–425
Digestive system, 72–74, 73, 85
Dilation, 368, 381, 381
Dining programs, 302
Direction terms, 46, 46
Director of nursing, 4
Direct questions, 56
Disability, 397, 401
Disaster, 91
Disease; see specific diseases
Disinfection, 123, 128
Disorientation, 3
Displacement, 427
Disputes, 7
Distal, 46, 46
Diverticular disease, 424, 424
Diverticulitis, 424
Diverticulosis, 424, 424
Diverticulum, 424
Doctor's orders
  to nursing assistants, 13
  for restraints, 110
Dogs, hearing assistance (guide), 415
"Do Not Resuscitate" order, 461
Dorsal, 46, 46
Dorsal recumbent position, 144
Dorsiflexion, 350, 353
Drainage systems, for urinary
      elimination, 269–271, 270
Drawsheets, 187–188, 192
Dressing and undressing
  procedures for, 246–254, 248, 250–252
  in rehabilitation and restorative care,
      398, 399
Dressings, 378, 378–380
Drinking water, 306
Drug-resistant microorganisms, 123
Drug side effects, 91
Dry heat, 382, 383
Duodenum, 73, 73
Durable power of attorney, 461
Dying, 459–465
  attitudes about, 459–460
  family in, 461
  focus on person in, 465
  hospice care for, 461
  legal issues in, 461
  physical needs in, 460–461
  psychological, social and spiritual
      needs in, 460
  signs of death in, 462
  stages of, 460
Dysphagia, 85, 291, 299, 411
Dyspnea, 85, 389
Dysuria, 257

E

Ear, 68, *69*
Eating devices, 398, *398*
Edema, 291, 299
Eggcrate-like mattress, 372, *373*
Ejaculatory duct, 74, *75*
Elastic bandages, 376, 377, *377*
Elastic stockings, 374, *374*, 375, *376*
Elbow
  exercise for, 355, *357*
  protectors for, 372, *372*
Elder abuse, 19–20
Elderly, 81–89, 91. *see also* Older persons
Electronic thermometers, 317, *318*, 319
Elimination
  bowel, 276–289, *277* (*see also* Bowel
    elimination)
  urinary, 256–275 (*see also* Urinary
    elimination)
Emboli, pulmonary, 374, *374*
Emergency care, 445
  basic life support in, 445–453 (*see also*
    Basic life support [BLS])
  fainting in, 455, *456*
  focus on person in, 456
  hemorrhage in, 453–455, *454*
  seizures in, 455
  shock in, 455
  stroke in, 456
Emergency Medical Services (EMS)
  system, 445
Emphysema, 420, *420*
Employers, 24–25
Endocardium, 70, *70*
Endocrine disorders, 423–424
Endocrine system, *77*, 77–78
Endometrium, 76
Enemas, 277, 280–286
  cleansing, 281–283, *283*
  oil-retention, 286
  overview of, *280*, 280–281
  small-volume, *284*, 284–285
Enteral nutrition, 291, 306, *306–308*, 307
Environment, 8
Epidermis, 62, *63*
Epididymis, 74, *75*
Epiglottis, 72, *72*
Epinephrine, 78
Epithelial tissue, 61
Ergonomics, 146
Erythrocytes, 69
Esophagus, 73, *73*
Estrogen, 76, 78
Ethics, 12. *see also* Work ethics
Evaluation step, 43
Exercise and activity, 349–365
  ambulation in, 359–364 (*see also*
    Ambulation)
  bedrest in, 350–351, *350–352*
  focus on person in, 365
  range-of-motion exercises in, 353–356,
    357–359
Exhalation, 71
Expiration, 71
Expressive aphasia, 413
Expressive-receptive aphasia, 413
Extension, 350, *353*
External rotation, 350, *353*

Eye, 68, *68*
Eye contact, 56
Eye disorders, 417–420
  blindness, *418*, 418–419, *419*
  cataract, 417, *417*
  corrective lenses for, 418, *418*
  glaucoma, 417, *417*
Eyeglasses, 418, *418*

F

Face mask, simple, 393, *394*
Facial expressions, *55*
Fainting, 445, 455, *456*
Fallopian tube, 76, *76*
False imprisonment, 12, 18, 110
Family, 8
  in Alzheimer's and dementia care, 441
  dying and, 461
Family visits, 58, *58*
Fats, 295
Fecal impaction, 277, 278
Fecal incontinence, 277, 278
Feces, 74, 277. *see also* Elimination, bowel
Feeding persons, 303–305
Fertilization, 77
Fetus, 76
Financial exploitation, 20
Finger exercises, 355, *358*
Flatulence, 277, 279
Flatus, 277
Flexion, 350, *353*
Floatation pads, 372, *373*
Floor cushions, *108*, 109
Flow rate, 291, 308, *308*
  of oxygen, *392*, 394
Flow sheets, 34, *37*
Fluid balance chart, *328*
Fluids; see Nutrition and fluids
Focus on the person
  in assessment, 334
  in bowel elimination, 288
  in comfort assistance, 201
  with common health problems, 429
  in confusion and dementia, 442
  in dying, 465
  in emergencies, 456
  in exercise and activity, 365
  in grooming, 254
  in heat and cold applications, 386
  in hygiene, 232
  in infection prevention, 141
  in older person care, 87, 88
  in oxygen needs, 395
  in positioning and body mechanics,
    176, 177
  in rehabilitation and restorative care,
    402
  in restraint use, 120
  in safety procedures, 103
  in specimen collection, 347
  in urinary elimination, 274
  in whole person caring, 51, *51*
Food; see Nutrition and fluids
Food practices, 296
Footboards, 351, *351*
Foot care, 243–246, *244*, *246*
Footdrop, 350, 351
Foot exercises, 356, *359*

Forearm exercises, 355, *357*
Foreign-body airway obstruction,
  450–453. *see also* Airway obstruction,
  foreign-body
Fowler's position, 144, 180, 182, *182*
  for deep-breathing exercises, 391
  semi-, 180, 182, *182*, 307
Fractures, 405, 408–410, *409*, *410*
  hip, 410, *410*, *411*
  traction for, 408–410, *409*
  types of, 408
Fraud, 12, 18
Friction, 144, 146
Fruits, *293*, 294
Frustration, in rehabilitation and
  restorative care, 402
Function
  of body, 60–80 (*see also* Body, structure
    and function of)
  optimal level of, 51
Functional incontinence, 257, 264
Functional nursing, 5
Fundus, 76, *76*
Furniture, in personal unit, *181*, 181–185
  bathroom, 185
  bed, 181–182, *181–182*
  bedside stand, 183, *183*
  call system, 183–185, *184*, *185*
  chairs, 183
  closet and drawer space, 185
  other equipment, 185
  overbed table, *180*, 182
  privacy curtains, 183
  safety and comfort with, 185

G

Gallbladder, 73, *73*
Gastrointestinal system, 72
Gastrotomy tube, 306, *307*
Gavage, 291
Generalized seizures, 455
Generalized tonic-clonic seizures, 455
Geriatrics, 81
Gerontology, 81
Gestational diabetes, 423
Glass thermometers, 312–316
  reading of, 313, *314*
  safety and comfort with, 314, 315
  types of, *313*, 314
  use of, 314–316, *317*
Glaucoma, 417, *417*
Glomerulus, 74, *75*
Glucocorticoids, 78
Glucosuria, 337, 341
Glycosuria, 337, 341
Gonads, 78
Gossip, 23, 28
Graduate, 329, *329*
Grains, 291–292, 293t
Grandeur, delusion of, 428
Grand mal seizure, 455
Graphic sheet, 34, *35*
Grievances, 7
Grooming, 234–255
  changing gowns and clothing in,
    246–254, *248*, *250–252*
  focus on person in, 254
  hair care in, 234–240 (*see also* Hair care)

Grooming (*Continued*)
  for job interview, 26, *26*
  nail and foot care in, 243–246, *244, 246*
  of nursing assistant, 24
  in rehabilitation and restorative care, 398, *398*
  shaving in, 241–242, *243*
Group insurance, 5
Groups, 8
Growth and development, 82, *83*

H

Hair, 62, *63*
  aging on, 84
Hair care, 234–240
  brushing and combing in, 236, *237, 238*
  overview of, 235
  shampooing in, 238, *239*, 240
Hallucinations, 428, 433, 436, 439
Handgrips, 351, *352*
Handrolls, 351, *352*
Harassment, 23
Hazardous substance
  biohazardous waste as, 123, 138, *139*
  definition of, 91
  safe handling for, 97, *99*, 99–100
Health care, paying for, 5
Health maintenance organization (HMO), 6
Health team, 2, 5, *6*
  communicating with, 33–49 (*see also* Communication with health team)
  health, hygiene, and appearance of, 23, 24
Hearing aids, 415, *416*
Hearing assistance (guide) dogs, 415
Hearing-impaired persons, 91, 415
Hearing loss, 414–416, *416*
Heart, 70, *70*
Heart failure, 423
Heat
  dry, 382, *383*
  moist, 382, *383*
Heat and cold applications, 381–386
  application rules for, 385, 386
  cold applications in, 382, *384*
  focus on person in, 386
  heat applications in, 381, *381*, 382, *383*, *384*
  safety and comfort for, 384
  temperature ranges for, *385*
Heel elevators, 372, *372*
Height, measurement of, 331–332, *332*
Heimlich maneuver, 450, *452*
Hematuria, 257, 337, 341
Hemiplegia, 405
Hemorrhage, 445, 453–455, *454*
  pressure and pressure points for, 454, *454*
Hepatitis, 425
Hip abduction wedges, 351, *352*
Hip exercises, 356, *358*
Hip fractures, 410, *410, 411*
Hip protector, *108*
Hirsutism, 235
Hormones, 77–78
Hospice care, 2, 3, 461

Hospitals
  organization of, 4, *4*
  patient care in, 51
  services provided by, 2
Hygiene, 203–233
  back massage in, 225, *226, 227*
  bathing in, 213–225 (*see also* Bathing)
  daily care in, 204–205
  focus on person in, 232
  oral, 205–212 (*see also* Oral hygiene)
  perineal care in, 228–231, *230, 231*
  personal, 23
Hymen, *76*
Hyperextension, 350, *353*
Hyperglycemia, 424
Hypertension, 312, 325, 421
Hyperventilation, 389
Hypoglycemia, 424
Hypotension, 312, 325
Hypotension, orthostatic, 350, 359
Hypoventilation, 389
Hypoxia, 389, *389*

I

Ice bag, 382, *384*
Ileostomy, 277, 286, *287*
Ileum, 73, *73–74*
Illness, 2. *see also specific illnesses*
Immune system, 78–79, *79*
Immunity, 78
Implementation step, 42
Income, reduced, 82
Incontinence
  fecal, 277, 278
  functional, 257, 264
  overflow, 257, 264
  reflex, 257, 264
  stress, 257, 264
  urge, 257, 264
  urinary, 257, 264–265, *265*
Infarction, myocardial, 422
Infection, 122–142
  bloodborne pathogen standard for, 139–140
  chain of, 123, *124*
  definition of, 123
  focus on person in, 141
  hand hygiene for, 125, *126, 127*
  isolation precautions for, 128, *130–132*, 132
  medical asepsis for, 124
  medical supplies and equipment asepsis in, 128, *128, 129*
  in older persons, 124
  signs and symptoms of, 123
  transmission of, 124, *125*
Infection, protective measures for, 132–133
  bagging items in, 138, *139*
  eyewear and face shields in, 137
  gloves in, 133, *133, 134*
  gowns in, 137, *138*
  masks in, 132, *132*, 135, *136*
  personal needs in, 139
Informed consent, 18, 110
Inhalation, 71
Insomnia, 180, 200
Inspiration, 71
Insulin, 78

Insurance, 5
Intake and output assessment, 328, 328–330, *329*
Integumentary system, 62–63, *63*
  aging on, 84
  hygiene for, 213–225 (*see also* Bathing)
  moving persons in bed and, 146, *147*
Intentional tort, 18–19
Interdisciplinary care planning, 43
Internal rotation, 350, *353*
Intervention, 40
Interview, 26, 26–27, *27*
Intestines, 73, *73–74*
Intravenous (IV) therapy, 291, 308, *308, 309*
Invasion of privacy; see Privacy
Involuntary muscles, 64

J

Jacket restraint, 117
Jejunum, 73, *73–74*
Job description, 12
Jobs, 23–27
  acceptance of, 27
  applications for, 24, *25*
  finding, 23
  interview for, 26, 26–27, *27*
  losing of, 30, *30*
  new employee orientation in, 27
  resigning from, 30
  teamwork on, 28–30, *30*
  traits needed for, 23–24, *25*
Joint movements, *353. see also* Range-of-motion exercises
Joint replacement, total, 407
Joints, 63, *64*

K

Ketone, 337, 341, *342*
Kidneys, 74, *74*
Kidney stones, 423
Knee exercises, 356, *358*

L

Labia majora/minora, 76, *76, 77*, 230, *230*
Language, 29
Larynx, 72, *72*
Lateral, 46, *46*
Lateral position, 144
Lateral position, 30–degree, 370, *372*
Law, 12, 18
Lenses, corrective, 418, *418*
Leukocytes, 69
Libel, 12
Lice, 235
Licensed practical nurse (LPN), 2, 4–5
Licensed vocational nurse (LVN), 2, 4–5
Life-long residents, 3
Life support, basic, 445–453. *see also* Basic life support (BLS)
Lighting
  with dementia, 181
  in personal unit, 181
Linens, *187*, 187–188
Liquid oxygen system, 392, *393*
Listening, 55–56, *56*
Living will, 461
Logrolling, 144
Long-term care centers, 2

Love and belonging needs, 52, *52*
Lung metastasis, 405, *406*
Lung tumor, 405, *406*
Lymphocytes, 78

M

Major depression, 428
Maladaptive behavior, 428
Malignant tumor, 405, *405*
Malpractice, 12, 18
Mammary glands, 76, *77*
Managed care, 6, *6*
Massage, 225, 226, 227
    circulatory ulcers and, *374*
    pressure ulcers and, *370*
Masturbation, 87, *87*
Mattress; see Beds
Mattress, eggcrate-like, *373*
Meal breaks, 29
Meal preparation, 300
Meal trays, 302
Meat, *293*, 294–295
Medial, 46, *46*
Medicaid, 5
Medical asepsis
    definition of, 123
    hand hygiene in, 125, *126, 127*
    supplies and equipment in, 128, *128, 129*
Medical record, 35–37, 7, 33
Medical terminology, 44, *44–45*, 46
Medicare, 5
Memory loss, in Alzheimer's disease, 434
Menstruation, 76–77
Mental health, 426
Mental health disorders, 426–429
    affective, 428
    anxiety, 427
    bipolar, 428
    major depression, 428
    personality, 428
    schizophrenia, 428
Mental illness, 426
Mentally ill residents, 3
Metabolism, 78
Metastases, 405, *406*
Methicillin-resistant *Staphylococcus aureus*, 123
Microbe, 123
Microorganism, 123
Milk, *293*, 294
Mineralocorticoids, 78
Minerals, 295
Minimum data set, 39
Mistreatment, 8, 402
Mitral valve, 70, *70*
Mitt restraints, *116*
Mobility, impaired, 91. *see also* Rehabilitation and restorative care
Moist heat, 382, *383*
Mons pubis, 76, *76, 77*
Montgomery ties, 378, *378*
Mouth, 72–73
Mouth-to-mouth breathing, 446–447, *447*
Multiple sclerosis, 413
Muscles, 64–65, *65*
    atrophy of, 350, *351*
    contracture of, 350, *350*

Muscle tissue, 61
Musculoskeletal disorders, 406–411
    arthritis, 406–407
    fractures, 408–410, *409, 410*
    osteoarthritis, 406
    osteoporosis, 407
    rheumatoid arthritis, 407, *407*
    total joint replacement (arthroplasty) for, 407
Musculoskeletal system, 63–65, *64, 65*, 84
Myocardial infarction, 422
Myocardium, 70, *70*
My Pyramid Food Guidance System, 291–295, *292*, 293t

N

Nails
    aging on, 84
    care of, 243–246, *244, 246*
    function of, 62
Nasal cannula, 393, *394*
Nasogastric tube, 306, *306*
Neck exercises, 355, *357*
Needs, 51–52, *52*
Neglect, 8, 12, 19
Negligence, 12, 18
Nephrons, 74, *75*
Nerve tissue, 61
Nervous system, 66–68, *66–69*, 84–85
Nervous system disorders, 411–414
    from aging, 84–85
    multiple sclerosis, 413
    Parkinson's disease, 413, *413*
    spinal cord injuries, 413–414, *414*
    stroke, 411–413, *412*
Nitroglycerin, 422
Nocturia, 257
Noise
    dementia patients and, 181
    in personal unit, 181
Non-pathogen, 123
Nonverbal communication, 55, *55*
Norepinephrine, 78
Nose, 71
Nothing by mouth (NPO), 299
Nursing assistant, 12–21
    abuse reporting for, 19–20
    definition of, 2
    delegation and, 14, 17, *17*
    ethical aspects for, 18, *18*
    health, hygiene, and appearance of, 23, *24*
    job description for, 14, *15–17*
    legal aspects for, 18–19
    in nursing team, 5
    OBRA requirements for, 12–13
    role and responsibilities of, 13, *13*
Nursing care patterns, 5
Nursing care plan, 40
Nursing center, 3
    definition of, 2
    organization of, 4, *4*
Nursing diagnosis, 40, *41*
Nursing facility, 2, 3
Nursing history, 34
Nursing home, 2, 3
Nursing intervention, 40
Nursing process, *39–42, 39–43*

Nursing service, 4
Nursing team, 4–5
    communication with, 33–49 (*see also under* Communication)
    definition of, 2
Nutrients, 291, 295
Nutrition and fluids, 290–310
    between-meal nourishment in, 306
    calorie counts in, 306
    cultural food practices in, 296
    culture in, 295
    dining programs in, 302, *302*
    drinking water in, 306
    enteral nutrition in, 291, 306, *306–308*, 307
    factors in, 295
    feeding persons in, 303–305, *304*
    fluid balance in, 299
    focus on person in, 309
    illness on, 295
    meal preparation in, 300, 301
    meal trays in, 302, 303
    meeting food and fluid needs in, 300–306
    my pyramid in, 291–295, *292*, 293t
    nutrients in, 295
    OBRA dietary requirements for, 296, *296*
    religion on, 295
    special diets in, 297, 297t–298t, 298, *299*
    special needs in, 306–307, *306–308*

O

Objective data, 39
OBRA; see Omnibus Budget Reconciliation Act of 1987 (OBRA)
Observation, 39, *39–40*
Obsessive-compulsive disorder, 427
Odors, in personal unit, 180
Oil glands, 62, *63*
Oils, *293*, 295
Old, defined, 82
Older persons, 81–89
    growth and development in, 82, *83*
    nursing center care needs of, 85–86
    ombudsman program for, 87
    person-focused care for, 87, *88*
    physical changes in, 84–85
    sexuality of, 86, *86, 87*
    social changes in, 82, *83*
Old-old, defined, 82
Oliguria, 257
Ombudsman program, 87
Omnibus Budget Reconciliation Act of 1987 (OBRA), 2, 6
    abuse requirements of, 20
    comprehensive care plan in, 41
    dietary requirements of, 296, *296*
    minimum data set in, 39
    resident care conferences in, 43
    on resident dignity and privacy, *9*
    on restraint use, 107, 109
    training requirements of, 12–13
Open-ended questions, 56
Open fracture, 408
Open reduction, 408
Optimal level of functioning, 51
Oral cavity, 72–73

Oral hygiene, 205–212. *see also under* Hygiene
  benefits of, 205
  definition of, 204
  denture care in, *210,* 210–212, *212*
  flossing in, 206, *207*
  in rehabilitation and restorative care, 398
  teeth brushing in, 205–206, *206, 207*
  for unconscious persons, *207,* 207–209, *208*
Organs, 61, *62. see also specific organs*
Orthopnea, 389
Orthostatic hypotension, 350, 359
Osteoarthritis, 406
Osteoporosis, 407
Ostomy, 277
Ova, 76
Ovaries, 76, *76*
Overbed table, *180,* 182, 183
Overflow incontinence, 257, 264
Oxygen concentrator, 392, *393*
Oxygen devices, 393, *394*
Oxygen needs, 388–395
  altered respiratory function in, 389, *389*
  focus on person in, 395
  oxygen therapy in, 392–394, *392–394*
  promoting oxygenation in, 389–391, *390, 391*
Oxygen system, liquid, 392, *393*
Oxygen tank, 392, *392, 393*
Oxygen wall outlet, 392, *392*
Oxytocin, 78

P
Pain assessment, 333, *333, 334*
Pain rating scale, 333, *333*
Pancreas, *77,* 78
Panic disorder, 427
Paranoia, 428
Paranoid personality, 428
Paraplegia, 405, 414, *414*
Parkinson's disease, 413, *413*
Partial seizures, 455
Partner, death of, 82
Pathogen, 123
Patient's rights, 2
Payment systems, prospective, 5
Pediculosis, 235
Penis, *75, 75,* 231, *231*
Pericardium, 70, *70*
Perineal care, 204
Peripheral nervous system, 67
Peristalsis, 73
Persecution, delusion of, 428
Personal choice, 7, *7, 9*
  of foods, 295
  in rehabilitation and restorative care, 402
Personal hygiene, 23
Personality disorders, 428
Personal matters, 29
Personal possessions, 8
Person-focused care; see Focus on the person
Person's unit, *180,* 180–185
  bathroom in, 185
  call system in, 183–185, *184, 185*
  lighting in, 181
  maintenance of, 180

Person's unit *(Continued)*
  odors and noise in, 181
  room furniture and equipment in, 181, *181–183 (see also* Furniture, in personal unit)
  safety and comfort in, 185
  temperature and ventilation in, 180
pH, 341
Phagocytes, 78, *79*
Pharynx, 71, *72, 73*
Phobias, 427
Phone, answering of, 47, *47*
Physical activity, *293*
Physical needs, 52, *52*
Physical restraint, 107. *see also* Restraints
Pillows and pillowcases, 190, *193, 194*
Pituitary gland, *77,* 78
Planning, 40
Plantar flexion, 350, 351, *353*
Plasma, 69
Platelets, 69
Pleura, 72, *72*
Pneumonia, 420
Polyuria, 257
Portal of entry, 123–124, *125*
Posey quick-release tie, *113*
Positioning
  for aspiration prevention, 307
  for bedrest, 351, *351, 352*
  for bedsore prevention, *370, 372*
  body mechanics in, 172–176, *173–176*
  for deep-breathing exercises, 391
  to promote oxygenation, 389, *390*
Posterior, 46, *46*
Postmortem, 459
Postmortem care, 462–463, *464*
Postural hypotension, 350
Posture, 144
Power of attorney, durable, 461
Preferred provider organization (PPO), 6
Prefix, 46
Prehypertension, 421
Pressure and pressure points, for bleeding, 454, *454*
Pressure ulcers, 368–372, *369–373*
  causes of, 368, *370*
  definition of, 368, *369*
  persons at risk for, 368
  prevention and treatment of, *370,* 370–372, *372, 373*
  signs of, 368, *370, 371*
  sites of, *369,* 370
Primary nursing, 5
Priority, 23
Privacy
  curtains for, 183
  full visual privacy in, 180, 183
  invasion of, 12, 18, *18*
  in rehabilitation and restorative care, 402
  right to, 7, *7, 9*
  sexuality and, *87*
Private insurance, 5
Problem-focused conferences, 43
Progesterone, 76, 78
Progress notes, 34, *36*
Projection, 427
Pronation, 350, *353*
Prone position, 144

Prostate gland, 74–75, *75*
Prosthesis, 397, 400
Protein, 295
Proximal, 46, *46*
Pseudodementia, 433
Psychology, 401. *see also specific disorders*
Psychosis, 428
Pulmonary embolus, 374, *374*
Pulse, 320–323
  apical, 323, *323*
  definition of, 312, 320
  radial, 321, *321,* 322
  rate of, 320
  rhythm and force of, 321, *321*
  stethoscope for, *313,* 325, *325,* 326, *326*
Pyelonephritis, 423

Q
Quadriplegia, 405, 414, *414*
Quality of life, 8, 51, 402
Questions, 56

R
Range-of-motion exercises, 350, 353–356, *357–359*
  delegation guidelines in, 353
  joint movements in, *353*
  overview of, 353
  performing, *354,* 354–356, *357, 358*
  safety and comfort in, 354
Rationalization, 427
Reagent strips, 342, *342*
Receptive aphasia, 413
Recording, *43,* 43–44, *44*
Recovery position, 453, *453*
Rectum, *73, 74,* 229, *230*
Red blood cells, 69
Reduction, 408
Reflex incontinence, 257, 264
Refusing treatment, 7
Registered nurse (RN), 2, 4
Registry, 12
Regression, 427
Regurgitation, 291
Rehabilitation and restorative care, 396–403
  focus on person in, 402
  guidelines for, *401*
  psychological and social aspects of, 401
  quality of life in, 402
  rehabilitation team in, 401
  restorative nursing in, 397
  wheelchair transfers in, 398, *400*
  whole person in, 397, 398, *398–401*
Reincarnation, 459
Religion, 52, 295
Renal calculi, 423
Renal failure, 423
Renal pelvis, 74, *74*
Repetitive behaviors, in Alzheimer's disease, 437
Reporting, 43
Repression, 427
Reproductive system, 74–77, *75–77,* 85
Rescue breathing, 446, *447*
Resident care conferences, 43
Resident groups, 8
Residential care facility, 2, 3

Residents
behavior issues of, 52–53, *53*
caring for, 51, *52*
communicating with, 54–57
culture and religion of, 52, *53*
rights of, 7–8, *9*
types of, 2–3
visitors of, 58, *58*
Resource-related groups, 5
Respiratory arrest, 445, 446
Respiratory disorders, 420–421
Respiratory function
altered, 389, *389*
assessment of, 324
Respiratory system, 71–72, *72*, 85
Restlessness, in Alzheimer's disease, 436
Restorative aides, 397
Restorative nursing care, 397
Restraints, 106–121
alternatives to, 107, *108, 109*
definition of, 107
extra protection needs in, 107
focus on person in, 120
freedom from, 8
history of, 107
risks of, *107*
Restraint use, safe, 109–117
application in, 115, *115–117*, 117–119
comfort in, 117
complications in, *107*, 110
guidelines in, 110–111, *111–115*
legal aspects in, 110
physical and drug restraints in, 109–110, *110*
reporting and recording in, 115
Retirement, 82, *83*
Rheumatoid arthritis, 407, *407*
Rights, patient's, 2
Rigor mortis, 459, 462
Room furniture, 181–185, *181–185. see also* Furniture, in personal unit
Roots, 46
Rotation, 350, *353*
Ruptured blood vessel, 411

S

Safety, 91–105
accident risk factors in, 91
in ambulation, 359
in basic life support, 446
bed alarms in, *93, 94*
in bedmaking, 188
bed rails in, 94, *95*
beds and, 183
with binder application, 381
in blood pressure taking, 325
bomb threats in, 102
in bowel elimination, *278*
burn prevention in, 96
disasters in, 102
in dressings application, 379
with elastic bandages, 376
with elastic stockings, 375
in emergency care, 445
equipment accident prevention in, 96, *96, 97*
fall prevention in, 92, *92, 93*
fire prevention in, 100, *101*

Safety *(Continued)*
focus on person in, 103
food temperature in, 304
grab bars in, 94
hand rails in, 94, *95*
hazardous substance handling in, 97, *99*, 99–100
for heat and cold applications, 384
in height and weight measurement, 331
identification issues in, 91, *92*
in intake and output assessment, 329
material safety data sheets in, 100
before meals, 300
for meal trays, 302
with oxygen sources, 393
for oxygen therapy, *394*
in person's unit, 185
poisoning prevention in, 96
for range-of-motion exercises, 354
in rehabilitation and restorative care, 402
risk management in, 102–103
and security needs, 52, *52*
in sputum specimen collection, 345
in stool specimen collection, 343
suffocation prevention in, 96
in temperature taking, 314, 315
in urine specimen collection, 337
in urine specimen testing, 341
wheel chair and stretchers in, 97, *98, 99*
wheel locks in, 94, *95*
workplace violence in, 102
Salivary glands, 73, *73*
Schizophrenia, 428
Screaming, in Alzheimer's disease, 437
Scrotum, 74, *75*, 231, *231*
Seizure, 445, 455, *455*
Self-actualization needs, 52, *52*
Self-centered behavior, 53
Self-esteem needs, 52, *52*
Semen, 74
Semi-Fowler's position, 180, 182, *182*, 307
Seminal vesicle, 74, *75*
Sense organs, 67–68, *68, 69*, 84
Sexual behavior
in Alzheimer's disease, 437
inappropriate, 53
sexuality and, *86*, 86–87
Sexually transmitted diseases (STDs), 426
Shampooing, 238, *239*, 240
Shaving, 241–242, *243*
Shearing, 144, 146, *147*
Shock, 445, 455
Short-term residents, 3
Shoulder exercises, 355, *357*
Showers; see *under* Bathing
Shroud, applying, *464*
Sick care practices, 53
Side effects, of drugs, 91
Side-lying position, 144
Signal light, 183–185, *184, 185*
Sign language, 415, *416*
Signs, 39
Silence, 56, *57*
Simple face mask, 393, *394*
Simple fracture, 408
Sims' position, 144, 286
Sitz bath, *383*, 384
Skilled nursing facility, 2, 3

Skin, 62–63, *63*
aging on, 84
hygiene for, 213–225 (*see also* Bathing)
moving persons in bed and, 146, *147*
Slander, 12
Sleep
no comfort for, too, 100, 200–201
in dementia patients, 201
Sleep deprivation, 180, 200
Sleep walking, 180, 200
Smell, impaired, 91
Smoker's cough, 420
Social changes, 82, *83, 84*
Specimens, 336–348
collecting of, *337*
focus on person in, 347
overview of, 337
sputum, 345, 346, *347*
stool, 343–345, *344, 345*
urine, 337–342 (*see also* Urine specimens)
Speech, 29
Sperm cells, 74
Splint, 351, *353*
Sputum, 337
Sputum specimen collecting, 345, 346, *347*
Stasis ulcers, 373, *373. see also* Circulatory ulcers
Sterile, 123
Sterilization, 123, 128, *128*
Stoma, 277
Stomach, 73, *73*
Stones, kidney, 423
Stool, 277
Stool specimen collecting, 343–345, *344, 345*
Strangulation, 110, *114*
Stress incontinence, 257, 264
Stroke, 411–413, *412*, 445, *453*, 456
Subacute care, 2
Subjective data, 39
Suffix, 46
Suffocation, 91
Sugar, blood, 424
Sundowning, 433, 436, 438
Supination, 350, *353*
Supine position, 144
Suppository, 277, 279, *279*
Sweat glands, 62, *63*
Symptoms, 39
Systole, 70
Systolic pressure, 312, 325

T

Tachypnea, 389
Task, 12
Task delegation, 17, *17*
T-binders, 380, *381*
T cells, 78
Team nursing, 5
Teamwork, 23
Temperature
for heat and cold applications, 385t
in person's unit, 180
Temperature, body, 312–319. *see also* Body temperature
electronic thermometers for, 317, *318*, 319
glass thermometers for, 312–316 (*see also* Thermometers, glass)

Temperature, body (*Continued*)
    normal, 313t
    overview of, 312
    sites for reading of, *313, 317*
    tympanic membrane thermometers for, *317, 318*
Terminal illness, 2, 459
Terminally ill residents, 3
Terminology, medical, 44, *44–45*, 46
Testes, 74, *75*
Testosterone, 74, 78
Tetany, 78
Thermometers, electronic, *317, 318,* 319
Thermometers, glass, 312–316
    reading of, 313, *314*
    safety and comfort with, *314, 315*
    types of, *313, 314*
    use of, 314–316, *317*
Thermometers, tympanic membrane, 317, *318*
30–degree lateral position, *370, 372*
Thrombi (thrombus), *374, 374*
Thrombocytes, 69
Thumb exercises, 355, *357*
Thyroid gland, *77,* 78
Tissues, 61, *62*
Toe exercises, 356, *359*
Toilet transfers, 170, *170,* 171
Tongue-jaw lift maneuver, 452, *453*
Torts, 18–19
Total joint replacement, 407
Touch, 55, *55*
    impaired, 91
    in inappropriate sexual behavior, 53
Trachea, 72, *72*
Traction
    for fractures, 408–410, *409*
    for spinal cord injuries, 413
Transfer belts, 144, 160, 161, *161*
Transfers
    bed to chair, *162, 162–165, 164, 165*
    chair to bath, 398, *400*
    chair to bed, 165, 166, *167,* 398, *400*
    to toilet, 170, *170,* 171
Transportation, 28
Treatment refusal, 7
Trendelenburg's position, 180, 182, *182*
Trendelenburg's position, reverse, 180, 182, *183*
Tricuspid valve, 70, *70*
Trochanter rolls, 351, *351*
Tuberculosis (TB), 420–421
Tumor, 405
    benign, 405, *405*
    lung, 405, *406*
    malignant, 405, *405*
Tympanic membrane thermometers, 317, *318*

U

Ulcers
    arterial, 373
    circulatory, 368, 373–377 (*see also* Circulatory ulcers)
    decubitus, 368

Ulcers (*Continued*)
    pressure, 368–372, *369–373* (*see also* Pressure ulcers)
    stasis, 373, *373*
    vascular, 373
Unintentional tort, 18
Ureter, 74, *74*
Urethra, 74, *74, 75, 75*
Urge incontinence, 257, 264
Urinals, 261, *261,* 262
Urinary elimination, 256–275
    bladder training in, 274, *274*
    catheters for, *266, 266–268, 267, 269*
    condom catheters for, 271–273, *272*
    drainage systems for, 269–271, *270*
    focus on person in, 274
    normal urination in, 256–264 (*see also* Urination, normal)
    urinary incontinence in, 264–265, *265*
Urinary frequency, 257
Urinary incontinence, 257, 264–265, *265*
Urinary system, 74, *74,* 85
Urinary system disorders, 423
Urinary tract infections (UTIs), 423
Urinary urgency, 257
Urination, normal, 256–264
    bedpans for, *258, 258–260, 260, 261*
    commodes for, 263, *263,* 264
    definition of, 257
    observations or, 257
    rules for, 257
    urinals for, 261, *261,* 262
Urine, 74
Urine specimens, 337–342
    double-voided, 340, 341
    midstream, 338, 339, *340*
    random, 338, 339, *339*
    safety and comfort and, 337, 341
    testing of, 341, 342, *342*
Uterus, 76, *76*

V

Vagina, 76, *76*
Validation therapy, 441
Vancomycin-resistant *Enterococcus,* 123
Vascular ulcers, 373. *see also* Circulatory ulcers
Vas deferens, 74, *75*
Vegetables, *293,* 294
Veins, 71, *71*
Vena cava, 71, *71*
Ventilation, in personal unit, 180
Ventral, 46, *46*
Ventricles, 70, *70*
Ventricular fibrillation, 446, 453
Venules, 71
Verbal communication, 54, *54*
Vest restraint, *112,* 117
Violence, workplace, 91
Vision, impaired, 91, *418,* 418–419, *419*
Vital signs, 312–327
    blood pressure in, 325–327, *326*
    body temperature in, 312–319 (*see also* Body temperature)
    pulse in, 320–323 (*see also* Pulse)
    respiration in, 324

Vitamins, 295
Voiding, of urine, 257
Voluntary muscles, 64
Vomiting, 425
Vulva, 76, *76*

W

Walkers, 362, *364*
Walking aids, 362, *362–365,* 364
Wandering, in Alzheimer's disease, 435–436, 438
Weight measurement, 331–332, *332*
Wheelchairs
    bed to chair transfers in, *162, 162–165, 164, 165*
    chair to bath transfers for, 398, *400*
    chair to bed transfers for, 165, 166, *167,* 398, *400*
    positioning persons in, 174, *174–176,* 176
    restraint straps for, 113–115
White blood cells, 69
Whole person, 397, 398, *398–401. see also* Focus on the person
Will, living, 461
Withdrawal, 53
Work, by residents, 7
Work ethics, 22–32, *23*
    harassment and, 30
    health, hygiene, and appearance in, 23, *24*
    in job acceptance, 27
    job applications and, 24, *25*
    job finding and, 23
    job interview and, *26,* 26–27, *27*
    in job loss, 30, *31*
    in job resignation, 30
    in job teamwork, 28–30, *30*
    traits for, 23–24, *25*
    in work preparation, 27–28
Workplace violence, 91
Wound care, 368–387
    binders in, 380, 381, *381*
    circulatory ulcers in, 373–377, *374, 376–378* (*see also* Circulatory ulcers)
    dressings in, *378,* 378–380
    pressure ulcers in, 368–372, *369–373* (*see also* Pressure ulcers)
    skin tears in, 368
Wound care, heat and cold applications in, 381–386
    application rules for, 385, 386
    cold applications in, 382, *384*
    focus on person in, 386
    heat applications in, 381, *381,* 382, *383, 384*
    safety and comfort for, 384
    temperature ranges for, *385*
Wrist
    exercise for, 355, *357*
    restraints for, *115*

Y

Young-old, defined, 82